POCKET MANUAL

OF

HOMŒOPATHIC
MATERIA MEDICA

COMPRISING

THE CHARACTERISTIC AND GUIDING
SYMPTOMS OF ALL REMEDIES

[CLINICAL AND PATHOGENETIC]

By

WILLIAM BOERICKE, M. D.

First Professor of Homœopathic Materia Medica and Therapeutics a
the University of California; Author of "A Compend of the
Principles of Homœopathy;" Translator of the Sixth
Edition of Hahnemann's Organon.

NINTH EDITION

REVISED AND ENLARGED

WITH THE ADDITION OF A REPERTORY BY

OSCAR E. BOERICKE, A. B., M. D.

PUBLISHED BY

BOERICKE & RUNYON

Boericke & Tafel, Inc.

PHILADELPHIA, PA.

Volume 2

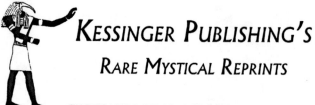
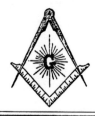

PRIMULA OBCONICA
(Primrose)

The poison of the Primrose occurs in its *glandular hairs,* which break easily and discharge an irritating fluid which is absorbed into the skin.

But skin symptoms of poisoning appear in sensitive patients even without coming in d'rect contact with the plant, mere nearness being sufficient, just like Poison ivy. Intermittency of symptoms; worse right side. Pain in liver and spleen. Deep infiltration and tension of tissues; blisters. *Paralyzed sensation. Weakness.* Pharyngeal soreness alternates with diminished facial irritation.

Face.—Moist eczema. Papular eruption on chin. Burns at night. Urticaria-like eruption. Eyelids swollen.

Extremities.—Eczema on arms, wrists, forearms, hands, papular and excoriated. Rheumatic pain around shoulder. Palms dry and hot. Cracking over joints and fingers. Eruption between fingers. Purple blotches on back of hands, palmar surface stiff. Blisters on fingers.

Skin.—*Great itching,* worse at night, red and swollen like erysipelas. Tumefied. *Small papules on a raised base.* Skin symptoms accompanied by febrile symptoms.

Relationship.—Compare: *Rhus; Fagopyrum* (Antidotal). *Humea Elegans,* similar skin symptoms.

PROPYLAMIN—TRIMETHYLAMINUM
(Distilled Herring-brine)

In acute rheumatism, dissipates fever and pain in a day or two. Rheumatic prosopalgia, and rheumatic metastases, especially heart lesions.

Extremities.—*Pain in wrists and ankles;* worse, slightest motion. [*Bry.*] Great restlessness and thirst. Rheumatism, needle held in fingers gets too heavy. *Tingling and numbness of fingers.* Pain in wrist and ankle, unable to stand.

Relationship.—(*Chenopodium vulvaria.* The plant has an odor of decaying fish and contains a large amount of Propylamine. Weakness in lumbar and lower dorsal region.)

Dose.—Ten to fifteen drops, in about six ounces of water; teaspoonful doses every two hours.

PRUNUS SPINOSA
(Black-thorn)

Special action on the urinary organs and head. Very valuable in certain neuralgias, anasarca, and especially œdema pedum. Ankle and foot feel sprained. *Ciliary neuralgia.* [*Spig.*]

Head.—Pressing-asunder pain beneath skull. *Shooting from right frontal bone through brain to occiput. Pain in right eyeball, as if it would burst.* Piercing toothache, as if teeth were pulled out; worse, taking anything warm.

Eyes.—*Ciliary neuralgia.* Bursting pain in right eyeball, shooting like lightning through the brain to occiput. *Sudden pain in left eye as if it would burst,* better by lachrymation. Irido-choroiditis. Opacity of vitreous humor. Eyes feel as if bursting.

Abdomen.—Ascites. Cramp-like pain in bladder region; worse, walking.

Rectum.—Hard, nodular stool, with rectal pain, as if angular body were pressed inward. Burning in anus after slimy diarrhœa.

Urine.—Tenesmus of bladder. Ineffectual effort to urinate. *Hurriedly impelled to urinate; the urine seems to pass as far as glans, and then returns and causes pain in urethra.* Neuralgic dysuria. *Must press a long time before urine appears.*

Respiratory.—Wheezing when walking. Oppression of chest; anxious, short respiration. Angina pectoris. Furious beating of heart; worse, slightest motion.

Skin.—Herpes zoster. *Dropsy.* Itching on tips of fingers, as if frozen.

Relationship.—Compare: *Lauroc.; Prunus padus*—Bird-cherry—(sore throat, pressure behind sternum and sticking pain in rectum); *Prunus Virginiana*—Wild Cherry—(*heart tonic;* relieves the flagging and distended ventricle; irritable heart; dilatation of right heart; *cough, worse at night on lying down;* weak digestion, especially in elderly people; chronic bronchitis; increases muscular tone); *Pyrus*—Mountain Ash—(irritation of eyes; constriction around waist; spasmodic pains in uterus, bladder, heart, cold-water sensation in stomach, coldness extends up œsophagus; neuralgic and gouty pains).

Dose.—Third to sixth potency.

PSORINUM
(Scabies Vesicle)

The therapeutic field of this remedy is found in so-called psoric manifestations. Psorinum is a cold medicine; wants the head kept warm, *wants warm clothing* even in summer. *Extreme sensitiveness to cold.* Debility, independent of any organic disease, especially the weakness remaining after acute disease. *Lack of reaction*, i. e., phagocytes defective; when well-chosen remedies fail to act. Scrofulous patients. Secretions *have a filthy smell*. Profuse sweating. Cardiac weakness. Skin symptoms very prominent. Often gives immunity from cold-catching. Easy perspiration when walking. Syphilis, inherited and tertiary. *Offensive discharges.*

Mind.—Hopeless; despairs of recovery. *Melancholy*, deep and persistent; religious. Suicidal tendency.

Head.—Awakens at night with pain as from blow on head. Chronic headaches; hungry during attacks; with vertigo. Hammering pain; brain feels too large; worse, change of weather. Dull, pressive pain in occiput. Humid eruption on scalp; hair matted. Hair dry.

Eyes.—Agglutinated. Blepharitis. *Chronic ophthalmia, that constantly recurs.* Edges of lids red. Secretion acrid.

Mouth.—Obstinate rhagades at corners. Tongue, gums ulcerated; tough mucus of foul taste adheres to soft palate.

Nose.—Dry, coryza, with stoppage of nose. Chronic catarrh; dropping from posterior nares. Acne rosacea.

Ears.—Raw, red, *oozing scabs around ears.* Sore pain behind ears. Herpes from temples over ears to cheeks. *Offensive discharge from eczema around ears. Intolerable itching.* Chronic otorrhœa. *Most fetid pus from ears*, brownish, offensive.

Face.—Swelling of upper lip. Pale, delicate. *Humid eruption on face.* Sickly.

Throat.—Tonsils greatly swollen; painful swallowing, with pain in ears. Profuse, offensive saliva; tough mucus in throat. Recurring quinsy. *Eradicates tendency to quinsy.* Hawking up of cheesy, pea-like balls of disgusting smell and taste. [*Agar.*]

Stomach.—Eructations like bad eggs. *Very hungry always; must have something to eat in the middle of the night.* Nausea: vomiting of pregnancy. Pain in abdomen after eating.

Stool.—Mucous, *bloody, excessively fetid, dark fluid.* Hard, difficult stool, with blood from rectum and burning piles. *Constipation of infants*, in pale, sickly scrofulous children.

Female.—*Leucorrhœa* fetid, lumpy, with much backache and *debility.* Mammæ swollen and painful. Pimples oozing an acrid fluid that burns and excoriates the glands.

Respiratory.—Asthma, with dyspnœa; worse, sitting up; better, lying down and keeping arms spread wide apart. Dry, hard cough, with great weakness in chest. *Feeling of ulceration under sternum.* Pain in chest; better, lying down. Cough returns every winter, from suppressed eruption. *Hay-fever returning irregularly every year.*

Extremities.—Weakness of joints, as if they would not hold together. *Eruption around finger-nails.* Fetid foot-sweats.

Skin.—Dirty, dingy look. Dry, lustreless, rough hair. *Intolerable itching.* Herpetic eruptions, especially on scalp and bends of joints with itching; worse, from warmth of bed. Enlarged glands. Sebaceous glands secrete excessively; oily skin. Indolent ulcers, slow to heal. Eczema behind ears. Crusty eruptions all over. Urticaria after every exertion. Pustules near finger-nails.

Fever.—Profuse, offensive perspiration; night-sweats.

Sleep.—Sleepless from intolerable itching. Easily startled.

Modalities.—*Worse*, coffee; Psorinum patient does not improve while using coffee. *Worse*, changes of weather, in hot sunshine, from cold. *Dread of least cold air or draft. Better*, heat, warm clothing, even in summer.

Relationship.—Complementary: *Sulphur.*

Compare: *Pediculus*—Head-louse—(psoric manifestations in children. Eruption on dorsum of hands, feet, neck. Prurigo; pellagra. Unusual aptitude for study and work). *Pediculus* (Cooties) transmit typhus and trench fever.) In lack of reaction compare *Calcarea* and *Natrum ars. Gaertner.* (Pessimistic, lack of confidence, subjective troublesome eye symptoms, fear of heights. Urticaria. Use 30th and 200th. (Wheeler.)

Dose.—Two hundredth and higher potencies. Should not be repeated too often. *Psorinum* requires something like 9 days before it manifests its action, and even a single dose may elicit other symptoms lasting for weeks. (Aegedi.)

PTELEA
(Wafer-ash)

Is a remarkable remedy in stomach and liver affections. The aching and heaviness in the region of the liver is *greatly aggravated by lying* on the left side. *Atonic states of stomach.* Asthma.

Head.—Feels dull and stupid. *Pain from forehead to root of nose; pressing-outward pain.* Frontal headache; worse, noise, motion, night, rubbing eyes, with acidity. Temples as if pressed together.

Mouth.—*Excess of saliva*, with dry *bitter taste.* Tongue coated white or yellow; feels rough, swollen. Papillæ *red and prominent.* [*Arg. n.*] Coating may be brownish-yellow.

Stomach.—Weight and fullness. Griping in epigastric region, with dryness of mouth. Eructations, nausea, vomiting. Constant sensation of corrosion, heat and burning in stomach. Stomach feels empty after eating. *Stomach and liver symptoms associated with pain in limbs.*

Abdomen.—Much weight and pain in right side; heavy, aching feeling, relieved by lying on right side. Liver sore, swollen, sensitive to pressure. Retraction of abdomen.

Respiratory.—Feeling of pressure on lungs and of suffocation, when lying on back. *Asthma;* dyspnœa; cramp-like pain in cardiac region.

Sleep.—Restless, with frightful dreams; nightmare, awakes languid and unrefreshed.

Modalities.—*Worse*, lying on left side; early morning. *Better*, eating sour things.

Relationship.—Compare: *Mercur.; Magn. mur.; Nux; Chelid.*

Dose.—First to thirtieth potency.

PULEX IRRITANS
(Common Flea)

Marked urinary and female symptoms.

Head.—Very impatient, cross, and irritable. Frontal headache, with *enlarged feeling of eyes. Face wrinkled and old-looking.*

Mouth.—Metallic taste. Sensation of a thread in throat. Thirsty, especially during headache.

Stomach.—Breath and taste foul. Intense nausea, with vomiting, purging, and faintness. Stool very offensive. Abdomen bloated.

Urine.—Scanty with frequent urging, with pressure on bladder and burning in urethra. Flow stops suddenly followed by pain. Urine foul. Cannot retain urine; must attend to the call without delay. Irritable bladder before menses.

Female.—Menses delayed. Increased flow of saliva during. Intense burning in vagina. Leucorrhœa, profuse, foul, staining a greenish yellow; stains of menses and leucorrhœa very hard to wash out. Backache. [*Oxal. ac.*]

Back.—Aches, weak; drawing of muscles below scapulæ.

Fever.—Feels a glow all over, like being over steam; *chilly,* while sitting beside the fire.

Skin.—Prickly itching. Sore spots all over. Skin emits foul odor.

Modalities.—*Better,* sitting or lying down. *Worse,* left side; moving about.

Dose.—The higher potencies.

PULSATILLA
(Wind Flower)

The weather-cock among remedies.

The disposition and mental state are the chief guiding symptoms to the selection of Pulsatilla. It is pre-eminently a female remedy, especially for mild, gentle, yielding disposition. Sad, crying readily; weeps when talking; *changeable,* contradictory. *The patient seeks the open air; always feels better there,* even though he is chilly. Mucous membranes are all affected. *Discharges thick, bland, and yellowish-green.* Often indicated after abuse of Iron tonics, and after badly-managed measles. *Symptoms ever changing. Thirstless, peevish, and chilly.* When first serious impairment of health is referred to age of puberty. Great sensitiveness. Wants the head high. Feels uncomfortable with only one pillow. Lies with hands above head.

Mind.—Weeps easily. Timid, irresolute. Fears in evening to be alone, dark, ghosts. Likes sympathy. Children like fuss and caresses. Easily discouraged. Morbid dread of the opposite sex. Religious melancholy. Given to extremes of pleasure and pain. Highly emotional. Mentally, an April day.

Head.—Wandering stitches about head; pains extend to face and teeth; vertigo; better in open air. Frontal and supra-orbital pains. Neuralgic pains, commencing in *right temporal region, with scalding lachrymation of affected side. Headache from overwork.* Pressure on vertex.

Ears.—Sensation as if something were being forced outward. Hearing difficult, as if the ear were stuffed. Otorrhœa. Thick, bland discharge; offensive odor. External ear swollen and red. Catarrhal otitis. Otalgia, worse at night. Diminishes acuteness of hearing.

Eyes.—*Thick, profuse, yellow, bland discharges.* Itching and burning in eyes. Profuse lachrymation and secretion of mucus. *Lids inflamed, agglutinated. Styes.* Veins of fundus oculi greatly enlarged. Ophthalmia neonatorum. Subacute conjunctivitis, with dyspepsia; worse, in warm room.

Nose.—Coryza; stoppage of right nostril, pressing pain at root of nose. Loss of smell. Large green fetid scales in nose. Stoppage in evening. Yellow mucus; abundant in morning. Bad smells, as of old catarrh. Nasal bones sore.

Face.—Right-sided neuralgia, with profuse lachrymation. Swelling of lower lip, which is cracked in middle. Prosopalgia towards evening till midnight; chilly, with pain.

Mouth.—Greasy taste. *Dry mouth, without thirst;* wants it washed frequently. Frequently licks the dry lips. *Crack in middle of lower lip. Yellow or white tongue, covered with a tenacious mucus.* Toothache; relieved by holding cold water in mouth. [*Coff.*] Offensive odor from mouth. [*Merc.; Aur.*] Food, especially bread, tastes bitter. Much *sweet* saliva. *Alterations of taste,* bitter, bilious, greasy, salty, *foul.* Loss of taste. Desire for tonics.

Stomach.—*Averse to fat food, warm food, and drink.* Eructations; *taste of food remains a long time;* after ices, fruits, pasty. *Bitter taste,* diminished taste of all food. Pain as from subcutaneous ulceration. *Flatulence.* Dislikes butter. [*Sang.*]

Heartburn. Dyspepsia, with great tightness after a meal; must loosen clothing. *Thirstlessness*, with nearly all complaints. Vomiting of food eaten long before. Pain in stomach an hour after eating. [*Nux.*] Weight as from a stone, especially in morning on awakening. Gnawing, hungry feeling. [*Abies c.*] Perceptible pulsation in pit of stomach. [*Asaf.*] All-gone sensation, especially in tea drinkers. Waterbrash, with foul taste in the morning.

Abdomen.—Painful, distended; loud rumbling. Pressure as from a stone. Colic, with chilliness in evening.

Stool.—Rumbling, watery; worse, night. *No two stools alike.* After fruit. [*Ars.; Chin.*] Blind hæmorrhoids, with itching and sticking pains. Dysentery; mucus and blood, with chilliness. [*Merc.; Rheum.*] *Two or three normal stools daily.*

Urine.—Increased desire; *worse when lying down.* Burning in orifice of urethra during and after micturition. Involuntary micturition at night, while coughing or passing flatus. After urinating, spasmodic pain in bladder.

Female.—Amenorrhœa. [*Cimicif.; Senec.; Polygon.*] Suppressed menses from wet feet, nervous debility, or chlorosis. Tardy menses. Too late, scanty, thick, dark, *clotted, changeable, intermittent.* Chilliness, nausea, downward pressure, painful, flow intermits. Leucorrhœa acrid, burning, creamy. Pain in back; tired feeling. Diarrhœa during or after menses.

Male.—Orchitis; pain from abdomen to testicles. Thick, yellow discharge from urethra; late stage of gonorrhœa. Stricture; urine passed only in drops, and stream interrupted. [*Clemat.*] *Acute prostatitis.* Pain and tenesmus in urinating, *worse lying on back.*

Respiratory.—Capricious hoarseness; comes and goes. *Dry cough in evening and at night; must sit up in bed to get relief; and loose cough in the morning,* with copious mucous expectoration. *Pressure upon the chest and soreness.* Great soreness of episgastrium. Urine emitted with cough. [*Caust.*] Pain as from ulcer in middle of chest. Expectoration bland, thick, bitter, greenish. Short breath, anxiety, and palpitation when lying on left side. [*Phos.*] Smothering sensation on lying down.

Sleep.—*Wide awake in the evening;* first sleep restless.

Wakes languid, unrefreshed. Irresistible sleepiness in afternoon. Sleeps with hands over head.

Back.—Shooting pain in the nape and back, between shoulders; in sacrum after sitting.

Extremities.—Drawing, tensive pain in thighs and legs, with restlessness, sleeplessness and *chilliness*. *Pain in limbs, shifting rapidly; tensive pain, letting up with a snap.* Numbness around elbow. Hip-joint painful. Knees swollen, with tearing, drawing pains. Boring pain in heels toward evening; *suffering worse from letting the affected limb hang down.* [*Vipera.*] Veins in forearms and hands swollen. Feet red, inflamed, swollen. Legs feel heavy and weary.

Skin.—Urticaria, after rich food, with diarrhœa, from delayed menses, worse undressing. *Measles.* Acne at puberty. Varicose veins.

Fever.—*Chilliness*, even in warm room, *without thirst.* Chilly with pains, in spots, worse evening. Chill about 4 p. m. Intolerable burning heat at night, with distended veins; heat in parts of body, coldness in other. One-sided sweat; pains during sweat. *External heat is intolerable, veins are distended.* During apyrexia, headache, diarrhœa, loss of appetite, nausea.

Modalities.—*Worse*, from heat, rich fat food, after eating, towards evening, warm room, lying on left or on painless side, when allowing feet to hang down. *Better*, open air, motion, cold applications, cold food and drinks. though not thirsty.

Relationship.—*Penthorum*, often indicated after Pulsatilla in later colds. *Ionesia Asoca*—Saraca indica—(*Amenorrhœa*, Menorrhagia—acts powerfully on female organs. Abdominal pain). *Atriplex* (Uterine symptoms, amenorrhœa; hysteria, coldness between shoulders, dislike of warm food, craves strange foods, palpitation, sleeplessness). *Pulsatilla Nuttaliana*, identical effects.

Compare: *Cyclamen; Kali bich.; Kali sulph.; Sulphur.*

Pimenta—Allspice—(one-sided neuralgias, parts of body hot and cold).

Anagyris (headache, amenorrhœa).

Complementary: *Coffea; Chamom.; Nux.*

Dose.—Third to thirtieth attenuation.

PYROGENIUM
(Artificial Sepsin)

This remedy was introduced by English Homœopathists, prepared from decomposed lean beef allowed to stand in the sun for two weeks and then potentized. The provings and most of the clinical experience have been obtained from this preparation. But, subsequently, Dr. Swan potentized some septic pus, which preparation has also been proved and clinically applied. There does not seem to be any marked difference in their effects.

Pyrogen is the great remedy for *septic states*, with intense restlessness. "In septic fevers, especially puerperal, Pyrogen has demonstrated its great value as a homœopathic dynamic antiseptic." (H. C. Allen.) Hectic, typhoid, typhus, ptomaine poisoning, diphtheria, dissecting wounds, sewer-gas poisoning, chronic malaria, after-effects of miscarriage, all these conditions at times may present symptoms calling for this unique medicine. *All discharges are horribly offensive*—menstrual, lochial, diarrhœa, vomit, sweat, breath, etc. Great pain and violent burning in abscesses. Chronic complaints that date back to septic conditions. Threatening heart failure in zymotic and septic fevers. Influenza, typhoid symptoms.

Mind.—Full of anxiety and insane notions. Loquacious. Thinks he is very wealthy. *Restless.* Feels if crowded with arms and legs. Cannot tell whether dreaming while awake or asleep.

Head.—Painless throbbing. Fan-like motion of alæ nasi. [*Lyc.; Phos.*] Bursting headache with restlessness.

Mouth.—Tongue red and *dry*, clean, cracked, smooth, as though varnished. Throat dry, articulation difficult. Nausea and vomiting. Taste terribly fetid. Breath horrible.

Stomach.—Coffee-grounds vomiting. Vomits water, when it becomes warm in stomach.

Abdomen.—Intolerable tenesmus of both bladder and rectum. Bloated, sore, cutting pain.

Stool.—Diarrhœa; horribly offensive, brown-black, painless, involuntary. Constipation, with complete inertia [*Opium*]; obstinate from impaction. Stools large, black, carrion-like, or small black balls.

Heart.—Tired feeling about heart. *Palpitation*. Sensation as if heart were too full. Always can hear her heart beat. Pulse abnormally rapid, *out of proportion to the temperature*. Pain in region of left nipple. Conscious of heart.

Female.—Puerperal peritonitis, with extreme fetor. Septicæmia following abortion. Menses horribly offensive. Uterine hæmorrhages. Fever at each menstrual period, consequent upon latent pelvic inflammation. *Septic puerperal infection*. Pelvic calculitis. Inflammatory exudate. Post-operative cases, with overwhelming sepsis.

Fever.—Coldness and chilliness. *Septic fevers*. Latent pyogenic condition. Chill begins in back. Temperature rises rapidly. Great heat with profuse hot sweat, but *sweating does not cause a fall in temperature*.

Extremities.—Throbbing in vessels of neck. Numbness of hands, arms, feet. Aching in all limbs and bones. *Bed feels too hard*. [*Arn*.] Great debility in the morning. Soreness; better by motion. [*Rhus*.] Rapid decubitus of septic origin.

Skin.—Small cut or injury becomes much swollen and inflamed—discolored. Dry.

Sleep.—Seems to be in semi-sleep. Dreams all night.

Modalities.—Relief from motion.

Relationship.—Compare: *Streptoccin* (anti-febrile action; septic symptoms in infectious diseases). Rapid in its action, especially in its effect on temperature;) *Staphyloccin* in diseases where the staphylococcus is the chief bacterial factor, as acne, abscess, furuncle; empyema, endocarditis, etc.); *Sepin* —A toxin of Proteus vulgaris, prepared by Dr. Shedd, same symptoms as Pyrogen, of which it is the main constituent; *Echinacea; Carbo; Ars.; Lach.; Rhus; Bapt.*

Complementary: *Bryon*.

Dose.—Sixth to thirtieth and higher potencies. Should not be repeated too frequently.

QUASSIA—PICRAENA EXCELSA
(Quassia-wood)

Acts on gastric organs as a tonic. [*Gentian; Hydr*.] Seems to possess marked action on eyes, producing amblyopia and cataract. Pain in right intercostal muscles above the liver. Pressure and stitches in liver, and sympathetically in spleen.

Stomach.—Atonic dyspepsia, with gas and acidity. Heartburn and gastralgia. Regurgitation of food. Abdomen feels empty and retracted. Dyspepsia after infectious diseases; especially grip, dysentery. Tongue dry or with brown sticky coating. Cirrhosis of liver with ascites.

Urinary.—Excessive desire—impossible to retain urine; copious micturition day and night. As soon as the child wakes up the bed is drenched.

Extremities.—Inclination to yawn and stretch. [*Rhus.*] Sensation of coldness over back. Prostration, with hunger. Cold extremities, with sensation of internal coldness. [*Heloderma.*]

Dose.—First to third potency, or spoonful doses of Aqua Quassiæ

QUERCUS GLANDIUM SPIRITUS
(Spirit distilled from Tincture of Acorn Kernels)

Used first by Rademacher for chronic spleen affections; *spleen-dropsy.* Antidotes effects of Alcohol. Vertigo; deafness, with noises in head. *Takes away craving for alcoholics;* give dose as below for several months. Dropsy and liver affections. Useful in gout, old malarial cases with flatulence.

Relationship.—Compare: *Angelica* (in tincture, five drops, three times daily, produces disgust for liquor; also for atony of different organs, dyspepsia, nervous headache, etc.; chronic bronchitis to increase expectoration.) *Ceanoth.; Lach.; Nat. mur.; Helianthus* (spleen enlarged and painful.)

Dose.—Ten drops to a teaspoonful of the distilled spirit three to four times a day. A passing diarrhœa often appears for a time when using it. Curative effect. Quercus acts well in trituration of the acorn 3x in splenic cases, flatulence, old malaria and alcoholic history. (Clark.)

QUILLAYA SAPONARIA
(Chile Soap-bark)

Produces and cures symptoms of acute catarrh, sneezing and sore throat. *Most effective in the beginning of coryza*, frequently checking its further development. Colds with sore throat; heat and dryness of throat. Cough with difficult expectoration. Squamous skin.

Relationship.—Compare: *Kali hyd.; Gels.; Cepa.; Squilla. Saponaria* (sore throat, involuntary urination). Senega.

Dose.—Tincture and first potency.

RADIUM
(Radium Bromide)

An important addition to the Materia Medica, especially since the provings by Diffenbach have precisionized its use. Radium brom. of 1,800,000 radio-activity was employed. Found effective in the treatment of rheumatism and gout, in skin affections generally, acne rosacea, nævi, moles, ulcers and cancers. Lowered blood pressure. *Severe aching pains all over*, with restlessness, better moving about. Chronic rheumatic arthritis. Lateness in appearance of symptoms. Ulcers due to Radium burns, take a long time to heal. Marked increase in the polymorphonuclear neutrophiles. Great weakness.

Mind.—Apprehensive, depressed; fear of being alone in the dark; great desire to be with people. Tired and irritable.

Head.—Vertigo, with pain in back of head, left when in bed. Occipital and vertex pain, accompanying severe lumbar aching. Severe pain over right eye, spreading back to occiput and to vertex, better in open air. Head feels heavy. Frontal headache. Both eyes ache. Itching and dryness of nasal cavities, better in open air. Aching pain in angle of right lower jaw. Violent trifacial neuralgia.

Mouth.—Dryness of mouth. Metallic taste. Prickling sensation on end of tongue.

Stomach.—Empty feeling in stomach. Warm sensation in stomach. Aversion to sweets, ice-cream. Nausea and sinking sensation, belching of gas.

Abdomen.—Pain, violent cramps, rumbling, full of gas; pain over McBurney's point, and at location of sigmoid flexure. Much flatulence. Alternating constipation and loose movements. Pruritus ani and piles.

Urinary.—Increased elimination of solids, particularly of chlorides. Renal irritation, albuminuria, granular and hyaline casts. Nephritis with rheumatic symptoms. Enuresis.

Female.—Pruritus vulvæ. Delayed and irregular menstruation and backache. Aching pains in abdomen over pubes when flow comes on. Right breast sore, relieved by hard rubbing.

Respiratory.—Persistent cough with tickling in suprasternal fossa. Dry, spasmodic cough. Throat dry, sore, chest constricted.

Back.—Aching in back of neck. Pain and lameness in cervical vertebræ, worse dropping head forward, better standing, or sitting erect. *Lumbar and sacral* backache, pain appears to be in *bone*, continued motion relieves. Backache between shoulders and lumbar-sacral region, better after walking.

Extremities.—Severe pain in all the limbs, *joints*, especially in knee and ankles, sharp pains in shoulders, arms, hands and fingers. Legs, arms and neck feel hard and brittle, as though they would break on moving. Arms feel heavy. Cracking in shoulder. *Pain in toes*, calves, hip-joint, popliteal spaces. Muscles of legs and hips sore. *Arthritis*, aching pains, *worse* at night. Dermatitis of the fingers. Trophic changes in the finger nails.

Skin.—Small pimples. Erythema and dermatitis, with itching, burning, swelling and redness. Necrosis and ulceration. *Itching all over body*, burning of skin, as if afire. Epithelioma.

Sleep.—Restless. Sleepiness with lethargy. Dreams vivid, busy. Dreams of fire.

Fever.—Cold sensation internally, with chattering of teeth until noon. Internal chilliness followed by heat of the skin, associated with bowel movements and flatulence.

Modalities.—*Better*, open air, continued motion, hot bath, lying down, pressure. *Worse*, getting up.

Relationship.—Compare: *Anacardium* (the ulceration produced by it is like *Radium*. It may appear elsewhere than on place of contact and appear late). Compare: *X-Ray; Rhus; Sepia; Uranium; Ars.; Pulsat.; Caustic.*

Antidotes: *Rhus ven.; Tellur.*

Dose.—Thirtieth and twelfth trituration.

RANUNCULUS BULBOSUS
(Buttercup)

Acts especially upon the muscular tissue and skin, and its most characteristic effects are upon the chest walls, like pleurodynia. *Bad effects of Alcohol; delirium tremens.* Spasmodic hiccough. Hydrothorax. Shocks throughout the whole body. Sensitive to air and touch. Chronic sciatica.

Head.—Irritable, pains in forehead and eyeballs. Creeping sensation in scalp. Pressing pain in forehead from within outward.

Eyes.—Day-blindness; mist before eyes; pressure and smarting in eyes, as from smoke. Pain over right eye; better, standing and walking. Herpes on cornea. Vesicles on cornea, with intense pain, photophobia, and lachrymation.

Chest.—Various kinds of pains and *soreness, as if bruised in sternum,* ribs, intercostal spaces, and both hypochondria. *Intercostal rheumatism. Chilliness in chest when walking in open air.* Stitches in chest, between shoulder-blades; worse, inspiring, moving. Rheumatic pain in chest, as from subcutaneous ulceration. *Tenderness of abdomen to pressure. Muscular pain along lower margin of the shoulder-blade;* burning in small spots from sedentary employment.

Skin.—*Burning and intense itching; worse, contact.* Hard excrescences. *Herpetic eruptions,* with great itching. *Shingles; bluish vesicles.* Itching in palms. Blister-like eruption in palms. Corns sensitive. Horny skin. Finger-tips and palms chapped. Vesicular and pustular eruptions.

Modalities.—*Worse,* open air, motion, contact, atmospheric changes, wet, stormy weather, evening. Cold air brings on all sorts of ailments.

Relationship.—Incompatible: *Sulph.; Staph.*

Compare: *Ranunc. acris* (pain in lumbar muscles and joints

by bending and turning body); *Ranunc. glacialis*—Reindeer flower Carlina—(Pulmonary affections; broncho-pneumonical Influenza—enormous weight in head with vertigo and sensation as of impending apoplexy; night-sweats—more on thighs); *Ranunc. repens* (crawling sensation in forehead and scalp in evening in bed); *Ranunc. flammula* (ulceration; gangrene of arm). Compare, also: *Bry.; Croton; Mez.; Euphorb.*

Antidotes: *Bry.; Camph.; Rhus.*

Dose.—Mother tincture, in ten to thirty drop doses in delirium tremens; third to thirtieth potency generally. Chronic sciatica, apply tincture to heel of affected leg (M. Jousset).

RANUNCULUS SCELERATUS
(Marsh Buttercup)

Is more irritating than others of this botanical family, as seen in the skin symptoms. *Boring, gnawing pain* very marked. *Pemphigus.* Periodical complaints. Fainting with pain in stomach.

Head.—Gnawing in one spot left of vertex. Frightful dreams about corpses, serpents, battles, etc. Fluent coryza, with sneezing and burning micturition.

Mouth.—Teeth and gums sensitive. *Tongue mapped.* Denuded patches. Mouth sore and raw. *Burning and rawness of tongue.*

Abdomen.—Sensation of a plug behind umbilicus. *Pain over region of liver, with sensation as if diarrhœa would set it.* Pressure as of a plug behind right false ribs; worse, deep inspiration.

Chest.—Integument sensitive. Bruised pain and weakness in the chest every evening. *Sore burning behind xiphoid cartilage.*

Skin.—*Vesicular eruption, with tendency to form large blisters. Acrid exudation, which makes surrounding parts sore.*

Extremities.—*Boring pain.* Sudden burning sticking *in right toe.* Corns, with burning and soreness, especially when feet hang down. Gout in fingers and toes.

Dose.—First to third potency.

RAPHANUS
(Black Garden Radish)

Produces pain and stitches in liver and spleen. Increases of bile and salivary secretion. Symptoms will not appear if salt is used with the Radish. Great accumulation and incarceration of flatulence. "Globus" symptoms. Seborrhœa, with greasy skin. Pemphigus. Hysteria; chilliness in back and arms. Sexual insomnia. [*Kali brom.*] Nymphomania. *Postoperative gas pains.*

Head.—Sadness, aversion to children, especially girls. Headache, brain feels tender and sore. Œdema of lower eyelids. Mucus in posterior nares.

Throat.—Hot-ball feeling from uterus to throat, stopping there. Heat and burning in throat.

Stomach.—Putrid eructations. Burning in epigastrium, followed by hot eructation.

Abdomen.—Retching and vomiting, loss of appetite. Distended, *tympanitic, hard. No flatus emitted upward or downward.* Griping about navel. Stool liquid, frothy, profuse, brown, with colic, and pad-like swelling of intestines. Vomiting of faecal matter.

Female.—Nervous irritation of genitals. Menses very profuse and long-lasting. *Nymphomania,* with aversion to her own sex and to children, and sexual insomnia.

Urine.—Turbid, with yeast-like sediment. Urine more copious, thick like milk.

Chest.—Pain in chest extends to back and to throat. Heavy lump and coldness in center of chest.

Relationship.—Compare: *Momordica* (worse, near splenic flexure); *Carbo; Anarc.; Arg. nit.; Brassica.*

Dose.—Third to thirtieth potency.

RATANHIA
(Krameria—Mapato)

The rectal symptoms are most important, and have received much clinical confirmation. It has cured pterygium. *Violent hiccough.* Cracked nipples. [*Graph.; Eup. ar.*] *Pin worms.*

Head.—Bursting in head after stool, and when sitting with head bent forward. Sensation as if scalp from nose to vertex were stretched.

Stomach.—Pain like knives cutting the stomach.

Rectum.—Aches, as if full of broken glass. Anus aches and burns for hours after stool. Feels constricted. Dry heat at anus, with sudden knife-like stitches. Stools must be forced with great effort; protrusion of hæmorrhoids. *Fissures of anus, with great constriction, burning like fire,* as do the hæmorrhoids; temporarily relieved by cold water. Fetid, thin diarrhœa; stools burn; burning pains before and after stools. Oozing at anus. *Pin-worms.* [*Sant.; Teuc.; Spig.*] Itching of anus.

Relationship.—Compare: *Pæon.; Croton* (rectal neuralgia); *Sanguin. nit.* (diseases of rectum); *Macuna prurens—Dolichos—* piles, *with* burning; hæmorrhoidal diathesis); *Silico-sulpho-calcite of Alumina; Slag*—blast iron furnace cinder—(anal itching, piles, and constipation; housemaid's knee); abdominal flatulent distension and lumbago. Analogue to Lycopod.

Dose.—Third to sixth potency. Locally, the Cerate has proved invaluable in many rectal complaints.

RHAMNUS CALIFORNICA
(California Coffee-tree)

One of the most positive remedies for rheumatism and *muscular pains.* Pleurodynia, lumbago, gastralgia. Vesical tenesmus; *dysmenorrhœa* of myalgic origin; pain in head, neck, and face. *Inflammatory rheumatism,* joints swollen, painful; tendency to metastasis; profuse sweat. Rheumatic heart (Webster).

Provings of students. 2x potency.

Mind.—Nervous, restless, irritable. Lassitude; mentally dull and dazed; unable to concentrate mind on studies.

Head.—*Dizzy* full feeling. Heavy bruised sensation; better, from pressure. *Bursting* feeling with every step. Soreness, especially in occiput and vertex, worse, bending over. Dull pain in left temple. Dull aching in frontal region (left), extending backwards and over forehead. Deep, right-sided frontal headache. Twitching eyelids.

Ears.—*Dullness of hearing.* Soreness, deep under right tragus on swallowing.

Face.—Flushed, hot and glowing. Outward pressure from malar processes.

Mouth.—Canker sore between gums and lips. Tongue coated, with clean, pink central patch.

Throat.—Dry, rough. Soreness on right side and tonsil.

Bowels.—*Constipation* with some flatus. Tenesmus and dry stool. Flatulent diarrhœa.

Genito-urinary.—Increased urination. Tickling in anterior urethra, small morning drop (no previous gonorrhœa). Sexual desire increased.

Respiratory.—Substernal oppression. Tenderness on pressure of right intercostal muscles.

Heart.—Variation of pulse. Slow pulse.

Extremities.—Unable to control muscular action. Legs sore. Walked like a drunken man.

Modality.—Symptoms worse in evening.

Relationship.—*Rhamnus cathartica* or *Rhamnus Frangula*—European Buckthorn—a rheumatic remedy—(abdominal symptoms, colic, diarrhœa; hæmorrhoids, especially chronic). *Rhamnus Purshiana—Cascara Sagrada*—(palliative in constipation, as an intestinal tonic, and dyspepsia dependent thereon. 10-15 drops of tincture).

Dose.—Tincture in 15-drop doses every four hours.

RHEUM
(Rhubarb)

Of frequent use in children with sour diarrhœa; difficult dentition. *Whole child smells sour.*

Mind.—Impatient and vehement; desires many things and cries. [*Cina.*]

Head.—Sweat on hairy scalp; constant and profuse. *Cool sweat on the face, especially about mouth and nose.*

Mouth.—Much saliva. Sensation of coolness in teeth. Difficult teething; restless and irritable. Breath smells sour. [*Cham.*]

Stomach.—Desire for various kinds of food, but soon tires of all. Throbbing in pit. Feels full.

Abdomen.—Colicky pain about navel. Colic when uncovering. Wind seems to rise up to chest.

Rectum.—Before stool, unsuccessful urging to urinate. *Stools smell sour*, pasty, with shivering and tenesmus, and burning in anus. Sour diarrhœa during dentition. Colicky, even ineffectual urging to evacuate altered fæcal stools.

Modalities.—*Worse*, uncovering, after eating, moving about.

Relationship.—Compare: *Mag. phos.; Hep.; Pod.; Cham.; Ipec.*

Antidotes: *Camph.; Cham.*

Complementary: *Mag. carb.*

Dose.—Third to sixth potency.

RHODIUM
(Metal Chemical Element)

(Proved by MacFarlan with the 200th potency.)

Nervous and tearful. Frontal headache; shocks through head. Fleeting neuralgic pains in head, over eyes, in ear, both sides of nose, teeth. Loose cold in head. Lips dry. Nausea especially from sweets. Dull headache. Stiff neck and rheumatic pain down left shoulder and arm. Itching in arms, palms and face. Loose stools with gripings in abdomen. Hyper-active peristalsis, tenesmus after stool. More urine passed. Cough scratchy, wheezy. Thick, yellow mucus from chest. Feels weak, dizzy and a tired feeling.

RHODODENDRON
(Snow-rose)

Rheumatic and gouty symptoms well marked. Rheumatism in the hot season. The modality (worse before a storm) is a true guiding symptom.

Mind.—Dread of a storm; particularly afraid of thunder. Forgetful.

Head.—Aching in temples. Tearing pain in bones. Headache; worse, wine, wind, cold and wet weather. Pain in eyes before a storm. *Ciliary neuralgia*, involving eyeball, orbit, and head. Heat in eyes when using them.

Eyes.—Muscular asthenopia; darting pains through eyes from head, worse before a storm.

Ears.—Difficult hearing, with whizzing and ringing in ears. Hearing better in the morning; noises come on after patient has been up a few hours.

Face.—Prosopalgia; violent jerking pain involving dental nerves, from temple to lower jaw and chin; *better, warmth and eating.* Toothache in damp weather and before a storm. Swollen gums. Stumps of teeth are loosened.

Chest.—Violent pleuritic pains running downward in left anterior chest. Breathless and speechless from violent pleuritic pains running down the anterior chest. Stitches in spleen from fast walking. Crampy pain under short ribs.

Male.—Testicles, worse left, swollen, painful, drawn up. Orchitis; glands feel crushed. Induration and swelling of testes after gonorrhœa. *Hydrocele.* [*Sil.*]

Extremities.—Joints swollen. Gouty inflammation of great toe-joint. *Rheumatic tearing in all limbs*, especially right side; worse, at rest and in stormy weather. Stiffness of neck. Pain in shoulders, arms, wrists; worse when at rest. Pains in bones in spots, and reappear by change of weather. *Cannot sleep unless legs are crossed.*

Modalities.—*Worse*, before a storm. *All symptoms reappear in rough weather*, night, towards morning. *Better*, after the storm breaks, warmth, and eating.

Relationship.—Compare: *Ampelopsis* (hydrocele and renal dropsy); *Dulc.; Rhus; Nat. sulph.*

Dose.—First to sixth potency.

RHUS AROMATICA
(Fragrant Sumach)

Renal and urinary affections, especially *diabetes*. Enuresis due to vesical atony; senile incontinence. Hæmaturia and cystitis come within the range of this remedy.

Urine.—*Pale*, albuminous. *Incontinence. Severe pain at beginning or before urination*, causing great agony in children. Constant dribbling. *Diabetes*, large quantities of urine of low specific gravity. [*Phos. ac.; Acet. ac.*]

Dose.—Tincture, in rather material doses.

RHUS GLABRA
(Smooth Sumach)

Epistaxis and *occipital headache*. *Fetid flatus*. Ulceration of mouth. *Dreams of flying through the air*. [*Sticta*.] *Profuse perspiration arising from debility*. [*China*.] It is claimed that this remedy will so disinfect the bowels that the flatus and stools will be free from odor. It acts well in putrescent conditions with tendency to ulceration.

Mouth.—Scurvy; nursing sore mouth. [*Veronica*.] Aphthous stomatitis.

Relationship.—Said to be antidotal to the action of Mercury, and has been employed in the treatment of secondary syphilis after mercurialization.

Dose.—Tincture. Usually locally to soft, spongy gums, aphthæ, pharyngitis, etc. Internally, first potency.

RHUS TOXICODENDRON
(Poison-ivy)

The effects on the skin, rheumatic pains, mucous membrane affections, and a typhoid type of fever, make this remedy frequently indicated. Rhus affects fibrous tissue markedly—joints, tendons, sheaths—aponeurosis, etc., producing pains and stiffness. Post-operative complications. *Tearing asunder pains*. Motion always "limbers up" the Rhus patient, and hence he feels better for a time from a change of position. Ailments from strains, overlifting, getting wet while perspiring. Septic conditions. Cellulitis and infections, carbuncles in early stages. [*Echinac*.] Rheumatism in the cold season. *Septicæmia*.

Mind.—Listless, sad. Thoughts of suicide. *Extreme restlessness, with continued change of position*. Delirium, with fear of being poisoned. [*Hyos*.] *Sensorium becomes cloudy. Great apprehension at night, cannot remain in bed*.

Head.—Feels as if a board were strapped on the forehead. Vertigo when rising. *Heavy* head. Brain feels loose and as if struck against skull on walking or rising. Scalp sensitive; worse on side lain on. Headache in occiput [*Rhus rad*.]; painful to touch. Pain in forehead and proceeds thence backward. Humid eruptions on scalp; itching greatly.

Eyes.—Swollen, red, œdematous; *orbital cellulitis. Pustular inflammations.* Photophobia; profuse flow of yellow pus. Œdema of lids, suppurative iritis. Lids inflamed, agglutinated, swollen. Old injured eyes. Circumscribed corneal injection. Intensive ulceration of the cornea. Iritis, after exposure to cold and dampness, and of rheumatic origin. Eye painful on turning it or pressing, can hardly move it, as in acute retrobulbar neuritis. Profuse gush of hot, scalding tears upon opening lids.

Ears.—Pain in ears, with sensation as if something were in them. Lobules swollen. Discharge of bloody pus.

Nose.—Sneezing; coryza from getting wet. Tip of nose red, sore, ulcerated. Swelling of nose. Nosebleed on stooping.

Face.—*Jaws crack when chewing.* Easy dislocation of jaw. [*Ign.; Petrol.*] *Swollen face*, erysipelas. Cheek bones sensitive to touch. Parotitis. Facial neuralgia, with chilliness; worse, evening. *Crusta lactea.* [*Calc.; Viol. tric.*]

Mouth.—Teeth feel loose and long; gums sore. Tongue red and cracked; *coated, except red triangular space at the tip;* dry and red at edges. Corners of mouth ulcerated; fever-blisters around mouth and chin. [*Nat. mur.*] *Pain in maxillary joint.*

Throat.—Sore, with *swollen glands.* Sticking pain on swallowing. Parotitis, left side.

Stomach.—Want of appetite for any kind of food, with unquenchable thirst. *Bitter taste.* [*Cupr.*] Nausea, vertigo, and bloated abdomen after eating. *Desire for milk.* Great thirst, with dry mouth and throat. Pressure as from a stone. [*Bry.; Ars.*] *Drowsy after eating.*

Abdomen.—Violent pains, relieved by lying on abdomen. Swelling of inguinal glands. Pain in region of ascending colon. Colic, compelling to walk bent. Excessive distention after eating. Rumbling of flatus on first rising, but disappears with continued motion.

Rectum.—Diarrhœa of blood, slime, and reddish mucus. Dysentery, with tearing pains down thighs. Stools of cadaverous odor. Frothy, painless stools. Will often abort a beginning suppurative process near the rectum. Dysentery.

Urinary.—Dark, turbid, high-colored, scanty urine, with white sediment. Dysuria, with loss of blood.

Male.—Swelling of glands and prepuce—dark-red erysipelatous; scrotum thick, swollen, *œdematous. Itching intense.*

Female.—Swelling, with intense itching of vulva. Pelvic articulations stiff when beginning to move. Menses early, profuse, and prolonged, acrid. *Lochia thin, protracted, offensive diminished* [*Puls.; Secale*], *with shooting upwards in vagina.* [*Sep.*]

Respiratory.—Tickling behind upper sternum. *Dry, teasing cough from midnight until morning, during a chill, or when putting hands out of bed.* Hæmoptysis from overexertion; blood bright red. Influenza, with aching in all bones. [*Eup. perf.*] Hoarseness from overstraining voice. [*Arn.*] Oppression of the chest, cannot get breath with sticking pains. Bronchial coughs in old people, worse on awaking and with expectoration of small plugs of mucus.

Heart.—Hypertrophy from overexertion. Pulse quick, weak, irregular, intermittent, with numbness of left arm. *Trembling and palpitation when sitting still.*

Back.—Pain between shoulders on swallowing. *Pain and stiffness in small of back; better, motion, or lying on something hard; worse, while sitting.* Stiffness of the nape of the neck.

Extremities.—Hot, painful swelling of joints. *Pains tearing in tendons, ligaments, and fasciæ.* Rheumatic pains spread over a large surface at nape of neck, loins, and extremities; better motion. [*Agaric.*] Soreness of condyles of bones. *Limbs stiff, paralyzed. The cold fresh air is not tolerated; it makes the skin painful.* Pain along ulnar nerve. Tearing down thighs. *Sciatica;* worse, cold, damp weather, at night. Numbness and formication, after overwork and exposure. Paralysis; trembling after exertion. Tenderness about knee-joint. Loss of power in forearm and fingers; crawling sensation in the tips of fingers. Tingling in feet.

Fever.—Adynamic; restless, trembling. Typhoid; tongue dry and brown; sordes; bowels loose; great restlessness. Intermittent; chill, with dry cough and restlessness. During heat, uticaria. Hydroa. Chilly, as if cold water were poured over him, followed by heat and inclination to stretch the limbs.

Skin.—Red, swollen; *itching intense.* Vesicles, herpes; *urticaria;* pemphigus; erysipelas; vesicular suppurative forms. Glands swollen. *Cellulitis.* Burning eczematous eruptions with tendency to scale formation.

Sleep.—*Dreams of great exertion.* Heavy sleep, as from stupor. Sleepless before midnight.

Modalities.—*Worse,* during sleep, cold, wet rainy weather and after rain; at night, *during rest,* drenching, when lying on back or right side. *Better,* warm, dry weather, motion; walking, change of position, rubbing, warm applications, from stretching out limbs.

Relationship.—Complementary: *Bry.; Calc. fluor. Phytol.* (Rheumatism). In urticaria follow with *Bovista.*

Inimical: *Apis.*

Antidotes: Bathing with milk and Grindelia lotion very effective. *Ampelopsis Trifolia*—Three-leaf Woodbine—(Toxic dermatitis due to vegetable poisons—30 and 200. Very similar to Rhus poisoning. Desensitizing against Ivy poisoning by the use of ascending doses of the tincture by mouth or by hypodermic injections is recommended by old school authorities, but is not as effective as the homœopathic remedies especially *Rhus* 30 and 200 and *Anacard.,* etc. *Anacard.; Croton.; Grindelia; Mezer.; Cyprip.; Plumbago* (eczema of vulva); *Graph.*

Compare: *Rhus radicans* (almost identical action); characteristics are, burning in tongue, tip feels sore, pains are often semilateral and in various parts, often remote and successive. Many symptoms are better after a storm has thoroughly set in, especially after an electric storm. Has pronounced *yearly* aggravation. [*Laches.*] *Rhus radicans* has headache in *occiput* even pain in nape of neck and from there pains draw over the head *forwards.) Rhus diversiloba*—California Poison-oak—(antidote to Rhus; violent skin symptoms, with frightful itching; much swelling of face, hands and genitals; skin very sensitive; eczema and erysipelas, great nervous weakness, tired from least effort; goes to sleep from sheer exhaustion); *Xerophyllum* (dysmenorrhœa and skin symptoms). Compare, also: *Arn.; Bapt.; Lach.; Ars.; Hyosc.; Op.* (stupefaction more profound). *Mimosa*—Sensitive Plant—(rheumatism. knee stiff, lancinating pains in back and limbs. Swelling of ankles Legs tremble).

Dose.—Sixth to thirtieth potency. The 200th and higher are antidotal to poisoning with the plant and tincture.

RHUS VENENATA
(Poison-elder)

The skin symptoms of this species of Rhus are most severe.

Mind.—Great melancholy; no desire to live, gloomy.

Head.—Heavy, frontal headache; worse, walking or stooping. Eyes nearly closed with great swelling. Vesicular inflammation of ears. Nose red and shiny. Face swollen.

Tongue.—Red at tip. Fissured in middle. Vesicles on under side.

Abdomen.—Profuse, watery, white stools in morning, 4 a. m., with colicky pains; expelled with force. Pain in hypogastrium before every stool.

Extremities.—Paralytic drawing in right arm, especially wrist, and extending to fingers.

Skin.—Itching; relieved by hot water. *Vesicles. Erysipelas; skin dark red.* Erythema nodosum, with nightly itching and pains in long bones.

Relationship.—Antidote: *Clematis.* The California Poison-oak (Rhus diversiloba) is identical with it. It antidotes *Radium* and follows it well. Compare: *Anacard.*

Dose.—Sixth to thirtieth potency.

RICINUS COMMUNIS—BOFAREIRA
(Castor-oil)

Has marked action on gastro-intestinal tract. *Increases the quantity of milk* in nursing women. Vomiting and purging. Languor and weakness.

Head.—Vertigo, occipital pain, congestive symptoms, buzzing in ears. Face pale, twitching of mouth.

Stomach.—Anorexia with great thirst, burning in stomach, pyrosis, nausea, *profuse vomiting*, pit of stomach sensitive. Mouth dry.

Abdomen.—Rumbling with contraction of recti muscles, colic, incessant diarrhœa with purging. Rice water stools with cramps and chilliness.

Stool.—Loose, incessant, painless, with painful cramps in muscles of extremities. Anus inflamed. Stools green, slimy, and bloody. Fever, emaciation, somnolence.

Relationship.—Compare: *Resorcin* (summer complaint with vomiting); destroys organic germs of putrifaction; *Cholos terrapina* (cramps of muscles). *Ars.; Verat.*

Dose.—Third potency. Five drops every four hours for increasing flow of milk; also locally a poultice of the leaves.

ROBINIA
(Yellow Locust)

The remedy for hperchlorhydria. In cases where albuminoid digestion is too rapid and starch digestion is perverted. The gastric symptoms with the most *pronounced acidity* are well authenticated, and are the guiding symptoms. The acidity of Robinia is accompanied by frontal headache. *Intensely acrid eructations.* Acrid and greenish vomiting, colic and flatulence, nightly burning pains in stomach and constipation with urgent desire.—*Acidity of children.* Stools and perspiration sour. Incarcerated flatus.

Head.—Dull, throbbing, frontal pain; worse, motion and reading. Gastric headache with acid vomiting.

Stomach.—Dull, heavy aching. Nausea; sour eructations; profuse vomiting of an *intensely sour* fluid. [*Sulph. ac.*] Great distention of stomach and bowels. Flatulent colic. [*Cham.; Diosc.*] Sour stools; child smells sour.

Female.—Nymphomania. Acrid, fetid leucorrhœa. Discharge of blood between menstrual periods. Herpes on vagina and vulva.

Relationship.—*Magnes. phos.; Arg. nit.; Orexine tannate.* (Hyperchlorhydria; deficient acid and slow digestion; 14 hourly doses).

Dose.—Third potency. Must be continued a long time.

ROSA DAMASCENA
(Damask Rose)

Useful in the beginning of hay-fever, with involvement of Eustachian tube.

Ear.—Hardness of hearing; tinnitus. *Eustachian catarrh.* [*Hydr.; Merc. dulc.*]

Relationship.—Compare: in hay-fever: *Phleum pratense*— Timothy grass—(Hay-fever with asthma; watery coryza, itching of nose and eyes; frequent sneezing, dyspnœa. Use 6-30 potency. Rabe.) *Succin. acid; Sabad.; Euph.; Psor.; Kali hyd.; Naphth.*

Dose.—Lower potencies.

RUMEX CRISPUS
(Yellow Dock)

Is characterized by pains, numerous and varied, neither fixed nor constant anywhere. Cough caused by an incessant tickling in the throat-pit, which tickling runs down to the bifurcation of the bronchial tubes. Touching the throat-pit brings on the cough. Worse from the least cold air; so that all cough ceases by covering up all the body and head with the bedclothes. Rumex diminishes the secretions of mucous membranes, and at the same time exalts sensibility of the mucous membranes of the larynx and trachea. Its action upon the skin is marked, producing an intense itching. *Lymphatics enlarged* and secretions perverted.

Stomach.—Tongue sore at edges; coated; sensation of hard substance in pit of stomach; hiccough, pyrosis, nausea; *cannot eat meat; it causes eructations, pruritus.* Jaundice after excessive use of alcoholics. Chronic gastritis; aching pain in pit of stomach and shooting in the chest; extends towards the throat-pit, worse any motion or talking. Pain in left breast after meals; *flatulence.*

Respiratory.—Nose dry. *Tickling in throat-pit causes cough. Copious mucous discharge* from nose and trachea. *Dry, teasing cough, preventing sleep. Aggravated by pressure, talking, and especially by inspiring cool air and at night.* Thin, watery, frothy expectoration by the mouthful; later, stringy and tough. Rawness of larynx and trachea. Soreness behind sternum, especially left side, in region of left shoulder. *Raw pain under clavicle.* Lump in throat.

Stool.—Brown, watery, diarrhœa *early in morning*, with cough, driving him out of bed. Valuable in advanced phthisis. [*Seneg.; Puls.; Lycop.; Ars.*] Itching of anus, with sensation as of a stick in rectum. Piles.

Skin.—Intense itching of skin, especially of *lower extremities; worse, exposure to cold air when undressing.* Urticaria; contagious prurigo.

Modalities.—Worse, in evening, from inhaling cold air; left chest; uncovering.

Relationship.—Compare: *Caust.; Sulph.; Bell.;* Rumex contains chrysophanic acid to which the skin symptoms correspond. *Rumex acetosa*—Sheep sorrel—(Gathered in June and dried, used locally for Epithelioma of face. (Cowperthwaite.) Dry, unremitting short cough, and violent pains in the bowels; uvula elongated; inflammation of œsophagus; also cancer); *Rumex obtusifolius—Lapathum*—Broad-leaf dock—(nosebleed and headache following; pain in kidneys; leucorrhœa).

Dose.—Third to sixth potency.

RUTA GRAVEOLENS
(Rue-bitterwort)

Acts upon the periosteum and cartilages, eyes and uterus. Complaints from straining *flexor tendons* especially. Tendency to the formation of deposits in the periosteum, tendons, and about joints, especially wrist. Overstrain of ocular muscles. All parts of the body are painful, *as if bruised.* Sprains (after *Arnica*). Lameness after sprains. Jaundice. *Feeling of intense lassitude, weakness and despair.* Injured "bruised" bones.

Head.—Pain as from a nail; after excessive intoxicating drinks. Periosteum sore. Epistaxis.

Eyes.—*Eye-strain followed by headache. Eyes red, hot, and painful from sewing or reading fine print.* [*Nat. mur.; Arg. nit.*] *Disturbances of accommodation.* Weary pain while reading. Pressure deep in orbits. Tarsal cartilage feels bruised. Pressure over eyebrow. Asthenopia.

Stomach.—Gastralgia of aching, gnawing character.

Urinary.—Pressure in neck of bladder after urinating; painful closure. [*Apis.*] Constant urging to urinate, feels bladder full.

Rectum.—*Difficult fæces*, evacuated only with straining. Constipation, alternating with mucous, frothy stools; discharge of blood with stool. When sitting, tearing stitches in rectum. *Carcinoma affecting lower bowel. Prolapsus ani* every time the bowels move, after confinement. Frequent, unsuccessful urging to stool. Protrusion of rectum when stooping.

Respiratory.—Cough with copious, thick, yellow expectoration; chest feels weak. Painful spot on sternum; short breath with tightness of chest.

Back.—Pain in nape, back and loins. Backache better pressure and lying on back. Lumbago worse morning before rising.

Extremities.—Spine and limbs feel bruised. Small of back and loins pain. Legs give out on rising from a chair, hips and thighs so weak. [*Phos.; Con.*] Contraction of fingers. Pain and stiffness in wrists and hands. Ganglia. [*Benzoic ac.*] Sciatica; worse, lying down at night; pain from back down hips and thighs. Hamstrings feel shortened. [*Graph.*] *Tendons sore.* Aching pain in tendo-Achilles. *Thighs pain when stretching the limbs.* Pain in bones of feet and ankles. Great restlessness.

Modalities.—*Worse*, lying down, from cold, wet weather.

Relationship.—Compare: *Ratanhia; Carduus.* Rectal (irritation); *Jaborandi; Phyt.; Rhus; Sil.; Arn.*

Antidote: *Camph.*

Complementary: *Calc. phos.*

Dose.—First to sixth potency. Locally, the tincture for ganglia and as a lotion for the eyes.

SABADILLA
(Cevadilla Seed. Asagræa Officialis)

Action on mucous membrane of the nose and the lachrymal glands, producing coryza and symptoms like *hay-fever*, which have been utilized homœopathically. *Chilliness;* sensitive to cold. Ascarides, with reflex symptoms (nymphomania; convulsive symptoms). Children's diarrhœa with constant cutting pains.

Mind.—Nervous, timid, easily startled. Has erroneous notions about himself. Imagines that he is very sick; that parts are shrunken; that she is pregnant; that she has cancer; delirium during intermittents.

Head.—Vertigo with sensation as though all things were turning around each other, accompanied by blackness before eyes and sensation of fainting. Dullness and oppression. Oversensitiveness to odors. *Thinking* produces headache and sleeplessness. *Eyelids red, burning. Lachrymation.* Difficult hearing.

Nose.—*Spasmodic sneezing, with running nose. Coryza,* with severe frontal pains and redness of eyes and lachrymation. Copious, watery, nasal discharge.

Throat.—Sore; *begins on left side.* [*Lach.*] Much tough phlegm. Sensation of a skin hanging loosely; must swallow it. *Warm food and drink relieve.* Empty swallowing most painful. Dry fauces and throat. Sensation of a lump in throat with *constant* necessity to swallow. Chronic sore throat; worse, from cold air. Tongue as if burnt.

Stomach.—Spasmodic pain in stomach with dry cough and difficult breathing. *No thirst.* Loathing for strong food. Canine appetite for sweets and farinaceous food. Pyrosis; copious salivation. Cold, empty feeling in stomach. *Desire for hot things. Sweetish* taste.

Female.—Menses too late; come by fits and starts. *Intermit* [*Kreos.; Puls.*] (due to transient and localized congestion of womb alternating with chronic anæmic state).

Fever.—*Chill predominates;* from below upwards. Heat in head and face; hands and feet icy cold, with chill. Lachrymation during paroxysm. Thirstless.

Extremities.—Cracking of skin under and beneath toes; inflammation under toe-nails.

Skin.—Dry, like parchment. Horny, deformed, *thickened nails.* Hot, burning, creeping, crawling sensation. Itching in anus.

Modalities.—*Worse,* cold and cold drinks, full moon. *Better,* warm food and drink, wrapped up.

Relationship.—Complementary: *Sepia.* Compare: *Vera-*

trina (is alkaloid of Sabadilla, *not* of Veratrum, locally in neuralgias, and for removal of dropsy. Five grains to two drams
Lanolin, rubbed on inside of thighs, causes diuresis). *Colch.;
Nux; Arundo* and *Pollatin. Phleum pratense*—Timothy—
Hay-fever—Potentized—12—specific to many cases and evi-
dently acts in a desensitizing manner. (Rabe.) *Cumarinum*
(hay-fever).

Antidotes: *Puls.; Lycop.; Conium; Lach.*

Dose.—Third to thirtieth potency.

SABAL SERRULATA
(Saw Palmetto)

Sabal is homœopathic to irritability of the genito-urinary
organs.

General and sexual debility. Promotes nutrition and tissue
building. Head, stomach, and ovarian symptoms marked. Of
unquestioned value in prostatic enlargement, *epididymitis*, and
urinary difficulties. Acts on membrano-prostatic portion of
urethra. Iritis, with prostatic trouble. *Valuable for undevel-
oped mammary glands. Fear of going to sleep.* Languor, apathy
and indifference.

Head.—Confused, full; dislikes sympathy; makes her angry.
Vertigo, with headache. Neuralgia in feeble patients. Pain
runs up from nose and centers in forehead.

Stomach.—Belching and acidity. Desire for milk. [*Rhus;
Apis.*]

Urinary.—Constant desire to pass water at night. *Enuresis;*
paresis of sphincter vesicæ. Chronic gonorrhœa. Difficult
urination. Cystitis with prostatic hypertrophy.

Male.—*Prostatic troubles;* enlargement; discharge of prostatic fluid. Wasting of testes and *loss of sexual power.* Coitus
painful at the time of emission. *Sexual neurotics.* Organs feel
cold.

Female.—Ovaries tender and enlarged; *breasts shrivel.* [*Iod.;
Kali iod.*] Young female neurotics; suppressed or perverted
sexual inclination.

Respiratory.—Copious expectoration, with catarrh of nose.
Chronic bronchitis. [*Stann.; Hep.*]

Relationship.—Compare: *Phosph. ac.; Stigmata maydis; Santal.; Apis.* In prostatic symptoms: *Ferr. pic.; Thuja; Picric acid* (more sexual erethism). *Populus tremul.;* (prostatic enlargement with cystitis).

Dose.—Mother tincture, ten to thirty drops. Third potency often better. The tincture must be prepared from the *fresh berries* to be effective.

SABINA
(Savine)

Has a special action on the uterus; also upon serous and fibrous membranes; hence its use in gout. *Pain from sacrum to the pubis. Hæmorrhages, where blood is fluid and clots together.* Tendency to miscarriage, especially at third month. *Violent pulsations;* wants windows open.

Mind.—*Music is intolerable,* produces nervousness.

Head.—Vertigo with suppressed menses. Bursting headache, suddenly coming and going slowly. Rush of blood to head and face. Drawing pains in masseter muscles. Teeth ache when chewing.

Stomach.—Heartburn. Desire for lemonade. Bitter taste. [*Rhus.*] Lancinating pain from pit of stomach across back.

Abdomen.—Bearing-down, constrictive pain. Colic, mostly in hypogastric region. Tympanitic distention.

Rectum.—Sense of fullness. Constipation. *Pain from back to pubis.* Hæmorrhoids, with bright red blood; bleed copiously.

Urine.—Burning and throbbing in region of kidneys. Bloody urine; much urging. Bladder inflamed with throbbing all over. Inflammation of urethra.

Male.—Inflammatory gonorrhœa, with pus-like discharge. Sycotic excrescences. Burning, sore pain in glans. Prepuce painful with difficulty in retracting it. Increased desire.

Female.—*Menses profuse, bright.* Uterine pains extend into thighs. Threatened miscarriage. Sexual desire increased. Leucorrhœa after menses, corrosive, offensive. Discharge of blood between periods, with sexual excitement. [*Ambr.*] Retained placenta; intense after-pains. Menorrhagia in women who aborted readily. Inflammation of ovaries and uterus after abortion. Promotes expulsion of moles from uterus. [*Canth.*] *Pain from sacrum to pubis, and from below upwards shooting up the vagina.* Hæmorrhage; partly clotted; worse *from least motion.* Atony of uterus.

Back.—*Pain between sacrum and pubis from one bone to another.* Paralytic pain in small of back.

Extremities.—Bruised pains in anterior portion of thighs. Shooting in heels and metatarsal bones. *Arthritic pain in joints.* Gout; worse, in heated room. Red, shining swelling. Gouty nodosities. [*Ammon. phos.*]

Skin.—Fig-warts, with intolerable itching and burning. Exuberant granulations. [*Thuj.; Nit. ac.*] *Warts.* Black pores in skin.

Modalities.—*Worse,* from least motion, heat, warm air. *Better,* in cool fresh air.

Relationship.—Complementary: *Thuja.*

Compare: *Sanguisorba* (Venous congestion and passive hæmorrhages; varices of lower extremities; dysentery. *Long lasting, profuse menses* with congestion to head and limbs in sensitive, irritable patients. *Climacteric* hæmorrhages. Use 2x attenuation.) *Sanguisuga*—The leech—(Hæmorrhages, especially bleeding from anus. Use 6x). *Rosmarinus* (menses too early; violent pains followed by uterine hæmorrhage. Head heavy, *drowsy.* Chilly with icy coldness of lower extremities without thirst, followed by heat. Memory deficient). *Croc.; Calc.; Trill.; Ipec.; Millef.; Erig.*

Antidote: *Puls.*

Dose.—Locally, for warts, tincture. Internally, third to thirtieth potency.

SACCHARUM OFFICINALE—SUCROSE
(Cane-sugar)

According to the great Dr. Hering, a large proportion of chronic diseases of women and children are developed by using too much sugar.

Sugar is an antiseptic. Combats infection and putrefaction; has a solvent action on fibrin and stimulates secretion by the intense osmotic changes induced, thus rinsing out the wound with serum from within outward, favoring healing. Leg ulcers.

Sugar must be considered a sustainer and developer of the musculature of the heart and hence useful in failure of compensation and a variety of cardio-vascular troubles. Acts as a nutrient and tonic, in wasting disorders, anæmia, neurasthenia, etc., increasing weight and power.

Opacity of cornea. Dim sight. *Acidity and anal itching.* Cold expectoration. Myocardial degeneration.

Fat, bloated, large-limbed children, who are *cross, peevish,* whining; capricious; want dainty things, tidbits, and refuse substantial food. Œdema of feet. Headache every seven days

Relationship.—Compare: *Saccharum lactis*—Sugar of milk—lactose—(diuresis; amblyopia; *cold pains,* as if produced by fine, icy cold needle with tingling, as if frost bitten; great physical exhaustion. *Sugar of milk* in large doses to develop the Bacillus acidophilus to correct putrefactive intestinal conditions and also constipation.)

Dose.—Thirtieth potency and higher. Locally in gangrene. One ounce of lump sugar morning and evening valuable adjunct in the treatment of obstinate cases of heart failure due to deficient heart muscle without valvular lesion. Epilepsy; blood with reduced sugar content irritates the nervous system with tending to convulsions.

Sugar as an oxytocic has its most suitable application towards the end of labor when there is no mechanical obstruction and delay is due to uterine inertia. 25 grammes dissolved in water, several times every half hour.

Compare: *Saccharin* (hinders both the salivary and peptic ferment actions with consequent dyspepsia. Prof. Lewin believes its action to be on the secretory cells themselves and it has caused pain (right hypogastrium), loss of appetite, diarrhœa and wasting).

SALICYLICUM ACIDUM

(Salicylic Acid)

The symptoms point to its use in rheumatism, dyspepsia, and *Meniere's disease.* Prostration after influenza; also tinnitus aurium and deafness. Hæmaturia.

Head.—Vertigo; tendency to fall to left side. Headache; confusion in head on rising suddenly. Incipient coryza. Piercing pain in temples.

Eyes.—Retinal hæmorrhage. Retinitis after influenza, also albuminuric.

Ears.—*Roaring and ringing in ears.* Deafness, with vertigo.

Throat.—Sore, red and swollen. Pharyngitis; swallowing difficult.

Stomach.—*Canker sores*, with burning soreness and fetid breath. *Flatulence; hot, sour belching.* Putrid fermentation. *Fermentative dyspepsia.* Tongue purplish, leaden-colored; foul breath.

Stools.—Putrid diarrhœa; gastro-intestinal derangements, especially in children; stools like green frog's spawn. [*Magn. carb.*] Pruritus ani.

Extremities.—Knees swollen and painful. Acute articular rheumatism; worse, touch and motion, profuse sweat. Pain shifts. Sciatica, burning pain; worse at night. Copious foot-sweat and ill affects where suppressed.

Skin.—Itching vesicles and pustules; better by scratching. Sweat without sleep. Urticaria. Hot and burning skin. Purpura. Herpes zoster. Necrosis and softening of bones.

Relationship.—Compare: *Salol* (rheumatic pain in joints, with soreness and stiffness, headache over eyes; urine violet-smelling); *Colch.; China; Lact. ac.* Spiræa and Gaultheria contain salicyl. acid.

Dose.—Third decimal trituration. In acute articular rheumatism, 5 grains every 3 hours. (Old school dose.)

SALIX NIGRA
(Black-willow)

Has a positive action on the generative organs of both sexes Hysteria and nervousness. Libidinous thoughts and lascivious dreams. Controls genital irritability. Moderates sexual passion. Satyriasis and erotomania. In acute gonorrhœa, with much erotic trouble; chordee. After masturbation; spermatorrhœa.

Face.—Red, swollen, especially the end of nose—eyes blood-shot and sore to touch and on motion. Roots of hair hurt. Epistaxis.

Female.—Before and during menses much nervous disturbance, pain in ovaries; difficult menstruation. Ovarian congestion and neuralgia. Menorrhagia. Bleeding with uterine fibroid. Nymphomania.

Male.—Painful movement of the testicles.

Back.—Pain across sacral and lumbar region. Unable to step out quickly.

Relationship.—Compare: *Yohimbin.; Canth.*

Dose.—Material doses of the tincture, thirty drops.

SALVIA OFFICINALIS
(Sage)

Controls excessive sweating when circulation is enfeebled; of less use in phthisis *with night-sweats* and suffocating tickling cough. Galactorrhœa. Exerts a tonic influence on the skin.

Respiratory.—Tickling cough, especially in consumption.

Skin.—Soft, relaxed, with enfeebled circulation and cold extremities. *Colliquative perspiration.*

Relationship.—Compare: *Chrysanthemum Leucanthemum*—Ox-eye Daisy. Has specific action on sudoriparous glands. Quiets nervous system like *Cypripedium.* Right sided tearing pain in bones of jaw and temple. Pain in teeth and gums, worse touch, better warmth. Irritable and tearful. Here use 12x. *Insomnia and night-sweats.* For colliquative sweating and hyperæsthesia of nervous system. Material doses of tincture.) *Phelland.; Tuberc.; Salvia sclerata* (tonic influence on nervous system; dose, teaspoonful to one pint hot water, as inhalent for sponging). *Rubia tinctorum*—Madder—A remedy for the spleen. [*Ceanothus.*] Chlorosis and amenorrhœa; tuberculosis. Anæmia; undernourished conditiòns; splenic anæmia. Dose, 10 drops of tincture).

Dose.—Tincture, in twenty-drop doses, in a little water. The effects manifest themselves quickly two hours after taking a dose, and they persist for from two to six days.

SAMBUCUS NIGRA
(Elder)

Acts especially on the respiratory organs. Dry coryza of infants, snuffles, œdematous swellings. *Profuse sweat* accompanies many affections.

Mind.—Sees images when shutting eyes. *Constant fretfulness.* Very easily frightened. Fright followed by suffocative attacks.

Face.—Turns blue with cough. Red, burning spots on cheeks. Heat and perspiration of face.

Abdomen.—Colic, with nausea and flatulence; frequent watery, slimy stools.

Urine.—Profuse urine with dry heat of skin. Frequent micturition, with scanty urine. Acute nephritis; dropsical symptoms, with vomiting.

Respiratory.—Chest oppressed with pressure in stomach, and nausea. Hoarseness with tenacious mucus in larynx. Paroxysmal, *suffocative cough, coming on about midnight*, with crying and dyspnœa. Spasmodic croup. Dry coryza. *Sniffles of infants;* nose dry and obstructed. Loose choking cough. When nursing child must let go of nipple, nose blocked up, cannot breathe. *Child awakes suddenly, nearly suffocating, sits up, turns blue. Cannot expire.* [*Meph.*] Millar's asthma.

Extremities.—Hands turn blue. Œdematous swelling in legs, insteps, and feet. Feet icy cold. Debilitating night-sweats. [*Salvia; Acet. ac.*]

Fever.—Dry heat while sleeping. *Dreads uncovering. Profuse sweat over entire body during waking hours.* Dry, deep cough precedes the fever paroxysm.

Skin.—Dry heat of skin during sleep. Bloated and swollen; general dropsy; *profuse sweat on waking.*

Modalities.—*Worse,* sleep, during rest, after eating fruit. *Better,* sitting up in bed, motion.

Relationship.—Compare: *Ipec.; Meph.; Opium; Sambucus Canadensis* (great vlaue in dropsies; large doses required—fluid extract, ¼ to 1 teaspoonful three times daily).

Antidotes: *Ars.; Camph.*

Dose.—Tincture, to sixth potency.

SANGUINARIA
(Blood Root)

Is a right-sided remedy pre-eminently, and affects chiefly the mucous membranes, especially of the respiratory tract. It has marked vaso-motor disturbances, as seen in the circumscribed redness of the cheeks, flashes of heat, determination of blood to head and chest, distention of temporal veins, burning in palms and soles, and has been found very applicable to climacteric disorders. *Burning* sensations, like from hot water. Influenzal coughs. Phthisis. *Sudden stopping of catarrh of respiratory tract followed by diarrhœa. Burning* in various parts is characteristic.

Head.—Worse *right* side, sun headache. Periodical sick headache; pain begins in occiput, spreads upwards, and *settles over eyes, especially right. Veins and temples are distended.* Pain better lying down and sleep. Headaches return at climacteric; every seventh day. [*Sulph.; Sabad.*] Pain in small spot over upper left parietal bone. Burning in eyes. Pain in the back of head "like a flash of lightning."

Face.—Flushed. Neuralgia; pain extends in all directions from upper jaw. *Redness and burning of cheeks. Hectic flush.* Fullness and tenderness behind angle of jaws.

Nose.—Hay-fever. Ozæna, with profuse, offensive yellowish discharges. *Nasal polypi.* Coryza, followed by diarrhœa. Chronic rhinitis; membrane *dry* and congested.

Ears.—Burning in ears. Earache with headache. Humming and roaring. Aural polypus.

Throat.—Swollen; worse, right side. Dry and constricted. Ulceration of mouth and fauces, with dry, burning sensation. Tongue white; feels scalded. Tonsillitis.

Stomach.—Aversion to butter. Craving for piquant things. Unquenchable thirst. Burning, vomiting. Nausea, with salivation. Sinking, faint all-gone feeling. [*Phos.; Sep.*] Spitting up of bile; gastro-duodenal catarrh.

Abdomen.—Diarrhœa as coryza improves. Pain over region of liver. Diarrhœa; bilious, liquid, gushing stool. [*Nat. sulph.; Lycop.*] Cancer of rectum.

Female.—Leucorrhœa fetid, corrosive. Menses offensive, profuse. Soreness of breasts. Uterine polypi. Before,menses, itching of axillæ. Climacteric disorders.

Respiratory.—Œdema of larynx. Trachea sore. Heat and tension behind the sternum. Aphonia. *Cough of gastric origin;* relieved by eructation. Cough, with burning pain in chest; worse, right side. Sputum tough, *rust-colored*, offensive, almost impossible to raise. Spasmodic cough after influenza and *after whooping-cough.* Cough returns with every fresh cold. Tickling behind sternum, causes a constant hacking cough; worse at night on lying down. Must sit up in bed. Burning soreness in right chest, through to right shoulder. Severe soreness under right nipple. Hæmoptysis from suppressed menses. *Severe dyspnœa* and constriction of chest. Offensive breath and purulent expectoration. Burning in chest as of hot steam from chest to abdomen. Fibroid phthisis. Pneumonia; better, lying on back. Asthma with stomach disorders. [*Nux.*] Valvular disease with lung development, phosphates in urine and loss of flesh. Sudden stoppage of catarrh of air passages brings on diarrhœa.

Extremities.—Rheumatism of right shoulder, left hip-joint and nape of neck. *Burning in soles and palms.* Rheumatic pains in places least covered by flesh; not in joints. Toes and soles of feet burn. Right-sided neuritis; better touching the part.

Skin.—Antidotes: *Rhus poisoning.* Red, blotchy eruptions; worse in spring. Burning and itching; worse by heat. Acne, with scanty menses. Circumscribed red spots over malar bones.

Modalities.—*Worse,* sweets, right side, motion, touch. Better, acids, sleep, darkness.

Relationship.—Complementary: *Tart. em.*

Compare: *Justicia* (bronchial catarrh, coryza, hoarseness; oversensitive). *Digitalis* (Migraine). *Bell.; Iris; Melil.; Lach.; Ferr.; Op.*

Dose.—Tincture in headaches; sixth potency in rheumatism.

SANGUINARINA NITRICA
(Nitrate of Sanguinarine)

Is of use in polypus of the nose. Acute and chronic catarrh. Acute pharyngitis. (*Wyethia*) Smarting and burning in throat and chest especially under sternum. *Influenza*. Lachrymation, pains in eyes and head, sore scalp; *sense of obstruction*. Chronic follicular pharyngitis.

Nose.—*Feels obstructed. Profuse, watery mucus, with burning pain.* Enlarged turbinates at beginning of hypertrophic process. Secretion scant, tendency to dryness. Small crust$_8$ which bleed when removed. Post-nasal secretions adherent to nasopharynx, dislodged with difficulty. Dry and burning nostrils; watery mucus, with pressure over root of nose. Nostrils plugged with thick, yellow, bloody mucus. *Sneezing*. Rawness and soreness in posterior nares.

Throat.—Rough, dry, *constricted, burning*. Right tonsil sore, swallowing difficult.

Mouth.—Ulceration on the *side* of the tongue.

Respiratory.—Short, hacking cough, with expectoration of thick, yellow, sweetish mucus. *Pressure behind center of sternum.* Dryness and burning in throat and bronchi. *Tickling cough.* Chronic nasal, laryngeal, and bronchial catarrh. Voice altered, deep, hoarse.

Relationship.—Compare: *Sanguin. tartaricum* (exophthalmos; *mydriasis;* dim vision); *Arum triph.; Psorin.; Kal. bich.*

Dose.—Third trituration.

SANICULA (AQUA)
(The Water of Sanicula Springs, Ottawa, Ill.)

Has been found a useful remedy in enuresis, seasickness, constipation, etc. Rickets.

Head.—Dread of downward motion. [*Borax.*] *Profuse sweat on occiput* and in nape of neck, during sleep. [*Calc.; Sil.*] Photophobia. Lachrymation in cold air or from cold application. Profuse scaly dandruff. Soreness behind ears.

Throat.—Thick, ropy, tenacious mucus.

Mouth.—Tongue large, flabby, burning; must protrude it to keep cool. Ringworm on tongue.

Stomach.—Nausea and vomiting from car-riding. Thirst; drink little and often. [*Ars.; Chin.*] Is vomited as soon as it reaches the stomach.

Rectum.—Stools large, heavy and painful. *Pain in whole perineum.* No desire until a large accumulation. After great straining only partially expelled; recedes, crumbles at verge of anus. [*Mag. mur.*] Very offensive odor. Excoriation of skin about anus, perineum, and genitals. Diarrhœa; changeable in character and color; after eating.

Female.—Bearing-down, as if contents of pelvis would escape; better, rest. Desire to support parts. Soreness of uterus. Leucorrhœa with *odor of fish-brine or old cheese.* [*Hepar.*] Vagina feels large.

Back.—Dislocated feeling in sacrum and better lying on right side.

Extremities.—Burning of soles of feet. [*Sulph.; Lach.*] *Offensive foot-sweat.* [*Sil.; Psor.*] Cold, clammy sweat of extremities.

Skin.—Dirty, greasy, brownish, wrinkled. Eczema, fissured hands and fingers. [*Petrol.; Graph.*]

Modalities.—*Worse, moving arms backward.*

Relationship.—Compare: *Abrot.; Alum.; Calc.; Sil.; Sulph.* Sanicula Aqua must not be confounded with the Sanicle (pool-root or wood marsh), also called *Sanicula.* This is used in various nervous affections, resembling Valeriana. It is used as a vulnerary, resolvent for sanguineous extravasations, and as an astringent. Has not been proved.)

Dose.—Thirtieth potency.

SANTONINUM
(Santonin)

Is the active principle of Santonica, the unexpanded flower heads of *Artemisia Maritima*—Cina., which see.

The eye stymptoms and those of the urinary tract are most prominent. It is of unquestioned value in the treatment of worm diseases, as gastro-intestinal irritation, *itching of nose*, restless sleep, twitching of muscles. Ascaris lumbricoides, and thread worms, but not tapeworms. *Night cough* of children. *Chronic cystitis.* Laryngeal crises and lightning pains of tabes.

Head.—Occipital headache, with *chromatic hallucinations.* *Itching of nose.* Bores into nostrils.

Eyes.—Sudden dimness of sight. *Color blindness;* Xanthopsia. Strabismus due to worms. Dark rings about eyes.

Mouth.—Fetid breath, depraved appetite; thirsty. Tongue deep-red. *Grinding of teeth.* Nausea; better after eating. Choking feeling.

Urinary.—Urine greenish if acid and reddish purple if alkaline. *Incontinence and dysuria. Enuresis.* Feeling of fullness of bladder. Nephritis.

Relationship.—Compare: *Cina; Teucr.; Napth.; Nat. phos.; Spigel.*

Dose.—Second to third trituration. Lower preparations are often toxic. Do not give to a child with fever or constipation.

SAPONARIA
(Soap Root)

Of great use in the treatment of acute colds, coryza, sore throat, etc. Will often "break up" a cold.

Mind.—Utter indifference to pain or possible death. Apathetic, *depressed, with sleepiness.*

Head.—Stitching pain, *supraorbital;* worse, left side, evening, motion. Throbbing over orbits. Congestions to head; tired feeling in nape. *Coryza.* Sensation of drunkenness with constant endeavor to go left-wards. Left-sided trigeminal neuralgia, especially supraorbital. Stopped up feeling in nose, also itching and sneezing.

Eyes.—Violent eye pains. Hot stitches deep in eyeball. Ciliary neuralgia; worse, left side. Photophobia. Exophthalmos, worse reading and writing. Increased intraocular pressure. Glaucoma.

Stomach.—Difficult swallowing. Nausea, heartburn; full feeling not relieved by eructation.

Heart.—Impulse weak; pulse less frequent. Palpitation with anxiety.

Modalities.—*Worse*, at night, mental exertion, left side.

Relationship.—Compare: *Saponin*—a glucosidal principle found in Quillaya, Yucca, Senega, Dioscorea and other plants. (Tired, indifferent. *Pain in left temple, eye*, photophobia, hot stitches deep in eye. Fifth nerve affections. Migraine. Much pain *before* the mentsrual flow; severe sore throat, worse right side; tonsils swollen, worse in warm room. Sharp burning taste and violent sneezing.)

Compare, also: *Verbasc.; Coccul.* (both containing Saponin). *Quillaya;* (Anagallis, *Agrostema*, Helonias, Sarsaparilla, Paris, Cyclamen and others contain Saponin).

SARCOLACTIC ACID

Is apparently formed in muscle tissue during the stage of muscle exhaustion. Differs from ordinary Lactic acid in its relation to polarized light.

It represents a much broader and more profoundly acting drug and its pathogenesis is quite dissimilar from the normal acid. Proved by Wm. B. Griggs, M. D., who found it of great value in the most violent form of *Epidemic influenza, especially with violent and retching and greatest prostration*, when Arsenic had failed. Spinal neurasthenia, muscular weakness, dyspnœa with myocardial weakness.

General Symptoms.—Tired feeling with *muscular prostration*, worse any exertion. Sore feeling all over, worse in afternoon. Restless at night. Difficulty in getting to sleep. Tired feeling in morning on getting up.

Throat.—Constriction in pharynx. Sore throat with tightness in naso-pharynx. Tickling in throat.

Stomach.—Nausea. Uncontrollable vomiting even of water followed by extreme weakness.

Back and Extremities.—Tired feeling in back and neck and shoulders. Paralytic weakness. Wrist tires easily from writing. Extreme weakness from climbing stairs. Stiffness of thigh and calves. Arms feel as if no strength in them. Cramp in the calves.

Dose.—Sixth to 30th potency. The 15x most marked action (Griggs).

SARRACENIA PURPUREA
(Pitcher-plant)

A remedy for variola. Visual disorders. Congestion to head, with irregular heart action. Chlorosis. Contains a very active proteolytic enzyme. Sick headache; throbbing in various parts, especially in neck, shoulders and head, which feels full to bursting.

Eyes.—Photophobia. Eyes feel swollen and sore. Pain in orbits. Black objects move with the eye.

Stomach.—Hungry all the time, even after a meal. Sleepy during meals. Copious, painful vomiting.

Back.—Pains shooting in *zig-zag* course from lumbar region to middle of scapula.

Extremities.—Limbs weak; bruised pain in knees and hip-joints. Bones in arm pain. *Weak between shoulders.*

Skin.—Variola, aborts the disease, arrests pustulation.

Relationship.—Compare: *Tartar. em.; Variol.; Maland.*

Dose.—Third to sixth potency.

SARSAPARILLA
(Smilax)

Renal colic; marasmus and periosteal pains due to venereal disease. Eruptions following hot weather and vaccinations; boils, and eczema. Urinary symptoms well marked.

Mind.—Despondent, sensitive, easily offended, ill humored and taciturn.

Head.—*Pains cause depression.* Shooting pain from above right temporal region. Pains *from occiput to eyes.* Words reverberate in ear to the root of nose. Periosteal pains due to venereal disease. Influenza. Scalp sensitive. *Eruptions on face and upper lip.* Moist eruption on scalp. Crusta lactea beginning in face.

Mouth.—Tongue white; *aphthæ; salivation;* metallic taste; no thirst. Fetid breath.

Abdomen.—Rumbling and fermentation. *Colic and backache at same time.* Much flatus; cholera infantum.

Urinary.—Urine scanty, slimy, flaky, sandy, *bloody.* Gravel. Renal colic. *Severe pain at conclusion of urination. Urine dribbles while sitting.* Bladder distended and tender. *Child screams before and while passing urine.* Sand on diaper. Renal colic and dysuria in infants. *Pain from right kidney downward.* Tenesmus of bladder; urine passes in thin, feeble stream. Pain at meatus.

Male.—Bloody, seminal emissions. Intolerable stench on genitals. Herpetic eruption on genitals. Itching on scrotum and perineum. Syphilis; squamous eruption and bone pains.

Female.—Nipples small, withered, *retracted. Before menstruation, itching and humid eruption of forehead.* Menses late and scanty. Moist eruption in right groin before menses.

Skin.—*Emaciated, shriveled, lies in folds* [*Abrot.; Sanic.*], dry, flabby. Herpetic eruptions; ulcers. Rash from exposure to open air; dry, itching; *comes on in spring;* becomes crusty. Rhagades; skin cracked on hands and feet. Skin hard, indurated. Summer cutaneous affections.

Extremities.—Paralytic, tearing pains. Trembling of hands and feet. Burning on sides of fingers and toes. Onychia, ulceration around ends of fingers, cutting sensation under nails. Rheumatism, bone pains; worse at night. Deep rhagades on fingers and toes; burn under nails. Tetter on hands; ulceration around ends of fingers. [*Psorin.*] Cutting sensation under nails. [*Petrol.*] Rheumatic pains after gonorrhœa.

Modalities.—*Worse,* dampness at night, after urinating, when yawning, in spring, before menses.

Relationship.—Complementary: *Merc.; Sep.*

Compare: *Berb.; Lycop.; Nat. m.; Petrol.; Sassafras; Saururus*—Lizard's tail—(Irritation of kidneys, bladder, prostate and urinary passages. Painful and difficult micturition; cystitis with strangury). *Cucurbita citrellus*—Watermellon. (Infusion of the seed acts promptly in painful urination with constriction and backache, relieves pain and stimulates flow.)

Antidote: *Bell.*

Dose.—First to sixth potency.

SCROPHULARIA NODOSA
(Knotted Figwort)

A powerful medicine whenever *enlarged glands* are present. Hodgkin's disease.

A valuable skin remedy. Has a specific affinity for the breast; very useful in the dissipation of breast tumors. *Eczema of the ear.* Pruritus vaginæ. Lupoid ulceration. *Scrofulous swellings.* [*Cistus.*] *Painful hæmorrhoids.* Tubercular testis. Ephithelioma. Nodosities in the breasts. [*Scirrhinum.*] Pain in all flexor muscles.

Head.—Vertigo felt in vertex, greater when standing; drowsiness; pain from forehead to back of head. Eczema behind ear. Crusta lactea.

Eyes.—Distressing photophobia. [*Conium.*] Spots before eyes. Stitches in eyebrow. Sore eyeballs.

Ears.—Inflammation about auricle. Deep ulcerated auricle. Eczema around ear.

Abdomen.—*Pain in liver* on pressure. Colic below navel. Pain in sigmoid flexure and *rectum. Painful.* bleeding, protruding *piles.*

Respiratory.—Violent dyspnœa, oppression of chest with trembling. Pain about bifurcation of trachea. Asthma in scrofulous patients.

Skin.—Prickling itching, worse back of hand.

Sleep.—*Great drowsiness;* in morning and before and after meals with weariness.

Modalities.—Worse lying on right side.

Compare: *Lobel. erinus; Ruta; Carcinosin; Conium; Asterias.*

Dose.—Tincture and first potency. Apply locally to cancerous glands also *Semper. viv.*

SCUTELLARIA LATERIFLORA
(Skullcap)

This is a nervous sedative, where *nervous fear* predominates. *Cardiac irritability. Chorea.* Nervous irritation and spasms of children, during dentition. *Twitching of muscles.* Nervous weakness after influenza.

Mental.—*Fear of some calamity.* Inability to fix attention. [*Æthus.*] Confusion.

Head.—*Dull, frontal headache.* Eyes feel pressed outwards. Flushed face. Restless sleep and frightful dreams. *Must move about.* Night terrors. Migraine; worse, over right eye; *aching in eyeballs.* Explosive headaches of school teachers with frequent urination; headaches in front and base of brain. Nervous sick headaches, worse noise, odor light, better night; rest, 5 drops of tincture.

Stomach.—Nausea; sour eructations; hiccough; pain and distress.

Abdomen.—Gas, fullness and distention, colicky pain and uneasiness. Light colored diarrhœa.

Male.—Seminal emissions and impotency, with fear of never being better.

Sleep.—Night-terrors; sleeplessness; sudden wakefulness; frightful dreams.

Extremities.—Twitchings of muscles; must be moving. Chorea. Tremors. Sharp stinging pains in upper extremities. Nightly restlessness. Weakness and aching.

Relationship.—Compare: *Cyprip.; Lycopus.*

Dose.—Tincture and lower potencies.

SECALE CORNUTUM—CLAVICEPS PURPUREA
(Ergot)

Produces contraction of the unstriped muscular fibers; hence a constringent feeling throughout the whole body. This produces an anæmic condition, coldness, numbness, petechiæ, mortification, gangrene. A useful remedy for old people with shriveled skin—thin, scrawny old women. All the Secale conditions are *better from cold;* the whole body is pervaded by a sense of great heat. Hæmorrhages; continued oozing; *thin,* fetid, watery black blood. *Debility, anxiety, emaciation, though appetite and thirst may be excessive.* Facial and abdominal muscles twitch. Secale decreases the flow of pancreatic juice by raising the blood pressure. (Hinsdale.)

Head.—Passive, congestive pain (rises from back of head), with pale face. Head drawn back. Falling of hair; dry and gray. *Nosebleed,* dark, oozing.

Eyes.—Pupils dilated. Incipient cataract, senile especially in women. *Eyes sunken and surrounded by a blue margin.*

Face.—*Pale, pinched, sunken.* Cramps commence in face and spread over whole body. Livid spots on face. *Spasmodic distortion.*

Mouth.—Tongue dry, *cracked; blood like ink exudes,* coated thick; viscid, yellowish, cold livid. *Tingling of tip of tongue, which is stiff.* Tongue swollen, paralyzed.

Stomach.—*Unnatural ravenous appetite; craves* acids. *Thirst* unquenchable. Singultus, nausea; vomiting of blood and coffee-grounds fluid. Burning in stomach and abdomen; tympanites. Eructations of bad odor.

Stool.—Cholera-like stools, with coldness and cramps. *Olivegreen, thin, putrid, bloody, with icy coldness and intolerance of being covered, with great exhaustion. Involuntary stools;* no sensation of passing fæces, anus wide open.

Urine.—Paralysis of bladder. Retention, with unsuccessful urging. Discharge of black blood from bladder. Enuresis in old people.

Female.—Menstrual colic, with coldness and intolerance of heat. Passive hæmorrhages in feeble, cachectic women. Burning pains in uterus. *Brownish, offensive leucorrhœa.* Menses irregular, copious, dark; *continuous oozing of watery blood* until next period. Threatened abortion about the *third* month. [*Sab.*] During labor no expulsive action, though everything is relaxed. After-pains. Suppression of milk; breasts do not fill properly. Dark, offensive lochia. Puerperal fever, putrid discharges, tympanitis, coldness, suppressed urine.

Chest.—Angina pectoris. Dyspnœa and oppression, with cramp in diaphragm. Boring pain in chest. Præcordial tenderness. Palpitation, with contracted and intermittent pulse.

Sleep.—Profound and long. Insomnia with restlessness, fever, anxious dreams. *Insomnia of drug and liquor habitues.*

Back.—Spinal irritation, tingling of lower extremities; can bear only slightest covering. *Locomotor ataxia.* Formication and numbness. Myelitis.

Extremities.—Cold, dry hands and feet of excessive smokers with feeling of fuzziness in fingers. Trembling, staggering gait.

Formication, pain and spasmodic movements. Numbness. Fingers and feet bluish, shriveled, *spread apart or bent backwards*, numb. *Violent cramps. Icy coldness of extremities.* Violent pain in finger-tips, tingling in toes.

Skin.—Shriveled, numb; mottled dusky-blue tinge. Scleræma and œdema neonatorum. Raynaud's disease. Blue color. *Dry gangrene*, developing slowly. *Varicose ulcers. Burning sensation;* better by cold; *wants parts uncovered*, though cold to touch. Formication; petechiæ. Slight wounds continue to bleed. Livid spots. Boils, small, painful, with green contents; mature slowly. *Skin feels cold to touch*, yet covering is not tolerated. *Great aversion to heat. Formication under skin.*

Fever.—*Coldness;* cold, dry skin; cold, clammy sweat; excessive thirst. Sense of internal heat.

Modalities.—*Worse*, heat, *warm covering. Better*, cold, *uncovering*, rubbing, stretching out limbs.

Relationship.—Compare: *Ergotin.* (Beginning arteriosclerosis progressing rather rapidly. Increased blood pressure: 2x trit. Edema, gangrene 'and purpura hæmorrhagia; when Secale, though indicated, fails); *Pedicularis Canadensis* (symptoms of locomotor ataxia; spinal irritation); *Brassica napus*—Rape-seed—(dropsical swellings, scorbutic mouth, voracious appetite, tympanitis, dropping of nails, gangrene); *Cinnamon.; Colch.; Ars.; Aurum mur.* 2x (locomotor ataxia); *Agrostema*—Corn-cockle—active constituent is *Saponin*, which causes violent sneezing and sharp burning taste; burning in stomach, extends to œsophagus, neck and breast; (vertigo, headache, difficult locomotion, burning sensation); *Ustilago; Carbo; Pituitrin* (dilated os, little pain, no progress. Dose, ½ c.c., repeat in half hour, if necessary. Hypodermically contraindicated in first stage of labor, valvular lesions or deformed pelvis).

Antidotes: *Camph.; Opium.*

Dose.—First to thirtieth potency. *Non-homœopathic use.*— In hæmorrhages of the puerperium, after the uterus is entirely emptied, when it fails to contract satisfactorily and in secondary puerperal hæmorrhage the result of incomplete involution of the uterus, give one-half to one dram of the fluid extract. Remember Pagot's law. "As long as the uterus contair. anything, be it child, placenta, membranes, clots, never administer Ergot."

SEDUM ACRE
(Small Houseleek)

Hæmorrhoidal pains, like those of anal fissures; constricting pains, worse few hours after stool. *Fissures.*

Relationship.—Compare: *Mucuna urens* (hæmorrhoidal diathesis and diseases depending thereon); *Sedum telephium* (uterine hæmorrhages, also of bowels and rectum; *menorrhagia, especially at climacteric*); *Sedum repens—S. alpestre—(cancer;* specific action on abdominal organs; pain, loss of strength).

Dose.—Tincture to sixth potency.

SELENIUM
(The Element Selenium)

Selenium is a constant constituent of bones and teeth.

Marked effects on the genito-urinary organs, and often indicated in elderly men, especially for prostatitis and sexual atony. *Great debility;* worse, heat. Easy exhaustion, mental and physical, in old age. Debility after exhausting diseases.

Mind.—Lascivious thoughts, with impotency. Mental labor fatigues. *Extreme sadness.* Abject despair, uncompromising melancholy.

Head.—Hair falls out. *Pain over left eye; worse, walking in sun, strong odors and tea.* Scalp feels tense. Headache from tea drinking.

Throat.—Incipient tubercular laryngitis. Hawking and raising transparent lumps of mucus every morning. *Hoarseness.* Cough in morning, with expectoration of bloody mucus. Hoarseness of singers. Much clear, starchy mucus. [*Stann.*]

Stomach.—Desire for brandy and other strong drink. Sweetish taste. Hiccough and eructations after smoking. After eating, pulsation all over, especially abdomen.

Abdomen.—Chronic liver affections; liver painful, *enlarged, with fine rash over liver region.* Stool constipated, hard and accumulated in rectum.

Urinary.—Sensation in the tip of urethra as if a biting drop were forcing its way out. Involuntary dribbling.

Male.—Dribbling of semen during sleep. Dribbling of prostatic fluid. Irritability after coitus. *Loss of sexual power*, with lascivious fancies. *Increases desire, decreases ability.* Semen thin, odorless. Sexual neurasthenia. On attempting coition, penis relaxes. *Hydrocele.*

Skin.—Dry, scaly eruption in palms, with itching. *Itching about the ankles* and folds of skin, between fingers. Hair falls out from brows, beard, and genitals. Itching about finger-joints and between fingers; in palms. Vesicular eruption between fingers. [*Rhus; Anac.*] Seborrhœa oleosa; comedones *with an oily surface of the skin;* alopecia. Acne.

Extremities.—Paralytic pains in small of back in the morning. Tearing pain in hands, at night.

Sleep.—*Sleep prevented by pulsation in all vessels,* worse abdomen. Sleepless until midnight, awakens early and always same hour.

Modalities.—*Worse,* after sleep, in hot weather, from Cinchona, draught of air, coition.

Relationship.—Incompatible: *China; Wine.*

Compare: *Agnus; Calad.; Sulphur; Tellur.; Phosph. acid.* Antidotes: *Ign.; Puls.*

Dose.—Sixth to thirtieth potency. Colloidal Selenium injection for inoperable cancer. Pain, sleeplessness, ulceration and discharge are markedly diminished.

SEMPERVIVUM TECTORUM
(Houseleek)

Is recommended for herpes, zoster and *cancerous tumors.* Scirrhous induration of tongue. Mammary carcinoma. Ringworm. Hæmorrhoids.

Mouth.—Malignant ulcers of mouth. Cancer of tongue. [*Galium.*] Tongue has ulcers; *bleed easily,* especially at night; much soreness of tongue with *stabbing* pains. Whole mouth very tender.

Skin.—Erysipelatous affections. *Warts* and corns. Aphthæ. Flushed surface and stinging pains.

Relationship.—Compare: *Sedum acre*—small Houseleek— (scorbutic conditions; ulcers, intermittent fever). [*Galium;*

Kali cyanat.] *Oxalis acetosella*—Wood sorrel—(The inspissated juice used as a cautery to remove cancerous growths of the lips). *Cotyledon. Ficus Carica*—(Fig)—The milky juice of the freshly broken stalk applied to warts; causes their disappearance.

Dose.—Tincture and 2 decimal, also fresh juice of plant. Locally for bites of insects, stings of bees, and poisoned wounds, *warts.*

SENECIO AUREUS
(Golden Ragwort)

Its action on the female organism has been clinically verified. Urinary organs also affected in a marked degree. Backaches of congested kidneys. Early cirrhosis of liver.

Mind.—Inability to fix mind upon any one subject. Despondent. Nervous and irritable.

Head.—Dull, stupefying headache. *Wavelike dizziness* from occiput to sinciput. *Sharp pains over left eye, and through left temple.* Fullness of nasal passages; burning; *sneezing;* profuse flow.

Face.—Teeth very sensitive. *Sharp, cutting pain* left side. *Dryness* of fauces, throat, and mouth.

Stomach.—Sour eructations; nausea.

Throat.—Dry mouth, throat, and fauces. Burning in pharynx, raw feeling in naso-pharynx, must swallow, though painful.

Abdomen.—Pain around umbilicus; spreads all over abdomen; better, stool. Thin, watery stool, intermingled with hard lumps of fæces. [*Ant. crud.*] *Straining at stool; thin, dark, bloody, with tenesmus.*

Urinary.—Scanty, high-colored, *bloody,* with much mucus and *tenesmus. Great heat and constant urging.* Nephritis. Irritable bladder of children, with headache. Renal colic. [*Pareira; Ocim.; Berb.*]

Male.—Lascivious dreams, with involuntary emissions. *Prostate enlarged.* Dull, heavy pain in spermatic cord, extending to testicles.

Female.—*Menses retarded,* suppressed. *Functional amenorrhœa of young girls* with backache. Before menses, inflammatory conditions of throat, chest, and bladder. After menstruation commences, these improve. Anæmic dysmenorrhœa with

urinary disturbances.   Premature and too profuse menses.
[*Calc.; Erig.*]

Respiratory.—Acute inflammatory conditions of upper respiratory tract. Hoarseness. *Cough loose,* with labored inspiration. Chest sore and raw. Dyspnœa on ascending. [*Calc.*]
Dry teasing cough, stitching chest pains.

Sleep.—Great drowsiness, with unpleasant dreams. Nervousness and sleeplessness.

Relationship.—Compare: *Senecio Jacobæa* (cerebro-spinal irritation, rigid muscles, chiefly of neck and shoulders; also, in cancer); *Aletris; Caulop.; Sep.*

Dose.—Tincture, to third potency. *Senecin,* first trituration·

SENEGA
(Snakewort)

Catarrhal symptoms, especially of the respiratory tract, and distinct eye symptoms of a paralytic type, are most characteristic. Circumscribed spots in chest left after inflammations.

Mind.—Suddenly remembers unimportant regions which he saw long ago. Inclined to quarrel.

Head.—Dullness, with pressure and weakness of eyes. Pain in temples. *Bursting* pain in forehead.

Eyes.—Hyperphoria, better by bending head backwards. Acts on the rectus superior. Blepharitis; lids dry and crusty. [*Graph.*] Dryness, with sensation *as if too large for orbits.* Staring. Lachrymation. Flickering; must wipe eyes frequently. Objects look shaded. Muscular asthenopia. [*Caust.*] Double vision; better only by bending head backward. Opacities of the vitreous humor. Promotes absorption of fragments of lens, after operation.

Nose.—Dry. Coryza; much watery mucus and sneezing. Nostrils feel peppery.

Face.—Paralysis of left side of face. Heat in face. Burning vesicles in corners of mouth and lips.

Throat.—Catarrhal inflammation of throat and fauces, with scraping hoarseness. Burning and rawness. Sensation as if membrane had been abraded.

Respiratory.—Hoarseness. Hurts to talk. Bursting pain in back on coughing. Catarrh of larynx. Loss of voice. Hacking cough. Thorax feels too narrow. *Cough often ends in a sneeze. Rattling in chest.* [*Tart. emet.*] Chest oppressed on ascending. Bronchial catarrh, *with sore chest walls;* much mucus; sensation of oppression and weight of chest. *Difficult raising of tough, profuse mucus,* in the aged. Asthenic bronchitis of old people with chronic interstitial nephritis or chronic emphysema. Old asthmatics with congestive attacks. *Exudations in Pleura.* Hydrothorax. [*Merc. sulph.*] Pressure on chest as though lungs were forced back to spine. Voice unsteady, vocal cords partially paralyzed.

Urinary.—Greatly diminished; loaded with shreds and mucus; scalding before and after urinating. *Back,* bursting distending pain in kidney region.

Modalities.—*Worse,* walking in open air, during rest. *Better,* from sweat; *bending head backwards.*

Relationship.—Compare: *Caust.; Phos.; Saponin; Ammon.; Calc.; Nepeta cataria*—Catnip (to break up a cold; infantile colic: hysteria).

Dose.—Tincture, to thirtieth potency.

SENNA
(Cassia Acutifolia)

Is of much use in infantile colics when the child seems to be *full of wind.* Oxaluria, with excess of urea; increased specific gravity. Where the system is broken down, bowels constipated, muscular weakness, and waste of nitrogenous materials, Senna will act as a tonic. Ebullitions of blood at night. *Acetonæmia,* prostration, fainting, constipation with colic and flatulence. Liver enlarged and tender.

Stool.—Fluid yellowish, with pinching pains before. Greenish mucus; never-get-done sensation. [*Merc.*] Burning in rectum, with strangury of bladder. *Constipation,* with colic and flatulence. Liver enlarged and tender, stools hard and dark, with loss of appetite, coated tongue, bad taste, and *weakness.*

Urine.—Specific gravity and density increased; hyperazoturia, oxaluria, phosphaturia, and acetonuria.

Relationship.—Compare: *Kali carb.; Jalapa.*

Antidotes: *Nux; Cham.*

Dose.—Third to sixth potency.

SEPIA
(Inky Juice of Cuttlefish)

Acts specially on the portal system, with venous congestion. Stasis and thereby ptosis of viscera and weariness and misery. Weakness, yellow complexion, bearing-down sensation, especially in women, upon whose organism it has most pronounced effect. Pains extend down to back, chills easily. Tendency to abortion. Hot flashes at menopause with weakness and perspiration. Upward tendency of its symptoms. Easy fainting. "Ball" sensation in inner parts. Sepia acts best on brunettes. All pains are from below up. One of the most important uterine remedies. Tubercular patients with chronic hepatic troubles and uterine reflexes. *Feels cold* even in warm room. Pulsating headache in cerebellum.

Mind.—*Indifferent* to those loved best. Averse to occupation, to *family.* Irritable; easily offended. Dreads to be alone. *Very sad.* Weeps when telling symptoms. Miserly. Anxious toward evening; indolent.

Head.—Vertigo, with sensation of something rolling round in head. Prodromal symptoms of apoplexy. Stinging pain from within outward and upward mostly left, or in forehead, with nausea, vomiting; worse indoors and when lying on painful side. Jerking of head backwards and forwards. Coldness of vertex. Headache in *terrible shocks* at menstrual nisus, with scanty flow. Hair falls out. Open fontanelles. Roots of hair sensitive. Pimples on forehead near hair.

Nose.—*Thick, greenish discharge;* thick plugs and crusts. *Yellowish saddle across nose.* Atrophic catarrh with greenish crusts from anterior nose and pain at root of nose. Chronic nasal catarrh, especially post-nasal, dropping of heavy, lumpy discharges; must be hawked through the mouth.

Eyes.—Muscular asthenopia; black spots in the field of vision; asthenic inflammations, and in connection with uterine trouble. Aggravation of eye troubles morning and evening. Tarsal tumors. Ptosis, ciliary irritation. Venous congestion of the fundus.

Ears.—*Herpes behind ears on nape of neck.* Pain as if from sub-cutaneous ulceration. Swelling and eruption of external ear.

Face.—Yellow blotches; pale or sallow; yellow about mouth. Rosacea; saddle-like brownish distribution on nose and cheeks.

Mouth.—Tongue white. Taste salty, putrid. Tongue foul, but clears during menses. Swelling and cracking of lower lip. Pain in teeth from 6 p. m. till midnight; worse on lying.

Stomach.—*Feeling of goneness; not relieved by eating.* [*Carb. an.*] Nausea at smell or sight of food. Nausea worse lying on side. *Tobacco dyspepsia.* Everything tastes too salty. [*Carbo veg.; Chin.*] Band of pain about four inches wide encircling hypochondria. *Nausea in morning before eating.* Disposition to vomit after eating. Burning in pit of stomach. Longing for *vinegar*, acids, and pickles. Worse, after milk, especially when boiled. Acid dyspepsia with bloated abdomen, sour eructations. Loathes fat.

Abdomen.—*Flatulent*, with headache. *Liver sore and painful; relieved by lying on right side.* Many brown spots on abdomen. Feeling of relaxation and bearing-down in abdomen.

Rectum.—Bleeding at stool and fullness of rectum. Constipation; large, hard stools; *feeling of a ball in rectum;* cannot strain; with great tenesmus and pains shooting *upward*. Dark-brown, round balls glued together with mucus. Soft stool, difficult. Prolapsus ani. [*Pod.*] *Almost constant oozing from anus.* Infantile diarrhœa, *worse from boiled milk,* and rapid exhaustion. *Pains shoot up* in rectum and vagina.

Urinary.—Red, *adhesive,* sand in urine. Involuntary urination, *during first sleep.* Chronic cystitis, slow micturition, with bearing-down sensation above pubis.

Male.—Organs cold. Offensive perspiration. Gleet; discharge from urethra only during night; no pain. Condylomata surround head of penis. Complaints from coition.

Female.—Pelvic organs relaxed. *Bearing-down sensation as if everything would escape through vulva* [*Bell.; Kreoso; Lac c.; Lil. t.; Nat. c.; Pod.*]; must cross limbs to prevent protrusion, or press against vulva. Leucorrhœa yellow, greenish: with much itching. Menses *too late and scanty*, irregular; *early and profuse;* sharp clutching pains. Violent stitches upward in the vagina, from uterus to umbilicus. *Prolapse* of uterus and vagina. Morning sickness. Vagina painful, especially on coition.

Respiratory.—Dry, fatiguing cough, apparently coming from stomach. Rotten-egg taste with coughing. Oppression of chest morning and evening. Dyspnœa; worse, after sleep; better, rapid motion. Cough in morning, with profuse expectoration, tasting salty. [*Phos.; Ambr.*] Hypostatic pleuritis. Whooping-cough that drags on. Cough excited by tickling in larynx or chest.

Heart.—Violent, intermittent palpitation. Beating in all arteries. Tremulous feeling with flushes.

Back.—*Weakness in small of back. Pains extend into back.* Coldness between shoulders.

Extremities.—Lower extremities lame and stiff, tension as if too short. Heaviness and bruised feeling. *Restlessness in all limbs*, twitching and jerkings night and day. Pain in heel. Coldness of legs and feet.

Fever.—Frequent flushes of heat; sweat from least motion. General lack of warmth of body. Feet cold and wet. Shivering, with thirst; worse, towards evening.

Skin.—Herpes circinatus in isolated spots. Itching; not relieved by scratching; worse in bends of elbows and knees. Chloasma; herpetic eruption on lips, about mouth and nose. Ringworm-like eruption every spring. Urticaria on going in open air; better in warm room. Hyperidrosis and bromidrosis. Sweat on feet, worse on toes; intolerable odor. Lentigo in young women. Ichthyosis with offensive odor of skin.

Modalities.—*Worse,* forenoons and evenings; washing, laundry-work, dampness, left side, after sweat; cold air, before thunder-storm. *Better,* by *exercise*, pressure, warmth of bed, hot applications, drawing limbs up, cold bathing, after sleep.

Relationship.—Complementary: *Nat. mur.; Phosph. Nux* intensifies action. *Guaiacum* often beneficial after *Sepia.*

Inimical: *Lach.; Puls.*

Compare: *Lil.; Murex· Silica; Sulph.; Asperula*—Nacent

oxygen—Distilled water charged with the gas—(leucorrhœa of young girls and uterine catarrh); *Ozonum* (*sacral* pain; tired feeling through pelvic viscera and perineum); *Dictamnus*— Burning Bush—(Soothes labor pains); (metrorrhagia, leucor- rhœa, and constipation; also somnambulism). *Lapathum.* (Leucorrhœa with constriction and expulsive effort through womb and pain in kidneys).

Dose.—Twelfth, 30th and 200th potency. Should not be used too low or be repeated too frequently. On the other hand Dr. Jousset's unique experience is that it should be continued for some time in strong doses. 1x twice a day.

SERUM ANGUILLAR ICHTHYOTOXIN
(Eel Serum)

The *serum of the eel* has a toxic action on the blood, rapidly destroying its globules. The presence of albumin and renal elements in the urine, the hemoglobinuria, the prolonged anuria (24 and 26 hours), together with the results of the autopsy, plainly demonstrate its elective action on the kidneys. Secon- darily, the liver and the heart are affected, and the alterations observed are those usually present in infectious diseases.

From all these facts it is easy to infer, *a priori*, the therapeu- tical indications of the *serum of the eel.* Whenever the kidney becomes acutely affected, either from cold or infection or intoxi- cation, and the attack is characterized by *oliguria, anuria* and *albuminuria,* we will find the *eel's serum* eminently efficacious to re-establish diuresis, and in rapidly arresting albuminuria. When during the course of *heart-disease,* the kidney, previously working well, should suddenly become affected and its function inhibited; and when besides we observe cardiac irregularities and a marked state of asystolia, we may yet expect good results from this serum. But to determine here the choice of this remedy is not an easy matter. While *digitalis* presents in its indications, the well-known symptomatic trilogy: *arterial hyper- tension, oliguria and œdema;* the *serum of the eel* seems better adapted to cases of *hypertension and oliguria, without œdema.* We should bear in mind that the elective action of the eel's serum is on the kidney, and I believe we can well assert that if *digitalis* is a cardiac, the *eel's serum* is a renal remedy. So far, at least, the clinical observations published seem to confirm this distinction. The serum of the eel has given very small results in attacks of asystolia; but it has been very efficacious in *cardiac uremia*. There, where *digitalis* is powerless, the *serum of the eel* has put an end to the renal obstruction and produced an abundant diuresis. But its really specific indication seems to be for *acute nephritis a frigori*. (Jousset.)

Subacute nephritis. Heart diseases, in cases of failure of compensation and impending asytole. The experiments of Dr. Jousset have amply demonstrated the rapid hæmaturia, albuminuria and oliguria caused by it. In the presence of acute nephritis with threatening uræmia we should always think of this serum. Very efficacious in functional heart diseases. Mitral insufficiency, asystolia with or without œdema, dyspnœa and difficult urinary secretion.

Relationship.—Great analogy exists between eel serum and the venom of the *Vipera*.

Compare, also: *Pelias; Lachesis*.

Dose.—Attenuations are made with glycerine or distilled water, the lower 1x to 3 in heart disease, the higher in sudden renal attacks.

SILICEA

(Silica. Pure Flint)

Imperfect assimilation and consequent defective nutrition. It goes further and produces neurasthenic states in consequence, and increased susceptibility to nervous stimuli and exaggerated reflexes. Diseases of bones, caries and necrosis. Silica can stimulate the organism to re-absorb fibrotic conditions and scar-tissue. In phthisis must be used with care, for here it may cause the absorption of scar-tissue, liberate the disease, walled in, to new activities. (J. Weir.) Organic changes; it is deep and slow in action. Periodical states; abscesses, quinsy, headaches, spasms, epilepsy, feeling of coldness before an attack. Keloid growth. Scrofulous, rachitic children, with large head, open fontanelles and sutures, distended abdomen, slow in walking. *Ill effects of vaccination. Suppurative processes.* It is related to all fistulous burrowings. Ripens abscesses since it promotes suppuration. Silica patient is cold, chilly, hugs the fire, wants plenty warm clothing, hates drafts, hands and feet cold, worse in winter. Lack of vital heat. Prostration of mind and body. Great sensitiveness to taking cold. *Intolerance of alcoholic stimulants.* Ailments attended with *pus formation.* Epilepsy. *Want of grit,* moral or physical.

Mind.-Yielding, *faint-hearted, anxious.* Nervous and excitable. *Sensitive* to all impressions. Brain-fag. Obstinate, headstrong children. Abstracted. Fixed ideas; thinks only of *pins,* fears them, searches and counts them.

Head.—Aches from fasting. Vertigo from looking up; *better, wrapping up warmly; when lying on left side.* [*Magnes. mur.; Strontia.*] *Profuse sweat of head,* offensive, and extends to neck. Pain begins at occiput, and spreads over head and settles over eyes. Swelling in the glabella.

Eyes.—Angles of eyes affected. *Swelling of lachrymal duct.* Aversion to light, especially daylight; it produces dazzling, sharp pain through eyes; eyes tender to touch; worse when closed. Vision confused; letters run together on reading. *Styes.* Iritis and irido-choroiditis, with pus in anterior chamber. *Perforating* or sloughing ulcer of cornea. Abscess in cornea after traumatic injury. Cataract in office workers. After-effects of keratitis and ulcus corn æ, clearing the opacity. Use 30th potency for months.

Ears.—Fetid discharge. Caries of mastoid. Loud pistol-like report. Sensitive to noise. *Roaring in ears.*

Nose.—Itching at point of nose. Dry, hard crusts form, *bleeding when loosened.* Nasal bones sensitive. Sneezing in morning. Obstructed and loss of smell. Perforation of septum.

Face.—Skin cracked on margin of lips. Eruption on chin. Facial neuralgia, throbbing, tearing, face red; worse, cold damp.

Mouth.—*Sensation of a hair on tongue.* Gums sensitive to cold air. Boils on gums. Abscess at root of teeth. Pyorrhœa. [*Merc. cor.*] Sensitive to cold water.

Throat.—Periodical quinsy. *Pricking as of a pin in tonsil.* Colds settle in throat. *Parotid glands swollen.* [*Bell.; Rhus; Calc.*] Stinging pain on swallowing. Hard, cold swelling of cervical glands.

Stomach.—Disgust for meat and *warm food.* On swallowing food, it easily gets into posterior nares. Want of appetite; thirst excessive. Sour eructations after eating. [*Sepia; Calc.*] Pit of stomach painful to pressure. Vomiting after drinking. [*Ars.; Verat.*]

Abdomen.—Pain or painful cold feeling in abdomen, better external heat. Hard, bloated. Colic; cutting pain, with constipation; yellow hands and blue nails. Much rumbling in bowels. Inguinal glands swollen and painful. Hepatic abscess.

Rectum.—Feels paralyzed. *Fistula in ano.* [*Berb.; Lach.*] Fissures and hæmorrhoids, *painful, with spasm of sphincter. Stool comes down with difficulty; when partly expelled, recedes again.* Great straining; rectum stings; closes upon stool. Fæces remain a long time in rectum. *Constipation always before and during menses;* with irritable sphincter ani. Diarrhœa of cadaverous odor.

Urinary.—Bloody, involuntary, with red or yellow sediment. Prostatic fluid discharged when straining at stool. Nocturnal enuresis in children with worms.

Male.—Burning and soreness of genitals, with eruption on inner surface of thighs. Chronic gonorrhœa, with thick, fetid discharge. Elephantiasis of scrotum. Sexual erethism; nocturnal emissions. Hydrocele.

Female.—A milky [*Calc.; Puls.; Sep.*], acrid leucorrhœa, during urination. Itching of vulva and vagina; very sensitive. Discharge of blood between menstrual periods. Increased menses, with paroxysms of *icy coldness over whole body.* Nipples very sore; ulcerated easily; drawn in. Fistulous ulcers of breast. [*Phos.*] Abscess of labia. Discharge of blood from vagina every time child is nursed. Vaginal cysts. [*Lyc.; Puls.; Rhod.*] Hard lumps in breast. [*Conium.*]

Respiratory.—Colds fail to yield; sputum persistently muco-purulent and profuse. Slow recovery after pneumonia. Cough and sore throat, with expectoration of little granules like shot, which, when broken, smell very offensive. Cough with expectoration in day, bloody or purulent. Stitches in chest through to back. *Violent cough when lying down, with thick, yellow lumpy expectoration;* suppurative stage of expectoration. [*Bals. Peru.*]

Back.—Weak spine; very susceptible to draughts on back. Pain in coccyx. Spinal irritation after injuries to spine; diseases of bones of spine. Potts' disease.

Sleep.—*Night-walking;* gets up while asleep. Sleeplessness, with great orgasm of blood and heat in head. Frequent starts in sleep. Anxious dreams. Excessive gaping.

Extremities.—Sciatica, pains through hips, legs and feet. Cramp in calves and soles. Loss of power in legs. Tremulous hands when using them. Paralytic weakness of forearm. *Affections of finger nails*, especially if white spots on nails. Ingrowing toe-nails. *Icy cold and sweaty feet. The parts lain on go to sleep. Offensive sweat on feet,* hands, and axillæ. Sensation in tips of fingers, as if suppurating. Panaritium. Pain in knee, as if tightly bound. Calves tense and contracted. Pain beneath toes. Soles sore. [*Ruta.*] *Soreness in feet from instep through to the sole. Suppurates.*

Skin.—*Felons, abscesses, boils, old fistulous ulcers.* Delicate, pale, waxy. Cracks at end of fingers. Painless swelling of glands. Rose-colored blotches. Scars suddenly become painful. Pus offensive. *Promotes expulsion of foreign bodies from tissues.* Every little injury suppurates. Long lasting suppuration and fistulous tracts. Dry finger tips. Eruptions itch only in daytime and evening. *Crippled nails.* Indurated tumors. Abscesses of joints. After impure vaccination. Bursa. Lepra, nodes, and coppery spots. *Keloid growths.*

Fever.—Chilliness; very sensitive to cold air. Creeping, shivering over the whole body. Cold extremities, even in a warm room. Sweat at night; worse towards morning. *Suffering parts feel cold.*

Modalities.—*Worse*, new moon, in morning, from washing, during menses, uncovering, lying down, damp, lying on left side, cold. *Better*, warmth, wrapping up head, summer; in wet or humid weather.

Relationship.—Complementary: *Thuja; Sanic.; Puls.; Fluor. ac.* Mercurius and Silica do not follow each other well.

Compare: *Black Gunpowder* 3x. (Abscesses, boils, carbuncles, limb purple. Wounds that refuse to heal; accident from bad food or water.—Clarke.) . *Hep.; Kali phos.; Pic. ac.; Calc.; Phos.; Tabasheer; Natrum silicum* (tumors, hæmophilia, arthritis; dose, three drops three times daily, in milk); *Ferrum cyanatum* (epilepsy; neuroses, with irritable weakness and hyper-sensitiveness, especially of a periodical character). *Silica marina*—Sea-sand—(Silica and Natrum mur. symptoms. *Inflamed glands* and commencing suppuration. Constipation. Use for some time 3x trit.) *Vitrum—Crown glass—*(Potts' disease, after Silica, necrosis, discharge thin, watery, fetid. Much pain, fine *grinding* and *grating* like grit.) *Arundo donax* (acts on excretory and generative organs; suppuration, especially chronic, and where the ulceration is fistulous, especially in long bones. Itching eruption on chest, upper extremities and behind eard).

Dose.—Sixth to thirtieth potency. The 200th and higher of unquestioned activity. In malignant affections, the lowest potencies needed at times.

SILPHIUM
(Rosin-weed)

Is used in various forms of asthma and chronic bronchitis Catarrh of bladder. Catarrhal influenza. Dysentery; attack preceded by constipated stools covered with white mucus.

Respiratory.—Cough with expectoration *profuse*, stringy, forthy, light-colored. Excited by sense of mucus rattling in chest and worse by drafts of air. Constriction of lungs. Catarrh, with copious, stringy, mucous discharges. Desire to hawk and scrape throat. Irritation of posterior nares, involving mucous membranes of nasal passages with constriction of supra-orbital region.

Relationship.—Compare: *Aral.; Copaiv.; Tereb.; Cubeb.; Samb.; Silphion cyrenaicum* (phthisis pulmonum, with incessant cough, profuse night-sweats, emaciation, etc.); *Polygonum aviculare* (has been found useful in phthisis, when given in material doses of the mother tincture); *Salvia* (tickling cough). *Arum dracontium* (loose cough at night on lying down). *Justicia adhatoda* (bronchial catarrh, hoarseness, oversensitive).

Dose.—Third **potency.** Lower *triturations* preferred by some.

SINAPIS NIGRA—BRASSICA NIGRA
(Black Mustard)

Is of use in hay-fever, coryza, and pharyngitis. Dry nares and pharynx, with thick, lumpy secretion. Small-pox.

Head.—Scalp hot and itches. *Sweat on upper lip and forehead.* Tongue feels blistered.

Nose.—Mucus from posterior nares feels *cold*. Scanty, *acrid* discharge. *Stoppage of left nostril all day,* or in afternoon and evening. Dry, hot, with lachrymation, sneezing; hacking cough; better lying down. *Nostrils alternately stopped.* Dryness of anterior nares.

Respiratory.—Cough is relieved by lying down.

Throat.—Feels scalded, hot, inflamed. Asthmatic breathing. Loud coughing-spells with barking expiration.

Stomach.—*Offensive breath,* smelling like onions. [*Asaf.*; *Armorac.*] Burning in stomach, extending up œsophagus, throat, and mouth, which is full of canker sores. Hot sour eructations. *Colic; pains come on while bent forward; better, sitting up straight.* Sweat better when nausea comes on.

Urinary.—Pain in bladder, frequent *copious* flow day and night.

Back.—Rheumatic pain in intercostal and lumbar muscles; sleeplessness from pain in back and hips.

Relationship.—Compare: *Sulph.*; *Capsic.*; *Colocy.*; *Sinapis alba*—White Mustard—(throat symptoms marked, especially *pressure and burning, with obstruction in œsophagus;* sensation of a lump in œsophagus behind the Manubrium Sterni and with much eructation; similar symptoms in rectum). *Mustard oil* by inhalation (acts on the sensory nerve endings of the trigeminal. Relieves pain in middle ear disease and in painful conditions of nose, nasal cavities, and tonsils.)

Dose.—Third potency.

SKATOL

Represents the ultimate end of proteid decomposition and is a constituent of human fæces.

Acne with auto-intoxication dependent upon intestinal decomposition.

Stomach and abdominal symptoms and frontal headache. Sluggishness with no ambition. Desire to curse and swear.

Mind.—Lack of concentration; impossible to study; *despondent;* desire to be with people. Irritable. Felt mean towards everyone.

Head.—Frontal headache, worse over left eye, in the evening, *better by short sleep.*

Gastric.—Tongue coated, *foul taste.* Salty taste to all cereals. *Belching.* Appetite increased. Light, yellow, narrow, *very offensive* stool. Intestinal dyspepsia.

Urinary.—Frequent, scanty, burning, difficult.

Sleep.—Increased desire to sleep; wakes unrefreshed, half doped feeling.

Relationship.—Compare: *Indol.; Baptis.; Sulph.*

Dose.—Sixth potency.

SKOOKUM-CHUCK

Chuck—Water and Skookum—Strong
(Salts from Water from Medical Lake near Spokane, Wash.)

Has strong affinity for skin and mucous membranes—An anti-psoric medicine.

Otitis media. Profuse, ichorous, cadaverously smelling discharge. Lithæmia. *Catarrh.* Urticaria. *Skin affections. Eczema. Dry skin. Hay-fever.* Profuse coryza and constant sneezing.

Relationship.—*Saxonite*—(appears to have remarkable cleansing, deodorizing and soothing properties for the skin. (Cowperthwaite.) Eczema, scalds, burns, sores and hæmorrhoids).

Dose.—Third trituration.

SOLANUM LYCOPERSICUM—
LYCOPERSICUM ESCULENTUM
(Tomato)

Marked symptoms of rheumatism and influenza. Severe aching pains all over body. *Pains left after influenza.* Head always shows signs of acute congestion. Hay-fever, with marked aggravation from breathing the least dust. Frequent urination and profuse watery diarrhœa.

Head.—Bursting pain, beginning in occiput and spreading all over. Whole head and scalp feels sore, bruised, after pain has ceased.

Eyes.—Dull, heavy; pupils contracted; eyeballs feel contracted; aching in and around eyes. Eyes suffused.

Nose.—Profuse, watery coryza; drops down throat. Itching in anterior chamber; worse, breathing any dust; better, indoors.

Heart.—Decided decrease in pulse rate with anxiety and apprehensiveness.

Respiratory.—Voice husky. Pain in chest, extending to head. Hoarseness; constant desire to clear throat. Expulsive cough, deep and harsh. Chest oppressed; dry, hacking cough coming on at night and keeping one awake.

Urine.—Constant dribbling *in open air*. Must rise at night to urinate.

Extremities.—Aching through back. Dull pain in lumbar region. *Sharp pain in right deltoid and pectoralis muscles.* Pain deep in middle of right arm. Rheumatic pain in right elbow and wrist, and hands of both sides. Intense aching in lower limbs. Right crural neuralgia. Tingling along right ulnar nerve.

Modalities.—*Worse*, right side, open air, continued motion, jars, noises. *Better*, warm room, tobacco.

Relationship.—Compare: *Bellad.* (follows well); *Eup. perf.; Rhus; Sanguin.; Caps.*

Dose.—Third to thirtieth potency.

SOLANUM NIGRUM
(Black Nightshade)

Used with success in ergotism, with tetanic spasms and stiffness of whole body, with mania. Marked action on head and eyes. *Meningitis.* Chronic intestinal toxæmia. Brain irritation during dentition. Restlessness of a violent and convulsive nature. Formication with contraction of extremities.

Head.—Furious delirium. Vertigo; terrible headache and complete cessation of the mental faculties. Night terrors. *Congestive* headache.

Nose.—Acute coryza; *profuse, watery discharge from right nostril;* left stopped up, with chilly sensation, alternating with heat.

Eyes.—Pain over both eyes. Alternate dilatation and contraction of pupils; weak sight; floating spots.

Respiratory.—Constrictive feeling in chest, with difficult breathing; cough with tickling in throat. Expectoration *thick, yellow.* Pain in *left* chest, sore to touch.

Fever.—Alternation of coldness and heat. Scarlet fever; eruption in spots, large and vivid.

Relationship.—Compare: *Bellad.; Solanum Carolinense*—Horse-nettle—(convulsions and epilepsy, twenty to forty-drop doses; is of great value in grand mal of idiopathic type, where the disease has begun beyond age of childhood; hystero-epilepsy, also in whooping-cough); *Solan. mammosum*—Apple of Sodom—(pain in left hip-joint); *Solan. oleraceum* (swelling of mammary gland, with profuse secretion of milk); *Solan. tuberosum* (cramps in calves and contraction of fingers; spitting through closed teeth); *Solan. vesicarium* (recommended in facial paralysis); *Solaninum aceticum* (threatening paralysis of the lungs in the course of bronchitis in the aged and children must cough a long time before able to raise expectoration; *Solan. pseudocaps.* (acute pains, in lower abdomen); *Solan. tuberos. ægrotans*—Diseased potato—(prolapse of the rectum, patulous anus; offensive breath and odor of body; tumors of rectum look like decayed potato; dreams of pools of blood); *Solanum tuberosum*—Potato berries—(cramps in the calves of the legs and fingers).

Dose.—Second to thirtieth potency.

SOLIDAGO VIRGA
(Golden-rod)

Inhalation of the pollen has caused hæmorrhage from the lungs in phthisis. *Repeated colds of tuberculosis* (2x). *Feeling of weakness,* chilliness alternating with heat; naso-pharyngeal catarrh, burning in throat, pains in limbs and thoracic oppression. Pain in region of kidneys, with dysuria. *Kidneys sensi-*

tive to pressure. Bright's disease. Hay-fever when Solidago is the exciting cause. Here give 30th potency or higher.

Eyes.—Injected, watery, burning, stinging.

Nose.—Nares irritated with abundant mucus secretion; paroxysms of sneezing.

Stomach.—Bitter taste, especially at night; coated tongue with very scanty brown and sour urine.

Respiratory.—Bronchitis, cough with much purulent expectoration, blood-streaked; oppressed breathing. Continuous dyspnœa. Asthma, with nightly dysuria.

Female.—Uterine enlargement, organ pressed down upon the bladder. *Fibroid tumors.*

Urine.—Scanty, reddish brown, thick sediment, dysuria, gravel. *Difficult and scanty.* Albumen, blood, and slime in urine. Pain in kidneys extend forward to abdomen and bladder. [*Berb.*] *Clear and offensive urine.* Sometimes makes the use of the catheter unnecessary.

Back.—Backache of congested kidneys. [*Senec. aur.*]

Skin.—Blotches, especially on lower extremities; *itch.* Exanthema of lower extremities, with urinary disturbances, dropsy and threatened gangrene.

Relationship.—*Iodoform* 2x antidotes poison of Golden-rod. *Arsenic. Agrimonia.* (Pain in region of kindeys.)

Dose.—Tincture, to third potency. Oil of Solidago, 1 oz. to 8 oz. Alcohol. 15 drops doses to promote expectoration in bronchitis and bronchial asthma in old people. (Eli G. Jones.)

SPARTIUM SCOPARIUM—CYSTISUS SCOPARIUS

(Broom)

Spartein sulphate increases the strength of the heart, slows it and reduces the blood pressure. It continues the good effects of Veratrum and Digitalis without any of the undesirable effects of either. (Hinsdale.)

The effect of spartein sulphate (the alkaloid of Broom) is to cause a *lowering* of the systolic and diastolic pressures of the provers. Sphygmograms also show a condition of lowered blood-pressure. It depresses the heart by poisonous action exerted on the myocardium and this, with the stimulating action of the drug upon the vagus, accounts for the lowered blood pressure and reduced pulse rate. It weakens the cardiac contraction. The total amount of urine is increased. The drug has, therfore, diuretic properties and is useful in dropsy.

Albuminuria. Cheyne-Stokes respiration. Irregular heart following grip and various infections. Hypotension. Used palliatively in physiological dosage to combat arterial hypertension, arterio-sclerosis. Very useful hypodermically 1/10 to 1/4 grain in sustaining heart after stopping habit of Morphia. Spartium is indicated when primarily the muscles of the heart and especially the nervous apparatus is affected. Acts rapidly and lasts three to four days. Does not disturb digestion. Nephritis.

Heart.—Tobacco heart. Angina pectoris. Irregular action, disturbed rhythm due to gas, etc., feeble in nervous hysterical patients. Myocardial degeneration, failing compensation. Hypotension. Spartein in 2 gr. doses for water-logged cases, cannot lie down. Here it produces much comfort. Has specific action upon the kidneys, enabling them to eliminate and relieve the distress upon the heart.

Stomach.—Great accumulation of gas in gastro-intestinal canal, with mental depression.

Urinary.—Burning along urinary tract or in pudendum. *Profuse flow of urine.*

Dose.—For non-homœopathic use (palliative as above), one to two grains t. i. d. by mouth, exerts a definite action upon the kidneys that will enable them to relieve the distress upon the heart. It is a safe drug and prompt in its action. Hypodermically, not less than 1/4 of a grain. Doses as high as 2 grains by mouth three times a day are safe (Hinsdale).

Homœopathically. First to third trituration.

SPIGELIA
(Pinkroot)

Spigelia is an important remedy in pericarditis and other diseases of the heart, because the provings were conducted with the greatest regard for objective symptoms and the subjective symptoms are by innumerable confirmations proved to be correct (C. Hering).

Has marked elective affinity for the eye, heart, and nervous system. Neuralgia of the fifth nerve is very prominent in its effects. Is especially adapted to anæmic, debilitated, rheumatic, and scrofulous subjects. Stabbing pains. Heart affections and neuralgia. *Very sensitive to touch. Parts feel chilly; send shudder through frame.* A remedy for symptoms due to the presence of worms. *Child refers to the navel as the most painful part.* [*Granat.; Nux mosch.*]

Mind.—Afraid of sharp, pointed things, pins, needles, etc.

Head.—*Pain beneath frontal eminence and temples, extending to eyes.* [*Onos.*] Semi-lateral, involving left eye; pain violent, throbbing; worse, making a false step. Pain as if a band around head. [*Carbol. ac.; Cact.; Gels.*] Vertigo, hearing exalted.

Eyes.—Feel too large; *pressive pain on turning them.* Pupils dilated; photophobia; rheumatic ophthalmia. *Severe pain in and around eyes, extending deep into socket.* Ciliary neuralgia, a true neuritis.

Nose.—Forepart of nose always dry; *discharge through posterior nares. Chronic catarrh,* with post-nasal dropping of bland mucus.

Mouth.—Tongue fissured, painful. Tearing toothache; worse, after eating and cold. *Foul odor from mouth.* Offensive taste.

Face.—*Prosopalgia, involving eye, zygoma, cheek, teeth, temple,* worse, stooping, touch, from morning until sunset.

Heart.—Violent palpitation. Præcordial pain and great aggravation from movement. Frequent attacks of palpitation, especially with foul odor from mouth. Pulse weak and irregular. Pericarditis, with sticking pains, palpitation, dyspnœa. Neuralgia extending to arm or both arms. Angina pectoris. Craving for hot water which relieves. Rheumatic carditis, trembling pulse; whole left side sore. *Dyspnœa; must lie on right side with head high.*

Rectum.—Itching and crawling. Frequent ineffectual urging to stool. Ascarides.

Fever.—Chilliness on the slightest motion.

Modalities.—*Worse,* from touch, motion, noise, turning, washing, concussion. *Better,* lying on right side with head high; inspiring.

Relationship.—Compare: *Spigelia Marylandica* (maniacal excitement, paroxysmal laughing and crying, loud, disconnected talking, vertigo, dilated pupils, congestions); *Acon.; Cact.; Cimicif.; Arnica* (Spigela is a chronic Arnica); *Cinnab.* (supra-orbital pain); *Naja; Spong. (heart)*; *Sabad.; Teucr.; Cina* (worm symptoms).

Antidote: *Pulsat.*

Dose.—Sixth to thirtieth potency for neuralgic symptoms; second to third potency for inflammatory symptoms.

SPIRAEA ULMARIA
(Hardhack)

Burning and pressure in œsophagus, feels contracted but not made worse by swallowing. *Morbidly conscientious.* Relieves irritation of the urinary passages; influences the prostate gland; checks gleet and prostatorrhœa; has been used for eclampsia, epilepsy, and hydrophobia. Bites of mad animals. Heat in various parts. (Salicylic acid is found in Spiræa.)

SPIRANTHES
(Lady's Tresses)

Has been used for milk-flow in nursing women, lumbago and rheumatism, colic, with drowsiness and spasmodic yawning. Is an anti-phlogistic remedy akin to Acon. its symptoms showing congestion and inflammation. Acidity and burning in œsophagus with eructation.

Female.—Pruritus; vulva red; dryness and burning in vagina. Burning pain in vagina during coition. Leucorrhœa, bloody.

Extremities.—Sciatic pain, especially right side. Pain in shoulders. Swelling of veins of hands. Pain in all articulations of hands. Coldness of feet and toes.

Fever.—Flushes of heat. Sweat on palms. Hands alternately hot and cold.

Dose.—Third potency.

SPONGIA TOSTA

(Roasted Sponge)

A remedy especially marked in the symptoms of the respiratory organs, cough, croup, etc. Heart affections and often indicated for the tubercular diathesis. Children with fair complexion, lax fiber; swollen glands. *Exhaustion and heaviness of the body after slight exertion, with orgasm of blood to chest, face. Anxiety and difficult breathing.*

Mind.—Anxiety and fear. Every excitement increases the cough.

Head.—Rush of blood; bursting headache; worse, forehead.

Eyes.—Watering; gummy or mucus discharge.

Nose.—Fluent coryza, alternating with stoppage. Dryness; chronic, dry, nasal catarrh.

Mouth.—Tongue dry and brown; full of vesicles.

Throat.—Thyroid gland swollen. Stitches and dryness. Burning and stinging. Sore throat; worse after eating sweet things. Tickling causes cough. Clears throat constantly.

Stomach.—Excessive thirst, *great hunger.* Cannot bear tight clothing around trunk. Hiccough.

Male.—*Swelling of spermatic cord and testicles, with pain and tenderness. Orchitis.* Epididymitis. Heat in parts.

Female.—Before menses, pain in sacrum, hunger, *palpitation. During menses*, wakes with suffocative spells. [*Cupr.; Iod.; Lach.*] Amenorrhœa, with asthma. [*Puls.*]

Respiratory.—Great dryness of all air-passages. *Hoarseness; larynx dry, burns, constricted.* Cough, *dry, barking, croupy;* larynx senstive to touch. *Croup; worse, during inspiration and before midnight.* Respiration short, panting, *difficult; feeling of a plug in larynx. Cough abates after eating or drinking,* especially warm drinks. The dry, chronic sympathetic cough or organic heart disease is relieved by Spongia. [*Naja.*] Irrepressible cough from a spot deep in chest, as if raw and sore. Chest weak; can scarcely talk. Laryngeal phthisis. Goitre, with suffocative spells. Bronchial catarrh, with wheezing, asthmatic cough, worse cold air, with profuse expectoration and suffocation; worse, lying with head low and in hot room. Oppression and heat of chest, with sudden weakness.

Heart.—Rapid and violent palpitation, with dyspnœa; cannot lie down; also feels best resting in horizontal position. *Awakened suddenly after midnight with pain and suffocation;* is flushed, hot, and frightened to death. [*Acon.*] Valvular insufficiency. Angina pectoris; faintness, and anxious sweat. Ebullition of blood, veins distended. *Surging of heart into chest, as if it would force out upward.* Hypertrophy of heart, especially right, with asthmatic symptoms.

Skin.—*Swelling and induration of glands;* also exophthalmic; cervical glands swollen with tensive pain on turning head, painful on pressure; goitre. Itching; measles.

Sleep.—*Awakes in a fright, and feels as if suffocating.* Generally worse after sleep, or sleeps into an aggravation. [*Lach.*]

Fever.—*Attacks of heat with anxiety;* heat and redness of face and perspiration.

Modalities.—*Worse,* ascending, wind, before midnight. *Better,* descending, lying with head low.

Relationship.—Compare: *Acon.; Hep.; Brom.; Lach.; Merc. prot.; Iod.* (Goitre.)

Dose.—Second trituration, or tincture to third potency.

SQUILLA MARITIMA
(Sea-onion)

A slow acting remedy. Corresponds to ailments requiring several days to reach their maximum. Persistent, dull, rheumatic pains permeate the body. A spleen medicine; stitches under left free ribs. Important heart and kidney medicine. *Broncho-pneumonia.*

Acts especially on mucous membranes of the respiratory and digestive tracts, and also upon the kidneys. Valuable in chronic bronchitis of old people with mucous rales, dyspnœa, and scanty bronchitis of old people with mucous rales, dyspnœa, and scanty urine.

Eyes.—Feel irritable; child bores into them with fists. Sensation as if swimming in cold water.

Stomach.—Pressure like a stone.

Respiratory.—Fluent coryza; margins of nostrils feel sore. Sneezing; throat irritated; short, dry cough; must take a deep breath. *Dyspnœa and stitches in chest,* and painful contraction of abdominal muscles. *Violent,* furious, exhausting cough, with much mucus; profuse, salty, slimy expectoration, and with *involuntary spurting of urine and sneezing. Child rubs face with fist during cough.* [*Caust.; Puls.*] Cough provoked by taking a deep breath or cold drinks, from exertion, change from warm to cold air. Cough of measles. Frequent calls to urinate at night, passing large quantities. [*Phos. ac.*] *Sneezing with coughing.*

Heart.—A cardiac stimulant affecting the peripheral vessels and coronary arteries.

Urinary.—Great urging; *much watery urine. Involuntary* spurting of urine when coughing. [*Caustic; Puls.*]

Skin.—Small, red spots over body, with prickling pain.

Extremities.—Icy cold hands and feet, with warmth of the rest of the body. [*Menyanthes.*] Feet get sore from standing. Tender feet with shop girls.

Modalities.—*Better,* rest; *worse,* motion.

Relationship.—Compare: *Digit.; Strophant.; Apocyn. can.; Bry.; Kali carb.* Squilla follows *Digitalis,* if this fails to relieve water-logged cases.

Dose.—First to third potency.

STANNUM
(Tin)

Chief action is centered upon the nervous system and respiratory organs. Debility is very marked when Stannum is the remedy, especially the debility of chronic bronchial and pulmonary conditions, characterized by profuse muco-purulent discharges upon tuberculosis basis. *Talking causes a very weak feeling in the throat and chest. Pains that come and go gradually,* call unmistakably for Stannum. Paralytic weakness; spasms; paralysis.

Mind.—Sad, anxious. *Discouraged.* Dread of seeing people.

Head.—Aching in temples and forehead. Obstinate acute coryza and influenza with cough. Pain worse motion; *gradually increasing and decreasing* as if constricted by a band; forehead feels pressed inwards. Jarring of walking resounds painfully in head. Drawing pains in malar bones and orbits. Ulceration of ringhole in lobe of ear.

Throat.—Much adhesive mucus, difficult to detach; efforts to detach cause nausea. Throat dry and stings.

Stomach.—Hunger. *Smell of cooking causes vomiting.* Bitter taste. Pain better pressure, but sore to touch. Sensation of *emptiness in stomach.*

Abdomen.—Cramp-like colic around navel, with a feeling of emptiness. *Colic relieved by hard pressure.*

Female.—*Bearing-down sensation.* Prolapsus, with *weak, sinking feeling in stomach.* [*Sep.*] *Menses early and profuse.* Pain in vagina, upward and back to spine. Leucorrhœa, with great debility.

Respiratory.—Hoarse; mucus expelled by forcible cough. Violent, dry cough in evening until midnight. Cough excited by *laughing,* singing, talking; worse lying on right side. During day, with *copious green, sweetish,* expectoration. Chest feels sore. *Chest feels weak;* can hardly talk. Influenzal cough from noon to midnight with scanty expectoration. Respiration short, oppressive; stitches in left side when breathing and lying on same side. *Phthisis mucosa. Hectic fever.*

Sleep.—Sleeps with one leg drawn up, the other stretched out.

Extremities.—Paralytic weakness; drops things. Ankles swollen. Limbs suddenly *give out when attempting to sit down.* Dizziness and weakness *when descending.* Spasmodic twitching of muscles of forearm and hand. Fingers jerk when holding pen. Neuritis. Typewriters' paralysis.

Fever.—Heat in evening; *exhausting night-sweats,* especially towards morning. Hectic. Perspiration, principally on forehead and nape of neck; debilitating; smelling musty, or offensive.

Modalities.—*Worse,* using voice (*i. e.,* laughing, talking, singing), lying on right side, warm drinks. *Better,* coughing or expectorating, hard pressure.

Relationship.—Complementary: *Puls.*

Compare: *Stann. iod.* 3x. (Valuable in chronic chest diseases characterized by plastic tissue changes. Persistent inclination to cough, excited by tickling dry spot in the throat, apparently at root of tongue. Dryness of throat. Trachial and bronchial irritation of smokers. Pulmonary symptoms; cough, loud, hollow, ending with expectoration. [Phellandrium.] State of purulent infiltration. *Advanced* phthisis sometimes when Stann. jod has not taken effect, an additional dose of Iodine in milk caused the drug to have its usual beneficial effect. (Stonham.) Compare: *Caust.; Calc.; Sil.; Tuberc.; Bacil.; Helon. Myrtus chekan* (chronic bronchitis, cough of phthisis, emphysema, with gastric catarrhal complications and thick, yellow difficult sputum. Old persons with weakened power of expectoration.)

Dose.—Third to thirtieth potency.

STAPHYSAGRIA
(Stavesacre)

Nervous affections with marked irritability, diseases of the genito-urinary tract and skin, most frequently give symptoms calling for this drug. Acts on teeth and alveolar periosteum. Ill effects of anger and insults. *Sexual sins and excesses. Very sensitive.* Lacerated tissues. Pain and nervousness after extraction of teeth. Sphincters lacerated or stretched.

Mind.—Impetuous, *violent outbursts of passion*, hypochondriacal, sad. *Very sensitive* as to what others say about her. Dwells on sexual matters; prefers solitude. Peevish. Child cries for many things, and refuses them when offered.

Head.—Stupefying headache; passes off with yawning. Brain feels squeezed. Sensation of a ball of lead in forehead. Itching eruption above and behind ears. [*Oleand.*]

Eyes.—Heat in eyeballs, dims spectacles. *Recurrent styes. Chalazœ.* [*Platanus.*] Eyes sunken, with blue rings. Margin of lids itch. Affections of angles of eye, particularly the inner. Lacerated or incised wounds of cornea. Bursting pain in eyeballs of syphilitic iritis.

Throat.—*Stitches flying to the ear on swallowing, especially left.*

Mouth.—Toothache during menses. *Teeth black and crumbling.* Salivation, spongy gums, bleed easily. [*Merc.; Kreos.*] Submaxillary glands swollen. After eating feels sleepy. Pyorrhœa. [*Plantago.*]

Stomach.—Flabby and weak. Desire for stimulants. Stomach feels relaxed. *Craving for tobacco.* Canine hunger, even when stomach is full. Nausea after abdominal operations.

Abdomen.—Colic after anger. Hot flatus. Swollen abdomen in children, with much flatus. Colic, with pelvic tenesmus. *Severe pain following an abdominal operation.* Incarcerated flatus. Diarrhœa after drinking cold water, with tenesmus. *Constipation* (2 drops tincture night and morning), hæmorrhoids, with enlarged prostate.

Male.—Especially after self-abuse; persistent dwelling on sexual subjects. Spermatorrhœa, with sunken features; guilty look; emissions, with backache and weakness and sexual neurasthenia. Dyspnœa after coition.

Female.—*Parts very sensitive,* worse sitting down. [*Berb.; Kreos.*] *Irritable bladder in young married women.* Leucorrhœa. Prolapsus, with sinking in the abdomen; aching around the hips.

Urinary.—*Cystocele* (locally and internally). Cystitis in lying-in patients. Ineffectual urging to urinate in *newly married* women. Pressure upon bladder; feels as if it did not empty. *Sensation as if a drop of urine were rolling continuously along the channel.* Burning in urethra during micturition. Prostatic troubles; frequent urination, burning in urethra *when not urinating.* [*Thuja; Sabal; Ferr. pic.*] Urging and pain *after* urinating. Pain after lithotomy.

Skin.—Eczema of head, ears, face, and body; thick scabs, dry, and itch violently; *scratching changes location of itching.* Fig-warts pedunculated. [*Thuja.*] Arthritic nodes. Inflammation of phalanges. Night-sweats.

Extremities.—Muscles, especially of calves, feel bruised. *Backache; worse in morning before rising.* Extremities feel beaten and painful. Joints stiff. *Crural neuralgia.* Dull aching of nates extending to hip-joint and small of back.

Modalities.—Worse, anger, indignation, grief, mortification, loss of fluids, onanism, sexual excesses, tobacco; least touch on affected parts. *Better,* after breakfast, warmth, rest at night.

Relationship.—Inimical: *Ranunc. bulb.*

Complementary: *Caust.; Colocy.*

Compare: *Ferrum pyrophos.* (tarsal cysts); *Colocy.; Caust.; Ign.; Phos. ac.; Calad.*

Antidote: *Camph.*

Dose.—Third to thirtieth potency.

STELLARIA MEDIA
(Chickweed)

Induces a condition of stasis, congestion, and sluggishness of all functions. Morning aggravation.

Sharp, *shifting*, rheumatic pains in all parts very pronounced. *Rheumatism;* darting pains in almost every part; stiffness of joints; parts sore to touch; worse, motion. *Chronic rheumatism. Shifting pains.* [*Puls.; Kali sulph.*] Psoriasis. Enlarged and inflamed gouty finger joints.

Head.—General irritability. Lassitude, indisposition to work. Smarting and burning in eyes, feel protruded. Dull, frontal headache; worse in morning and left side with sleepiness. Neck muscles stiff and sore. Eyes feel protruded.

Abdomen.—*Liver engorged, swollen, with stitching pain and sensitive to pressure.* Clay-colored stools. Hepatic torpor. Constipation or alternating constipation and diarrhœa.

Extremities.—Rheumatoid pains in different parts of the body. Sharp pain in small of back, over kidneys, in gluteal region, extending down thigh. Pain in shoulders and arms. *Synovitis.* Bruised feeling. Rheumatic pains in calves of legs.

Modalities.—*Worse*, mornings, warmth, tobacco. *Better*, evenings, cold air, motion.

Relationship.—Compare: *Pulsat.* (similar in rheumatism, pains shifting, worse rest, warmth; better cold air).

Dose.—Tincture, externally. Internally, 2x potency.

STERCULIA
(Kola-nut)

Neurasthenia. Regulates the circulation, is tonic and anti-diarrhœic, regulates cardiac rhythm and acts diuretically. Weak heart.

The remedy for the drinking habit. It promotes the appetite and digestion, and lessens the craving for liquor. *Asthma.* Gives power to endure prolonged physical exertion without taking food and without feeling fatigued.

Relationship.—*Coca.*

Dose.—Three to ten drops, even one dram doses, three times a day.

STICTA
(Lungwort)

Offers a set of symptoms like coryza, bronchial catarrh and influenza, together with nervous and *rheumatic* disturbances. There is a general feeling of dullness and malaise, as when a cold is coming on; dull, heavy pressure in forehead, catarrhal conjunctivitis, etc. *Rheumatic stiffness of neck.*

Mind.—*Feels as if floating in air.* [*Datura arborea.; Lac. Can.*] Confusion of ideas; *patient must talk.*

Head.—Dull headache, with dull heavy pressure in forehead and *root of nose. Catarrhal headache before discharge appears.* Burning in eyes and soreness of balls. Sensation as if scalp were too small. Burning in eyelids.

Nose.—*Feeling of fullness at the root of the nose.* [*Nux.*] Atrophic rhinitis. [*Calc. fluor.*] *Dryness of nasal membrane. Constant need to blow the nose, but no discharge.* Dry scabs, especially in evening and night. *Hay-fever;* incessant sneezing. [*Sabad.*]

Female.—Scanty flow of milk.

Abdomen.—Diarrhœa; stools profuse, frothy; worse, morning. Urine increased, with soreness and aching in bladder.

Respiratory.—Throat raw; dropping of mucus posteriorly. *Dry, hacking cough during night; worse, inspiration.* Tracheitis, facilitates expectoration. Loose cough in morning. Pain through chest from sternum to spinal column. Cough after measles [*Sang.*]; *worse towards evening and when tired. Pulsation from right side of sternum down to abdomen.*

Extremities.—Rheumatic pain in right shoulder joint, deltoid, and biceps. Swelling, heat, redness of joints. *Spot of inflammation and redness over affected joint.* Pain severe and drawing. Chorea-like spasms; legs feel floating in air. *Housemaid's knee.* [*Rhus; Kali hyd.; Slag.*] Shooting pains in knees. Joints and neighboring muscles red, swollen, painful. Rheumatic pains precede catarrhal symptoms.

Modalities.—*Worse,* sudden changes of temperature.

Relationship.—Compare: *Datura arborea—Bougmancia candida* (cannot concentrate thoughts; brain floats in thousands of problems and grand ideas. Floating sensation as if ideas were floating outside of brain. Headache, heartburn. Burning sensation around cardiac end of stomach, extending to œsophagus with sense of constriction. Heat and fullness over liver region.) *Cetraria*—Iceland Moss (chronic diarrhœa, phthisis, bloody expectoration. Is used as a decoction and boiled with milk as an expectorant and nutrient in bronchorrhœa, catarrh, etc.) Also compare: *Eryng.; Dros.; Stilling.; Rumex; Sambuc.*

Dose.—Tincture, to sixth potency.

STIGMATA MAYDIS—ZEA
(Corn-silk)

Has marked urinary symptoms, and has been used with success in organic heart disease, with much œdema of lower extremities and scanty urination. Enlarged prostate and retention of urine. Uric and phosphatic Gonorrhœa. Cystitis.

Urinary.—Suppression and *retention*. Dysuria. Renal lithiasis; nephritic colic; blood and red sand in urine. Tenesmus after urinating. Vesical catarrh. Gonorrhœa. Cystitis.

Shucks (as a decoction used for chronic malaria, teaspoonful doses freely. Dr. E. C. Lowe, England).

Dose.—Tincture in ten-to fifty-drop doses.

STILLINGIA
(Queen's Root)

Chronic periosteal rheumatism, syphilitic and scrofulous affections. Respiratory symptoms well marked. Torpor of lymphatics; torpid liver, with jaundice and constipation.

Mind.—*Gloomy forebodings;* depressed.

Respiratory.—Dry, spasmodic cough. Larynx constricted, with stinging in fauces. Trachea feels sore when pressed. *Hoarseness* and chronic laryngeal affections of public speakers.

Urinary.—Urine colorless. *Deposits white sediment;* urine milky and thick.

Extremities.—Aching pains in *bones* of extremities and back

Skin.—Ulcers; chronic eruptions on hands and fingers. *Enlarged cervical glands*. Burning, itching of legs; worse, exposure to air. Exostosis. Scrofuloderma; syphilis, secondary eruption and later symptoms. Valuable for intercurrent use.

Modalities.—*Worse*, in afternoons, damp air, motion. *Better*, in morning, dry air.

Relationship.—Compare: *Staphis.; Mercur.; Syphil.; Aur.; Corydalis* (syphilitic nodes).

Dose.—Tincture and first potency.

STRAMONIUM
(Thorn-apple)

The entire force of this drug seems to be expended on the brain, though the skin and throat show some disturbance. Suppressed secretions and excretions. Sensation as if limbs were separated from body. Delirium tremens. Absence of pain and muscular mobility especially of muscles of expression and of locomotion. Gyratory and graceful motions. Parkinsonism.

Mind.—*Devout, earnest, beseeching and ceaseless talking.* Loquacious, garrulous, laughing, singing, swearing, praying, rhyming. Sees ghosts, hears voices, talks with spirits. Rapid changes from joy to sadness. Violent and lewd. Delusions about his identity; thinks himself tall, double, a part missing. Religious mania. Cannot bear solitude or darkness; *must have light and company.* Sight of water or anything glittering brings on spasms. Delirium, with desire to escape. [*Bell.; Bry.; Rhus.*]

Head.—*Raises head frequently from the pillow.* Pain in forehead and over eyebrows, beginning at 9 a. m.; worse until noon. Boring pain, preceded by obscure vision. Rush of blood to head; staggers, with tendency to fall forward and to the left. Auditory hallucinations.

Eyes.—Seem prominent, *staring wide open;* pupils dilated. Loss of vision; complains that it is dark, *and calls for light. Small objects look large.* Parts of the body seem enormously swollen. Strabismus. All objects look black.

Face.—Hot, red; circumscribed redness of cheeks. Blood rushes to face; distorted. *Expression of terror.* Pale face.

Mouth.—Dry; dribbling of viscid saliva. Aversion to water. *Stammering.* Risus sardonicus. Cannot swallow on account of spasm. Chewing motion.

Stomach.—Food tastes like straw. Violent thirst. Vomiting of mucus and *green* bile.

Urine.—*Suppression*, bladder empty.

Male.—*Sexual erethism*, with indecent speech and action. Hands constantly kept on genitals.

Female.—*Metrorrhagia*, with *loquacity*, *singing*, praying. Puerperal mania, with characteristic mental symptoms and profuse sweatings. Convulsions after labor.

Sleep.—Awakens terrified; screams with fright. Deep snoring sleep. Sleepy, but cannot sleep. [*Bell.*]

Extremities.—*Graceful, rhythmic motions.* Convulsions of upper extremities and of isolated groups of muscles. *Chorea;* spasms partial, constantly changing. *Violent pain in left hip.* Trembling, twitching of tendons, staggering gait.

Skin.—Shining red flash. *Effects of suppressed eruption in scarlatina*, with delirium, etc.

Fever.—Profuse sweat, which does not relieve. Violent fever.

Modalities.—*Worse*, in dark room, when alone, looking at bright or shining objects, after sleep, on swallowing. *Better*, from bright light, company, warmth.

Relationship.—Compare especially: *Hyoscy.* and *Bellad.* It has less fever than *Bellad.*, but more than *Hyos.* It causes more functional excitement of the brain, but never approaches the true inflammatory condition of *Bellad.*

Antidotes: *Bellad.; Tabac.; Nux.*

Dose.—Thirtieth potency and lower.

STRONTIA

(Carbonate of Strontia)

Rheumatic pains, chronic sprains, stenosis of œsophagus. Pains make patient faint or sick all over. Chronic *sequelæ of hæmorrhages*, after operations with much cozing of blood and coldness and prostration. Arterio-sclerosis. High blood pressure with flushed face pulsating arteries, threatened apoplexy. Violent involuntary starts. Affections of bones, especially femur. Restlessness at night, smothering feeling. *For shock after surgical operations. Neuritis*, great sensitiveness to cold.

Head.—*Vertigo with headache and nausea.* Distensive pressure. Aches from nape of neck, spreading upwards; better wrapping head up warmly. [*Sil.*] Flushes in face; violent pulsating. Supraorbital neuralgia; pains increase and decrease slowly. [*Stann.*] Bloody crusts in nose. Face red; burns, itches. Itching, redness and burning of nose.

Eyes.—Burning and redness of eyes. Pain and lachrymation on using eyes, with dancing and chromatic alterations of objects looked at.

Stomach.—Loss of appetite, aversion to meat, craves bread and beer. Food tasteless. Eructations after eating. Hiccough causes chest pains; cardialgia.

Abdomen.—Sticking in abdominal ring. Diarrhœa; *worse at night; continuous urging;* better towards morning. Burning in anus lasts a long time after stool. [*Ratanh.*] Uncomfortable fullness and swelling of abdomen.

Extremities.—Sciatica with œdema of ankle. Rheumatic pain in right shoulder. Rheumatism with diarrhœa. Gnawing as if in marrow of bones. Cramps in calves and soles. *Chronic spasms, particularly of ankle-joint.* Œdematous swelling. Icy-cold feet. Rheumatic pains, especially in joints. Veins of hands engorged.

Fever.—Heat, with aversion to uncover or undress.

Skin.—Moist, itching, burning eruption; better in open air, especially warm sunshine. *Sprains of ankle-joint, with œdema.* Violent perspiration at night.

Modalities.—*Better* immersing in *hot water; worse,* change of weather; from being quiet; when beginning to move; great sensitiveness to cold.

Relationship.—Compare: *Arnica; Ruta; Sil.; Baryta c.; Carbo.; Stront. jodat.* (arterio-sclerosis.) *Strontium brom.* (often gives excellent results where a bromide is indicated. Vomiting of pregnancy. Nervous dyspepsia. It is anti-fermentative and neutralizes excessive acidity.) *Stront. nit.* (Morbid cravings; headache and eczema behind ears.)

Dose.—Sixth trituration and thirtieth potency.

STROPHANTHUS HISPIDUS
(Kombe-seed)

Strophanthus is a muscle poison; it increases the contractile power of all striped muscles. Acts on the heart, *increasing the systole and diminishes the rapidity.* May be used with advantage to tone the heart, and run off dropsical accumulations. In small doses for weak heart; it feels enlarged. In mitral regurgitation, where œdema and dropsy have supervened. [*Digit.*] Strophantus occasions no gastric distress, has no cumulative effects, is a greater diuretic, and is safer for the aged, as it does not affect the vaso-motors. In pneumonia and in severe prostration from hæmorrhage after operations and acute diseases. After the long use of stimulants; *irritable heart* of tabacco-smokers. Arterio-sclerosis; rigid arteries of aged. Restores tone to a *brittle* tissue, especially of the heart muscle and valves. Especially useful in failing compensation dependent upon fatty heart. *Hives.* Anæmia with palpitation and breathlessness. Exophthalmia goitre. Corpulent persons.

Head.—Temporal pains with double vision, impaired sight; brilliant eyes, flushed face. Senile vertigo.

Stomach.—Nausea with special disgust for alcohol and so aids in treatment of dipsomania. Seven drops of tincture.

Urinary.—Increased secretion; scanty and albuminous.

Female.—Menorrhagia; uterine hæmorrhage; uterus heavily congested. Aching pain through hips and thighs during climacteric.

Respiratory.—*Dyspnœa,* especially on ascending. Lungs congested. Œdema of lungs. Bronchial and cardiac asthma.

Heart.—Pulse quickened. Heart's action weak, rapid, irregular, due to muscular *debility;* and *insufficiency.* Cardiac pain.

Skin.—Urticaria, especially more chronic forms.

Extremities.—Swollen, dropsical. Anasarca.

Relationship.—Compare: *Digit.* (but is slower than *Strophant.* in its action); *Phos. ac.* (weak heart, irregular pulse, fluttering sensation in cardiac region, palpitation during sleep, fainting).

Dose.—Tincture and 6x potency. In more acute cases, five to ten drops of the tincture three times a day.

STRYCHNINUM

(Alkaloid of Nux Vomica)

Its primary function is to stimulate the motor centers and the reflex action of the spinal cord. Homœopathic to spasms of muscles, cramps from an undue reflex excitability of the cord, spasms of the bladder, etc. Strychnin stimulates the central nervous system, mental activities, special senses rendered more acute. Respiration increased. All reflexes are made more active. Stiffness in muscles and face and neck. Opisthotonos. Tetanic convulsions with opisthotonos. The muscles relax between paroxysms; worse slightest touch, sound, odor. Influences more directly the spinal cord and is less appropriate in visceral derangements than Nux. *Tetanus*. Explosive nervousness. The pains and sensations come *suddenly* and return at *intervals*.

Head.—Restless. *Over-irritability*. Full and bursting headache, with heat in eyes. Vertigo, with roaring in ears. Jerking of head forwards. Scalp sore. Itching of scalp and nape.

Eyes.—Hot, painful, protruding, staring. Pupils dilated. Sparks before eyes. Spasmodic contraction of ocular muscles; twitching and trembling of lids.

Ears.—Hearing very acute; burning, itching, and roaring in ears.

Face.—Pale, anxious, livid. Jaws stiffened; lower jaw spasmodically closed.

Throat.—Dry, contracted; feeling of a lump. Deglutition impossible. Burning along and spasms of œsophagus. Violent itching in roof of mouth.

Stomach.—Constant retching. Violent vomiting. Nausea of pregnancy.

Abdomen.—Sharp pain in abdominal muscles, griping pain in bowels.

Rectum.—Fæces discharged involuntarily during spasms. Very obstinate constipation.

Female.—Desire for coitus. [*Canth.; Camph.; Fl. ac.; Lach.; Phos.; Plat.*] Any touch on body excites a voluptuous sensation.

Respiratory.—*Spasm of muscles* about larynx. Excessive

dyspnœa. Sharp, contractive pains in muscles of chest. Persistent cough, recurring after influenza.

Back.—*Rigidity of cervical muscles.* Sharp pain in nape and down spine. *Back stiff;* violent jerks in spinal column. *Icy sensation down spine.*

Extremities.—Limbs stiff. Rheumatism with stiff joints. *Violent jerking, twitching, and trembling.* Tetanic convulsions and opisthotonos; spasms provoked by slightest touch and attempt to move. Shocks in the muscles. *Cramp-like pains.*

Fever.—Cold chills down spine. Perspiration in a stream down head and chest. Lower extremities cold.

Skin.—Itching of whole body, especially nose. Icy sensation down the spine.

Modalities.—*Worse,* morning; touch; noise; motion; after meals. *Better,* lying on back.

Relationship.—Compare: *Eucalyptus* (neutralizes ill effects of *Strychnin*). *Strych. ars.* (Paresis in the aged, relaxed musculature. Prostration. Psoriasis; chronic diarrhœa with paralytic symptoms: compensatory hypertrophy of heart with beginning fatty degeneration; marked dyspnœa when lying down; œdema of lower extremities, urine scanty, high specific gravity, heavily loaded with glucose. Diabetes. 6x trit.). *Strych. et Ferr. cit.* (chlorotic and paralytic conditions; dyspepsia, with vomiting of ingesta; 2x and 3x trit.); *Strychnin. nit.* (2x and 3x. Said to remove craving for alcohol. Use for two weeks); *Strychnin. sulph.* (Gastric atony); *Strych. valerin.* (exhaustion of brain-power; women of high nervous erethism; 2x trit.). Compare: *Cicuta; Arnica* (tetanus).

Dose.—Third to thirtieth potency. For non-homœopathic use, to produce its direct physiological effects in paralysis the dose will range from one-fiftieth to one-twentieth of a grain, repeated three times a day. Under twelve years of age, one-fiftieth to one two-hundredth of a grain. *Strych.,* hypodermically, is capable of arresting progressive muscular atrophy, and is a certain stimulant to the respiratory centers, and is useful in embarrassed breathing, in the course of pneumonia especially. Is an antidote to Chloral, used in asphyxia from gas and chloroform and early stages of Opium poisoning. Dose, one one-hunddredth to one-sixtieth grain every three hours.

STRYCHNIA PHOSPHORICA
(Phosphate of Strychnin)

This drug acts through the cerebro-spinal system upon muscles, causing twitching, stiffness, weakness and loss of power; upon circulation, producing irregularity of pulse, and upon the mind, producing lack of control, *uncontrollable desire to laugh* and disinclination to use the brain. Very irregular pulse. Tachycardia. Rapid and weak pulse. Useful in chorea, hysteria, acute asthenia after acute fevers. Symptoms *worse* motion, *better* rest and in open air. An excellent remedy in anæmia of spinal cord; paralysis; burning, aching, and weakness of spine; pain extends to front of chest; tenderness on pressure in mid-dorsal region; cold, clammy feet; *hands and axillæ covered with clammy perspiration.* Atelectasis and break in the compensation of a hypertrophied heart; the beginning of fatty degeneration of the heart muscle. (Royal.)

Dose.—Third trituration.

SUCCINUM
(Electron. Amber)—(A Fossil Resin)

Nervous and hysterical symptoms. Asthma. Affections of spleen.

Head.—Fear of trains and close places. Headache, lachrymation, sneezing.

Respiratory.—Asthma, incipient phthisis, chronic bronchitis, pains in chest. Whooping-cough.

Relationship.—Compare: Do not confound with Ambergris (Ambra). *Succinic acid.* (Hay-fever. Paroxysmal sneezing, dropping of watery mucus from nostrils; asthma. Inflammation through respiratory tract; causing asthma, chest pains, etc.; itching of eyelids and canthi and nose worse drafts. Use 6 to 30th potency). Compare: *Arundo, Wyethia, Sabadilla, Sinapis.*

Dose.—Third trituration. Five drop doses of the oil.

SULFONAL
(A Coal-tar Product)

Vertigo of cerebral origin, cerebellar disease, ataxic symptoms, and chorea, present a field for the homœopathic employment of this drug. *Profound weakness*, gone, faint feeling, and despondency. Loss of control of sphincter. Muscular inco-ordination.

Mind.—Mental confusion, incoherency, illusions; apathetic. *Alternation of happy, hopeful states with depression and weakness.* Extreme irritability.

Head.—Dropsy, stupid; pain on attempting to raise head. Double vision; heavy look about eyes; tinnitus, aphasia; *tongue as if paralyzed. Eyes bloodshot and restless.* Vertigo, unable to rise. Double vision; ptosis; tinnitus; dysphagia, difficult speech.

Urinary.—Albuminuria, with casts. Scanty. Pink color. Constant desire to urinate; scanty, brownish red. Hæmatoporphyrinuria.

Respiratory.—Congestion of lungs; stertorous breathing. Sighing dyspnœa.

Extremities.—Ataxic movements, *staggering gait;* cold, weak, trembling; legs seem too heavy. Extreme restlessness; muscular twitchings. Knee-jerks disappear. Stiffness and paralysis of both legs. Anæsthesia of legs.

Sleep.—Fidgety, wakeful, drowsy. Insomnia.

Skin.—Itching, bluish purpura. Erythema.

Relationship.—*Trional;* insomnia associated with physical excitement; (vertigo, loss of equilibrium, ataxia, nausea, vomiting, diarrhœa, stertorous breathing, cyanosis, tinnitus, hallucinations).

Dose.—Third trituration.

Non-Homœopathic Uses.—As a hypnotic. Dose, ten to thirty grains in hot water. Takes about two hours to act.

SULPHUR
(Sublimated Sulphur)

This is the great Hahnemannian anti-psoric. Its action is centrifugal—from within outward—having an elective affinity for the skin, where it produces heat and *burning*, with itching; made worse by heat of bed. Inertia and relaxation of fiber; hence feebleness of tone characterizes its symptoms. *Ebullitions of heat, dislike of water, dry and hard hair and skin, red orifices, sinking feeling at stomach about* 11 a. m., *and cat-nap sleep;* always indicate Sulphur homœopathically. *Standing* is the worst position for sulphur patients, it is always uncomfortable. Dirty, filthy people, prone to skin affections. Aversion to being washed. *When carefully-selected remedies fail to act, especially in acute diseases,* it frequently arouses the reactionary powers of the organism. *Complaints that relapse. General offensive character of discharge and exhalations.* Very red lips and face, flushing easily. Often great use in beginning the treatment of chronic cases and in finishing acute ones.

Mind.—Very forgetful. Difficult thinking. Delusions; thinks rags beautiful things—that he is immensely wealthy. Busy all the time. Childish peevishness in grown people. Irritable. Affections vitiated; *very selfish,* no regard for others. Religious melancholy. Averse to business; loafs—too lazy to arouse himself. Imagining giving wrong things to people, causing their death. Sulphur subjects are nearly always irritable, depressed, thin and weak, even with good appetite.

Head.—Constant *heat on top of head.* [*Cup. sulph.; Graph.*? Heaviness and fullness, pressure in temples. Beating headache; worse, stooping, and with vertigo. Sick headache recurring periodically. Tinea capitis, dry form. *Scalp dry,* falling of hair; worse, washing. *Itching; scratching causes burning.*

Eyes.—*Burning* ulceration of margin of lids. Halo around lamp-light. Heat and *burning in eyes.* [*Ars.; Bell.*] Black motes before eyes. First stage of ulceration of cornea. Chronic ophthalmia, with much burning and itching. Parenchymatous keratitis. Cornea like ground glass.

Ears.—Whizzing in ears. Bad effects from the suppression of an otorrhœa. Oversensitive to odors. Deafness, preceded by exceedingly sensitive hearing; catarrhal deafness.

Nose.—Herpes across the nose. Nose stuffed indoors. Imaginary foul smells. *Alæ red and scabby. Chronic dry catarrh; dry scabs and readily bleeding.* Polypus and adenoids.

Mouth.—Lips dry, *bright red*, burning. *Bitter taste* in morning. Jerks through teeth. Swelling of gums; throbbing pain. Tongue white, with red tip and borders.

Throat.—Pressure as from a lump, as from a splinter, as of a hair. Burning, redness and dryness. Ball seems to rise and close pharynx.

Stomach.—Complete loss of, or excessive appetite. Putrid eructation. Food tastes too salty. Drinks much, eats little. *Milk disagrees.* Great desire for sweets. [*Arg. nit.*] *Great acidity*, sour eructation. Burning, painful, weight-like pressure. *Very weak and faint about* 11 a. m.; must have something to eat. Nausea during gestation. Water fills the patient up.

Abdomen.—Very sensitive to pressure; internal feeling of rawness and soreness. Movements as of something alive. [*Croc.; Thuj.*] Pain and soreness over liver. Colic after drinking.

Rectum.—Itching and burning of anus; piles dependent upon abdominal plethora. Frequent, unsuccessful desire; hard, knotty, insufficient. Child afraid on account of pain. *Redness around the anus*, with itching. *Morning diarrhœa, painless, drives out of bed*, with prolapsus recti. Hæmorrhoids, oozing and belching.

Urine.—Frequent micturition, especially at night. *Enuresis*, especially in scrofulous, untidy children. Burning in urethra during micturition, lasts long after. Mucus and pus in urine; *parts sore over which it passes. Must hurry*, sudden call to urinate. *Great quantities of colorless urine.*

Male.—Stitches in penis. Involuntary emissions. Itching of genitals when going to bed. Organs cold, relaxed and powerless.

Female.—Pudenda *itches. Vagina burns.* Much offensive perspiration. Menses too late, short, scanty, and difficult; thick, black, *acrid, making parts sore.* Menses preceded by headache or suddenly stopped. Leucorrhœa, burning, excoriating. Nipples cracked; smart and burn.

Respiratory.—Oppression and burning sensation in chest. *Difficult respiration; wants windows open.* Aphonia. Heat, throughout chest. Red, brown spots all over chest. Loose cough; worse talking, morning, greenish, purulent, sweetish expectoration. *Much rattling of mucus.* Chest feels heavy; stitches, with heart feeling too large and palpitating. *Pleuritic exudations.* Use Tinctura sulphuris. Stitching pains shooting through to the back, worse lying on back or breathing deeply. Flushes of heat in chest rising to head. *Oppression, as of a load on chest. Dyspnœa* in middle of night, relieved by sitting up. *Pulse more rapid in morning* than in evening.

Back.—Drawing pain between shoulders. Stiffness of nape. Sensation as if vertebræ glided over each other

Extremities.—Trembling of hands. *Hot, sweaty hands.* Rheumatic pain in left shoulder. Heaviness; paretic feeling. Rheumatic gout, with itching. *Burning in soles and hands at night.* Sweat in armpits, smelling like garlic. Drawing and tearing in arms and hands. Stiffness of knees and ankles. Cannot walk erect; *stoop-shouldered.* Ganglion.

Sleep.—Talks, jerks, and twitches during sleep. Vivid dreams. Wakes up singing. Wakes frequently, and becomes wide awake suddenly. *Catnaps;* slightest noise awakens. Cannot sleep between 2 and 5 a. m.

Fever.—*Frequent flashes of heat. Violent ebullitions of heat throughout entire body.* Dry skin and great thirst. Night sweat, on nape and occiput. Perspiration of single parts. Disgusting sweats. Remittent type.

Skin.—*Dry, scaly, unhealthy; every little injury suppurates.* Freckles. *Itching, burning; worse scratching and washing.* Pimply eruption, pustules, rhagades, hang-nails. Excoriation, especially in folds. [*Lyc.*] Feeling of a band around bones. Skin affections after local medication. *Pruritus,* especially from warmth, in evening, often recurs in spring-time, in damp weather.

Modalities.—*Worse,* at rest, when standing, *warmth in bed,* washing, bathing, in morning, 11 a. m., night, from alcoholic stimulants, periodically. *Better, dry, warm weather,* lying on right side, from drawing up affected limbs.

Relationship.—Complementary: *Aloe; Psorin.; Acon.; Pyrarara* (a fish caught in the Amazon, clinically used for various skin affections). Lepra, tuberculides, syphilides, varicosities, etc.

Compare: *Acon.* (Sulph. often follows in acute diseases); *Mercur.* and *Calcarea* are frequently useful *after* Sulphur, not before. Lyc.; Sep.; Sars.; Puls.; *Sulphur hydrogenisatum* (delirium, mania, asphyxia); *Sulphur terebinthinatum* (chronic rheumatic arthritis; chorea); *Tannic acid* (Nasal hæmorrhage; elongated uvula; gargle; constipation). *Magnes. artiflcialis* (great hunger in evening, profuse sweat on face, bruised pain in joints, rectal constriction after stool).

Magnetis polus Articus (anxious, *coldness of eyes as if a piece of ice lay in orbit*, increased flow of saliva, constipation, sopor, trembling, abdominal flatulence).

Magnetis polus Australis (dryness of lids, easy dislocation of ankle, *ingrowing toe-nails*, aching in patella, shooting in soles).

Compare in adenoids: *Agraphis.*

Dose.—Acts in all potencies from the lowest to the highest. Some of the best results are obtained from the higher, and not too frequent doses. The twelfth potency is a good one to begin treatment with, going higher or lower according to the susceptibility of the patient. In chronic diseases, 200th and upward. In *torpid* eruptions the *lowest* potencies.

SULPHUR IODATUM
(Iodide of Sulphur)

Obstinate skin affections, notably in *barber's itch* and *acne*. Weeping eczema.

Throat.—Uvula and tonsils enlarged and reddened. Swollen. Tongue thick. Parotid hypertrophied.

Skin.—Itching on ears, nose, and in urethra. Papular eruption on face. Cold-sores on lips. Boils on neck. Barber's itch. *Acne*. Lichen planus. Arms covered with itching rash. Hair feels as if erect.

Dose.—Third trituration.

SULPHURICUM ACIDUM
(Sulphuric Acid)

The "debility" common to acids shows itself here, especially in the digestive tract, giving a very relaxed feeling in the stomach, with craving for stimulants. *Tremor and weakness;* everything must be done in a hurry. *Hot flushes,* followed by perspiration, with trembling. Tendency to gangrene following mechanical injuries. Writer's cramp. Lead poisoning. Gastralgia and hypochlorrhydria. Purpura hæmorrhagia.

Mind.—Fretful, impatient. Unwilling to answer questions; hurried.

Head.—Right-sided neuralgia; painful shocks; skin feels pinched. Sensation as if brain was loose in forehead and falling from side to side. [*Bell.; Rhus.*] Concussion of brain where skin is cold, body bathed in cold sweat. Compressive pain in side of occiput; *relieved by holding the hands near the head.* Pain of outer parts, as if there were subcutaneous ulceration; painful to touch. *Thrust in right temple as if plug were pressed in.*

Eyes.—Intra-ocular hæmorrhage following traumatism. Great chemosis of conjunctiva, with aching and sharp pain.

Mouth.—Aphthæ; gums bleed readily. Offensive breath. Pyorrhœa.

Stomach.—Heartburn; *sour eructations; sets teeth on edge.* [*Robin.*] *Craving for alcohol. Water causes coldness of stomach;* must be mixed with liquors. *Relaxed feeling in stomach.* Averse to smell of coffee. Sour vomiting. Desire for fresh food. *Hiccough.* Coldness of stomach relieved by applied heat. Nausea with chilliness.

Abdomen.—Weak feeling, with dragging into the hips and small of back. *Feeling as if hernia would protrude,* especially left side.

Rectum.—Piles; oozing dampness. Rectum feels as if it had a big ball. Diarrhœa, fetid, black, with sour odor of body, and empty faint feeling in abdomen.

Female.—Menstruation early and profuse. Erosion of cervix in the aged; easily bleeding. Acrid, burning leucorrhœa, often of bloody mucus.

Respiratory.—Respiration rapid with shooting in cervical muscles and movement of wings of nose; *larynx moves up and down violently.* Bronchitis in children with short, teasing cough.

Extremities.—Cramp-like paralytic contraction in arms, hands; jerking of fingers while writing.

Skin.—Bad effects from mechanical injuries, with bruises and livid skin. Ecchymosis. Petechiæ. *Purpura hæmorrhagica.* Livid, red, itching blotches. Hæmorrhage of black blood from all outlets. Cicatrices turn red and blue and become painful. Chilblains with gangrenous tendency. Carbuncles, boils and other staphylococcic and streptococcic infections.

Modalities.—*Worse,* from excess of heat or cold in forenoon and evening. *Better,* from warmth, and lying on affected side.

Relationship.—Complementary: *Puls.*

Compare: *Arn.; Calend.; Led.; Sep.; Calc.*

Dose.—Sulphuric acid mixed with three parts of alcohol, ten to fifteen drops three times daily for several weeks, has been successfully used to subdue the craving for liquor. For homœopathic purposes second to thirtieth potency.

SULPHUROSUM ACIDUM

(Sulphurous Acid. $H_2 S O_3$)

Sulphurous acid, (tonsillitis (as a spray), acne rosacea, *ulcerative stomatitis,* pityriasis versicolor).

Head.—Anxious, furious, disposed to fight. Headache better by vomiting. Ringing in ears.

Mouth.—Ulcerative inflammation of mouth. Tongue red or bluish-red. Coated.

Stomach.—Loss of appetite. Obstinate constipation.

Respiratory.—Persistent choking cough with copious expectoration. Hoarseness, constriction of chest. Difficult breathing.

Female.—Fluor albus. Debility.

Dose.—As a spray in tonsillitis. According to Ringer, ten to fifteen minims taken ten minutes before each meal will remedy pyrosis and prevent fermentation and flatulence. It also removes thrush. Homœopathically, third attenuation.

SUMBUL—FERULA SUMBUL
(Musk-root)

Has many hysterical and nervous symptoms, and is of use in neuralgic affections and anomalous, functional, cardiac disorders. *Numbness on becoming cold.* Numbness on left side. *Insomnia* of delirium tremens (fifteen drops of tincture). Sensation as if water dropped down spine. Asthma. A tissue remedy for sclerosed arteries.

Head.—Emotional and fidgety. Dull in morning, clear in evening. Mistakes in writing and adding. Comedones. Tenacious, yellow, mucus in nose.

Throat.—Choking constriction; constant swallowing. Belching of gas from stomach. Spasm of pharyngeal muscles. Tenacious mucus in throat.

Heart.—*Nervous palpitation.* Neuralgia around left breast and left hypochondriac region. *Cardiac asthma.* Aching in left arm, heavy, numb and weary. Loses breath on any exertion. Pulse irregular.

Female.—Ovarian neuralgia. *Abdomen full, distended, and painful.* Climacteric flushes.

Urinary.—*Oily pellicle on surface of urine.*

Modalities.—*Worse,* active exercise; left side.

Relationship.—Compare: *Asaf.; Mosch.*

Dose.—Tincture, to third potency. Dr. W. McGeorge advises the 2x every 3 hours for arterio-sclerosis.

SYMPHORICARPUS RACEMOSA
(Snowberry)

This drug is highly recommended for the persistent *vomiting of pregnancy.* Gastric disturbances, fickle appetite, nausea, waterbrash, bitter taste. *Constipation.* Nausea during menstruation. Nausea, *worse any motion. Averse to all food. Better,* lying on back.

Dose.—Second and third potency.

200th has proved curative.

SYMPHYTUM
(Comfrey—Knitbone)

The root contains a crystalline solid, that stimulates the growth of epithelium on ulcerated surfaces. It may be administered internally in the treatment of gastric and duodenal ulcers. Also in gastralgia, and externally in pruritus ani. Injuries to sinews, tendons and the periosteum. Acts on joints generally. Neuralgia of knee.

Of great use in wounds penetrating to perineum and bones, *and in non-union of fractures;* irritable stump after amputation, irritable bone at point of fracture. Psoas abscess. *Pricking pain* and soreness of periosteum.

Head.—Pain in occiput, top and forehead; changing places. Pain comes down bone of nose. Inflammation of inferior maxillary bone, hard, red, swelling.

Eye.—*Pain in eye after a blow of an obtuse body.* For traumatic injuries of the eyes no remedy equals this.

Relationship.—Compare: *Arn.; Calc. phos.*

Dose.—Tincture.

Externally as a dressing for sores and ulcers and pruritus ani.

SYPHILINUM
(The Syphilitic Virus—A Nosode)

[Utter prostration and debility in the morning.

Shifting rheumatic pains. Chronic eruptions and rheumatism.

Ichthyosis. Syphilitic affections. Pains from darkness to daylight; decrease and increase gradually. Hereditary tendency to alcoholism. *Ulceration of* mouth, nose, genitals, skin. *Succession of abscesses.*

Mind.—Loss of memory; remembers everything previous to his illness. Apathetic; *feels as if going insane or being paralyzed. Fears the night,* and the suffering from exhaustion on awakening. Hopeless; *despairs of recovery.*

Head.—Linear pains from temple across, or from eyes backward; cause sleeplessness and delirium at night. *Falling of the hair.* Pain in bones ot head. Top of head feels as if coming off. Stupefying cephalalgia.

Eyes.—*Chronic, recurrent, phlyctenular inflammation of cornea;* successive crops of phyctenules and abrasions of epithelial layer of cornea; photophobia intense, lachrymation profuse. Lids swollen; *pain intense at night;* ptosis. Tubercular iritis. Diplopia; one image seen below the other. Feeling of cold air blowing on eye. [*Fluor. ac.*]

Ears.—Caries of ossicles in ear of syphilitic origin.

Nose.—Caries of nasal bones, hard palate and septum, with perforation; ozæna.

Mouth.—Teeth decay at gum; edges serrated, dwarfed. Tongue coated, teeth-indented; deep longitudinal cracks. Ulcers smart and burn. *Excessive flow of saliva; it runs out of mouth when sleeping.*

Stomach.—*Craves alcohol.*

Rectum.—Feels tied up with strictures. Enemas very painful. Fissures, prolapse.

Extremities.—Sciatica; worse at night; better about daybreak. Rheumatism of shoulder-joint, at insertion of deltoid. Run-around. Severe pain in long bones. Redness and rawness between toes. [*Sil.*] Rheumatism, muscles are caked in hard knot or lumps. *Always washing the hands.* Indolent ulcers. Muscles contracted in hard knots.

Female.—Ulcers on labia. Leucorrhœa *profuse, thin, watery, acrid,* with sharp, knife-pain in ovaries.

Respiratory.—Aphonia; chronic asthma in summer, wheezing and rattling. [*Tart. emet.*] Cough dry, hard; worse at night; windpipe sensitive to touch. [*Lach.*] Lancinating pains from base of heart to apex at night.

Skin.—Reddish-brown eruption, with a disagreeable odor. Extreme emaciation.

Relationship.—Compare: *Merc.; Kal. hyd.; Nit. ac.; Aur.; Alum.*

Modalities.—*Worse,* at night, sundown to sunrise, seashore, in summer. *Better,* inland and mountains, during day, moving about slowly.

Dose.—The highest potencies only, and in infrequent doses.

SYZYGIUM JAMBOLANUM
(Jambol Seeds—Enlexing, active principle)

Has an immediate effect of increasing the blood sugar, glycosuria results.

A most useful remedy in diabetes mellitus. *No other remedy causes in so marked degree the diminution and disappearance of sugar in the urine. Prickly heat in upper part of the body;* small red pimples itch violently. Great thirst, weakness, emaciation. Very large amount of urine, specific gravity high. Old ulcers of skin. Diabetic ulceration. The seeds powdered, ten grains three times a day; also, the tincture.

Relationship.—Compare: *Insulin*—An aqueous solution of an active principle from pancreas which affects sugar metabolism. If administered at suitable intervals in diabetes mellitus, the blood sugar is maintained at a normal level and the urine remains free of sugar. Overdosage is followed by weakness and fatigue and tremulousness and profuse sweating.

TABACUM
(Tobacco)

The symptomatology of Tabacum is exceedingly well marked. The nausea, giddiness, death-like pallor, vomiting, icy coldness, and sweat, with the intermittent pulse, are all most characteristic. Has marked antiseptic qualities, antidotal to cholera germs. Complete prostration of the entire muscular system. Collapse. Gastralgia, enteralgia, *seasickness*, cholera infantum; cold, but *wants abdomen uncovered.* Vigorous peristaltic activity. diarrhœa. Produces high tension and arteriosclerosis of the coronary arteries. Should prove the most homœopathic drug for angina pectoris, with coronaritis and high tension (Cartier). Constriction of throat, chest, bladder, rectum. Pallor, breathlessness, hard-cordlike pulse.

Mind.—Sensation of excessive wretchedness. *Very despondent.* Forgetful. Discontented.

Head.—Vertigo on *opening eyes;* sick headache, with deathly nausea; periodical. Tight feeling as from a band. Sudden pain, as if struck by a hammer. Nervous deafness. Secretion from eyes, nose and mouth increased.

Eyes.—Dim sight; sees as through a veil; strabismus. *Amaurosis;* muscæ volitantes. Central scotoma. Rapid blindness without lesion, followed by venous hyperæmia and atrophy of optic nerve.

Face.—Pale, blue, pinched, sunken, collapsed, covered with cold sweat. [*Ars.; Verat.*] Freckles.

Throat.—Nasopharyngitis and tracheitis, *hemming,* morning cough, sometimes with vomiting. Hoarseness of public speakers.

Stomach.—Incessant nausea; worse, smell of tobacco smoke [*Phos.*]; vomiting on least motion, sometimes of fecal matter. *during pregnancy with much spitting. Seasickness; terrible faint, sinking feeling at pit of stcmach.* Sense of relaxation of stomach, with nausea. [*Ipec.*] Gastralgia; pain from cardiac end extending to left arm.

Abdomen.—Cold. *Wants abdomen uncovered.* It lessens the nausea and vomiting. Painful distension. Incarcerated hernia.

Rectum.—Constipation; rectum paralyzed, prolapsed. Diarrhœa, sudden, watery, with nausea and vomiting, prostration, and cold sweat; discharges look like sour milk, thick, curdled, watery. Rectal tenesmus.

Urinary.—Renal colic; violent pain along ureter, left side.

Heart.—Palpitation when lying on left side. Pulse intermits, feeble, imperceptible. Angina pectoris, pain in præcordial region. Pain radiates from center of sternum. Tachycardia. Bradycardia. *Acute dilatation* caused by shock or violent physical exertion (Royal).

Respiratory.—Difficult, violent constriction of chest. Præcordial oppression, with palpitation and pain between shoulders. Cough followed by hiccough. Cough dry, teasing, must take a swallow of cold water [*Caust.; Phos.*]. Dyspœna, with tingling down left arm when lying on left side.

Extremities.—Legs and hands icy cold; limbs tremble. Paralysis following apoplexy. [*Plumb.*] Gait shuffling, unsteady. Feebleness of arms.

Sleep.—Insomnia with dilated heart, with cold, clammy skin and anxiety.

Fever.—Chills, with *cold sweat.*

Modalities.—*Worse*, opening eyes; evening; extremes of heat and cold. *Better*, uncovering, open fresh air.

Relationship.—Compare: *Hydrobromic acid; Camph.; Verat.; Ars.* Compare: *Nicotinum* (Alternate tonic and clonic spasms, followed by general relaxation and trembling; nausea, cold sweat, and speedy collapse; head drawn back, contraction of eyelids and masseter muscles; muscles of neck and back rigid; hissing respiration from spasm of laryngeal and bronchial muscles).

Antidote: Vinegar; sour apples. *Camphor* in the physiological antagonist. *Ars.* (chewing tobacco); *Ign.;* (smoking); *Sep.* (neuralgia and dyspepsia); *Lycop.* (impotency); *Nux* (bad taste due to tobacco); *Calad.* and *Plantag.* (cause aversion to tobacco); *Phosph.* (tobacco heart, sexual weakness).

Dose.—Third to thirtieth and higher potencies.

TANACETUM VULGARE
(Tansy)

Abnormal lassitude. Nervous and tired feeling. "Half dead, half alive feeling" all over. Of use in chorea and reflex spasms (worms). Said to be a specific against effects of poison ivy.

Head.—Heavy, dull, confused. Headache with least exertion.

Mental.—Irritable, sensitive to noise. Mental fatigue, nausea and vertigo, worse in a closed room.

Ears.—Roaring and ringing; voice sounds strange; *ears seem to close up suddenly.*

Abdomen.—Pain in bowels; relieved by stool. Desire for stool immediately after eating. *Dysentery.*

Female.—Dysmenorrhœa, with bearing-down pains, tenderness, drawing in groins. Menses suppressed; later, profuse.

Respiratory.—Hurried, labored, stertorous respiration. Frothy mucus obstructs the air-passages.

Relationship.—Compare: *Cimicif.; Cina; Absinth. Nux* follows well.

Dose.—Tincture, to third potency.

TANNIC ACID
Tannin—(Digallic Acid)

Mostly used locally against excessive secretion of mucous membranes, to contract tissue and check hæmorrhage. In Osmidrosis, corrects fetor of the perspiration. Obstinate nervous coughs. Hæmaturia. Obstinate constipation. Pain in abdomen, sensitive to pressure. Intestines can be felt like cylindrical enlargements. One-half per cent solution.

Relationship.—Gallic acid q. v.

TARENTULA CUBENSIS
(Cuban Spider)

A toxæmic medicine, septic conditions. *Diphtheria.* Adapted to the most severe types of inflammation and pain, early and persistent prostration. Various forms of malignant suppuration. Purplish hue and burning, stinging pains. Bubo. It is the remedy for *pain of death; soothes the last struggles. Pruritus, especially about genitals.* Restless feet. Intermittent septic chills. Bubonic plague. As a curative and preventive remedy especially during the period of invasion.

Head.—Dizziness after heat and hot perspiration. Dull ache on top of head. Shooting pain through left eye across frontal region.

Gastric.—Stomach feels hard, sore. Loss of appetite, except for breakfast.

Back.—Itches across kidney region.

Extremities.—Hands tremble, turgid with blood.

Urinary.—Retention. Cannot hold urine on coughing.

Skin.—Red spots and pimples. Feels puffed all over. *Carbuncles,* burning, stinging pains. Purplish hue. Gangrene. Abscesses, where pain and inflammation predominate. Scirrhus of breasts. "Senile" ulcers.

Sleep.—Drowsiness. Sleep restless. Sleep prevented by harsh cough.

Relationship.—Compare: *Ars.; Pyrog.; Crotal.; Echin.; Anthrac.; Bellad.; Apis.*

Modalities.—*Better,* smoking. *Worse,* night.

Dose.—Sixth to thirtieth potency.

TARENTULA HISPANIA
(Spanish Spider)

Remarkable nervous phenomena; hysteria with chlcrosis; *chorea*, dysmenorrhœa, spinal irritability. Bladder tenesmus. *Constriction* sensations. Formication. *Extreme restlessness; must keep in constant motion even though walking aggravates.* Hysterical epilepsy. Intense sexual excitement.

Mind.—Sudden alteration of mood. Foxy. Destructive impulses; *moral relaxation.* Must constantly busy herself or walk. *Sensitive to music.* Averse to company, but wants some one present. Ungrateful, discontented. Guided by whims.

Head.—Intense pain, as if thousands of needles were pricking into brain. *Vertigo.* Wants hair brushed or head rubbed.

Male.—Sexual excitement; lasciviousness reaching almost to insanity; seminal emissions.

Heart.—Palpitation; præcordial anguish, sensation as if heart twisted and turned around.

Female.—Vulva dry and hot, with much itching. Profuse menstruation, with frequent erotic spasms. *Pruritus vulvæ; nymphomania.* Dysmenorrhœa, with very sensitive ovaries.

Extremities.—Weakness of legs; choreic movements. Numbness of legs. Multiple sclerosis, with trembling. *Twitching and jerking.* Yawning with uneasiness of legs, must move them constantly. Extraordinary contractions and movements.

Modalities.—*Worse*, motion, contact, noise. *Better*, in open air, *music*, bright colors, rubbing affected parts. *Worse*, seeing others in trouble.

Relationship.—Compare: *Agar.; Ars.; Cupr.; Mag. phos.* Antidotes: *Lach.*

Dose.—Sixth to thirtieth potency.

TARAXACUM
(Dandelion)

For gastric headaches, bilious attacks, with characteristically mapped tongue and jaundiced skin. Cancer of bladder. Flatulence. *Hysterical tympanites.*

Head.—Sensation of great heat on top of head. *Sterno-mastoid* muscle very painful to touch.

Mouth.—Mapped tongue. Tongue covered with a white film; feels raw; comes off in patches, leaving *red, sensitive spots.* Loss of appetite. Bitter taste and eructations. Salivation.

Abdomen.—Liver enlarged and indurated. Sharp stitches in left side. Sensation of bubbles bursting in bowels. Tympanites. Evacuation difficult.

Extremities.—Very restless limbs. *Neuralgia of knee; better, pressure.* Limbs painful to touch.

Fever.—Chilliness after eating, worse drinking; *finger tips cold. Bitter taste.* Heat without thirst, in face, *in toes.* Sweat on falling asleep.

Skin.—*Profuse night-sweats.*

Modalities.—*Worse,* resting, lying down, sitting. *Better,* touch.

Relationship.—Compare: *Choline,* a constituent of Taraxacum root, has given encouraging results in the treatment of cancer. Choline is closely related to *Neurin,* it is the "Cancronie" of Prof. Adamkiewicz (E. Schlegel.) *Bry.; Hydrast.; Nux. Tela aranea* (nervous asthma and sleeplessness).

Dose.—Tincture, to third potency. In cancer 1-2 drams fluid extract.

TARTARICUM ACIDUM
(Tartaric Acid)

Found in grapes, pineapple, sorrel and other fruits. It is an antiscorbutic antiseptic, stimulating the mucous and salivary secretions.

Dullness and lassitude. Great weakness, with diarrhœa, with dry and brown tongue. Pain in heels. [*Phytol.*]

Stomach.—Excessive thirst, continued vomiting burning in throat and stomach. Dyspepsia with copious secretion of mucus.

Abdomen.—Pain around umbilicus and region of loins. Stool color of coffee-grounds (worse at night), with brown and dry tongue, and dark-green vomiting.

Dose.—Third trituration. The pure acid 10-30 grains dissolved in water.

TAXUS BACCATA
(Yew)

In pustular diseases of skin and night-sweats. Also in gout and chronic rheumatism.

Head.—Supra-orbital and temporal pain on right side, with lachrymation. Pupils dilated. Face puffy and pale.

Stomach.—*Saliva hot*, acrid. Nausea. Pain in pit of stomach and region of navel. After eating, cough. Feeling of pins and needles at pit of stomach; of *emptiness*, must eat frequently (compare the coniferæ).

Skin.—Large, flat, itching pustules. Badly smelling night-sweats. Podagra. Erysipelas.

Dose.—Tincture, to third potency.

TELLURIUM
(The Metal Tellurium)

Marked skin (herpes circinatus), spinal, eye and ear symptoms. Very *sensitive back*. Pains all over body. Offensive discharges. Slow development of symptoms. [*Radium.*] Sacral and sciatic pains.

Head.—Neglectful and forgetful. Pain in left side of head and in forehead above left eye. Distortion and twitching of left facial muscles; when speaking left angle of mouth drawn upwards and to left. Fear of being touched in sensitive places. Congestion to head and nape of neck, followed by weakness and faintness in stomach. Itching of scalp; red spots.

Eyes.—Lids *thickened, inflamed*, itching. Pterygium; pustular conjunctivitis. Cataract, following ocular lesions; aids the absorption of infiltrations in iris and choroid.

Ears.—*Eczema behind ear. Catarrh of middle ear, discharge acrid, smells like fish-pickle. Itching, swelling, throbbing in meatus.* Deafness.

Nose.—Coryza, lachrymation and hoarseness; better in open air. [*Cepa.*] Obstructed; hawks salty phlegm from posterior nares.

Stomach.—Craving for apples. Empty and weak feeling. Heartburn.

Rectum.—Prutitus ani et perinei after every stool.

Back.—Pain in sacrum. *Pain from last cervical to fifth dorsal vertebra*, very sensitive; worse touch. [*Chin. s.; Phosph.*] *Sciatica;* worse right side, *coughing, straining*, and at night, with sensitive vertebral column. *Contraction of tendons in bends of knees.*

Skin.—Itching of hands and feet. Herpetic spots; *ringworm.* [*Tuberc.*] *Ring-shape lesions*, offensive odors from affected parts. Barber's itch. Stinging in skin. *Fetid exhalations.* [*Sulph.*] Offensive foot-sweat. Eczema, back of ears and occiput. Circular patches of eczema.

Modalities.—*Worse*, while at rest at night, cold weather, from friction, coughing, laughing, lying on painful side, touch.

Relationship.—Compare: *Radium; Selenium; Tetradymite* —crystals from Georgia and North Carolina containing *Bismuth, Tellurium* and *Sulphur*—(coccygodynia, ulceration of nails; pains in hands, in small spots, ankles, heels, and tendo-Achilles); *Sep.; Ars.; Rhus.*

Dose.—Sixth potency and higher. Takes long time to develop its action, which is very prolonged.

TEREBINTHINA
(Turpentine)

Has a selective affinity for *bleeding mucous surfaces.* Tympanites and urinary symptoms very marked. Inflammation of kidneys, with hæmorrhages—dark, passive, fetid. Bright's disease preceded by dropsy (Goullon). Drowsiness and strangury. Coma. *Unbroken chilblains.*

Head.—Dull pain like from a band around the head. [*Carb. ac.*] Vertigo, with vanishing of vision. Disturbed sense of equilibrium. Tired and difficult concentration of thoughts. Cold in head with sore nostrils with disposition to bleed.

Eyes.—Ciliary neuralgia over right eye. Intense pain in eye and side of head. Amblyopia from alcohol.

Ears.—Own voice sounds unnatural; humming as of a seashell, talking loudly is painful. Otalgia.

Mouth.—Tongue *dry, red sore, shining;* burning in tip, with prominent papillæ. [*Arg. n.; Bell.; Kali b.; Nux m.*] Breath cold, foul. Choking sensation in throat. Stomatitis. Dentition.

Stomach.—Nausea and vomiting; heat in epigastric region.

Abdomen.—*Enormous distention.* Diarrhœa; stools watery, greenish, fetid, bloody. Pain before flatus with and relief after stool. Hæmorrhage from bowels. Worms; lumbrici. Abdominal dropsy; pelvic peritonitis. Fainting after every stool. Entero-colitis, with hæmorrhage and ulceration of bowels.

Urinary.—*Strangury, with bloody urine.* Scanty, suppressed, *odor of violets.* Urethritis, with painful erections. [*Canthar.*] Inflamed kidneys following any acute disease. Constant tenesmus.

Female.—Intense *burning in uterine region.* Metritis; puerperal peritonitis. Metrorrhagia with burning in uterus.

Respiratory.—Difficult breathing; lungs feel distended; hæmoptysis. Bloody expectoration.

Heart.—Pulse rapid, small, thready, intermittent.

Back.—*Burning pain in region of kidneys.* Drawing in right kidney extending to hip.

Skin.—Acne. Erythema; itching pustular, vesicular eruption; urticaria. Purpura, ecchymosis, dropsies. Scarlatina. Chilblains; with excessive itching and pulsative pains. Aching soreness of the muscles.

Fever.—Heat, with violent thirst, dry tongue, profuse cold, clammy sweat. Typhoid with tympanites, hæmorrhages, stupor, delirium. Prostration.

Relationship.—Compare: *Alumen; Secale; Canth.; Nit. ac. Terebene* 1x; (chronic bronchitis and winter coughs; subacute stages of inflammation of respiratory tract. Loosens secretion, relieves tightened feeling, makes expectoration easy). *Neurotic coughs.* Huskiness of public speakers, and singers. Cystitis when urine is alkaline and offensive.)

Ononis spinosa—Rest Harrow—(Diuretic, Lithontriptic. Chronic nephritis; diuretic effects like *Juniper*; calculus nosebleed, worse washing face).

Antidote: *Phos.*

Dose.—First to sixth potency.

TEUCRIUM MARUM
(Cat-thyme)

Nasal and rectal symptoms marked. *Polypi*. Affections of children. Suitable after too much medicine has been taken. Oversensitiveness. *Desire to stretch*. A remedy of first importance in chronic nasal catarrh with atrophy; large, offensive crusts and clinkers. *Ozæna. Loss of sense of smell.*

Head.—Excited, tremulous feeling. Frontal pain; worse, stooping. Strengthens brain after delirium tremens.

Eyes.—Smarting in canthi; lids red and puffy; tarsal tumor. [*Staph.*]

Ears.—Hissing and ringing otalgia.

Nose.—Catarrhal condition of both anterior and posterior nostrils. *Mucous polypus.* Chronic catarrh; *discharge of large, irregular clinkers.* Foul breath. *Crawling in nostrils*, with lachrymation and sneezing. Coryza, with stoppage of nostrils.

Stomach.—Vomiting of large quantities of dark-green masses. Constant hiccough, attended with pain in back. Unnatural appetite. Hiccough on eating, after nursing.

Respiratory.—Dry cough, tickling in trachea; *mouldy taste in throat* when hawking up mucus, expectoration profuse.

Extremities.—Affection of finger-tips and joints of toes. Tearing pains in arms and legs. *Pain in toe-nails*, as if they had grown into flesh.

Rectum.—*Itching of anus, and constant irritation in the evening in bed. Ascarides, with nightly restlessness.* Crawling in rectum after stool.

Sleep.—Restless, with twitching, choking, and starting up frightened.

Skin.—Itching causes tossing about all night. Very dry skin. Suppurating grooves in the nails.

Relationship.—Compare: *Teucrium scorodonia*—Wood-sage (in tuberculosis with muco-purulent expectoration; dropsy; orchitis and *tuberculous epidymitis; especially* in young, thin individuals with tuberculosis of lungs, glands; bones and urogenitals, 3x). *Cina; Ignat.; Sang.; Sil.*

Dose.—First to sixth potency. Locally for polypi, dry powder.

THALLIUM
(The Metal Thallium)

Thallium seems to influence the endocrines, especially the hyroid and adrenalin. Most horrible neuralgic, spasmodic, shooting pains. Muscular atrophy. Tremors. Relieves the violent pains in locomotor ataxia. *Paralysis of lower limbs.* Pain in stomach and bowels, like electric shocks. Paraplegia. *Alopecia* following acute, exhausting diseases. Night sweats. Polyneuritis. Dermal trophic lesions.

Extremities.—*Trembling.* *Paralytic feeling.* Lancinating pains, like electric shocks. Very tired. Chronic myelitis. Numbness in fingers and toes, with extension up lower extremities, involving lower abdomen and perineum. *Paralysis of lower limbs.* Cyanosis of extremities. Formication, beginning in fingers and extending through pelvis, perineum and inner thighs to feet.

Relationship.—Compare: *Lathyr.; Caust.; Arg. nit.; Plumbum.*

Dose.—Lower trituration to thirtieth potency.

THASPIUM AUREUM—ZIZIA
(Meadow Parsnip)

Hysteria, epilepsy, chorea, hypochondirasis, come within the sphere of this remedy.

Mind.—Suicidal; depressed; laughing and weeping moods alternate.

Head.—Pressure on top, in right temple, associated with backache.

Male.—Great lassitude following coitus. Sexual power increased.

Female.—Intermittent neuralgia of left ovary. Acrid, profuse leucorrhœa, with retarded menses.

Respiratory.—Dry cough, with stitches in chest. Dyspnœa.

Extremities.—Unusual tired feeling. *Chorea, especially during sleep. Fidgety legs.* [*Tarant.*] Lameness in arms and spasmodic twitching.

Modalities.—Worse, *during sleep*.

Relationship.—Compare: *Agar.; Stram.; Tarant.; Cicuta, Æthusa.*

Dose.—Tincture, to third potency.

THEA
(Tea)

Nervous sleeplessness, heart troubles, palpitation, and dyspepsia of old tea-drinkers. Produces most of the sick headaches Tabacum antidotal (Allen).

Head.—Temporary mental exaltation. Ill-humored. Sick headache radiating from one point. Sleepless and restless. Hallucinations of hearing. Cold damp feeling at back of head.

Stomach.—Sinking sensation at epigastrium. *Faint, gone feeling.* [*Sep.; Hyd.; Oleand.*] Craves acids. Sudden production of wind in large quantities.

Abdomen.—Borborygmi. Liability to hernia.

Female.—Soreness and tenderness in ovaries.

Heart.—Anxious oppression. Præcordial distress. Palpitation; unable to lie on left side. Fluttering. Pulse rapid, irregular, intermittent.

Sleep.—Sleepy in daytime; sleepiness at night, with vascular excitement and restlessness, and dry skin. Horrible dreams cause no horror.

Modalities.—*Worse*, night, on walking in open air, after meals. *Better* warmth; warm bath.

Relationship.—Antidote: *Kali hypophos.; Thuja; Ferr.; Kali hyd.* (Material doses for tea-taster's cough.)

Dose.—Third to thirtieth potency.

Theine ¼-½ grain hypodermically for sciatica and supraorbital neuralgia.

THERIDION
(Orange-spider)

Nervous hyperæsthesia. Has affinity for the tubercular diathesis. Vertigo, sick headache, peculiar pain around heart region, phthisis florida, scrofula have all been treated successfully with this remedy. *Sensitive to noise; it penetrates the body, especially teeth.* Noises seem to strike on painful spots over the body. Rachitis, caries, necrosis. Phthisis, stitch high up in left apex. [*Anthrax.*] Where the indicated remedy does not hold long.

Mind.—Restless; finds pleasure in nothing. Time passes too quickly.

Head.—Pain worse anyone walking over floor. *Vertigo, with nausea and vomiting on least motion,* particularly when closing eyes.

Eyes.—Luminous vibrations before eyes; sensitive to light. Pressure behind eyeballs. Throbbing over left eye.

Nose.—Discharge yellowish, thick, offensive; ozæna. [*Puls.; Thuja.*]

Stomach.—Seasickness. Nausea and vomiting when closing eyes and on motion. [*Tabac.*] Stinging pain on left side over anterior aspect of spleen. Burning in liver region.

Respiratory.—Pain in upper left chest. [*Myrt.; Pix.; Anis.*] *Pain in left floating ribs. Cardiac anxiety and pain.* Pinching in left pectoral muscle.

Back.—Sensitiveness between vertebræ; avoids pressure on spine. Stinging pains.

Skin.—*Stinging thrusts everywhere.* Sensitive skin in thighs. Itching sensations.

Modalities.—*Worse,* touch; pressure; on shipboard; riding in carriage; closing eyes; jar; noise: coitus; left side.

Dose.—Thirtieth potency.

THIOSINAMINUM—RHODALLIN
(A Chemical Derived from Oil of Mustard-seed)

A resolvent, externally and internally, for *dissolving scar tissue,* tumors, enlarged glands; lupus, strictures, adhesions. Ectropion, opacities of cornea, cataract, ankylosis, fibroids, scleroderma. Noises in ear. Suggested by Dr. A. S. Hard for retarding old age. A remedy for Tabes dorsalis, improving the lightning pains. Gastric, vesicle and rectal crises. Stricture of rectum, 2 grains twice daily.

Ear.—Arterio-sclerotic *vertigo. Tinnitus.* Catarrhal deafness with cicatricial thickening. Subacute suppurative otitis media, formation of fibrous bands impeding free movement of the ossicles. Thickened drum. Deafness due to some fibrous change in the nerve.

Dose.—Inject under skin, or, into the lesion a 10 per cent. solution in glycerine and water, 15-30 drops twice a week. Internally in capsules ½ grain daily. Obstinate arterio-sclerotic ailments in doses of ½ grain, never more, 3 times a day. Vertigo and arthritis (Bartlett). 2x attenuation.

THLASPI BURSA PASTORIS—CAPSELLA
(Shepherd's Purse)

Is an anti-hæmorrhagic and anti-uric-acid remedy. Albuminuria during gestation. Chronic neuralgia. Renal and vesical irritation. Hæmorrhage from uterine fibroid with aching in back or general bruised soreness. Aching between scapulæ. Uterine hæmorrhage, with cramps and expulsion of clots. Craves buttermilk. Effects of suppressed uterine disease. (Burnett.)

Head.—Eyes and face puffy. Frequent epistaxis. Vertigo; worse, rising. Frontal pain; worse toward evening. Scaly eruption behind ears. Tongue white, coated. Mouth and lips cracked. Sharp pain over right eye drawing eye upwards.

Nose.—Bleeding in nasal operations. Especially passive hæmorrhage.

Male.—Spermatic cord sensitive to concussion of walking or riding.

Female.—Metrorrhagia; too frequent and copious menses. Hæmorrhage, with violent uterine colic. Every alternate period very profuse. Leucorrhœa before and after menses; bloody, dark, offensive; *stains indelibly. Sore pain in womb on rising.* Scarcely recovers from one period before another begins.

Urinary.—Frequent desire; urine *heavy*, phosphatic. Chronic cystitis. Dysuria and spasmodic retention. Hæmaturia. Accumulation of gravel. Renal colic. *Brick-dust sediment.* Urethritis; urine runs away in little jets. Often replaces the use of the catheter.

Relationship.—Compare: *Urtica; Croc.; Trill.; Millefol.*

Dose.—Tincture, to sixth potency.

THUJA OCCIDENTALIS
(Arbor vitæ)

Acts on skin, blood, gastro-intestinal tract, kidneys, and brain. Its relation to the production of pathological vegetations condylomate, warty excrescences, spongy tumors is very important. Moist mucous tubercles. Bleeding fungus growths. Nævus. Excess of venosity.

The main action of Thuja is on the skin and genito-urinary organs, producing conditions that correspond with Hahnemann's sycotic dyscrasia, whose chief manifestation is the formation of wart-like excrescences upon mucous and cutaneous surfaces—fig-warts and condylomata. Has a specific antibacterial action, as in gonorrhœa and vaccination. Suppressed gonorrhœa, salpingitis. *Ill-effects of vaccination.* Sycotic pains, i. e., tearing in muscles and joints, worse at rest, better in dry weather, worse damp humid atmosphere; lameness. *Hydrogenoid constitutions*, whose blood is morbidly hydroscopic, so that damp air and water are inimical. Complaints from moonlight. *Rapid exhaustion and emaciation.* Left-sided and chilly medicine. Variola, aborts the pustule and prevents the suppurating fever. *Vaccinosis*, viz., inveterable skin troubles, neuralgia, etc.

Mind.—*Fixed ideas*, as if a strange person were at his side; as if soul and body were separated; as if something alive in abdomen. [*Croc.*] Emotional sensitiveness; music causes weeping and trembling.

Head.—Pain as if pierced by a nail. [*Coff.; Ign.*] Neuralgia from tea. [*Selen.*] Left-sided headache. White, scaly dandruff; hair dry and falling out. Greasy skin of face.

Eyes.—Ciliary neuralgia; iritis. Eyelids agglutinated at night; dry, scaly. Styes and tarsal tumors. [*Staph.*] Acute and subacute inflammation of sclera. Sclera raised in patches, and looks bluish-red. Large, flat phlyctenules; *indolent*. Recurring episcleritis. Chronic scleritis.

Ears.—Chronic otitis; discharge purulent. Creaking when swallowing. Polypi.

Nose.—Chronic catarrh; thick, green mucus; blood and pus. On blowing nose, pain in teeth. Ulceration within the nostrils. Dryness of nasal cavities. Painful pressure at root.

Mouth.—Tip of tongue very painful. *White blisters on side close to root, painfully sore.* Teeth decay next to gums; very sensitive; gums retract. Drinks fall audibly into stomach. Ranula; varicose veins on tongue and mouth. Pyorrhœa alveolaris.

Stomach.—Complete loss of appetite. Dislike for fresh meat and potatoes. Rancid eructations after fat food. Cutting pain in epigastrium. Cannot eat onions. Flatulence; pain after food; sinking sensation in epigastrium before food; thirst. Tea-drinking dyspepsia.

Abdomen.—Distended; indurations in abdomen. Chronic diarrhœa, worse after breakfast. Discharges forcibly expelled; gurgling sound. Brown spots. *Flatulence and distention; protruding here and there.* Rumbling and colic. Constipation, with violent rectal pain, causing stool to recede. [*Sil.; Sanic.*] Piles swollen; pain worse sitting, with stitching, burning pains at the anus. Anus fissured; painful to touch, with warts. *Movements as of something living* [*Crocus*], without pain.

Urinary.—Urethra swollen, inflamed. Urinary stream split and small. Sensation of trickling after urinating. Severe cutting *after.* [*Sars.*] Frequent micturition accompanying pains. Desire sudden and urgent, but cannot be controlled. Paralysis sphincter vesicæ.

Male.—Inflammation of prepuce and glans; pain in penis. Balanitis. *Gonorrhœal rheumatism. Gonorrhœa.* Chronic induration of testicles. Pain and burning felt near neck of bladder, with frequent and urgent desire to urinate. Prostatic enlargement. [*Ferr. pic.; Thiosinaminum; Iod.; Sabal.*]

Female.—Vagina *very sensitive.* [*Berb.; Kreos.; Lyssin.*] Warty excrescences on vulva and perineum. Profuse leucorrhœa; thick, greenish. Severe pain in left ovary and left inguinal region. Menses scanty, retarded. *Polypi;* fleshy excrescences. Ovaritis; worse left side, at every menstrual period. [*Lach.*] Profuse perspiration before menses.

Respiratory.—Dry, hacking cough in afternoon, with pain in pit of stomach. Stitches in chest; worse, cold drinks. *Asthma in children.* [*Nat. sulph.*] Papilloma of larynx. Chronic laryngitis.

Extremities. —When walking, limbs feel as if made of wood or glass, and would break easily. Tips of fingers swollen, red, feel dead. Muscular twitchings, weakness and trembling. Cracking in joints. Pain in heels and tendo-Achilles. Nails brittle. Ingrowing toe nail.

Skin.—Polypi, tubercles, *warts* epithelioma, næva, carbuncles; ulcers, especially in ano-genital region. Freckles and blotches. Perspiration sweetish, and strong. Dry skin, with brown spots. Zona; herpetic eruptions. Tearing pains in glands. Glandular enlargement. Nails crippled; brittle and soft. *Eruptions only on covered parts;* worse after scratching. Very sensitive to touch. Coldness of one side. Sarcoma; polypi. *Brown spots on hands and arms.*

Sleep.—Persistent insomnia.

Fever.—Chill, beginning in thighs. Sweat *only on uncovered parts,* or all over except head, when sleeping; profuse, sour, smelling like honey. Orgasm of blood in the evening, with throbbing in the blood-vessels.

Modalities.—*Worse,* at night, from heat of bed; at 3 a. m. and 3 p. m., from cold, damp air; after breakfast; fat, coffee; vaccination. *Better,* left side; while drawing up a limb.

Relationship.—Compare: (Hydrogenoid constitution: *Calcar.; Silica; Nat. sulph.; Aranea; Apis; Pulsat.*) *Cupressus australis* (sharp, prickling pain; general feeling of warmth; rheumatism and gonorrhœa). *Cupressus Lawsoniana* (acts like Thuja; *terrible pains in the stomach*). *Sphingurus* (falling out of hair from beard; pain in jaw-joint and zygoma); *Sil.; Maland.* (vaccination); *Medorrh.* (suppressed gonorrhœa); *Merc.; Cinnab.; Terebinth.; Juniperus; Sabin.; Sil.; Canth.; Cannab.; Nit. ac.; Puls.; Ant. tart.; Arborin* is a non-alcoholic preparation of *Thuja.*

Antidotes: *Merc.; Camph.; Sabin.* (warts).

Complementary: *Sabina; Ars.; Nat. sulph.; Silica.*

Dose.—Locally, for warts and excrescences, tincture, or cerate. Internally, tincture to thirtieth potency.

THYMOL
(Thyme Camphor)

A remedy having a wide field in genito-urinary diseases. It is indicated in pathological emissions, priapism and prostatorrhœa. The provings show an action limited to the sexual organs, producing a typical sexual neurasthenia. Specific for hookworm disease. [*Chenopodium.*]

Mental.—Irritable, arbitrary, must have his own way. Craves company. Energy gone.

Back.—Tired, aching throughout lumbar region. Worse, mental and physical labor.

Male.—Profuse, nightly, seminal emissions with lascivious dreams of a perverted character. Priapism. Urinary burning and subsequent dribbling of urine. Polyuria. Urates increased. Phosphates decreased.

Sleep.—Awakes tired and unrefreshed. Lascivious and fantastic dreams.

Relationship.—Compare: *Carbon Tetrachloride* as a remedy for Hookworms, according to Dr. Lambert, Suva, Fiji who employed it in 50,000 cases.

"1. Carbon tetrachloride is a vermifuge and vermicide of great potency, and has shown itself to be the best vermifuge for the treatment of hookworm in a country where the disease predominates.

"2. It gives little discomfort to the patient, is palatable, required no preparation of the patient, and when pure is apparently not toxic—all of which features are of advantage in a popular campaign.

"W. G. Smillie, and S. B. Pessoa, of Sao Paulo, Brazil, also have found carbon tetrachloride to be extremely efficient in removing hookworms. A single dose of 3 Cc. given to adults has been proved to remove 95 per cent. of all the hookworms harbored."

Modalities.—Thymol. *Worse*, mental and physical labor.

Dose.—Sixth attenuation.

THYMUS SERPYLLUM
(Wild Thyme)

Respiratory infections of children; dry nervous asthma, whooping-cough, severe spasms but little sputum.

Ringing in ears with feeling of pressure in head. Burning in pharynx, sore throat worse empty swallowing; blood vessels distended, dark.

Dose.—Tincture.

THYROIDINUM
(Dried Thyroid Gland of the Sheep)

Thyroid produces anæmia, emaciation, muscular weakness, sweating, headache, nervous tremor of face and limbs, tingling sensations, paralysis. Heart rate increased, exophthalmus and dilatation of pupils. *In myxœdema and cretinism* its effects are striking. Rheumatoid arthritis. Infantile wasting. Rickets. Delayed union of fractures. In half grain doses twice a day over a considerable period said to be *effective in undescended testicle* in boys. Thyroid exercises a general regulating influence over the mechanism of the organs of nutrition, growth and development. Thyroid weakness causes decided craving for large amount of sweets.

Of use in psoriasis; and *tachycardia.* Arrested development in children. Improves the memory. *Goitre.* Excessive obesity. Acts better with pale patients, rather than those of high color. Amblyopia. *Mammary tumor. Uterine fibroid.* Great weakness and hunger, yet loses flesh. *Nocturnal enuresis. Agalactea.* Begin treatment early in pregnancy. Dose 1½ gr. 2 to 3 times daily. *Vomiting of pregnancy* (give early in morning before patient gets up). *Fibroid tumors of the breast,* 2x trit. Dilates arterioles. [*Adrenalin contracts them.*] Sensation of faintness and nausea. Marked sensitiveness to cold Hypothyroidism after acute diseases, i. e., weakness. Easy fatigue, weak pulse, tendency to fainting, palpitation, cold hands and feet, low blood pressure, chilliness and sensitive to cold. (Thyroid 1x 3 times daily.) Has a powerful diuretic action in myxodema and various types of œdema.

Mind.—Stupor, alternating with restless melancholy. Irritable, worse least opposition; goes into a rage over trifles.

Head.—Feeling of lightness in brain. *Persistent frontal* headache. Eyeballs prominent. Face flushed; lips burn. Tongue thickly coated. Fullness and heat. Face flushed. Bad taste in mouth.

Heart.—Weak, frequent pulse, with inability to lie down. *Tachycardia.* [*Naja.*] Anxiety about chest, *as if constricted.* *Palpitation from least exertion.* Severe heart pain. Ready excitability of heart. Heart's action weak, with numbness of fingers.

Eyes.—Progressive diminution of sight with central scotoma. [*Carbon. sulf.*]

Throat.—Dry, congested, raw, burning; worse left side.

Stomach.—Desire for sweets and thirst for cold water. Nausea worse riding in car. Flatulence, much flatus in abdomen.

Urinary.—Increased flow; polyuria; some albumen and sugar. *Enuresis* in weakly children who are nervous and irritable (½ gr. night and morning). Urine smells of violets, burning along urethra, increase of uric acid.

Extremities.—Rheumative arthritis with tendency to obesity, coldness and cramps of extremities. Peeling of skin of lower limbs. Cold extremities. Aching pains. Œdema of legs. Trembling of limbs and entire body.

Respiratory.—Dry, painful cough with scanty, difficult expectoration and burning in pharynx.

Skin.—*Psoriasis* associated with adiposity (*not* in developing stage). Skin *dry*, impoverished. Cold hands and feet. *Eczema.* Uterine fibroids. *Browny swelling.* Swelling of glands of stony hardness. Sluggish cases. Jaundice with prutitus. Ichthyosis, lupus. Itching without eruption, worse night.

Relationship.—Compare: *Spongia; Calc.; Fucus; Lycopus; Iodothyrine,* (the active principle isolated from thyroid gland, a substance rich in Iodine and nitrogen, affects metabolism, reducing weight, may produce glycosuria. Use cautiously in obesity, for a fatty heart may not be able to maintain the accelerated rhythm. Milk contains the internal secretion of the thyroid.) *Thymus gland extract* (arthritis deformans; metabolic osteoarthritis, 5-grain tablets 3 times daily). High potencies very efficient in exophthalmic goitre.

Dose.—Crude Thyroid at times; better sixth to thirtieth potency. If the crude Thyroid is taken (two to three grains or more daily); the pulse should be watched. Must not be given in physiological doses where with feeble heart there is high blood pressure and not in tubercular patients.

TILIA EUROPA
(Linden)

Of value in muscular weakness of the eye; hæmorrhage o thin, pale blood. Puerperal metritis. Diseases of the antrum. [*Kali hyd.; Chelid.*]

Head.—*Neuralgia* (first right, then left side), *with veil before eyes.* Confusion, with dimness of vision. Much sneezing, with fluent coryza. Bleeding from nose.

Eyes.—Sensation as of gauze before eyes. [*Calc.; Caust.; Nat. m.*] Binocular vision imperfect.

Female.—*Intense sore feeling about uterus;* bearing-down, with hot sweat, but without relief. Much slimy leucorrhœa when walking. [*Bov.; Carb. an.; Graph.*] Soreness and redness of external genitals. [*Thuj.; Sulph.*] Pelvic inflammation, tympanites, abdominal tenderness and hot sweat which does not relieve.

Skin.—Urticaria. Violent itching, and burning like fire after scratching. Eruption of small, red itching pimples. *Sweat warm and profuse* soon after falling asleep. Sweat increases as rheumatic pains increase.

Modalities.—*Worse,* in afternoon and evening; in warm room, heat of bed. *Better,* cool room, motion.

Relationship.—Compare: *Lilium; Bellad.*

Dose.—Tincture, to sixth potency.

TITANIUM
(The Metal)

Is found in the bones and muscles. Has been used in lupus and tuberculosis processes externally, also in skin disease, nasal catarrh, etc. Apples contain 0.11 per cent. of Titan. Imperfect vision, the peculiarity being that *half an object* only could be seen at once. Giddiness with *vertical hemiopia.* Also sexual weakness, with *too early ejaculation* of semen in coitus' Bright's disease. Eczema, lupus, rhinitis.

Dose.—Lower and middle potencies.

TONGO—DIPTRIX ODORATA
(Seeds of Coumarouna—a tree in Guiana)

Useful in neuralgia; pertussis.

Head.—Tearing pain in supra-orbital nerve, with heat and throbbing pain in head and epiphora. Confused, especially the occiput, with somnolence and a sort of intoxication. Trembling in right upper lid. Coryza; nose stopped, must breathe through mouth.

Extremities.—Tearing pains in hip-joints, femur, and knee, especially left side.

Relationship.—*Melilotus. Anthoxanthum, Asperula,* and *Tonga* contain *Coumarin,* the active principle. Compare them in hay-fever; also, *Trifol.; Napth.; Sabad.*

Dose.—Tincture and lower potencies.

TORULA CEREVISIAE
(Saccharomyces) (Yeast Plant)

Introduced by Drs. Lehman and Yingling. Not proved, hence clinical symptoms only but many have been verified. Sycotic remedy Anaphylactic states produced by proteins and enzymes (Yingling).

Head.—Aching back of head and neck. Headache and sharp pains all over. Worse from constipation. Sneezing and wheezing. Catarrhal discharge from posterior nares. Irritable and nervous.

Stomach.—Bad taste. Nausea. Poor digestion. Belching of gas in stomach and abdomen. Soreness all over abdomen. Sense of fulness. Rumbling, pains shift, flatulence. *Constipation.* Sour, yeasty, mouldy odor from discharges.

Extremities.—Backache, tired and weak from elbows and knees down. Hands cold like ice and go to sleep easily.

Sleep.—Disturbed with much restlessness.

Skin.—Boils, recurrent. Itching eczema around ankles. Tinea versicolor.

Dose.—Pure yeast cake or potencies from 3rd to high. Yeast poultices are much used in skin diseases, boils and swelling.

TRIBULUS TERRESTRIS
(Ikshugandha)

An East Indian drug useful in urinary affections, expecially dysuria, and in debilitated states of the sexual organs, as expressed in seminal weakness, ready emissions and impoverished semen. Prostatitis, calculous affections and sexual neurasthenia. It meets the auto-traumatism of masturbation, correcting the emissions and spermatorrhœa. Partial impotence caused by overindulgence of advancing age, or when accompanied by urinary symptoms, incontinence, painful micturition, etc.

Dose.—Ten to twenty drops of the tincture three times daily.

TRIFOLIUM PRATENSE
(Red Clover)

Produces most marked ptyalism. Feeling of fullness with congestion of salivary glands, followed by increased copious flow of saliva. Feeling as if mumps were coming on. *Crusta lactea;* dry, scaly crusts. Stiff neck. *Cancerous diathesis.*

Head.—Confusion and headache on awaking. Dullness in anterior brain. Mental failure, loss of memory.

Mouth.—*Increased flow of saliva.* [*Merc.; Syphil.*] Sore throat, with hoarseness.

Respiratory.—Coryza like that which precedes hay-fever; thin mucus, with much irritation. *Hoarse and choking; chills with cough at night.* Cough on coming into the open air. Hay-fever. Spasmodic cough; *whooping cough,* paroxysms; worse at night.

Back.—Neck stiff; cramp in sterno-cleido muscles; relieved by heat and irritation.

Extremities.—Tingling in palms. Hands and feet cold. Tibial ulcers,

Relationship.—Compare: *Trifolium repens*—White clover—
(Prophylactic against mumps, feeling of congestion in salivary
glands, pain and hardening, especially submaxillary; worse,
lying down. Mouth filled with watery saliva, *worse lying down*.
Taste of blood in mouth and throat. Sensation as if heart would
stop, with great fear, better sitting up or moving about; worse,
when alone, with cold sweat on face.)
Dose.—Tincture.

TRILLIUM PENDULUM
(White Beth-root)

A general hæmorrhagic medicine, *with great faintness* and
dizziness. Chronic diarrhœa of bloody mucus. Uterine hæmorrhage. Threatened abortion. *Relaxation of pelvic region.*
Cramp-like pains. Phthisis with purulent and copious expectoration and spitting of blood.

Head.—Pain in forehead; worse, noise. Confused; eyeballs
feel too large. Vision blurred; everything looks bluish. *Nosebleed.* [*Millef.; Melilot.*]

Mouth.—Hæmorrhage from gums. *Bleeding after tooth
extraction.*

Stomach.—Heat and burning stomach rising up in œsophagus. Hæmatemesis.

Rectum.—Chronic diarrhœa; discharge bloody. Dysentery;
passage almost pure blood.

Female.—Uterine hæmorrhages, *with sensation as though hips
and back were falling to pieces; better tight bandages.* Gushing
of bright blood on least movement. Hæmorrhage from fibroids.
[*Calc.; Nitr. ac.; Phos.; Sulph. ac.*] Prolapse, with great
bearing-down. Leucorrhœa copious, yellow, stringy. [*Hydras.;
Kali b.; Sabin.*] Metrorrhagia at climacteric. *Lochia suddenly becomes sanguinous.* Dribbling of urine after labor.

Respiratory.—Cough, with spitting of blood. Copious, purulent expectoration. Hæmoptysis. Aching at end of sternum.
Suffocative attack of irregular breathing with sneezing. Shooting pains through chest.

Relationship.—Compare: *Trillium cernum* (eye symptoms)
everything looks bluish; greasy feeling in mouth); *Ficus*

(hæmorrhages; menorrhagia, hæmaturia, epistaxis, hæmatemesis, bleeding piles); *Sanguisuga*—Leech—(hæmorrhages; bleeding from anus). *Ipec.; Sab.; Lach.; Hamam.*

Dose.—Tincture and lower potencies.

TRIOSTEUM PERFOLIATUM
(Fever-root)

Triosteum is a very valuable remedy in diarrhœa attended with colicky pains and nausea, *numbness of lower limbs after stool,* and increased flow of urine; also in influenza. Quiets nervous symptoms. [*Coffea.; Hyos.*] Biliousness. Bilious colic.

Head.—Occipital pain, with nausea on rising, followed by vomiting. Influenza, with aching pains all over, and heat in the limbs. *Ozæna;* frontal pain.

Stomach.—Loathing of food; nausea on rising, followed by vomiting and cramps. Stools watery, frothy.

Extremities.—Stiffness of all joints; calves numb; aching in bones. Rheumatic pain in back. Pains in limbs.

Skin.—Itching welts. *Urticaria* from gastric derangement.

Dose.—Sixth potency.

TRINITROTOLUENE
(T.N.T.)

Symptoms found in munition workers handling T.N.T. who inhale and ingest it and also absorb some through the skin. They were compiled by Dr. Conrad Wesselhoeft and published in the December, 1926 number of the Journal of the American Institute of Homœopathy.

The destructive action of T.N.T. on the red blood corpuscles is responsible for the anemia and the jaundice with their secondary symptoms. The hemoglobin is changed so it cannot act satisfactorily as an oxygen carrier and as a result we have breathlessness, dizziness, headache, faintness, palpitation, undue fatigue, muscle cramps and cyanosis; also drowsiness, depression and insomnia. Later stages of the poisoning produce toxic jaundice and aplastic anemia. The jaundice is the result of cellular destruction in contrast to obstructive jaundice.

Head.—Depression and headache (frontal). Aversion to company, apathetic and weeps easily. Faintness, dizziness, mental sluggishness; delirium, convulsions, coma. Face very dark.

Respiratory.—Nose dry with stuffed sensation. Sneezing, coryza, burning of trachea, choking weight on chest; dry, convulsive cough, raising mucous plugs.

Gastro-Intestinal.—Bitter taste, much thirst, sour regurgitation; dull burning behind the ensiform; nausea, vomiting, constipation followed by diarrhœa with cramps.

Cardio Vascular.—Palpitation, tachycardia, bradycardia, intermittent pulse.

Urinary.—High colored urine, burning on urination, sudden desire, incontinence and retention.

Skin.—Hands stained yellow. Dermatitis, nodular erythema, vesicles, itching and burning; puffiness. *Tendency to hæmorrhage* under the skin and from the nose. *Tired pain in back of knees.*

Modalities.—*Worse*, alcohol (falls after one or two drinks of whisky). *Tea* (marked aversion).

Relationship.—Compare: *Zinc.; Phosph.; Cina; Ars.; Plumbum.*

Dose.—Thirtieth potency has been used with success.

TRITICUM—AGROPYRON REPENS
(Couch-Grass)

An excellent remedy in excessive irritability of the bladder, dysuria, cystitis, gonorrhœa.

Nose.—Always blowing nose.

Urinary.—Frequent, *difficult*, and painful urination. [*Pop.*] Gravelly deposits. Catarrhal and purulent discharges. [*Pareira.*] Strangury, pyelitis; enlarged prostate. Chronic cystic irritability. Incontinence; constant desire. Urine is dense and causes irritation of the mucous surfaces.

Relationship.—Compare: *Tradescantia;* (Hæmorrhage from ear and upper air passages; painful urination, urethral discharge; scrotum inflamed). *Chimaph.; Senecio; Populus trem.; Buchu; Uva.*

Polytrichum Juniperinum—Ground Moss—(Painful urination of old people; dropsy, urinary obstruction and suppression).

Dose.—Tincture or infusion by boiling two ounces in a quart of water until it is reduced to a pint. To be taken in four doses in 24 hours.

TROMBIDIUM
(Red acarus of the fly)

Has a specific place in the treatment of dysentery. Symptoms *are worse by food and drink.*

Abdomen.—Much pain before and after stool; stool only after eating. Griping in hypochondrium in morning. Congestion of the liver, with urgent, loose, stools on rising. Brown, thin, bloody stools, with tenesmus. During stool, sharp pain in left side, shooting downward. Burning in anus.

Dose.—Sixth to thirtieth potency.

TUBERCULINUM
(A Nucleo-protein, a Nosode from Tubercular Abscess)

Tuberculinum is indicated in renal affections, but caution is necessary, for where skin and intestines do not perform normally even high potencies are dangerous. In chronic cystitis, brilliant and permanent results. (Dr. Nebel Montreux.)

Of undoubted value in the treatment of *incipient tuberculosis.* Especially adapted to the light-complexioned, narrow-chested subjects. Lax fiber, low recuperative powers, and very susceptible to changes in the weather. Patient always tired; motion causes intense fatigue; aversion to work; wants constant changes. When *symptoms are constantly changing and well-selected remedies fail to improve, and cold is taken from the slightest exposure.* Rapid emaciation. Of great value in epilepsy, neurasthenia and in nervous children. Diarrhœa in children running for weeks, extreme wasting, bluish pallor, exhaustion. Mentally deficient children. Enlarged tonsils. Skin affections, *acute articular rheumatism.* Very sensitive, mentally and physically. General exhaustion. Nervous weakness. Trembling. Epilepsy. Arthritis.

Mind.—Contradictory characteristics of Tuberculinum are mania and melancholia; insomnia and sopor. Irritable, especially when awakening. *Depressed*, melancholy. *Fear of dogs. Animals especially.* Desire to use foul language, curse and swear.

Head.—Subject to deep brain headaches and intense neuralgias. Everything seems strange. Intense pain, as of an iron band around head. Meningitis. When critical discharges appear, sweat, polyuria, diarrhœa, exanthema, repeating the dose only when crises come on. Nocturnal hallucinations, awakes frightened. Plica polonica. [*Vinca.*] Crops of small boils, intensely painful, successively appear in the nose; *green, fetid pus.*

Ears.—Persistent, offensive otorrhœa. *Perforation in membrana tympani, with ragged edges.*

Stomach.—Averse to meat. All-gone, hungry sensation. [*Sulph.*] Desire for cold milk.

Abdomen.—Early-morning, sudden diarrhœa. [*Sulph.*] Stools dark-brown, offensive, discharged with much force. Tabes mesenterica.

Female.—*Benign mammary tumors.* Menses too early, too profuse, long-lasting. *Dysmenorrhœa. Pains increase with the establishment of the flow.*

Respiratory.—*Enlarged tonsils.* Hard, dry cough during sleep. Expectoration thick, easy; profuse bronchorrhœa. Shortness of breath. Sensation of suffocation, even with plenty of fresh air. Longs for cold air. Broncho-pneumonia in children. Hard, hacking cough, profuse sweating and loss of weight, rales all over chest. Deposits begin in apex of lung. (Repeated doses.)

Back.—Tension in nape of neck and down spine. Chilliness between shoulders or up the back.

Skin.—Chronic eczema; itching intense; worse at night. *Acne* in tuberculous children. Measles; psoriasis [*Thyroid.*]

Sleep.—Poor; wakes early. Overpowering sleepiness in daytime. Dreams vivid and distressing.

Fever.—Post-critical temperature of a remittent type. Here repeat dose every two hours. (MacFarlan.) Profuse sweat. General chilliness.

Modalities.—*Worse*, motion, music; before a storm; standing; dampness; from draught; early morning, and after sleep. *Better*, open air.

Relationship.—Compare: *Koch's lymph* (*acute and chronic parenchymatous nephritis;* produces pneumonia, bronchopneumonia, and congestion of the lungs in tuberculous patients, and is a remarkably efficacious remedy in lobular pneumonia—*broncho-pneumonia*); *Aviare*—Tuberculin from birds—(acts on the apices of the lungs; has proved an excellent remedy in influenzal bronchitis; symptoms similar to tuberculosis; relieves the debility, diminishes the cough, improves the appetite, and braces up the whole organism; acute broncho-pulmonary diseases of children; itching of palms and ears; *cough*, acute, inflammatory, irritating, incessant, and tickling; loss of strength and appetite); *Hydrast.* (to fatten patients after Tuberc.): *Formic acid* (tuberculosis, chronic nephritis, malignant tumors; pulmonary tuberculosis, not in third stage, however; lupus; carcinoma of breast and stomach; Dr. Krull uses injections of solutions corresponding to the third centesimal potency; these must not be repeated before six months). Compare: *Bacil.; Psorin.; Lach. Kalagua* (tuberculosis; garlicky odor of all secretions and breath). *Teucrium scoradonia.* Compare: *Thuja.* (Vaccinosis may block the way of action of *Tuberculin* until Thuja has been given and then acts brilliantly. (Burnett.)
Complementary: *Calcarea; China; Bryon.*

Dose.—*Tuberculin* needs more frequent repetition in children's complaints than nearly every other chronic remedy. (H. Fergie Woods.) Thirtieth and much higher, in infrequent doses. When Tuberculinum fails *Syphilinum* often follows advantageously, producing a reaction.

"The use of Tuberculinum in phthisis pulmonalis demands attention to the following points: In apyretic purely tubercular phthisis results are marked, provided the eliminative organs are in good order, but nothing below the 1000th should be used, unless absolutely necessary. With patients where strepto-staphylo-pneumococci are in the bronchi; where also after washing the sputum, a pure "t. b." bacilli-mass remains, the same treatment is indicated. With mixed infection—found in the majority of cases—where the sputum swarms with virulent micro-organisms in addition to the "t. b.," other procedure is necessary. If the heart is in good shape, a single dose of Tuberculinum 1000-2000 is given, provided there are no marked indications for other remedies. With due attention to temperature and possible excretions, the dose is allowed to work until effects are no longer observed, eight days to eight weeks. Usually a syndrome then presents, permitting the accurate choice of an antipsoric Silica, Lycopodium, Phosphorus, etc. After a while the picture again darkens and now a high potency of the isopathic remedy corresponding to the most virulent and prominent micro-organism found in the sputum is given: Staphylo-, Strepto-, or Pneumococcin. The accurate bacteriological analysis of the sputum is absolutely essential; the choice of the ison again clears the picture, and so, proceeding on the one side etiologically (where these isopathica have not yet been proved); on the other side symptomatically with antipsoric remedies, the disease is dominated.

My own experience warns, in the case of mixed infection, against the use of Strepto-, Staphylo-, or Pneumococcin below the 500th. I use them only from 2000 to 1000, having seen terrible aggravations from the 30, 100, 200, with a lowering temperature from 104 to 96. Hence the admonition, which need not concern scoffers, but those alone who wish to avail themselves of a potent weapon. The toxins used as remedies are, like Tuberculinum, prepared from pure and virulent cultures.

And cases, seemingly condemned to speedy death, are brought in a year or two back to normal temperature, though, of course, sacrificing a large portion of lung tissue. This result is sure when the patient can and will take care of himself, where the heart has withstood the toxin and the stomach and liver are in good function. Further, climatic variations must be avoided. With the great mineral metabolism of the phthisic, diet regulation is imperative, and should be preponderately vegetable, together with the addition of psysiological salts in low potency, Calcarea carb., 3x, 5x, Calcarea phos., 2x, 6x, and intercurrently according to indications organ-remedies as Cactus Tr. 30, Chelidonium Tr. 30, Taraxacum Tr., Nasturtium Tr., Urtica urens Tr., Tussilago farfara Tr., Lysimachia numularia Tr., for short periods.

The first dose of Tuberculinum in any difficult case is, however, the most weighty prescription. The remedy should not be given without a most careful cardiac examination. As the surgeon before the anæsthetic, so must the physician know the heart before administering this drug, especially to children, and seniles—and to young seniles. He who observes this rule will have fewer clinical reproaches on his conscience. When Tuberculinum is contraindicated, recourse must be had to the nearest antipsoric.

The above caution applies also to asthma, pleuritis, peritonitis in scrofulous (tuberculous) subjects." [Dr. Nebel Montreux.]

TURNERA
(Damiana)

Said to be of use in sexual neurasthenia; impotency. Sexual debility from nervous prostration. Incontinence of old people. Chronic prostatic discharge. Renal and cystic catarrh; *frigidity of females*. Aids the establishment of normal menstrual flow in young girls.

Dose.—Tincture and fluid extract—ten- to forty-drop doses.

TUSSILAGO PETASITES
(Butter-burr)

Has some action on the urinary organs, and found useful in gonorrhœa. Affections of pylorus.

Urinary.—Crawling in urethra.

Male.—Gonorrhœa; yellowish, thick discharge. Erections, with urethral crawling. Pain in spermatic cord.

Relationship.—Compare: *Tussilago fragrans* (pylorus pain, plethora and corpulency); *Tussilago farfara* (coughs); as an intercurrent medicine in phthisis pulmonalis. (See Tuberculinum.)

Dose.—Tincture.

UPAS TIENTE
(Upas-tree—Strychnos Tiente)

Produces *tonic spasms, jetanus, and asphyxia.*

Head.—Disinclined for mental work. Irritable. Dull headache deep in brain.

Eyes.—*Pain in eyes and orbits, with conjunctivitis.* Dull sunken eyes. Styes.

Mouth.—Herpes on lips. Burning on the tongue. Pain in mouth, as from a splinter. [*Nit. ac.*]

Male.—Desire increased, with loss of power. *Dull backache, as after excessive coitus.*

Chest.—Lancinating pain throughout right lung toward the liver, stopping breathing. Violent palpitation; sensation of heaviness in stomach.

Skin.—Numb hands and feet. Hangnails inflamed; itching and redness of roots of nails.

Relationship.—Compare: *Upas antiaris*—resinous exudation of *Antiarus toxicaria,* (a deadly poison to the muscular system. It suspends both voluntary muscular action and that of the heart without causing convulsions. Used in Java as an arrow poison (Merrell). Differs in producing *clonic spasms,* violent vomiting, diarrhœa, great prostration). *Oxal. ac. Upas* when Bryonia fails (typhoid).

Antidote: *Curare.*

Dose.—Third to sixth potency.

URANIUM NITRICUM
(Nitrate of Uranium)

Causes glycosuria and increased urine. Is known to produce nephritis, diabetes, degeneration of the liver, high blood pressure and dropsy. Its therapeutic keynote is *great emaciation, debility and tendency to ascites and general dropsy.* Backache and delayed menses. Dry mucous membranes and skin.

Head.—Ill-tempered; dull, heavy pain. Nostrils sore, with purulent, acrid discharge. Mental depression.

Eyes.—Lids inflamed and agglutinated; *styes.*

Stomach.—Excessive thirst; nausea; *vomiting. Ravenous appetite;* eating followed by flatulence. *Boring pain in pyloric region. Gastric and duodenal ulcers.* Burning pain. *Abdomen bloated.* Gas, second only to Lycop.

Urinary.—Copious urination. *Diuresis.* Incontinence of urine. *Diabetes.* Emaciation and tympanites. *Burning in* *urethra,* with very acid urine.   *Unable to* retain urine without pain.   *Enuresis.   [Mullein oil.]*

Male.—Complete impotency, with nocturnal emissions. Organs cold, relaxed, sweaty.

Relationship.—Compare: *Syzygium; Phos. ac.; Lact. ac.; Arg. nit.; Kali bich.; Ars.; Phloridzin* (a glucosidal principle obtained from the bark of the root of the apple and other fruit trees.   Produces diabetes and fatty degeneraion of the liver; intermittent fever.   Daily doses, 15 grains.   Phlorizin causes glycosuria.   No hyperglycemia results.   It compels the secretory epithelium of the kidney to break down serum albumin into sugar.   There is no increase in blood sugar.)

Dose —Second trituration.

UREA
(Carbamide)

Tuberculosis.   Lumps.   Enlarged glands.   Renal dropsy, with symptoms of general intoxication.   Gouty eczema.   Albuminuria, diabetes; uræmia.   Urine thin and of low specific gravity. A hydrogogue diuretic in the treatment of dropsies.   10 grains every 6 hours.

Relationship.—Compare: *Uric acid* (gout, gouty eczema, rheumatism, lipoma);   *Urinum* (acne, boils, scurvy, dropsy); *Urtica; Tubercul.; Thyroid.*

URTICA URENS
(Stinging-nettle)

A remedy for agalactia and *lithiasis.*   Profuse discharge from mucous surfaces.   Enuresis and urticaria.   Spleen affections. *Antidotes ill-effects of eating shellfish.*   Symptoms return at the same time every year.   Gout and uric acid diathesis.   Favors elimination.

Rheumatism associated with urticaria-like eruptions.   Neuritis.

Head.—Vertigo, headache with spleen pains.

Abdomen.—Diarrhœa chronic disease of large intestine characterized by large secretion of mucus.

Male.—Itching of scrotum, keeps him awake; **scrotum swollen.**

Female.—*Diminished secretion of milk.* Uterine hæmorrhage. Acid and excoriating leucorrhœa. *Pruritus vulvæ, with stinging, itching,* and œdema. Arrests flow of milk after weaning. Excessive swelling of breasts.

Extremities.—Pain in acute gout deltoid; pain in ankles, wrists.

Skin.—*Itching blotches. Urticaria,* burning heat, with formication; violent itching. Consequences of suppressed nettle-rash. Rheumatism alternates with nettle-rash. Burn confined to skin. Urticaria nodosa. [*Bov.*] Erythema, with burning and stinging. *Burns and scalds. Chicken-pox.* [*Dulc.*] Angioneurotic œdema. Herpes labialis with sensation of heat and itching. Itching and stinging of scrotum.

Fever.—General heat in bed with soreness over abdomen. Fever of gout. Tropical fever.

Modalities.—*Worse,* from snow-air; water, cool moist air, touch.

Relationship.—Compare: *Medusa; Nat. mur.; Lac. can.; Ricin* (diminished mammary secretion); *Bombyx; Rhus; Apis; Chloral.; Astac.; Puls.* (urticaria); *Boletus luridus* and *Anacard.* (urticaria tuberosa); *Lycop.* and *Hedeoma* (uric acid conditions); *Formica.*

Dose.-Tincture and lower potencies.

USNEA BARBATA
(Tree-moss)

Is a remedy in some forms of congestive headache; sunstroke.

Head.—Bursting feeling, *as if temples would burst, or the eyes burst out of the sockets.* Throbbing carotids.

Relationship.—Compare: *Glonoine; Bellad.*

Dose.—Tincture, drop doses.

USTILAGO MAYDIS
(Corn-smut)

Flabby condition of uterus. Hæmorrhage. Congestion to various parts, especially at climacteric. Crusta lactea. [*Viola tric.*]

Head.—Very depressed. Full feeling. Nervous headache from menstrual irregularities. Aching in eyeballs, with much lachrymation.

Male.—Uncontrollable masturbation. Spermatorrhœa, with erotic fancies and amorous dreams. Emissions, with irresistible tendency to masturbation. Dull pain in lumbar region, with great despondency and mental irritability.

Female.—Vicarious menstruation. Ovaries burn, pain, swell. Profuse menses after miscarriage; discharge of blood from slightest provocation; bright red; partly clotted. Menorrhagia at climaxis. [*Calc. c.; Lach.*] Oozing of dark blood, clotted, forming long black strings. Uterus hypertrophied. *Cervix bleed easily.* Postpartum hæmorrhage. Profuse lochia.

Fever.—Abundant sweat. Pulse at first accelerated then enfeebled. Palpitations.

Extremities.—Muscular debility, *sensation of boiling water along the back.* Clonic and tetanic movements. Muscular contractions, especially of lower limbs.

Skin.—Alopecia. Tendency to small boils. Skin dry; eczema; copper-colored spots. Pruritus; sunburn. Psoriasis. (Internally and externally.)

Relationship.—Compare: *Secale; Sabin.; Zea Italica.* (Possess curative properties in skin diseases, particularly in psoriasis and eczema rubrum. Mania for bathing. Impulse to suicide, particularly by drowning. Easily angered. Appetite increased, voracious, alternating with disgust for food. Pyrosis, nausea, vomiting, better drinking wine.)

Dose.—Tincture, to third potency.

UVA URSI
(Bearberry)

Urinary symptoms most important. Cystitis, with bloody urine. Uterine hæmorrhage. Chronic vesical irritation, with pain, tenesmus, and catarrhal discharges. *Burning after the discharge of slimy urine.* Pyelitis. Calculous inflammation. Dyspnœa, nausea, vomiting, pulse small and irregular. Cyanosis. Urticaria without itching.

Urinary.—Frequent urging, with severe spasms of bladder;

burning and tearing pain. Urine contains blood, pus, and much tenacious mucus, with clots in large masses. Involuntary; green urine. Painful dysuria.

Relationship.—Compare: *Arbutin* (a crystallized glucoside of Uva; found also in Kalmia, Gaultheria and other genera of the family of *Eriaceæ;* given in doses of 3 to 8 grains with sugar three times a day. Used as an urinary antiseptic and diuretic. *Arctosphylos manzanita* (acts on renal and reproductive organs. Gonorrhœa, vesical catarrh, diabetes, menorrhagia. Tincture of leaves). *Vaccinum myrtillus*—Huckleberries—(dysentery; typhoid, keeps intestines aseptic and prevents absorption and reinfection).

Dose.—Tincture, five to thirty drops. In pyelitis a trituration of the leaves.

VACCININUM
(Nosode—From vaccine matter)

Vaccine poison is capable of setting up a morbid state of extreme chronicity, named by Burnett Vaccinosis, symptoms like those of Hahnemann's Sycosis. Neuralgias, inveterate skin eruptions, chilliness, indigestion with great flatulent distension (Clark). Whooping-cough.

Mind.—Irritable, impatient ill-humored, nervous.

Head.—Frontal headache. Forehead and eyes feel as if split. Inflamed and red lids.

Skin.—Hot and dry. Pimples and blotches. Eruption like variola.

Relationship.—Compare: anti-vaccinal remedies; *Variolin; Malandrinum;* Thuja, powerful adjuvants in treatment of malignant disease.

Dose.—Sixth to 200th potency.

VALERIANA
(Valerian)

Hysteria, over-sensitiveness, nervous affections, when apparently well-chosen remedies fail. Hysterical spasms and affections generally. *Hysterical flatulency.*

Mind.—Changeable disposition. Feels light, as if floating in air. Over-sensitiveness. [*Staph.*] Hallucinations at night. *Irritable.* Tremulous.

Head.—Sensation of great coldness. Pressure in forehead. Feeling of intoxication.

Ears.—*Earache from exposure to draughts and cold.* Nervous noises. Hyperæsthesia.

Throat.—*Sensation as if a thread were hanging down throat.* Nausea felt in throat. Pharynx feels constricted.

Stomach.—Hunger, with nausea. Erucatations foul. Heart-burn with gulping of rancid fluid. Nausea, with faintness. *Child vomits curdled milk in large lumps after nursing.*

Abdomen.—Bloated. Hysterical cramps. Thin, watery diarrhœa, *with lumps of coagulated milk, with violent screaming in children.* Greenish, papescent, bloody stool. Spasms in bowels after food and at night in bed.

Respiratory.—Choking on falling asleep. Spasmodic asthma; convulsive movements of the diaphragm.

Female.—Menses late and scanty. [*Puls.*]

Extremities.—Rheumatic pains in limbs. *Constant jerking.* Heaviness. Sciatica; *pain worse standing and resting on floor* [*Bell.*]; better walking. Pain in heels *when sitting.*

Sleep.—Sleepless, with nightly itching and muscular spasms. Worse on waking.

Fever.—Long lasting heat, often with sweat on face. *Heat predominates.* Sensation of icy coldness. [*Heloderma; Camp.; Abies c.*]

Relationship.—Compare: *Asaf.; Ign.; Croc.; Castor.; Amm. valer.* (in neuralgia, gastric disturbance, and great nervous agitation). Insomnia especially during pregnancy and menopause. Feeble, hysterical nervous patients.

Dose.—Tincture.

VANADIUM
(The Metal)

Its action is that of an oxygen carrier and a catalyzer, hence its use in wasting diseases. Increases amount of hæmoglobin, also combines its oxygen with toxines and destroys their virulence. Also increases and stimulates phagocytes.

A remedy in degenerative conditions of the liver and arteries. Anorexia and symptoms of gastro intestinal irritation; albumen, casts and blood in urine. Tremors; vertigo; hysteria and melancholia; neuro-retinitis and blindness. Anæmia, emaciation. Cough dry, irritating and paroxysmal, sometimes with hæmorrhages. Irritation of nose, eyes and throat. Tuberculosis, chronic rheumatism, diabetes. *Acts as a tonic to digestive function* and in early tuberculosis. Arterio-sclerosis, sensation as if heart was compressed, as if blood had no room in the aorta. Anxious pressure on whole chest. Fatty heart. Degenerative states, has brain softening. Atheroma of arteries of brain and liver. Compare: *Ars.; Phos. Ammon. vanad.* (fatty degeneration of liver.)

Dose.—6-12 potency. The best form is Vanadiate of Soda, 2 mg. daily, by mouth.

VANILLA—PLANIFOLIA
(Vanilla)

Marked skin irritation resembling milk Poison-oak; is sometimes produced by handling the beans, also by local use of vanilla essence in a hair wash. Vanilla is supposed to stimulate the brain and sexual propensities. Do not use the synthetic Vanilla extract. Various disorders of the nervous system and circulation are produced in workers with Vanilla. Is an emmagogue and aphrodisiac. Menses prolonged.

Dose.—Vanilla, 6th to 30th, has been found effective in curing the skin affection.

VARIOLINUM
(Lymph from Small-pox Pustule)

Used for "internal vaccination." Seems to be efficacious in protecting against, modifying and aiding in the cure of small-pox.

Head.—Morbid fear of small-pox. Deafness. Pain in occiput. Inflamed eyelids.

Respiratory.—Oppressed breathing. Throat feels closed. Cough with thick viscid, bloody mucus. Feeling of a lump in right side of throat.

Relationship.—*Excruciating backache. Aching in legs.* Tired all over with restlessness. Wrists pain. Pains shift from back to abdomen.

Fever.—Hot fever, with intense radiating heat. Profuse, bad-smelling sweat.

Skin.—Hot, dry. Eruption of pustules. *Shingles.*

Relationship.—Compare: *Vaccin.* (same action); *Malandrinum*—the morbid product of the grease of the horse (a prophylactic of small-pox and a remedy for the ill-effects of vaccination; chronic eczema following vaccination).

Dose.—Sixth to thirtieth potency.

VERATRUM ALBUM
(White Hellebore)

A perfect picture of *collapse*, with *extreme coldness, blueness, and weakness,* is offered by this drug. Post-operative shock with cold sweat on forehead, pale face, rapid, feeble pulse. *Cold perspiration on the forehead,* with nearly all complaints. *Vomiting, purging, and cramps in extremities.* The *profuse,* violent retching and vomiting is most characteristic. Surgical shock. Excessive dryness of all mucous surfaces. *"Coprophagia"* violent mania alternates with silence and refusal to talk.

Mind.—Melancholy, with stupor and mania. Sits in a stupid manner; notices nothing; *Sullen indifference.* Frenzy of excitement; shrieks, curses. Puerperal mania. Aimless wandering from home. *Delusions of impending misfortunes.* Mania, with desire to cut and tear things. [*Tarant.*] Attacks of pain, with delirium driving to madness. Cursing, howling all night.

Head.—Contracted features. *Cold sweat on forehead. Sensation of a lump of ice on vertex.* Headache, with nausea, vomiting, diarrhœa, pale face. Neck too weak to hold head up.

Eyes.—Surrounded by dark rings. Staring; turned upwards. without lustre. Lachrymation with redness. Lids dry heavy.

Face.—Features sunken. *Icy coldness of tip of nose and face.* Nose grows more pointed. Tearing in cheeks, temples, and eyes. *Face very pale, blue, collapsed, cold.*

Mouth.—Tongue pale, cold; cool sensation, as from peppermint. Dry in center not relieved by water. Salty saliva. Toothache, teeth feel heavy as if filled with lead.

Stomach.—*Voracious* appetite. *Thirst for cold water, but is vomited as soon as swallowed.* Averse to warm food. Hiccough. *Copious vomiting and nausea; aggravated by drinking and least motion.* Craves fruit, juicy and cold things, ice, salt. Anguish in pit of stomach. Great weakness after vomiting. Gastric irritability with *chronic* vomiting of food.

Abdomen.—Sinking and empty feeling. *Cold feeling* in stomach and abdomen. Pain in abdomen preceding stool. Cramps, knotting abdomen and legs. Sensation as if hernia would protrude. [*Nux.*] Abdomen sensitive to pressure, swollen with terrible colic.

Rectum.—Constipation from inactivity of rectum, with heat and headache. Constipation of babies, and when produced by very cold weather. *Stools large, with much straining until exhausted, with cold sweat.* Diarrhœa, very painful, watery, *copious, and forcibly evacuated,* followed by great prostration. Evacuations of cholera morbus and true cholera when vomiting accompanies the purging.

Respiratory.—Hoarse, weak voice. Rattling in chest. Much mucus in bronchial tubes, that cannot be coughed up. Coarse rales. Chronic bronchitis in the aged. [*Hippozanin.*] Loud, barking, stomach cough, followed by eructation of gas; worse, warm room. Hollow cough, tickling low down, with blue face. Cough comes on from drinking, especially cold water; urine escapes when coughing. Cough on entering warm room from cold air. [*Bryonia.*]

Heart.—Palpitation with anxiety and rapid audible respiration. Pulse irregular, feeble. Tobacco heart from chewing. Intermittent action of heart in feeble persons with some hepatic obstruction. One of the best heart stimulants in homœop. doses. (J. S. Mitchell.)

Female.—Menses too early; profuse and exhausting. *Dysmenorrhœa, with coldness,* purging, *cold sweat. Faints from least exertion.* Sexual mania precedes menses.

Extremities.—Soreness and tenderness of joints. Sciatica;

pains like electric flashes. *Cramps in calves.* Neuralgia in brachial plexus; arms feel swollen, cold, paralytic.

Skin.—Blue, cold, clammy, inelastic; *cold as death.* Cold sweat. Wrinkling of skin of hands and feet.

Fever.—Chill, *with extreme coldness* and thirst.

Modalities.—*Worse,* at night; wet, cold weather. *Better,* walking and warmth.

Relationship.—Compare: *Veratrinum*—alkaloid from seeds of Sabadilla.—(electric pains, electric shocks in muscles, fibrillary twitchings); *Cholos terrepina* (cramps in calves); *Camph.; Cupr.; Ars.; Cuprum ars.* (*intermittent, cold, clammy sweat*); *Narcissus poeticus* (gastro-enteritis with much griping and cutting pain in bowels. Fainting, trembling, cold limbs, small and irregular pulse); *Trychosanthes*—(diarrhœa, pain in liver, dizziness after every stool); *Agaric. emetic.* (vertigo; longing for ice-cold water; burning pains in stomach); *Agaric. phalloides* (cholera, cramps in stomach, cold extremities, urine suppressed). *Veratrine* (Increased vascular tension. It relaxes it and stimulates the elimination of toxins by skin, kidneys, and liver).

Dose.—First to thirtieth potency. In diarrhœa, not below the sixth.

VERATRUM VIRIDE
(White American Hellebore)

Paroxysms of auricular fibrillation. Induces fall of both systolic and diastolic blood pressure. Congestions, especially to lungs, base of brain, with nausea and vomiting. Twitchings and convulsions. Especially adapted to full-blooded, plethoric persons. Great prostration. Rheumatism of heart. *Bloated, livid face.* Furious delirium. Effects of sunstroke. *Œsophagitis.* (Farrington.) *Verat. vir,* will raise the opsonic index against the *diploccus pneumonia,* 70 to 109 per cent. Congestive stage and early manifestations of hepatization in pneumonia. Zigzag temperature. Clinically, it is known that such diseases as Tiegel's contracture, Thompson's Disease, athetosis and pseudo-hypertrophic muscular paralysis present a symptomatology quite like that produced by Veratrum vir. upon muscular tissue. (A. E. Hinsdale, M.D.)

Mind.—Quarrelsome and delirious.

Head—Congestion intense, almost apoplectic. Hot head,

bloodshot eyes. Bloated, livid face. Hippocratic face. Head retracted, *pupils dilated*, double vision. Meningitis. *Pain from nape of neck;* cannot hold head up. Sunstroke; head full, throbbing arteries. [*Bell.; Glon.; Usnea.*] *Face flushed.* Convulsive twitching of facial muscles. [*Agaricus.*] Vertigo with nausea.

Tongue.—White or yellow, *with red streak down the middle.* Feels scalded. Increased saliva.

Stomach.—Thirsty. Nausea and vomiting. Smallest quantity of food or drink immediately rejected. Constrictive pain; increased by warm drinks. *Hiccough;* excessive and painful, with *spasms of œsophagus.* Burning in stomach and œsophagus.

Abdomen.—Pain above pelvis, with soreness.

Respiratory.—Congestion of lungs. Difficult breathing. Sensation of a heavy load on chest. Pneumonia, with faint feeling in stomach and violent congestion. *Croup.* Menstrual colic before the appearance of the discharge with strangury.

Urine.—Scanty with cloudy sediment.

Female.—Rigid os. [*Bell.; Gels.*] Puerperal fever. Suppressed menstruation, with congestion to head. [*Bell.*] Menstrual colic before the appearance of the discharge with strangury.

Heart.—Pulse *slow, soft, weak,* irregular, intermittent. Rapid pulse, low tension. [*Tabac.; Dig.*] Constant, dull, burning pain in region of heart. Valvular diseases. *Beating of pulses throughout body,* especially in right thigh.

Extremities.—Aching pain in back of neck and shoulders. Severe pain in joints and muscles. Violent electric-like shocks in limbs. Convulsive twitchings. *Acute rheumatism. Fever.*

Skin.—Erysipelas, with cerebral symptoms. Erythema. Itching in various parts. *Hot sweating.*

Fever.—Hyperthermy in the evening and hypothermy in the morning. Suppurative fevers with great variation of temperature.

Relationship.—Compare: *Gels.; Bapt.; Bell.; Acon.; Ferr. phos.* Antidotes Strychnin—fluid extract, 20-40 drops.

Dose.—First to sixth potency.

VERBASCUM
(Mullein)

Has a pronounced action on the inferior maxillary branch of the fifth pair of the cranial nerves; on the ear; and respiratory tract and bladder. *Catarrhs*, and colds, *with periodical proso-palgia*. Quiets nervous, and bronchial, and urinary irritation, and cough.

Face.—Neuralgia affecting zygoma, temporo maxillary joint, and ear [*Menyanth.*], particularly of left side, with lachryma-tion, coryza, and sensation *as if parts were crushed with tongs.* Talking, sneezing, and change of temperature aggravate the pains; also, pressing teeth together. Pains seem to come in flashes, excited by least movement, occurring periodically at same hour in morning and afternoon each day.

Ears.—Otalgia, with a sense of obstruction. Deafness. Dry, scaly condition of meatus (use locally).

Abdomen.—Pain extends deep down, causing contraction of sphincter ani.

Rectum.—Many movements a day, with twisting about navel. Hæmorrhoids, with obstructed, hardened stool. Inflamed and painful piles.

Respiratory.—*Hoarse;* voice deep, harsh; sounds like a trumpet; "basso profundo." Cough; worse at night. Asthma. Soreness in pharynx, cough during sleep.

Urinary.—Constant dribbling. *Enuresis.* Burning urination. Increase with pressure in bladder.

Extremities.—Cramp-like pain in soles, right foot, and knee. Lower extremities feel heavy. Thumb feels numb. Neuralgic pain in left ankle. Stiffness *and soreness of joints of lower ex-tremities.*

Modalities.—*Worse*, change of temperature, talking, sneezing, biting hard (inferior dental nerve): from 9 a. m. to 4 p. m.

Relationship.—Compare: *Rhus arom.; Caust.; Platin.; Sphingurus* (pain in zygoma).

Dose.—*Mullein oil*, (locally, for earache and dry, scaly con-dition of meatus. Also for teasing cough at night or lying down. Internally, tincture and lower potencies. *Enuresis,* five-drop doses night and morning.

VERBENA
(Blue Vervain)

Affects the skin and *nervous system*. Nervous depression, weakness and irritation and spasms. Promotes the absorption of blood and allays pain in bruises. Vesicular erysipelas. Passive congestion and intermittent fever. One of the remedies for Poison-oak. *Epilepsy*, insomnia, mental exhaustion. In epilepsy, it *brightens up the patient's mental powers* and helps the constipation.

Dose.—Single dose of the tincture. In epilepsy must be continued for a long time. Verbena in the form of a tea as a diuretic drink is used by Vannier (Paris) to aid elimination in tubercular therapy.

VESPA CRABRO
(Live Wasp)

Skin and female symptoms marked. Indurated feeling. Vasomotor symptoms of skin and mucous membranes.

Dizzy, better lying on back. Fainting. Numbness and blindness. Nausea and vomiting, followed by creeping chills from feet upward. Cramping pain in bowels. Axillary glands swollen with soreness of upper arms. Perspiration on parts laid on with itching.

Face.—Painful and swollen. Erysipelatous inflammation of lids. *Chemosis of conjunctiva.* Swelling of mouth and throat, with violent burning pains.

Urinary.—*Burning* with micturition; also itching.

Female.—Menstruation, preceded by depression, pain, pressure, and constipation. *Left ovary markedly affected,* with *frequent burning, micturition;* sacral pains extending up back. *Erosion around external os.*

Skin.—Erythema; *intense itching;* burning. *Boils;* stinging and soreness, relieved by bathing with vinegar. Wheals, macules and swellings with burning, stinging and soreness. Erythema multiforme, *relieved* by bathing with vinegar.

Relationship.—Compare: *Scorpio* (salivation; strabismus; tetanus); *Apis.*

Antidote: *Sempervivum tector.,* locally.

Dose.—Third to thirtieth potency.

VIBURNUM OPULUS
(High Cranberry)

A general remedy for cramps. Colicky pains in pelvic organs. Superconscious of internal sexual organs. Female symptoms most important. *Often prevents miscarriage.* False labor-pains. Spasmodic and congestive affections, dependent upon ovarian or uterine origin.

Head.—Irritable. Vertigo; feels as if falling forward. Severe pain in temporal region. Sore feeling in eyeballs.

Stomach.—Constant nausea; relieved by eating. No appetite.

Abdomen.—*Sudden cramps and colic pains.* Tender to pressure about umbilicus.

Female.—Menses *too late, scanty, lasting a few hours,* offensive in odor, with crampy pains, cramps extend down thighs. [*Bell.*] Bearing-down pains before. Ovarian region feels heavy and congested. Aching in sacrum and pubes, with pain in anterior muscles of thighs [*Xanthox.*]; *spasmodic and membranous dysmenorrhœa.* [*Borax.*] Leucorrhœa, excoriating. Smarting and itching of genitals. Faint on attempting to sit up. *Frequent and very early miscarriage,* causing seeming sterility. Pains from back to loins and womb worse early morning.

Urinary.—Frequent urging. Copious, pale, light-colored urine. Cannot hold water on coughing or walking.

Rectum.—Stools large and hard, with cutting in rectum and soreness of anus.

Extremities.—Stiff, sore feeling in nape of neck. Feels as if back would break. Sacral backache. Lower extremities weak and heavy.

Modalities.—*Worse,* lying on affected side, in warm room, evening and night. *Better,* in open air and resting.

Relationship.—Compare: *Virburnum prunifolium*—Black Haw—(habitual miscarriage; *after-pains;* cancer of the tongue; obstinate hiccough; supposed to be a uterine tonic. Morning sickness; menstrual irregularities of sterile females with uterine displacements.) *Cimicif.; Cauloph.; Sep.; Xanthox.*

Dose.—Tincture, and lower potencies.

VINCA MINOR
(Lesser Periwinkle)

A remedy for skin affections, eczema, and especially plica polonica; also for hæmorrhages and diphtheria.

Head.—Tearing pain in vertex, ringing and whistling in ears. Whirling vertigo, with flickering before eyes. *Spots on scalp, oozing moisture, matting hair together. Corrosive itching of scalp.* Bald spots. *Plica polonica.* Irresistible desire to scratch.

Nose.—Tip gets red easily. Moist eruption on septum. Stoppage of one nostril. *Sores in nose.* Seborrhœa upper lip and base of nose.

Throat.—Difficult swallowing. Ulcers. Frequent hawking. *Diphtheria.*

Female.—Excessive menstruation with great weakness. *Passive uterine hæmorrhages.* [*Ust.; Trill.; Secale.*] Menorrhagia; continuous flow, particulary at climacteric. [*Lach.*] Hæmorrhages from fibroids.

Skin.—Corrosive itching. *Great sensitiveness of skin, with redness and soreness* from slight rubbing. Eczema of head and face; pustules, itching, burning, and offensive odor. Hair matted together.

Relationship.—Compare: *Oleand.; Staph.*

Dose.—First to third potency.

VIOLA ODORATA
(Violet)

Has a specific action on the ear. Affects especially dark-haired patients; supra-orbital and orbital regions; rheumatism in upper parts of the body when on the *right* side. *Worm affections* in children. [*Teuc.*] Locally, for pain due to uterine fibroids. Also against snake-bites, bee-stings. *Tension* extends to upper half of face and ears.

Head.—*Burning of the forehead.* Vertigo; everything in head seems to whirl around. Heaviness of head, with sensation of weakness in muscles of nape of neck. *Scalp tense; must knit the brows. Tendency to pain immediately above eyebrows.* Throbbing under eye and temple. *Headache across the fore-*

head. Acts upon frontal sinuses. Hysterical attacks in tuberculous patients.

Eyes.—Heaviness of lids. Eyeball feels compressed. Flames before eyes. Myopia. Choroiditis. Illusions of vision; fiery, serpentine circles.

Ears.—Shooting in ears. Aversion to music. Roaring and tickling. Deep stitches beneath ears. Deafness; *otorrhœa.* Ear affections with pain in eyeballs.

Respiratory.—Torpor in the end of nose, as from a blow. Dry, short, spasmodic cough and dyspnœa; worse in daytime. Oppression of chest. Pertussis, with hoarseness. *Dyspnœa during pregnancy.* Difficult breathing, anxiety and palpitation, with hysteria.

Extremities.—Rheumatism of the deltoid muscle. Trembling of limbs. *Pressing pain in right carpal and metacarpal joints.* [*Ulmus.*]

Urinary.—*Milky urine;* smells strong. Enuresis in nervous children.

Modalities.—*Worse,* cool air.

Relationship.—Compare: *Ulmus* (formication in feet, numb, creeping pain in legs and feet; rheumatic pains above wrists; numbness, tingling, and full soreness where gastrocnemius gives off its tendon); *Chenopodium* (*ears; serous or bloody effusion in the labyrinth;* chronic otitis media; progressive *deafness to the voice, but sensitive to sounds* of passing vehicles and other sounds; buzzing; absent or deficient bone conduction; a consciousness of the ear; hearing better for shrill, high-pitched sounds than for low ones); *Aur.; Puls.; Sep.; Ign.; Cina; Cauloph.* (in rheumatism of small joints.)

Dose.—First to sixth potency.

VIOLA TRICOLOR
(Pansy)

The principal uses of this remedy are for eczema in childhood and nocturnal emission accompanied by very vivid dreams.

Head.—Heavy, pressing-outward pain. Eczema of scalp, with swollen glands. Face hot and sweating after eating.

Throat.—Much phlegm, causing hawking; worse in the air. Swallowing difficult.

Urinary.—Copious; disagreeable, cat-like odor.

Male.—Swelling of prepuce, burning in glans. Itching. Involuntary, seminal emissions at stool.

Skin.—*Impetigo.* Intolerable itching. Eruptions, particularly over face and head, with burning, itching; worse at night. Thick scabs, which crack and exude a tenacious yellow pus. Eczema impetigonoides of the face. Sycosis.

Modalities.—*Worse*, winter; 11 a. m. Compare: *Lycop.*

Relationship.—Compare: *Rhus; Calc.; Sepia.*

Dose.—Lower potencies.

VIPERA
(The German Viper)

Viper poisoning causes a temporary increase in reflexes, paresis supervenes, a paraplegia of the lower extremities extending upwards. Resembles acute ascending paralysis of Landry. (Wells.) Has special action on kidneys and induces hæmaturia. Cardiac dropsy.

Indicated in inflammation of veins with great swelling; *bursting sensation. Enlargement of liver.* Ailments of menopause. Œdema of glottis. Poly-neuritis, polio-myelitis.

Face.—Excessively swollen. Lips and tongue swollen, livid, protruding. Tongue dry, brown, black. Speech difficult.

Liver.—Violent pain in enlarged liver, with jaundice and fever; extends to shoulder and hip.

Extremities.—Patient is obliged to keep the extremities elevated. *When they are allowed to hang down, it seems as if they would burst, and the pain is unbearable.* [*Diad.*] *Varicose veins* and acute phlebitis. Veins swollen, sensitive; bursting pain. Severe cramps in lower extremities.

Skin.—Livid. Skin peels in large plates. Lymphangioma, boils, carbuncles, with *bursting* sensation, relieved by elevating parts.

Relationship.—*Pelius berus*—Adder. (Prostration and fainting, faltering pulse, skin yellow, *pain about navel.* Swelling of arm, tongue, right eye; giddiness, nervousness, faintness, sickness, compression of chest, could not breathe properly or take a deep breath; aching and stiffness of limbs, joints stiff, collapsed feeling, great thirst.) *Eel serum* (heart and kidney diseases. Failure of compensation and impending asystole).

Dose.—Twelfth potency.

VISCUM ALBUM
(Mistletoe)

Lowered blood pressure. Dilated blood vessels but does not act on the centers in the medulla. Pulse is slow due to central irritation of the vagus.

The symptoms point especially to rheumatic and gouty complaints; neuralgia, especially sciatica. Epilepsy, *chorea*, and metrorrhagia. *Rheumatic deafness. Asthma.* Spinal pains, due to uterine causes. Rheumatism with *tearing pains.* Hypertensive albuminuria. Valvular disease, with disturbances in sexual sphere. Symptoms like epileptic aura and petit mal.

Head.—Feeling as if whole vault of skull were lifted up. Blue rings around eyes. Double vision. Buzzing and stopped-up feeling in ear. Deafness from cold. Facial muscles in constant agitation. Persistent vertigo.

Respiratory.—Dyspnœa; *feeling of suffocation when lying on left side.* Spasmodic cough. *Asthma*, if connected with gout or rheumatism. Stertorous breathing.

Female.—Hæmorrhage, with pain; blood partly clots and bright red. Climacteric complaints. [*Lach.; Sulph.*] Pain from sacrum into pelvis, with tearing, shooting pains from above downwards. Retained placenta. [*Secale.*] Chronic endometritis. Metrorrhagia. Ovaralgia, especially left.

Heart.—Hypertrophy with valvular insufficiency; pulse small and weak; unable to rest in a reclining position. Palpitation during coitus. Low tension. Failing compensation, dyspnœa worse lying on left side. Weight and oppression of heart; as if a hand were squeezing it; tickling sensation about heart.

Extremities.—Pains alternate in the knee and ankle with shoulder and elbow. *Sciatica. Tearing*, shooting pains in both thighs and upper extremities. A *glow* rises from the feet to the head; seems to be on fire. Periodic pains from sacrum into pelvis, *worse in bed*, with pains into thighs and upper extremities. General tremor, as if all muscles were in state of fibrillary contraction. Dropsy of extremities. Sensation of a spider crawling over back of hand and foot. Itching all over. Compressing pain in feet.

Modalities.—*Worse,* winter, cold, stormy weather; in bed. Movement; lying on left side.

Relationship.—Compare: *Secale; Convallar.; Bry.; Puls.; Rhodod. Guipsine*—active principle—(exalts the hypotensive properties of Viscum). *Hedera Helix*—Ivy—(Intercranial pressure).

Dose.—Tincture and lower potencies.

WYETHIA
(Poison-weed)

Has marked effects on the throat, and has proven an excellent remedy in *pharyngitis,* especially the follicular form. Irritable throats of singers and public speakers. Useful also in hæmorrhoids. Hay-fever symptoms; *itching in posterior nares.*

Head.—Nervous, uneasy, depressed. Dizzy. Rush of blood to head. Sharp pain in forehead.

Mouth.—Feels as if scalded; sensation of heat down œsophagus. Itching of the palate.

Throat.—Constant clearing and hemming. *Dry,* posterior nares; no relief from clearing. *Throat feels swollen;* epiglottis dry and burning. Difficult swallowing. Constant desire to swallow saliva. Uvula feels elongated.

Stomach.—Sense of weight. Belching of wind alternating with hiccough. Nausea and vomiting.

Abdomen.—Pain below ribs of right side.

Stool.—Loose, dark, at night. Itching of anus. Constipation, *with hæmorrhoids;* not bleeding.

Respiratory.—*Dry, hacking cough,* caused by tickling of the epiglottis. Burning sensation in the bronchial tubes. Tendency to get hoarse talking or singing; throat hot, dry. Dry asthma.

Female.—Pain in left ovary, shooting down to knee. Pain in uterus; could outline its contour.

Extremities.—Pain in back; extends to end of spine. Pain right arm, stiffness of wrist and hand. Aching pains all over.

Fever.—Chill at 11 a. m. Thirst for ice-water during chill. No thirst with heat. Profuse sweat all night. Terrific headache during sweat.

Relationship.—Compare: *Arum; Sang.; Lach.*

Dose.—First to sixth potency.

XANTHOXYLUM
(Prickly Ash)

Its specific action is on the nervous system and mucous membranes. Paralysis, especially *hemiplegia*. Painful hæmorrhages, after-pains, *neuralgic dysmenorrhœa*, and rheumatic affections, offer a therapeutic field for this remedy, especially in patients of spare habit and nervous, delicate organization. Indigestion from over-eating or from too much fluid. Sluggish capillary circulation. Neurasthenia, poor assimilation, insomnia, occipital headache. Increases mucous secretion of mouth and stimulates the secretion from all glands with ducts opening in the mouth.

Mind.—Nervous, frightened. Mental depression.

Head.—Feels full. Weight and pain on vertex. Pain over eyes, throbbing pressure over nose, pressure in forehead; head seems divided; ringing in ears. Occipital headache. Sick headache with dizziness and flatulence.

Face.—Neuralgia of lower jaw. Dryness of mouth and fauces. Pharyngitis. [*Wyethia.*]

Abdomen.—Griping and diarrhœa. Dysentery, with *tympanites*, tenesmus; inodorous discharges.

Female.—Menses too early and painful. Ovarian neuralgia, with pain in loins and lower abdomen; worse, *left side*, extending down the thigh, along genito-crural nerves. *Neuralgic dysmenorrhœa*, with neuralgic headaches; pain in *back and down legs*. Menses thick, almost black. *After-pains*. [*Arnica; Cup.; Cham.*] Leucorrhœa at time of menses. Neurasthænic patients who are thin, emaciated; poor assimilation with insomnia and occipital headache.

Respiratory.—Aphonia. Constant desire to take a long breath; oppression of chest. Dry cough, day and night.

Extremities.—Paralysis of left side following spinal disorders. Numbness of left side; impairment of nerves of motion. Hemiplegia. Pain in nape, extending down back. Sciatica; worse, hot weather. Anterior, crural neuralgia. [*Staph.*] Left arm numb. Neuralgic shooting pain, as from electricity, all over limbs.

Sleep.—Hard and unrefreshing; dreams of flying. Sleeplessness in neurasthenics.

Relationship.—Compare: *Gnaph.; Cimicif.; Staph.; Mezer.; Piscidia*—White dogwood—(a nerve sedative. *Insomnia due to worry*, nervous excitement, spasmodic coughs; pains of irregular menstruation; regulates the flow. Neuralgic and spasmodic affections. Use tincture in rather material doses.)

Dose.—First to sixth potency.

XEROPHYLLUM

(Tamalpais Lily. Basket Grass Flower)

Should prove curative in eczematous conditions, poison-oak, early typhoid states, etc.

Mind.—Dull, cannot concentrate mind for study; forgets names; *writes last letters of words first;* misspells common words.

Head.—Feels full, stuffed up, pain across forehead and above eyes. Great pressure at root of nose. Bewildered. Loss of consciousness. Pulsating headache.

Eyes.—Painful, as of sand, smarting; difficult to focus for close work. Eyes feel sore, burn.

Nose.—Stuffed; tightness at bridge of nose; acute nasal catarrh.

Face.—Bloated in morning. Puffy under eyes.

Throat.—Stitching pain upon swallowing.

Stomach.—Feels full and heavy. Eructations sour; offensive, an hour after luncheon and dinner. Vomiting at 2 p. m.

Abdomen.—Intestinal flatulence. In morning rumbling in bowels, with desire for stool.

Rectum.—Constipation, stools hard, small lumps. Difficult, soft stools, with much straining. Much flatus. Bearing-down pain in rectum.

Urine.—Difficulty of retaining; dribbling when walking. Frequent urination at night.

Female.—Bearing-down sensation. Vulva inflamed, with furious itching. Increased sexual desire, with ovarian and uterine pains and leucorrhœa.

Respiratory.—Posterior nares raw; discharge thick, yellow mucus. Sneezing. Trachea sore; lumps feel constricted.

Back.—Feels hot from sacrum to scapulæ. Backache, extending down legs. Pain over kidneys. Heat deep in spine.

Extremities.—Muscular lameness, trembling. Pain in knees. Limbs feel stiff. [*Rhus.*]

Skin.—Erythema, with vesication and intense itching, stinging, and burning. Blisters, little lumps. Skin rough and cracked; feels like leather. Dermatitis, especially around knees. Inflammation resembling poison-oak. Inguinal glands and behind knee swollen.

Modalities.—*Worse*, application of cold water, in afternoon and evening. *Better*, application of hot water, in morning, moving affected part.

Relationship.—Compare: *Rhus; Anacard.; Grindelia.*

Dose.—Sixth potency or higher.

X-RAY

(Vial containing alcohol exposed to X-Ray)

Repeated exposure to Roentgen (X-ray) has produced skin lesions often followed by cancer. Distressing pain. Sexual glands are particularly affected. Atrophy of ovaries and testicles. Sterility. Changes take place in the blood lymphatics and bone marrow. Anæmia and leukæmia. Corresponds to stubbornness as in burns, they refuse to heal. Psoriasis.

Has the property of stimulating cellular metabolism. Arouses the reactive vitality, mentally and physically. Brings to the surface suppressed symptoms, especially sycotic and those due to mixed infections. Its homœopathic action is thus centrifugal, towards the periphery.

Head.—Sticking pains in different parts of head and face. Dull pain in right upper jaw. Stiff neck. Sudden cricks in neck, pains more severe behind ears. Pain in muscles of neck when lifting head from pillow. Fullness in ears, ringing in head.

Mouth.—Tongue dry, rough, sore. Throat painful on swallowing. Nausea.

Male.—Lewd dreams. Sexual desire lost. Re-establishes suppressed gonorrhœa.

Extremities.—Rheumatic pains. General tired and sick feeling. Palms rough and scaly.

Skin.—Dry, itching eczema. Erythema around roots of nails. Skin dry, wrinkled. Painful cracks. Warty growths. Nails thicken. Psoriasis.

Modalities.—*Worse*, in bed, afternoon, evening and night; open air.

Dose.—Twelfth potency and higher.

Compare: *Electricitas.*—Sugar of milk saturated with the current. (Anxiety, nervous tremors, restlessness, palpitation, headaches. Dreads approach of thunder-storms; heaviness of limbs.)

Magnetis Poli Ambo.—The Magnet.—Sugar of milk or distilled water exposed to influence of entire mass. (Burning lancinations throughout the body; pains as if broken in joints, when cartilages of two bones touch; shooting and jerkings; headache as if a nail were driven in; tendency of old wounds to bleed afresh.)

Magnetis Polus Arcticus.—North pole of the magnet.—(Disturbed sleep, somnambulism, cracking in cervical vertebræ, sensation of coldness; toothache.)

Magnetis Polus Australis.—South pole of the magnet.—(Severe pain in inner side of nail of the big toe, *ingrowing toenail;* easy dislocation of joints of foot; feet are painful when letting them hang down.)

YOHIMBINUM

(Coryanthe Yohimbe)

Excites sexual organs and acts on central nervous system and respiratory centre. An aphrodisiac, used in physiological doses, but contraindicated in all acute and chronic inflammations of abdominal organs. Homœopathically, should be of service in congestive conditions of the sexual organs. Causes hyperæmia of the milk glands and stimulates the function of lactation. Menorrhagia.

Head.—Agitation, with flying sensations of heat in face. Disagreeable, metallic taste. Copious salivation. Nausea and eructation.

Sexual.—*Strong and lasting erections.* Neurasthenic impotence. Bleeding piles. Intestinal hæmorrhage. Urethritis.

Fever.—Rigor; intense heat, waves of heat and chilliness, tendency to sweat.

Sleep.—*Sleepless.* Thoughts of events of whole past life keep him awake.

Dose.—As a sexual stimulant, ten drops of a one per cent. solution, or hypodermic tablets of 0.005 gm. Homœopathic dose, third potency.

YUCCA FILAMENTOSA
(Bear-grass)

So-called bilious symptoms, with headache. Despondent and irritable.

Head.—Aches as if top of head would fly off. Arteries of forehead throb. Nose red.

Face.—Yellow; tongue yellow, coated, taking imprint of teeth. [*Merc.; Pod.; Rhus.*]

Mouth.—Taste as of rotten eggs. [*Arnica.*]

Throat.—Sensation as if something hung down from posterior nares; cannot get it up or down.

Abdomen.—Deep pain in right side over liver, going through back. Stool yellowish brown, with bile.

Male.—Burning and swelling of the prepuce, with redness of meatus. Gonorrhœa. [*Cann.; Tussil.*]

Skin.—Erythematous redness.

Dose.—Tincture, to third potency.

ZINCUM METALLICUM
(Zinc)

The provings picture cerebral depression. The word "fag" covers a large part of zinc action. Tissues are worn out faster than they are repaired. Poisoning from suppressed eruptions or discharges. The nervous symptoms of most importance. Defective vitality. Impending brain paralysis. *Period of depression in disease.* Spinal affections. Twitchings. Pain, as if between skin and flesh. Great relief from discharges. Chorea, from fright or suppressed eruption. *Convulsions, with pale face and no heat.* Marked anæmia with profound prostration. It causes a decrease in the number, and destruction of red blood corpuscles. Repercussed eruptive diseases. In chronic diseases with brain and spinal symptoms, trembling, convulsive twitching and fidgety feet are guiding symptoms.

Mind.—Weak memory. *Very sensitive to noise.* Averse to work, to talk. *Child repeats everything said to it.* Fears arrest on account of a supposed crime. Melancholia. *Lethargic, stupid.* Paresis.

Head.—Feels as if he would fall to left side. Headache from the smallest quantity of wine. Hydrocephalus. Rolls head from side to side. Bores head into pillow. *Occipital* pain, with weight on vertex. Automatic motion of head and hands. Brain-fag; headaches of overtaxed school children. *Forehead cool; base of brain hot.* Roaring in head. Starting in fright.

Eyes.—Pterygium; smarting, lachrymation, itching. Pressure as if pressed into head. Itching and soreness of lids and *inner angles.* Ptosis. *Rolling of eyes.* Blurring of one-half of vision; worse, stimulants. *Squinting.* Amaurosis, with severe headache. Red and inflamed conjunctiva; *worse, inner canthus.*

Ears.—Tearing, stitches, and external swelling. Discharge of fetid pus.

Nose.—Sore feeling high up; pressure upon root.

Face.—*Pale* lips, and corners of mouth cracked. Redness and itching eruption on chin. Tearing in facial bones.

Mouth.—Teeth loose. Gums bleed. Gnashing of teeth. Bloody taste. Blisters on tongue. Difficult dentition; child weak; cold and restless feet.

Throat.—Dry; constant inclination to hawk up tenacious mucus. Rawness and dryness in throat and larynx. Pain in muscles of throat when swallowing.

Stomach.—Hiccough, nausea, vomiting of bitter mucus. Burning in stomach, heartburn from sweet things. *Cannot stand smallest quantity of wine. Ravenous hunger* about 11 a. m. [*Sulph.*] Great greediness when eating; cannot eat fast enough. Atonic dyspepsia, feeling as if stomach were collapsed.

Abdomen.—Pain after a light meal, with tympanitis. Pain in spot beneath navel. Gurgling and griping; distended. Flatulent colic, with retraction of abdomen. [*Plumb.*] Enlarged, indurated sore liver. Reflex symptoms from floating kidney. *Griping after eating.*

Urine.—Can only void urine when sitting bent backwards. Hysterical retention. Involuntary urination when walking, coughing or sneezing.

Rectum.—Hard, small, constipated stool. *Cholera infantum,* with tenesmus; green mucous discharges. Sudden cessation of diarrhœa, followed by cerebral symptoms.

Male.—Testicles swelled, drawn up. Erections violent. Emissions with hypochondriasis. Falling off of hair (pubic). Drawing in testicles up to spermatic cord.

Female.—Ovarian pain, *especially left; can't keep still.* [*Viburn.*] Nymphomania of lying-in women. Menses too late, suppressed; lochia suppressed. [*Puls.*] Breasts painful. Nipples sore. 'Menses flow more at night. [*Bov.*] Complaints all *better during menstrual flow.* [*Eupion; Lach.*] *All the female symptoms are associated with restlessness, depression, coldness, spinal tenderness and restless feet.* Dry cough before and during menses.

Respiratory.—Burning pressure beneath sternum. Constriction and cutting in chest. Hoarseness. Debilitating, spasmodic cough; worse, eating sweet things. Child grasps genitals during cough. Asthmatic bronchitis, with constriction of chest. *Dyspnœa better as soon as expectoration appears.*

Back.—Pain in small of back. Cannot bear back *touched.* [*Sul.; Therid.; Cinch.*] Tension and stinging between shoulders. Spinal irritation. *Dull aching about the last dorsal or first lumbar vertebræ; worse sitting. Burning along spine. Nape of neck weary from writing or any exertion.* Tearing in shoulder-blades.

Extremities.—Lameness, *weakness, trembling and twitching* of various muscles. Chilblains. [*Agar.*] *Feet in continued motion; cannot keep still. Large varicose veins on legs.* Sweaty. Convulsions, *with pale face. Transverse pains,* especially in upper extremity. *Soles of feet sensitive.* Steps with entire sole of foot on floor.

Sleep.—Cries out during sleep; body jerks; wakes frightened, stared. Nervous motion of feet when asleep. Loud screaming out at night in sleep without being aware of it. Somnambulism. [*Kali phos.*]

Skin.—*Varicose veins*, especially of lower extremities. [*Puls.*] Formication of feet and legs as from bugs crawling over the skin, preventing sleep. Eczema, especially in the anæmic and neurotic. Itching of thighs and *hollow of knees. Retrocession of eruptions.*

Fever.—Frequent, febrile shiverings down back. Cold extremities. Night-sweat. Profuse sweat on feet.

Modalities.—*Worse*, at menstrual period, from touch, between 5 to 7 p. m.; after dinner, from wine. *Better*, while eating, discharges, and appearance of eruptions.

Relationship.—Compare: *Agaric.; Ign.; Plumb.; Argent.; Puls.; Helleb.; Tuberc.* Inimical: *Nux; Cham.* Compare in amelioration by secretions: *Lach.; Stan.; Mosch.*

Compare: *Zincum aceticum* (effects of night-watching and erysipelas; brain feels sore; *Rademacher's solution*, five-drop doses three times a day in water, *for those who are compelled to work, on an insufficient amount of sleep*); *Zinc, bromatum* (dentition, chorea, hydrocephalus; *Zinc. oxydatum.* (Nausea and sour taste. Sudden vomiting in children. Vomiting of bile and diarrhœa. Flatulent abdomen. Watery stools with tenesmus. Debility after grip. Fiery red face, *great drowsiness* with dream-like unrefreshing sleep. Similar to effect of night watching. Mental and physical exertion (Rademacher). *Zinc. Sulph.*, not repeated frequently (high potency) will clear up opacities of the cornea (McFarland). Corneitis; granular lids; tongue paralyzed; cramps in arms and legs; trembling and convulsions. Hypochrondriasis due to masturbation; nervous headaches); *Zinc. cyanatum* (as a remedy for meningitis and cerebro-spinal meningitis, paralysis agitans, chorea, and hysteria, it has received some attention); *Zinc. ars.* (chorea, anæmia, *profound exhaustion* on slight exertion. Depression and marked involvement of lower extremities); *Zinc. carb.* (post-gonorrhœal throat affections, tonsils swollen, bluish superficial spots); *Zinc. phos.* (herpes zoster 1x); *Zinc. muriat.* (disposition to pick the bedclothes; sense of smell and taste perverted; bluish-green tint of skin; cold and sweaty); *Zinc. phos.* (neuralgia of head and face; lightning-like pains in locomotor ataxia, brain-fag, nervousness, and vertigo; sexual excitement and sleeplessness); *Ammon. valerian* (violent neuralgia, with great nervous agitation); *Zinc. picricum* (facial paralysis; brain-fag, headache in Bright's disease; seminal emissions; loss of memory and energy). Oxide of zinc is used locally as an astringent and stimulant application to unhealthy ulcers, fissures, intertrigo, burns, etc.

Dose.—Second to sixth potency.

ZINCUM VALERIANUM
(Valerinate of Zinc)

A remedy for *neuralgia*, hysteria, angina pectoris, and other *painful* affections, notably in *ovarian affections*. Epilepsy without aura. Hysterical heart-pain. *Facial* neuralgia, violent in left temple and inferior maxillary. Sleeplessness in children. Obstinate *hiccough*.

Head.—Violent, neuralgic, *intermittent headaches*. Becomes almost insane with pain, which is piercing and stabbing. Uncontrollable sleeplessness from pain in head with melancholy.

Female.—*Ovaralgia; pain shoots down limbs,* even to foot.

Extremities.—Severe pain in neck and spine. Cannot sit still; must keep legs in constant motion. Sciatic neuralgia.

Dose.—First and second trituration. Must be continued for some time in treatment of neuralgia.

ZINGIBER
(Ginger)

States of debility in the digestive tract, and sexual system and respiratory troubles, call for this remedy. Complete cessation of function of kidneys.

Head.—Hemicrania; sudden glimmering before eyes; feels confused and empty. Pain over eyebrows.

Nose.—Feels obstructed and dry. Intolerable itching; red pimples.

Stomach.—Taste of food remains long, especially of bread and toast. Feels heavy, like from a stone. *Complaints from eating melons and drinking impure water. Acidity.* [*Calc.;*

Robinia.] Heaviness in stomach on awakening with wind and rumbling, great thirst and emptiness. Pain from pit to under sternum, worse eating.

Abdomen.—Colic, diarrhœa, extremely loose bowels. Diarrhœa from drinking bad water, with much flatulence, cutting pain, relaxation of sphincter. Hot, sore, painful anus during pregnancy. Chronic intestinal catarrh. Anus red and inflamed. Hæmorrhoids hot, painful, sore. [*Aloe.*]

Urinary.—Frequent desire to urinate. Stinging, burning in orifice. Yellow discharge from urethra. Urine thick, turbid, of strong odor, suppressed. Complete suppression after typhoid. After urinating, continues to ooze in drops.

Male.—Itching of prepuce. Sexual desire excited; painful erections. Emissions.

Respiratory.—Hoarseness. *Smarting below larynx;* breathing difficult. *Asthma,* without anxiety, *worse* toward morning. Scratching sensation in throat; stitches in chest. Cough dry, hacking; copious morning sputa.

Extremities.—Very weak in all joints. Back lame. Cramps in soles and palms.

Relationship.—Compare: *Calad.*

Antidote: *Nux.*

Dose.—First to sixth potency.

REPERTORY

MIND

AWKWARD—Lets things fall from hand: Æth.; *Apis; Bov.;* Helleb.; Ign.; Lach.; *Nat. m.;* Nux v.; Tar. h.

BRAIN-FAG—*Æth.;* Ail.; Alfal.; *Anac.;* Anhal.; *Arg. n.;* Avena; Bapt.; *Calc. e.; Calc. p.;* Coca; *Cocc.;* Cupr. m.; *Gels.;* Kali br.; *Kali p.;* Lecith.; Nat. m.; Nux v.; *Phos. ac.; Phos.; Picr. ac.;* Sil.; *Strych. p.;* Zinc. m.; *Zinc. p.; Zinc. picr.* See Neurasthenia (Nervous System).

CATALEPSY—Trance: Acon.; Art. v.; Camph. monobr.; *Can. ind.;* Cham.; Cic.; *Crot. casc.;* Cur.; Gels.; Graph.; Hydroc. ac.; Hyos.; Lach.; Merc.; *Morph.; Mosch.;* Nux m.; *Op.;* Sabad.; Stram.

CLAIRVOYANCE—*Acon.; Anac.;* Anhal.; Can. ind.; Nabulus; Nux m.; *Phos.* See Hallucinations.

COMPREHENSION—Difficult: Agn.; *Ail.; Anac.;* Bapt.; Cocc.; *Gels.; Helleb.;* Lyc.; Nat. c.; *Nux m.;* Oleand.; *Op.; Phos. ac.;* Phos.; Plumb. m.; Xerophyl.; *Zinc. m.* See Memory.

COMPREHENSION—Easy: Bell.; *Coff.;* Lach.

CONSCIOUSNESS—Loss: Absinth.; *Ail.;* Arn.; Atrop.; *Bell.; Can. ind.;* Carb. ac.; *Cic.;* Cupr. ac.; Gels.; Glon.; *Helleb.; Hydroc. ac.; Hyos.;* Mur. ac.; Nux m.; Œnanthe; *Op.;* Stram.; Xerophyl.; *Zinc. m.*

CRETINISM—Imbecility, Idiocy: Absinth.; *Æth.; Anac.;* Arn.; Bac.; *Bar. c.;* Bar. m.; *Bufo;* Calc. p.; Helleb.; Ign.; Iod.; Lol.; Nat. c.; Oxytrop.; Phos. ac.; Plumb. m.; Sul.; *Thyr.*

DELIRIUM—Alcoholic (delirium tremens): Acon.; *Agar.;* Ant. t.; *Atrop.; Bell.; Can. ind.;* Caps.; Chin. s.; Cim.; Dig.; Hyos.; *Hyosc. hydrobr.; Kali br.;* Kali p.; Lach.; Lupul.; *Nux v.;* Op.; Passifl.; Pastin.; *Ran. b.; Stram.;* Strych. n.; Sumb.; Teucr.

Carphologia (picking at bed clothes, flocks)—Agar.; Atrop.; *Bell.;* Helleb.; *Hyos.;* Mur. ac.; Op.; *Stram.;* Zinc. mur.

Coma Vigil—Cur.; *Hyos.;* Mur. ac.; Op.; Phos.

Destructive (desire to bark, bite, strike, tear things)—*Bell.; Canth.;* Cupr. m.; Hyos.; Sec.; *Stram.; Ver. a.;* Ver. v.

Effort to escape from bed, or hide—Acon.; *Agar.; Bell.; Bry.;* Cupr. m.; Helleb.; *Hyos.;* Operc.; Op.; Rhus t.; *Stram.; Ver. a.*

Furor, frenzy, ravings—Acon.; Agar.; *Bell.; Canth.;* Cic.; Cupr. m.; *Hyos.;* Merc. cy.; Œnanthe; Solan. n.; *Stram.; Ver. a.*

Lascivious furor—*Canth.; Hyos.;* Phos.; Stram.; Ver. a.

Loquacity, talks incessantly—*Agar.;* Bell.; Can. ind.; *Cim.; Hyos.; Lach.;* Merc. cy.; Oper.; Op.; *Stram.;* Ver. a.

Merry, dancing, singing—Agar.; *Bell.; Hyos.;* Stram.; Ver. a.

Muttering, low, incoherently—Agar.; *Ail.;* Apis; Arn.; Bapt.; Bell.; Crot.; Helleb.; *Hyos.;* Lach.; *Mur. ac.; Phos. ac.;* Phos.; *Rhus t.;* Stram.; Ver. a.

Rapid answering—Cim.; *Lach.;* Stram.; Ver. a.

Slow answering, relapses—Arn.; Bapt.; Diph.; *Helleb.;* Hyos.; *Phos. ac.;* Phos.; Sul.

Sopor, stupor, coma—Æth.; Agar.; *Ail.;* Am. c.; *Ant. t.; Apis;* Arn.; *Bapt.;* Bell.; Benz. nit.; *Camph.; Carb.* ac.; Diph.; Gels.; *Helleb.; Hyos.;* Lach.; Laur.; Lob. purp.; Mur. ac.; Nitr. sp. d.; Nux m.; *Op.; Phos. ac.;* Phos.; Piloc.; *Rhus t.;* Stram.; Tereb.; Thyr.; Ver. a.; *Zinc. m.*

DEMENTIA—*Agar.; Anac.;* Apium v.; *Bell.;* Calc. c.; Calc. p.; Can. ind.; Con.; Helleb.; *Hyos.;* Ign.; *Lil t.;* Merc.; *Nat. sal.;* Op.; *Phos. ac.;* Phos.; *Picr. ac.;* Sul.; *Ver. a.*

Epileptic—Acon.; *Bell.;* Cim.; *Cupr. ac.;* Cupr. m.; Laur.; *Œnanthæ; Sil.;* Solan. c.; Stram.; Ver. v.

Masturbatic—*Agn.;* Calc. p.; Canth.; Caust.; Damiana; Nux v.; Op.; *Phos. ac.;* Phos.; Picr. ac.; *Staph.*

Paretic—*Acon.; Æsc. gl.;* Agar.; Ars.; *Bad.;* Bell.; Can. ind.; Cim.; Cupr. m.; Hyos.; Ign.; Iodof.; Merc.; *Phos.; Plumb. m.;* Stram.; Ver. v.; Zinc. m.

Senile—Anac.; *Aur. iod.;* Bar. ac.; *Bar. c.;* Calc. p.; Con.; Nat. iod.; Phos.; Sec.

Syphilitic—Aur. iod.; *Kali iod.;* Mercuries; Nit. ac.; Sul.

EMOTIONS—**Effects: Anger, bad news, disappointment, vexation:** Acon.; Apis; Ars.; Aur.; *Bry.;* Caust.; *Cham.;* Cocc.; Colch.; *Col.; Gels.;* Grat.; Hyos.; Ign.; Lach.; Nat. m.; *Nux v.;* Phos. ac.; Puls.; Sep.; *Staph.*

Fright, fear—*Acon.;* Apis; Aur.; Bell.; *Gels.;* Hyos.; Hyper.; Ign.; Nat. m., Morph.; *Op.;* Puls.; Samb.; Ver. a.

Grief, sorrow—Am. m.; Ant. c.; Apis; Aur. m.; Calc. p.; Caust.; *Cocc.;* Cycl.; Hyos.; *Ign.;* Lach.; Nat. m.; *Phos. ac.;* Plat.; Samb.

Jealousy—Apis; Hyos.; *Lach.;* Staph.

Joy, excessive—Caust.; *Coff.;* Croc.

Nostalgia (homesickness)—*Caps.;* Eup. purp.; Helleb.; *Ign.;* Mag. m.; *Phos. ac.;* Senec.

Shame, mortification, reserved displeasure—Aur.; Ign.; Nat. m.; *Staph.*

FEARS—**Dread: Being carried or raised:** *Bor.;* Bry.; Sanic.

Crossing streets, crowds, excitement—*Acon.;* Hydroc. ac.; Plat.

Dark, ghosts—*Acon.; Ars.;* Bell.; Carb. v.; Caust.; Hyos.; Lyc.; Med.; Op.; *Phos.; Puls.;* Radium; Rhus t.; *Stram.*

Death, fatal diseases, impending evil—*Acon.; Agn.;* Anac.; *Apis;* Arg. n.; *Ars.; Aur.; Cact.;* Calc. c.; Can. ind.; *Cim.; Dig.;* Gels.; Graph.; Hydr.; Ign.; Kali c.; Lac c.; *Lil. t.;* Med.; Naja; Nat. m.; *Nit. ac.; Nux v.;* Phaseol.; *Phos.; Plat.;* Pod.; *Psor.;* Puls.; Rhus t.; Sabad.; *Sec.;* Sep.; Stann.; Staph.; Still.; Syph.; Ver. a.

Downward motion, falling—*Bor.;* Gels.; Hyper.; *Sanic.*

Heart ceases beating, must move—Gels. (reverse Dig.).

Lectophobia—Can. s.

Loss of reason—*Acon.;* Alum.; *Arg. n.;* Calc. c.; Can. ind.; Chlorum; *Cim.;* Iod.; Kali br.; Lac c.; *Lil. t.;* Lyssin; *Mancin.;* Med.; Plat.; Sep.; Syph.; Ver. a.

Motion—*Bry.;* Calad.; Gels.; Mag. p.

Music—*Acon.; Ambra;* Bufo; *Nat. c.;* Nux v.; *Sab.;* Tar. h.; Thuya.

Noises—Acon.; *Asar.; Bell.; Bor.;* Calad.; *Cham.;* Cocc.; Ferr.; Ign.; Kali c.; Mag. m.; Med.; Nat. c.; Nit. ac.; *Nux v.; Phos.;* Sil.; Tanac.; Tar. h.; *Ther.;* Zinc. m.

People (anthropophobia)—*Acon.;* Ambra.; Anac.; *Aur.; Bar. c.;* Con.; Gels.; Ign.; Iod.; Kali p.; Lyc.; Meli.; Nat. c.; Nat. m.; *Sep.;* Stann.; *Staph.*

Places closed—Succin.

Pointed objects—Sil.; Spig.

Poison—*Hyos.;* Kali br.; Lach.; Rhus t.; Ver. v.

Rain—Naja.

Solitude, aversion to—Ant. t.; Ars.; *Bism.;* Con.; *Hyos.; Kali. c.;* Lac c.; Lil. t.; *Lyc.;* Naja; *Phos.;* Puls.; Radium; Sep.; *Stram.;* Thymol; Ver. a.

Solitude, desire for—Ambra; Aragal.; *Ars. m.;* Aur.; *Bar. c.;* Bry.; *Bufo;* Cact.; Caps.; *Carbo an.;* Cim.; *Coca;* Cycl.; *Gels.;* Ign.; Iod.; Nat. c.; Nat. m.; *Nux v.;* Oxytr.; Phos. ac.; *Staph.;* Thuya.

Space (agoraphobia)—*Acon.;* Arg. n.; Arn.; *Calc. c.;* Hydroc. ac.; Nux v.

Stage-fright—Anac.; Arg. n.; *Gels.*

Syphilis—Hyos.

Thunderstorms—Bor.; Electricitas; *Nat. c.; Phos.;* Psor.; Rhod.; Sil.

Touch, contact—*Acon.;* Angust. sp.; *Ant. c.;* Ant. t.; Apis; *Arn.; Bell.; Cham.;* Cina; *Cinch.; Colch.; Hep.;* Iod.; *Kali c.; Lach ;* Mag. p.; Nit. ac.; Nux m.; *Nux v.;* Phos.; *Plumb.;* Sanic.; Sep.; *Spig.;* Stram.; Sul.; *Tar. h.;* Thuya.

Water (hydrophobia)—Agave; Anag.; Ant. c.; *Bell.; Canth.;* Coccinel.; Fagus; *Hyos.; Lach.;* Laur.; *Lyssin;* Spirea; *Stram.;* Sul.; Tanac.; Ver. a.; Xanth. sp.

HYPOCHONDRIASIS—Alfal.; Aloe; Alum.; *Anac.; Arg. n.; Ars.; Aur. m.;* Aur. mur.; Avena; Cact.; *Calc. c.; Cim.;* Con.; Ferr. m.; Helon.; Hydroc. ac.; Hyos.; *Ign.;* Kali br.; *Kali p.; Lyc.;* Merc.; Nat. c.; *Nat. m.; Nux v.; Phos. ac.;* Plumb.; Pod.; Puls.; Stann.; *Staph.; Sul.;* Sumb.; Tar. h.; Thasp. a.; Thuya; Val.; *Ver. a.;* Zinc. m.; Zinc. oxy.

HYSTERIA—Acon.; Agn.; *Ambra;* Am. val.; Apis; Aquil.; *Asaf.;* Aster.; Bell.; Cact.; Cajup.; Camph. monobr.; Can. ind.; Castor.; Caul.; Cham.; *Cim.; Cocc.;* Con.; *Croc.; Eup. ar.; Gels.;* Hyos.; *Ign.; Kali p.;* Lil. t.; Mag. m.; *Mosch.;* Myg.; *Nux m.;* Orig.; Phos. ac.; *Phos.; Plat.;* Poth.; *Puls.;* Scutel.; Senec.; *Sep.;* Stram.; Strych. p.; *Sumb.;* Tar. h.; Ther.; *Val.; Zinc. v.*

IMAGINATION—**Fancies, hallucinations, illusions: Acute vivid:** *Absinth.;* Acon.; Agar.; Ambra; *Bell.; Can. ind.;* Dub.; *Hyos.;* Kali c.; *Lach.; Op.;* Rhus t.; Scopal.; *Stram.;* Sul.; *Ver. a.* See Hallucinations.

Away from home, must get there—*Bry.;* Calc. p.; Cim.; Hyos.; *Op.*

Bed occupied by another person—Petrol.

Bed sinking—Bapt.; Bell.; *Benz.;* Kali c.

Bed too hard—*Arn.; Bapt.;* Bry.; *Morph.; Pyr.;* Ruta.

Being abused or criticized—*Bar. c.;* Cocaine; Hyos.; Ign.; Pallad.; Staph.

Being assassinated—Absinth.; Kali br.; Plumb. m.
Being broken in fragments, scattered about—*Bapt.;* Daph.; *Petrol.;* Phos.; Stram.
Being crushed by houses—Arg. n.
Being dead—Apis; *Lach.;* Mosch.; *Op.*
Being demon, curses, swears—Anac.
Being doomed, lost to salvation—Acon.; Ars.; Aur.; Cycl.; Lach.; *Lil. t.;* Lyc.; Meli.; Op.; *Plat.;* Psor.; Puls.; Stram.; Sul.; *Ver. a.*
Being double, (dual personality)—*Anac.; Bapt.;* Can. ind.; Petrol.; *Stram.;* Thuya; Val.
Being enveloped in dark cloud, world black and sinister—Arg. n.; *Cim.; Lac c.;* Puls.
Being frightened by a mouse running from under a chair—*Æth.; Cim.;* Lac c.
Being guilty of some committed crime—Ars.; Cina; *Cycl.; Ign.;* Nux v.; Ruta; Staph.; *Ver. a.;* Zinc. m.
Being hollow in organs—*Cocc.;* Oxytr.
Being in strange surroundings—*Cic.;* Hyos., Plat.; Tub.
Being light, spirit-like, hovering in the air—*Asar.; Dat. arb.;* Hyper.; *Lac c.;* Latrod. has.; Nat. ars.; Op.; Rhus gl.; *Sticta; Val.*
Being made of glass, wood, etc.—Eupion; Rhus t.; *Thuya.*
Being occupied about business—*Bry.;* Op
Being persecuted by his enemies—*Anac.;* Cinch.; *Cocaine; Hyos.;* Kali br.; *Lach.;* Nux v.; Plumb. m.; Rhus t.; Stram.
Being poisoned—*Hyos.;* Lach.; Rhus t.; Ver. v.
Being possessed of two wills—*Anac.;* Lach.
Being possessed of brain in stomach—Acon.
Being possessed of two noses—Merc. per.
Being pregnant, or something alive in the abdomen—*Croc.;* Cycl.; *Op.;* Sabad.; Sul.; *Thuya;* Ver. a.
Being pursued—*Anac.;* Hyos.; Stram.
Being separated body and soul—*Anac.;* Nit. ac.; Thuya.
Being swollen—Acon.; *Aran.; Arg. n.;* Asaf.; Bapt.; *Bov.; Can. ind.;* Glon.; Op.; Plat.
Being under superhuman control—*Anac.; Lach.;* Op.; Plat.; Thuya.
Being very sick.—Ars.; Pod.; Sabad.
Being very wealthy—Phos.; *Plat.;* Pyr.; *Sul.;* Ver. a.
Dimensions of things larger—Acon.; Agar.; *Arg. n.;* Atrop.; Bov.; *Can. ind.; Gels.;* Glon.; *Hyos.;* Op.; Paris.
Dimensions of things reversed—Camph. monobr.
Dimensions of things smaller.—Plat.
Duration of time and space lost or confused—Anhal.; *Can. ind.;* Cic.; *Glon.;* Lach.
Duration of time changed, it passes too rapidly—*Cocc.;* Ther.
Duration of time changed, it passes too slowly—*Alum.;* Ambra; Anhal.; *Arg. n.; Can. ind.;* Med.; Nux m.; Nux v.
Hallucinations—Remedies in general: *Absinth.; Agar.;* Ambra; *Anac.;* Anhal.; *Antipyr.;* Ars.; Atrop.; *Bell.; Can. ind.;* Cantn.; Cham.;

Chloral; Cim.; Cocaine; *Crot. casc.; Hyos.;* Kali br.; Lach.; Nat. sal.; Nux v.; *Op.:* Phos.; *Stram.;* Sul.; Thea; Trion.; Zinc. mur.

Hallucinations, auditory (bells, music, voices)—Agar.; *Anac.; Antipyr.;* Ars.; Bell.; *Can. ind.;* Carbon. s.; *Cham.;* Cocaine; Elaps; Merc.; Naja; Nat. p.; Puls.; *Stram.;* Thea.

Hallucinations, olfactory—*Agn.; Anac.;* Ars.; Euph. amv.; *Op.;* Paris; Puls.; Zinc. mur.

Hallucinations, tactile—Anac.; Canth.; *Op.;* Stram.

Hallucinations, visual (animals, bugs, faces)—*Absinth.;* Agar.; Ambra; Anhal.; *Antipyr.;* Ars.; *Atrop.; Bell.;* Calc. c.; *Can. ind.;* Cim.; Cocaine; *Hyos.;* Kali br.; Lach.; *Morph.;* Nat. sal.; *Op.;* Pastin.; Phos.; Plat.; Puls.; Sant.: *Stram.;* Sul.; Val.; Ver. a.

INSANITY—See Mania, Melancholia, Dementia.

LOQUACITY—*Agar.;* Ambra; Bell.; Can. ind.; *Cim.;* Cocaine; Eug. j.; *Hyos.; Lach.;* Op.; Pastin.; Physal.; *Stram.;* Tar. h.; Val.; Ver. a.

MANIA—Remedies in general: Absinth.; *Acon.;* Agar.; *Anac.;* Arn.; Ars.; Atrop.; Bapt.; *Bell.;* Bry.; *Can. ind.; Canth.;* Chloral; *Cim.;* Cinch.; Croc.; *Crot. casc.;* Cupr. ac.; Cupr. m.; Glon.; *Hyos.;* Kali br.; *Lach.;* Laur.; Lil. t.; Lyc.; Merc.; Nat. m.; Nux v.; *Op.;* Orig.; Passifl.; Phos.; Picr. ac.; Piscidia; *Plat.;* Puls.; Rhus t.; Sec.; *Solan. n.;* Spig. mar.; Spong.; Sul. hydr.; Sul.: *Stram.;* Tar. h.; Ust.; *Ver. a.;* Ver. v.

Erotomania (nymphomania, satyriasis)—Ambra; Apis: Bar. m.; Calc. p.; *Can. ind.; Canth.;* Ferrula gl.; Ginseng; Grat.; *Hyos.;* Lil. t.; Mancin.; *Murex;* Orig.; *Phos.;* Picr. ac.; Plat.; Robin.; Salix n.; *Stram.;* Tar. h.; Ver. a.

Lypemania—Ars.; *Aur.;* Caust.: Cic.; *Ign.;* Nux v.; *Puls.*

Monomania (kleptomania, etc.)—*Absinth.;* Cic.; Hyos.; Oxytr.; Plat.; Tar. h.

Puerperal—Agn.; Bell.; *Cim.;* Hyos.; Plat.; Sec.; Senec.; *Stram.; Ver. a.; Ver. v.*

MELANCHOLIA—Remedies in general: Acon.; *Agn.;* Alum.; *Anac.;* Arg. n.; *Ars.; Aur.;* Bapt.; Bell.; Cact.; Calc. c.; Camph.; Caust.; *Cim.;* Cinch.; Coca; Coff.; *Con.; Cycl.;* Dig.; Ferr. m.; Gels.; Helleb.; *Helon.; Ign.;* Iod.; Kali br.; Lac c.; Lach.; *Lil. t.;* Lyc.; Merc.; *Nat. m.;* Nux m.; *Nux v.;* Op.; *Phos. ac.;* Phos.; Picr. ac.; *Plat.;* Plumb. ac.; Plumb. m.; Pod.; *Puls.; Sep.;* Sil.; Solan. c.; Stram.; Sul.; Tar. h.; Thuya; *Ver. a.;* Ver. v.; Zinc. m.

Pubertic—Ant. c.; *Helleb.;* Mancin.; Nat. m.

Puerperal—Agn.; Bell.; *Cim.;* Nat. m.; Plat.; *Ver. v.*

Religious—Ars.; *Aur. m.; Aur. mur.;* Kali br.; Lil. t.; Meli.; Plumb.; Psor.; Puls.; *Stram.; Sul.; Ver. a.*

Sexual—Agn.; Aur.; *Cim.;* Con.; *Lil. t.;* Nux v.; Picr. ac.; Plat.; Sep.

MEMORY—**Forgetful, weak or lost:** Absinth.; Acon.; *Æth.; Agn.; Alum.;* Ambra; *Anac.;* Anhal.; *Arg. n.;* Arn.; *Aur.;* Azar.; *Bar. c.;* Calad.; *Calc. c.;* Calc. p.;* Camph.; *Can ind.;* Carbo v.; Cocc.; *Con.;* Glycerin; Ichthy.; *Kali br.;* Kali c.; *Kali p.; Lac c.;* Lach.; Lecith.; *Lyc.;* Med.; Merc.; *Nat. c.; Nat. m.;* Nit. ac.; *Nux m.; Nux v.;* Oleand.;

Op.; *Phos. ac.; Phos.; Picr. ac.;* Plumb. m.; Rhod.; Rhus t.; *Selen.;* Sep.; Sil.; *Sul.;* Syph.; Tellur.; Thyr.; *Zinc. m.; Zinc. p.;* Zinc. picr.

Cannot remember familiar streets—Can. ind.; *Glon.;* Lach.; Nux m.

Cannot remember names—*Anac.;* Bar. ac.; *Chlorum; Euonym.;* Guaiac.; Hep.; Lyc.; Med.; *Sul.;* Syph.; Xerophyl.

Cannot remember right words (amnesic aphasia, paraphasia)—Agar.; Alum.; *Anac.;* Arag.; Arg. n.; Arn.; Calc. c.; Calc. p.; Can. ind.; Cham.; Cinch.; Diosc.; Dulc.; *Kali br.;* Lac c.; Lil. t.; *Lyc.; Nux m.;* Phos. ac.; *Plumb. m.;* Sumb.; Xerophyl.

Difficulty or inability of fixing attention—*Æth.;* Agar.; *Agn.;* Aloe; Alum.; *Anac.;* Apis; Arag.; Arg. n.; Bapt.; Bar. c.; Can. ind.; Caust.; *Con.;* Fagop.; *Gels.;* Glon.; Glycerin; Helleb.; Ichthy.; Indol; Irid.; Lac c.; Lyc.; Op.; Nat. c.; *Nux m.; Nux v.; Phos. ac.; Phos.; Picr. ac.;* Pituit.; Sep.; Sil.; Staph.; Sul.; Syph.; Xerophyl.; *Zinc. m.*

Omits letters, words—Benz. ac.; Cereus serp.; Cham.; *Kali br.;* Lac c.; Lach.; *Lyc.;* Meli.; *Nux m.;* Nux v.

Thoughts, rapid—Anac.; Bell.; *Can. ind.;* Cim.; Cinch.; *Coff.; Ign.;* Lac c.; Lach.; *Physost.*

Thoughts, slow—Agn.; Caps.; *Carbo v.;* Lyc.; Med.; *Nux m.;* Op.; *Phos. ac.; Phos.;* Plumb.; Sec.; Thuya.

Thoughts vanish while reading, talking, writing—*Anac.;* Asar.; Camph.; *Can. ind.;* Lach.; Lyc.; *Nux m.;* Picr. ac.; Staph.

Unable to think—Abies n.; *Æth.;* Alum.; *Anac.;* Arg. n.; Aur. m.; Bapt.; Calc. c.; Can. ind.; Caps.; *Con.;* Dig.; *Gels.;* Glycerin; *Kali p.;* Lyc.; *Nat. c.;* Nat. m.; *Nux m.; Nux v.;* Oleand.; Petrol.; *Phos. ac.; Phos.; Picr. ac.;* Rhus t.; Sep.; Sil.; Zinc. m.

Weak from sexual abuse—*Agn.; Anac.;* Arg. n.; Aur.; Cinch.; Nat. m.; Nux v.; *Phos. ac.; Staph.*

MIND—Absence: Acon.; *Agn.; Anac.;* Apis; Arag.; Arn.; Bar. c.; *Can. ind.; Kali br.;* Kreos.; *Lac c.;* Lach.; Merc.; Nat. m.; *Nux m.;* Phos. ac.; Poth.; Rhus t.; Tellur.; Zinc.

Absence of moral and will power—Abrot.; Acetan.; *Anac.;* Cereus serp.; *Coca; Cocaine;* Kali br.; *Morph.;* Op.; Picr. ac.; Strych. p.; *Tar. h.*

Cloudiness, confusion, depression, dullness—*Abies n.;* Acon.; Æsc.; Agar.; *Ail.;* Alfal.; Alum.; *Anac.; Apis;* Aragal.; Arg. n.; Arn.; *Bapt.;* Bar. c.; Bell.; Calc. c.; Can. ind.; Cann. s.; Carbon. s.; Cic.; Cocc.; Colch.; Euonym.; Ferr. m.; *Gels.; Glon.;* Glycerin; *Helleb.;* Hyos.; Hyper.; Indol; Irid.; Kali br.; Kali p.; Lac c.; Lecith.; Lyc.; Mancin.; Nat. c.; *Nux m.; Nux v.; Op.; Phos. ac.;* Phos.; Picr. ac.; Piscidia; *Rhus t.; Selen.;* Staph.; Stram.; Sulphon.; Xerophyl.; *Zinc. m.;* Zinc. v.

Excitement, exhilaration—Acon.; Agar.; *Bell.; Can. ind.; Canth.;* Coca; Cocaine; *Coff.;* Croc.; Eucal.; *Hyos.; Lach.;* Merc. cy.; Nux v.; Op.; Paul.; Physost.; Piscidia; *Stram.;* Thea; *Ver. a.*

MOOD—DISPOSITION—Anxiety felt during thunderstorm: Nat. c.; *Phos.* **Anxiety felt in stomach**—*Ars.; Dig.;* Ipec.; Kali c.; *Puls.;* Ver. a.

Anxious—*Acon.; Æth.; Agn.;* Amyl; Anac.; Ant. c.; Arg. n.; *Ars.;* Asaf.; Aur.; Bell.; *Bism.;* Bor.; Cact.; *Calc. c.;* Camph.; Can. ind.; Cham.; Cim.; Cinch.; Coff.; Con.; Cupr. m.; *Dig.;* Hep.; *Ign.; Kali* e.; *Lach.; Lil. t.;* Med.; Nat. c.; Nat. m.; Nit. ac.; *Nux v.;* Op.; *Phos.; Plat.;* Psor.; *Puls.;* Rhus t.; Sec.; *Sep.;* Sil.; Staph.; Stram.; Sul.; Tab.; *Ver. a.*

Apathetic, indifferent to everything—Agar.; Agn.; *Apis;* Arg. n.; Arn.; Ars.; *Bapt.;* Bry.; *Cim.; Cinch.;* Con.; Fluor. ac.; *Gels.;* Glycerin; *Helleb.;* Hydroc. ac.; *Ign.;* Indol; Laburn.; Lach.; Lil. t.; Merc.; Nat. m.; Nux m.; Nux v.; *Op.; Phos. ac.;* Phos.; Phyt.; *Picr. ac.;* Plat.; Puls.; Sec.; *Sep.; Staph.;* Thuya; *Ver. a.*

Aversion to mental and physical work—Agar.; Alfal.; *Aloe; Anac.;* Aragal.; Aur. mur.; Bapt.; *Bar. c.; Calc. c.; Caps.; Carb. ac.;* Caust.; *Cinch.;* Coca; Con.; Cycl.; *Gels.;* Glon.; Helleb.; Indol; *Kali p.;* Lecith.; Mag. p.; Nat. c.; Niccol. s.; Nit. ac.; *Nux v.;* Oxytr.; *Phos. ac.;* Phos.; *Picr. ac.;* Puls.; Rhamnus cal.; Selen.; Sep.; Sil.; Strych. p.; *Sul.;* Tanac.; Thymol; *Zinc m.*

Bashful, timid—*Ambra;* Aur.; *Bar. c.;* Calc. c.; Calc. sil.; Caust.; Coca; Con.; Graph.; *Ign.;* Kali p.; Lil. t.; Mancin.; Meli.; Phos.; *Puls.;* Sil.; *Staph.*

Complaining, discontented, dissatisfied—Aloe; *Ant. c.;* Ars.; Bism.; Bor.; Bry.; Caps.; *Cham.; Cina;* Colch.; Indol; Kali c.; Mag. p.; Nit. ac.; *Nux v.;* Plat.; Psor.; *Puls.;* Staph.; Sul.; Tab.

Despairing, hopeless, discouraged easily, lack of confidence—*Acon.; Agn.;* Alum.; *Anac.;* Ant. c.; Arg. n.; Arn.; *Ars.; Aur.;* Bar. c.; Calc. c.; Calc. sil.; Caust.; Con.; *Gels.;* Helleb.; *Ign.;* Iod.; Lil. t.; Nat. m.; Nit. ac.; Nux v.; Op.; *Phos. ac.;* Phos.; Picr. ac.; Psor.; *Puls.;* Ruta; Selen.; *Sep.;* Sil.; Staph.; Syph.; Thymol; *Ver. a.*

Fault-finding, finicky, cautious—Apis; *Ars.; Cham.;* Graph.; Helon.; Morph.; *Nux v.; Plat.;* Sep.; Staph.; Sul.; Tar. h.; Ver. a.

Fearlessness, daring—*Agar.;* Bell.; Cocaine; *Op.;* Sil.

Fretful, cross, irritable, peevish, quarrelsome, whining—Abrot.; *Acon.; Æsc.;* Æth.; Agar.; Alfal.; Anac.; *Ant. c.; Ant. t.;* Apis; Ars.; Aur.; *Bry.;* Bufo; Calc. br.; Calc. c.; *Caps.;* Caust.; *Cham.; Cina;* Cinch.; *Colch.; Col.;* Con.; Croc.; Ferr.; Helon.; Hep.; Iberis; *Ign.;* Indol; Ipec.; Kali c.; *Kali p.; Kreos.;* Lac c.; Lil. t.; Lyc.; *Nat. m.; Nit. ac.; Nux v.;* Plat.; Puls.; Radium; Rheum; Sars.; *Sep.;* Sil.; *Staph.;* Sulphon.; Sul.; Syph.; Thuya; Thymol; Tub.; *Val.;* Ver. a.; Ver. v.; Zinc. m.

Fretful day and night—*Cham.;* Ign.; Ipec.; Lac c.; *Psor.; Stram.*

Fretful day only—Lyc.

Fretful night only—Ant. t.; *Jal.;* Nux v.; Rheum.

Fretful, so that child cannot bear to be touched, looked at, or spoken to—Ant. c.; Ant. t.; *Cham.; Cina;* Gels.; *Nux v.;* Sanic.; *Sil.;* Thuya.

Fretful, so that child wants different things, but petulantly rejects them—Ant. t.; Bry.; *Cham.; Cina;* Ipec.; Kreos.; Rheum; *Staph.*

Gay, frolicsome, hilarious—Anag.; Bell.; *Can. ind.; Coff.; Croc.;* Cyprip.; Eucal.; *Formica; Hyos.;* Lach.; Nux m.; Plat.; Spong.; Stram.; Thea; Val.

Grieving, introspective, sighing—Ail.; Calc. p.; *Cim.;* Dig.; *Iberis; Ign.;* Lyc.; *Mur. ac.;* Nat. m.; *Phos. ac.;* Puls.

Haughty. arrogant, prideful—Bell.; Con.; Cupr. m.; Lach.; Lyc.; *Pall.;* Phos.; *Plat.;* Staph.; *Stram.;* Ver. a.

Haughty, contempt of others—Ipec.; *Plat.*

Haughty, contempt of self—*Agn.; Aur.;* Lac c.; Thuya.

Hypersensitive, cannot bear contradiction, vexed at trifles—Acon.; *Anac., Ant. c.;* Arn.; Ars.; Asaf.; Asar.; Aster.; *Aur.;* Bell.; *Bry.;* Canth.; *Caps.; Cham.; Cina;* Cinch.; Cocc.; *Colch.;* Col.; Con.; Ferr. m.; Glon.; Helleb.; Helon.; Hep.; *Ign.;* Lach.; Lyc.; Mez.; Morph.; Mur. ac.; *Nat. m.;* Nit. ac.; *Nux v.;* Pall.; Petrol.; Phos.: *Plat.;* Puls.; Sars.; *Sep.;* Sil.; *Staph.;* Thuya; Thyr.

Hysterical (changeable, vacillatory)—*Acon.; Alum.; Ambra; Asaf.;* Camph. monobr.; Cast.; Caust.; *Cim.;* Cob.; Cocc.; Coff.; *Croc.;* Gels.; *Ign.;* Kali p.; Lil. t.; Mang. ac.; *Mosch.;* Nat. m.; *Nux m.;* Phos.; *Plat.; Puls.;* Sep.; *Sumb.;* Tar. h.; Thasp.; *Val.; Zinc. v.*

Impatient, impulsive—Acon.; *Anac.;* Ant. c.; Arg. n.; *Cham.; Col.;* Hep.; Ign.; Ipec.; Med.; *Nat. m.; Nux v.;* Puls.; Rheum; Sep.; *Staph.;* Sul.

Impudent, insulting, malicious, revengeful, spiteful—*Anac.;* Ars.; Bufo; *Cham.;* Cinch.; Cupr.; Lac c.; Lyc.; *Nit. ac.; Nux v.;* Staph.; Tar. h.

Impudent, teasing, laugh at reproof—Graph.

Indecisive, irresolute—Arg. n.; Aur.; *Bar. c.; Calc. sil.;* Caust.; *Graph.; Ign.;* Nux m.; Nux v.; *Puls.*

Indolent, listless, lethargic, ambitionless—Alet.; Aloe; Anac.; *Apis;* Aur. m.; *Bapt.;* Bar. c.; Berb. aq.; *Bry.;* Calc. c.; *Caps.;* Carb. ac.; Carbo v.; Con.; Cycl.; Dig.; Euphras.; Ferr.; *Gels.;* Glon.; Helon.; Indol; Kali p.; Lecith.; Lil. t.; Merc.; Nat. m.; Nux v.; *Phos. ac.;* Phos.; *Picr. ac.;* Puls.; Ruta; Sarcol. ac.; *Sep.;* Stann.; Sul.; Thymol; Zinc.

Jealous—*Apis;* Hyos.; Ign.; *Lach.;* Nux v.

Melancholic, despondent, depressed, low-spirited, gloomy, apprehensive, "blues"—Abies n.; *Acon.; Æsc.; Agn.;* Alfal.; *Alum.;* Am. c.; Am. m.; *Anac.;* Ant. c.; Apis; Arg. m.; Arg. n.; *Ars.;* Ars. m.; *Aur.;* Bry.; But. ac.; Cact.; Calc. ars.; Calc. c.; Caust.; *Cim.; Cinch.;* Cocc.; *Con.;* Cupr. m.; *Cycl.;* Dig.; Euonym.; Euphras.; *Graph.;* Helleb.; *Helon.;* Hep.; *Hydr.;* Iberis; *Ign.; Indigo;* Indol; Iod.; Kali br.; Kali p.; Lac c.; Lac d.; Lach.; *Lil. t.; Lyc.;* Med.; Merc.; Myg.; Myr.; Naja; Nat. c.; *Nat. m.;* Nat. s.; Nit. ac.; Nux m.; *Nux v.; Phos. ac.; Phos.; Plat.; Plumb.;* Pod.; *Psor.; Puls.;* Radium; Rhus t.; Sarcol. ac.; Sars.; Senec.; *Sep.;* Sil.; Spig.; *Stann.; Staph.;* Still.; Sul.; **Tab.;** Thuya; *Tub.;* Ver. a.; Zinc. m.; Zinc. p.

Mild, gentle, yielding—Alum.; *Ign.;* Murex; Phos. ac.; *Puls.;* Sep.; Sil.

Misanthropic, miserly, selfish—Ars.; *Lyc.;* Pall.; Plat.; Sep.; *Sul.*

Nervous, excited, fidgety, worried—Absinth.; *Acon.; Ambra; Anac.;* Apis; Apium gr.; *Arg. n.; Ars.;* Asaf.; *Asar.;* Aur. m.; *Bell.; Bor.;* Bov.; But. ac.; Calc. br.; *Camph. monobr.;* Caust.; Ced.; *Cham.; Cim.;* Cina; *Coff.;* Con.; Ferr.; *Gels.;* Helon.; Hyos.; *Hyos. hydrobr.;* Iberis; *Ign.;* Kali br.; Kali p.; Lac c.; Lach.; Lil. t.; Mag. c.; Med.; Morph.; Nat. c.; Nux m.; *Nux v.; Phos.;* Psor.; Puls.; Sec.; *Sep.; Sil.;* Staph.; Stram.; *Sumb.;* Tar. h.; Thea; *Val.;* Zinc. m.; Zinc. p.; Zinc. v.

Obscene, amative—*Canth.;* Hyos.; Lil. t.; Murex; *Phos.;* Puls.; Staph.; Stram.; *Ver. a.*

Restless (mentally and physically)—Absinth.; *Acon.;* Agar.; Ambra; Arag.; *Ars.;* Aur. m.; Bell.; *Bism.;* Camph.; Can. ind.; Canth.; Caust.; Cenchris; *Cham.;* *Cim.;* *Coff.;* *Hyos.;* *Ign.;* Iod.; *Kali br.;* Lac c.; Lach.; Laur.; Lil. t.; Med.; *Morph.;* Mur. ac.; Myg.; Nat. c.; Nat. m.; Nux v.; Op.; *Phos.;* Phyt.; Plat.; Psor.; *Pyr.;* Radium; *Rhus t.;* Ruta; Sil.; *Stram.;* *Tar. h.;* Urt.; Val.; Ver. a.; Ver. v.; Zinc. m.; Zinc. v.

Sad, sentimental, sighing—*Agn.;* Am. c.; Am. m.; *Ant. c.;* *Aur.;* Cact.; Calc. p.; Carbo an.; Cim.; Cocc.; Con.; *Cycl.;* Dig.; *Graph.;* Iberis; *Ign.;* *Indigo;* Kali p.; Lach.; Lil. t.; Mur. ac.; Naja; Nat c.; *Nat. m.;* Nat. s.; Nit. ac.; Nux v.; Phos. ac.; Phos.; Plat.; Psor.; *Puls.;* Rhus t.; Sec.; *Selen.;* *Sep.;* *Stann.;* Staph.; Sul.; Thuya; Zinc. m.

Sad, weeping from music—Acon.; *Ambra;* *Graph.;* *Nat. c.;* Nat. s.; *Sab.;* Tar. h.; *Thuya.*

Slovenly, filthy—Am. c.; *Caps.;* Merc.; *Psor.;* *Sul.;* Ver. a.

Stubborn, obstinate, self-willed—Agar.; Ant. c.; *Bry.;* Caps.; *Cham.;* Cinch.; Kali c.; *Nit. ac.;* *Nux v.;* Sanic.; Sil.; *Staph.*

Stupid—Æsc. gl.; *Anac.;* *Apis;* Arn.; *Bapt.;* Bell.; Bry.; Cocc.; *Gels.;* *Helleb.;* Hyos.; Indol; Lach.; *Nux m.;* *Op.;* *Phos. ac.;* Phos.; Rhus t.; Sec.; Stram.; Ver. a.

Suicidal—Alum.; Anac.; *Ant. c.;* *Ars.;* *Aur.;* Cinch.; Fuligo; Ign.; Iod.; Kali br.; *Naja;* Nat. s.; Nit. ac.; *Nux v.;* Psor; Puls.; Rhus t.; Sec.; Sep.; Sil.; Ustil.; Ver. a.

Suspicious, mistrustful—*Anac.;* Anhal.; Caust.; *Cim.;* *Hyos.;* Lach.; Merc.; *Nux v.;* Puls.; *Staph.;* Ver. a.; Ver. v.

Sympathetic—*Caust.;* Cocc.; Puls.

Taciturn, disinclined to be disturbed, or answer questions—Agar.; *Ant. c.;* Ant. t.; Arn.; Bell.; *Bry.;* Cact.; Carbo an.; *Cham.;* Col.; *Gels.;* Helleb.; Ign.; Iod.; Mur. ac.; Naja; *Nat. m.;* Nat. s.; *Nux v.;* Oxytr.; *Phos. ac.;* Phos.; Sars.; Sil.; Sul.

Taciturn, morose, sulky, sullen, unsociable—*Ant. c.;* Ant. t.; Arn.; Aur.; *Bry.;* *Cham.;* Cim.; *Cinch.;* Col.; Con.; Cupr.; Ign.; Lyc.; Nat. m.; *Nux v.;* *Plat.;* Puls.; Sanic.; Sil.; Sul.; Tub.; *Ver. a.;* Ver. v.

Tearful, weeping—*Am. m.;* Ant. c.; *Apis;* Ars.; Aur.; Cact.; Calc. c.; Caust.; *Cim.;* Cocc.; Croc.; *Cycl.;* Dig.; *Graph.;* *Ign.;* Lac. c.; Lach.; Lil. t.; Lyc.; Mag. m.; *Nat. m.;* Nit. ac.; Nux m.; Phos. ac.; Plat.; *Puls.;* Rhus t.; *Sep.;* Sil.; *Stann.;* Sul.

NIGHT-TERRORS—Acon.; *Aur. br.;* Calc. c.; Cham.; Cic.; *Cina;* Chloral.; Cyprip.; *Kali br.;* Kali p.; Scutel.; Solan. n.; *Stram.;* Tub.; Zinc. m.

PROPENSITY—**To be abusive, curse, swear**—*Anac.;* Bell.; Canth.; Cereus serp.; *Lac c.;* Lil. t.; *Nit. ac.;* Pall.; *Stram.;* *Tub.;* Ver. a.

To be aimlessly busy—Absinth.; *Arg. n.;* Ars.; Canth.; *Lil. t.;* Sul.; Tar. h.

To be carried—Ant. t.; Ars.; Benz. ac.; *Cham.;* Cina; Ipec.

To be cruel, violent, inhuman—Abrot.; *Absinth.;* *Anac.;* Bell.; Bry.; Canth.; Croc.; *Nit. ac.;* *Nux v.;* Plat.; Staph.; *Stram.;* Tar. h.; Ver. a.

To be destructive, bite, strike, tear clothes—*Bell.;* Bufo; *Canth.;* Cupr. m.; *Hyos.;* Lil. t.; Sec.; *Stram.;* Tar. h.; *Ver. a.*

To be dirty, untidy, filthy—Caps.; *Psor.;* Sil.

To be magnetized—Calc. c.; *Phos.;* Sil.

To be obscene—Anac.; *Canth.; Hyos.;* Lach.; Lil. t.; *Phos.;* Plat.; Stram.; Ver. a.

To commit suicide—Alum.; *Ant. c.; Ars.; Aur.;* Caps.; Cim.; *Ign.;* Kali br.; Merc.; *Naja;* Nat. s.; *Nux v.;* Psor.; Puls.; Rhus t.; Thasp.; Ustil.; Ver. a.

To dance—*Agar.;* Bell.; Cic.; *Croc.;* Hyos.; Sticta; Stram.; *Tar. h.*

To do absurd things—Bell.; Can. ind.; Cic.; *Hyos.;* Lach.; Stram.; Tar. h.

To eat greedily—Lyc.; Zinc. m.

To handle organs—Bufo; Canth.; Hyos.; Ustil.; Zinc.

To hurry—Acon.; Alum.; Apis; *Arg. n.; Aur.;* Bell.; Coff.; Ign.; *Lil. t.;* Med.; Nat. m.; *Sul. ac.;* Thuya; Zinc v.

To hurry others—Arg. n.; Can. ind.; *Nux m.*

To kill beloved ones—Ars.; Cinch.; Merc.; *Nux v.; Plat.*

To laugh immoderately at trifles—Anac.; *Can. ind.; Croc.; Hyos.;* Ign.; *Mosch.;* Nux m.; *Plat.; Stram.; Strych. p.;* Tar. h.; Zinc. oxy.

To lie—*Morph.;* Op.; Ver. a.

To mutilate body—Agar.; *Ars.;* Bell.; Hyos.; Stram.

To perform great things—Cocaine.

To pray, beseech, entreat—Aur. m.; Puls.; *Stram.;* Ver. a.

To repeat everything—Zinc. m.

To scold—*Con.;* Dulc.; Lyc.; *Mosch.; Nux v.;* Pall.; *Petrol.;* Ver. a.

To sing—*Agar.;* Bell.; Can. ind.; Cic.; *Croc.; Hyos.;* Spong.; *Stram.;* Tar. h.; Ver. a.

To slide down in bed—Mur. ac.

To stretch and yawn incessantly—Amyl; Plumb. m.

To talk in rhymes, repeat verses, prophecy—Agar.; Ant. c.; Lach.; Stram.

To tear things—Agar.; *Bell.; Cimex;* Cupr. m.; *Stram.;* Tar. h.; *Ver. a.*

To tease, laugh at reproofs—Graph.

To theorize or meditate—*Can. ind.;* Cocc.; Coff.; *Sul.*

To touch different things—Bell.; Sul.; *Thuya.*

To wander from home—Arag.; *Bry.;* Elat.; Lach., Ver. a.

To work—Æth.; Aur.; Cereus; *Cocaine;* Coff.; *Eucal.;* Fluor. ac.; *Helon.; Lacertus;* Pedic.; Piscidia.

SCREAMS—Shrill, sudden, piercing—*Apis; Bell.;* Bor.; Bry.; Calc. c.; Cham.; *Cic.; Cina; Cinch.;* Cyprip.; Gels.; *Helleb.;* Iodof.; Kali br.; *Stram.;* Tub.; Ver. a.; *Zinc. m.*

SENSES—Dulled—Ail.; *Anac.; Bapt.;* Caps.; Dig.; *Gels.; Helleb.;* Phos. ac.; Rhus t.

Hyperacute—*Acon.;* Asaf.; *Asar.;* Atrop.; Aur.; *Bell.;* Bor.; *Cham.;* Cinch.; *Coff.; Colch.;* Ferr. m.; *Ign.;* Lyssin; Morph.; *Nux v.; Op.; Phos.;* Sil.; *Strych.;* Sul.; Tar. h.; Val.; Zinc. m.

SPEECH—Hurried—Anac.; Aur.; *Bell.; Bry.;* Cocc.; *Hep.; Hyos.;* Lil. t.; Merc.; *Ver. a.*

Lost or paralysis (aphasia)—Bar. ac.; *Bar. c.; Bothrops; Caust.;* Cham.; Chenop.; *Colch.;* Con.; Glon.; *Kali br.;* Kali cy.; Lach.; *Lyc.;* Mez.; Phos.; Plumb. m.; *Stram.;* Sulphon. See Nervous System.

Nasal—Bar. m.; Bell.; Lach.; Phos. ac.

Slow, difficult enunciation, inarticulate, stammering—*Æsc. gl.;* Agar.; Anac.; Anhal.; Atrop.; Bar. c.; Bell.; *Bothrops; Bov.;* Bufo; Can. ind.; *Can. s.; Caust.;* Cereus serp.; Cic.; *Cupr. m.;* Gels.; Hyos.; *Ign.;* Kali br.; Kali cy.; Lach.; Laur.; Merc.; Myg.; Naja; Nat. m.; Nux m.; Oleand.; *Op.; Phos.; Stram.;* Sulphon.; Thuya; Vip.

Slow, monotonous, economical—Mang. ac.; Mang. oxy.

SOMNAMBULISM—Acon.; *Art. v.; Can. ind.;* Cur.; Ign.; *Kali br.;* Kali p.; Phos.; *Sil.; Zinc. m.*

STARTLES—Easily frightened—*Acon.;* Agar.; Apis; *Asar.; Bell.; Bor.;* Calad.; Calc. c.; Carbo v.; *Cham.;* Cim.; Cyprip.; *Ign.; Kali br.:* Kali c.; Kali p.; Nat. c.; *Nux v.;* Op.; *Phos.;* Psor.; Samb.; *Seutel.;* Sep.; *Sil.; Stram.;* Sul.; *Tar. h.;* Ther.; Tub.; Zinc. m.

TAEDIUM VITAE (disgust of life)—*Ant. c.;* Ars.; *Aur.; Cinch.;* Hydr.; Lac c.; Lac d.; Kali br.; Naja; Nat. s.; Nit. ac.; *Phos.;* Plat.; Pod.; Rhus t.; Sul.; Tab.; *Thuya;* Ver. a.

HEAD

BRAIN—Abscess—Arn.; Bell.; Crot.; Iod.; Lach.; Op.; Vipera.

Anaemia—Alum.; *Ars.; Calc. p.;* Camph.; *Cinch.; Ferr. m.;* Ferr. p.·
Kali c.; *Kali p.; Nux v.; Phos.;* Sec.; Tab.; Ver. a.; *Zinc. m.*

Atrophy—*Aur.; Bar. c.;* Fluor. ac.; Iod.; *Phos.; Plumb. m.;* Zinc. m.

Concussion—*Acon.; Arn.; Bell.;* Cic.; Ham.; *Hyper.;* Kali iod.; *Nat. s. ;
Op.;* Sul. ac.

Congestion—(rush of blood to head)—Absinth.; *Acon.;* Act. spic.; Agar.;
Ambra; *Amyl;* Arn.; Aster.; Aur.; *Bell.; Bry.;* Cact.; Calc. ars.;
Carbo v.; Cham.; *Chin. s.;* Cinnab.; *Cinch.;* Coff.; Croc.; Cupr. ac.;
Cupr. m.; Ferr. p.; *Ferr. pyroph.;* Gels.; *Glon.;* Hyos.; Ign.; Iod.;
Lach.; Lyc.; *Meli.;* Nat. s.; *Nux v.; Op.;* Sang.; Sep.; Sil.; Solan.
lyc.; Stram.; *Sul.; Ver. v.*

Congestion, passive—Æsc.; Chloral.; *Cinch.;* Dig.; *Ferr. pyroph.; Gels.;*
Helleb.; *Op.;* Phos.

Inflammation (meningitis)—Cerebral (acute and chronic)—Acon.; Æth.;
Apis; Apoc. c.; Arn.; Ars.; Bapt.; *Bell.; Bry.;* Calc. br.; Calc. c.;
Calc. p.; Camph.; Carb. ac.; Chin. s.; Chrom. oxy.; *Cic.;* Cim.; Cinch.;
Crot.; *Cupr. ac.; Cupr. m.;* Dig.; Gels.; Glon.; *Helleb.;* Hydroc. ac.;
Hyper.; Iod.; Iodof.; Kali iod.; Kreos.; Lach.; Merc. c.; Merc. d.;
Mosch.; *Op.;* Ox. ac.; Physost.; Plumb. m.; Phos.; Rhus t.; *Sil.;*
Solan. n.; *Sul.; Stram.; Tub.;* Ver. v.; Vipera; *Zinc. m.* See Hydro-
cephalus.

Inflammation, basilar—*Cupr. cy.;* Dig.; Helleb.; Iod.; Sec.; Tub.; *Ver. v.*

Inflammation, cerebro-spinal—*Agar.;* Ail.; *Apis;* Arg. n.; Atrop.; *Bell.;*
Bry.; *Cic.; Cim.;* Cocc.; *Crot.; Cupr. ac.;* Echin.; *Gels.;* Glon.; *Helleb.;*
Hyos.; Ipec.; Kali iod.; Laburn.; Nat. s.; Op.; Oreodaph.; Physost.;
Sil.; Stram.; Sul.; Ver. v.; *Zinc. cy.;* Zinc. m.

Inflammation, traumatic—Acon.; *Arn.;* Bell.; *Hyper.;* Nat. s.; Sil.

Inflammation, tubercular—*Apis; Bac.;* Bell.; Bry.; Calc. c.; *Calc. p.;*
Cocc.; *Cupr. cy.;* Dig.; Glon.; *Helleb.;* Hyos.; Iod.; *Iodof.;* Kali iod.;
Op.; Stram.; *Sul.;* Tub.; *Ver. v.;* Zinc. m.; Zinc. oxy.

Paralysis—Alumen; Con.; Cupr. m.; Gels.; Helleb.; Lyc.; Op.; *Plumb.;*
Sec.; *Zinc. m.* See Apoplexy (Circulatory System).

Sclerosis (softening, degeneration)—Agar.; Arg. n.; *Aur.; Bar. c.;* Can.
ind.; Con.; Kali br.; Kali iod.; Kali p.; Lach.; Lyc.; Nux m.; Nux v.;
Phos.; Pier. ac.; *Plumb. m.;* Salam.; Vanad.; *Zinc. m.* See Arterio-
sclerosis (Circulatory System).

Tumors—Apomorph.; Arn.; *Bar. c.;* Bell.; Calc. c.; *Con.;* Glon.; Graph.;
Hydr.; *Kali iod.; Plumb. m.;* Sep.

CEREBELLAR DISEASE—Helod.; Sulphon.

FONTANELLES—Tardy closure—Apis; Apoc.; *Calc. c.; Calc. p.;* Merc.;
Sep.; *Sil.; Sul.;* Zinc. m.

HEADACHE (cephalalgia)—Cause: Altitude high: Coca.
Bathing—Ant. c.

Beer—Rhus t.

Bright's disease—Am. v.; Zinc. picr.

Candy, sweets—Ant. c.

Catarrh—*Cepa;* Hydr.; Merc.; Puls.; *Sticta.*

Catarrh suppressed—Bell.; *Kali bich.;* Lach.

Coffee—Arum; Ign.; *Nux v.;* Paul.

Constipation—*Aloe;* Alum.; *Bry.;* Collins.; Hydr.; Nit. ac.; *Nux v.;* Op.; Ratanh.

Dancing—Arg. n.

Diarrhoea alternating—*Aloe;* Pod.

Effete matter in system—Asclep. s.

Emotional disturbances—Acetan.; Arg. n.; Cham.; Cim.; Coff.; *Epiph.; Gels.; Ign.;* Mez.; Phos. ac.; *Picr. ac.;* Plat.; Rhus t.; Sil.

Eruptions suppressed—Ant. c.; Psor.; Sul.

Eye-strain—Acetan.; *Cim.; Epiph.; Gels.; Nat. m.; Onosm.;* Phos. ac.; *Ruta;* Tub.

Fasting—Ars.; Cact.; Lach.; *Lyc.;* Sil.

Gastralgia alternating or attending—Bism.

Gastro-intestinal derangements—*Ant. c.;* Bry.; Carbo v.; *Cinch.;* Ipec.; *Iris;* Nux m.; *Nux v.; Puls.;* Rham. c.; Robin.

Hair-cut—Bell.; Bry.

Hat, pressure—Calc. p.; Carbo v.; *Hep.;* Net. m.; Nit. ac.

Hæmorrhage, excesses or vital losses—Carbo v.; *Cinch.;* Ferr.; Ferr. pyroph.; Phos. ac.; Sil.

Hæmorrhoids—Collins.; Nux v.

Ice-water—Dig.

Influenza—Camph.; Lob. purp.

Ironing—*Bry.;* Sep.

Lemonade, tea, wine—Selen.

Liver derangements—Lept.; Nux v.; Ptelea.

Lumbago, alternating with it—Aloe.

Malaria—*Ars.;* Caps.; Ced.; *Chin. s.;* Cinch.; Cupr. ac.; *Eup. perf.; Gels.; Nat. m.*

Mental exertion or nervous exhaustion—Acetan.; Agar.; *Anac.; Arg. n.;* Aur. br.; Chionanth.; Cim.; Coff.; *Epiph.; Gels.;* Ign.; *Kali p.;* Mag. p.; *Nat. c.;* Niccol.; *Nux v.;* Phaseol.; Phos. ac.; *Picr. ac.;* Sabad.; Scutel.; Sil.; Zinc. m.

Mercury—Still.

Narcotics, abuse---Acet. ac.

Over-lifting—Calc. c.

Perspiration, suppressed—Asclep. s.; Bry.

Riding against wind—Calc. iod.; *Kali c.*

Riding in cars—*Cocc.;* Graph.; Med.; *Nit. ac.*

Sexual excitement, weakness—Cinch.; Nux v.; Onosm.; *Phos. ac.; Sil.*

Sleep, damp room—Bry.

Sleep, loss—Cim.; Cocc.; *Nux v.*

Spinal disease, chorea—Agar.

Spirituous liquors—Agar.; *Ant. c.;* Lob. infl.; *Nux v.;* Paul.; Rhod.; Ruta; *Zinc. m.*

Sunlight or heat—*Bell.;* Cact.; Ferr. p.; *Gels.; Glon.;* Kal.; Lach.; *Nat. c.;* Nux v.; Sang.; Stram.

Syphilis—Ars.; Aur. ars.; *Aur.;* Sars.; Still.; Syph.

Tea—Nux v.; Paul.; *Selen.;* Thuya.

Tobacco—Ant. c.; Calad.; Carb. ac.; *Gels.; Ign.;* Lob. infl.; Nux v.

Traumatism—*Arn.;* Hyper.; Nat. s.

Uraemia—Arn.; Bapt.; Can. ind.; *Glon.;* Hyper.; *Sang.*

Uterine disease, reflex—Aloe; Bell.; *Cim.;* Gels.; Ign.; Puls.; *Sep.;* Zinc. p.

Vaccination—Thuya.

Weather changes—*Calc. p.;* Phyt.

TYPE—Anaemic: Ars.; Calc. p.; *Cinch.;* Cycl.; Ferr. m.; *Ferr. p.;* Ferr. r.; Kal.; Nat. m.; *Phos. ac.;* Zinc. m.

Catarrhal—Ars.; *Bell.;* Bry.; Camph.; *Cepa;* Eup. perf.; Euphras.; *Gels.; Kali bich.;* Lyc.; Menthol; *Merc.;* Nux v.; *Puls.;* Sabad.; Sang.; *Sticta;* Sul.

Chronic—*Arg. n.;* Chin. s.; Cocc.; Lach.; *Nat. m.;* Phos.; Plumb.; *Psor.;* Sep.; *Sil.;* Thuya; Tub.; *Zinc. m.*

Chronic, old people—Bar. c.; Calc. p.; Iod.; Phos.

Chronic, school girls—*Calc. p.;* Kali p.; *Nat. m.; Phos. ac.; Picr. ac.;* Psor.; Tub.; Zinc. m.

Chronic, sedentary persons—Anac.; *Arg. n.;* Bry.; *Nux v.*

Climacteric—Amyl; Cact.; *Cim.;* Croc.; *Cycl.; Glon.;* Lach.; *Sang.;* Sul.

Congestive—*Acon.;* Amyl; Arg. n.; *Bell.;* Bry.; *Cact.;* Chin. s.; *Ferr. p.; Gels.; Glon.;* Glycerin; Jonosia; Lach.; *Meli.;* Nat. m.; Nux v.; Op.; Phaseol.; *Sang.;* Sil.; Solan. n.; Sul.; Usnea; *Ver. v.*

Congestive, passive—*Chin. s.;* Ferr. p.; *Ferr. pyroph.;* Gels.; Op.; Sil.

Gastric, bilious—Am. picr.; Anac.; *Arg. n.;* Bapt.; *Bry.;* Cham.; Chel.; *Chionanth.;* Cycl.; Eup. perf.; *Ipec.; Iris;* Lob. infl.; Merc. s.; *Nux v.;* Pod.; *Puls.;* Robin.; *Sang.;* Strych.; Tarax.

Hysterical (clavus)—Agar.; Aquil.; *Coff.;* Euonym.; Hep.; *Ign.;* Kali c.; Mag. m.; Nat. m.; Nux v.; *Plat.;* Puls.; Thuya.

Menstrual—Æth.; Avena; Bell.; Cact.; Can. ind.; Can. s.; Chionanth.; *Cim.;* Cinch.; Cocc.; *Croc.;* Cycl.; Ferr. m.; *Glon.;* Glycerin; Kali p.; Lac d.; Lach.; Lil. t.; *Nat. m.; Plat. mur.; Puls.; Sang.; Sep.;* Ustil.; Vib. op.; Xanth.

Migraine, megrim, nervous—Am. c.; Am. val.; *Anac.;* Anhal.; *Arg. n.;* Aspar.; Avena; *Bell.;* Bry.; Caff. citr.; *Calc. ac.;* Calc. c.; *Can. ind.;* Carb. ac.; Ced.; Chionanth.; *Cim.; Cocc.; Coff.;* Crot. casc.; *Cycl.; Epiph.; Gels.; Guar.; Ign.;* Indigo; *Iris;* Kali bich.; *Kali c.; Lac d.; Lach.; Meli.; Menisp.;* Nat. m.; Niccol.; *Nux v.; Onosm.;* Paul.; Plat. mur.; *Puls.; Sang.;* Saponin; *Scutel.; Sep.;* Sil.; Spig.; Stann.; Sul.; Tab.; Thea; Ther.; Verbasc.; Xanth.; *Zinc. sul.; Zinc. v.;* Zizia.

Neuralgic—*Aconitine; Æsc.;* Arg. n.; *Ars.; Bell.;* Bism.; *Ced.;* Cepa; Chel.; *Chin. s.;* Cim.; Col.; Derris; *Gels.; Mag. p.;* Meli.; Menthol; Oreodaph.; Pall.; Phos.; *Spig.;* Tar. h.; Zinc. v.

Rheumatic, gouty—Act. spic.; Bell.; Bry.; Calc. c.; Colch.; Col.; Derris;

Guaiac.; Hep.; Ipec.; Kali s.; Kal.; Lyc.; Nux v.; *Phyt.; Rhus t.;*
Sep.; Sil.; Sul.

Uraemic—Arn.; *Glon.;* Hyper.; Sang.

Utero-ovarian—Bell.; *Cim.; Gels.;* Helon.; Ign.; Jonosia; Lil. t.; Plat.;
Puls.; Sep.; Zinc.

LOCATION—Frontal: *Acon.;* Æsc.; Alfal.; Agar.; Ail.; *Aloe;* Am. c.;
Anac.; Antipyr.; Arg. n.; Ars.; Aur.; *Bell.; Bry.;* Calc. c.; Carb. ac.;
Ced.; *Cepa; Chin. s.;* Chionanth.; Eup. perf.; Euphras.; Gels.; *Glon.;*
Hydr.; Ign.; Indol; Iris; *Kali bich.; Lept.;* Meli.; Menisp.; Nat. m.;
Nux v.; Phos.; Picr. ac.; Prun. sp.; *Ptel.;* Puls.; Robin.; Rhus t.;
Scutel.; Sil.; Stellar.; Sticta; *Viola od.*

Frontal, extending to eyes, root of nose, face, etc.—Acon.; *Agar.; Aloe;*
Ars. m.; Bad.; *Bry.;* Caps.; Ced.; Cepa; Cereus; *Cim.;* Hep.; Ign.;
Kali iod.; *Lach.;* Mag. m.; Menthol; Onosm.; *Plat.;* Prun. sp.; *Ptel.;*
Spig.; Sticta.

Frontal, extending to occiput, nape of neck and spine—*Bry.;* Euonym.;
Gels.; Lac d.; Menisp.; Nux v.; *Oreodaph.;* Prun. sp.; Sep.; Tub.

Occipital—Æth.; Alfal.; Anac.; Avena; *Bry.;* Camph.; Can. ind.; Carbo
v.; *Cim.; Cocc.;* Euonym.; Eup. perf.; Ferr. m.; *Gels.;* Gins.; Jugl. c.;
Lac c.; Lach.; Lecith.; Niccol. s.; *Nux v.;* Onosm.; Oreodaph.; *Petrol.;*
Phos. ac.; *Picr. ac.;* Plat. mur.; Radium; *Rhus gl.; Sang.;* Sep.; *Sil.;*
Sul.; Xanth.; Zinc. m.

Occipital extending to eyes and forehead—Arundo; Bell.; Carbo v.; Cim.;
Cinch.; *Gels.;* Glycerin; Indol; Lac c.; Mag. m.; Onosm.; Phos. ac.;
Picr. ac.; *Rhus r.; Sang.; Sars.; Sil.;* Spig.

Semilateral (hemicrania)—Arg. n.; *Ars.; Bell.; Bry.;* Ced.; Cham.;
Coff.; Col.; *Cycl.;* Gins.; Glon.; *Ign.;* Jonosia; Kali bich.; Lach.;
Nat. m.; Ol. an.; *Onosm.;* Phos.; Prun. sp.; *Puls.; Sang.;* Sep.; *Sil.;*
Spig.; Stann.; Thuya.

Semilateral, left side—Nat. m.; Nux v.; *Onosm.;* Saponin; *Spig.*

Semilateral, right side—*Ced.;* Chel.; Iris; Kali bich.; Radium; *Sang.;* Sil.;
Tab.

Spinal and cervical—Bell.; *Cim.; Cocc.;* Dulc.; *Gels.; Gossyp.; Helleb.;*
Nat. m.; Nat. s.; Niccol. s.; *Oreodaph.; Phos. ac.; Picr. ac.;* Scutel.;
Sil.; Ver. v.

Supraorbital—Acon.; Aconit.; Aloe; *Ars.;* Carb. ac.; *Ced.;* Cereus; *Chin.
s.;* Cim.; Cinnab.; Col.; Glon.; Ign.; Indol; Iris; *Kali bich.;* Lyc.;
Meli.; Menthol; *Nux v.;* Phell.; Puls.; Viola od.

Supraorbital, left—Act. spic.; Arg. n.; Astrag.; Bry.; Carbo v.; *Ced.;*
Cocc.; Euonym.; Menthol; Nux v.; Oreodaph.; Sapon.; Selen.; Senec.;
Spig.; Tellur.; Xanth.

Supraorbital, right—Arundo; *Bell.; Bism.; Chel.; Iris;* Kali bich.; Meli.;
Plat.; Sang.; Sil.

Sutures, along—Calc. p.

Temples—*Acon.; Anac.;* Arn.; *Bell.; Bry.;* Caps.; Ced.; *Carb. ac.;*
Chin. s.; *Cinch.;* Epiph.; Gels.; *Glon.;* Ign.; Lach.; Naja; *Onosm.,*
Oreodaph.; *Phell.;* Phos. ac.; *Plat.;* Rhus t.; *Sang.; Senec.;* Sep.;
Spig.; *Stann.;* Sul. ac.; Usnea.

Temples, ear to ear—Antipyr.; Calc. ars.; Menthol; Pall.; Syph.

Vertex (crown of head)—Alumen; Anac.; Act. spic.; Ars.; *Cact.;* Calc. p.; *Cim.;* Cinch.; Gels.; Glon.; Hyper.; *Lach.; Menyanth.;* Naja; Nux v.; Pall.; *Phell.; Phos. ac.;* Plat.; Puls.; Radium; Sep.; *Sul.;* Ver. a.

CHARACTER OF PAIN—**Aching, dull:** Acon.; *Æsc.;* Alfal.; *Aloe;* Ant. c.; *Arg. n.;* Ars.; Azar.; Bapt.; Bell.; But. ac.; Caps.; Carb. ac.; Carbo v.; Card. m.; Cepa; *Cim.; Cinch.;* Cocc.; Eyonym.; *Gels.; Helleb.; Hydr.;* Ichthy.; *Ign.;* Indol; Iris; Kali bich.; *Lept.;* Lil. t.; Menthol; Myr.; Naja; Nat. ars.; *Nux v.; Nyctanth.;* Onosm.; Oreodaph.; *Phell.;* Picr. ac.; *Plumb. m.;* Scutel.; *Sil.; Stann.; Stellar.*

Boring, digging—*Arg. n.; Asaf.;* Aur.; Bell.; *Clem.; Col.; Hep.;* Nat. s.; Sep.; Stram.

Bruised, battered, sore—Arn.; *Bapt.;* Bellis; *Cinch.;* Coff.; Euonym.; *Eup. perf.; Gel.;* Guarea; *Ign.;* Ipec.; Lyc.; Menthol; *Nux v.;* Phell.; Phos. ac.; *Rhus t.;* Sil.; Tab.

Burning, heat—*Acon.;* Alumen; *Apis;* Arn.; *Ars.;* Aster.; Bell.; Calc. p.; *Glon.;* Helon.; *Lach.;* Lil. t.; Merc.; Ox. ac.; Phell.; *Phos.;* Sil.; Tongo; Ver. v.; Viola od.

Bursting, splitting—*Acon.;* Bell.; *Bry.;* Cact.; *Caps.; Cinch.;* Daphne; Gels.; *Glon.;* Mag. m.; Meli.; *Nat. m.;* Nux m.; Nux v.; Oleand.; Puls.; Sang.; Sep.; Solan. lyc.; Strych.; *Usnea;* Ver. a.

Constrictive, band-like, squeezing—Acon.; *Anac.; Ant. t.;* Antipyr.; *Cact.; Carb. ac.;* Carbo v.; Card. m.; Coca; Cocc.; Eup. perf.; *Gels.;* Glon.; Guano; Iod.; *Lept.;* Merc. per.; *Merc.; Nit. ac.;* Osm.; *Plat.;* Spig.; *Stann.; Sul.;* Tar. h.; Tub.

Distensive, full—*Acon.;* Amyl; Arg. n.; Bapt.; *Bell.;* Bov.; *Bry.;* Cact.; *Caps.;* Chin. ars.; Cim.; Cinch.; *Gels.; Glon.;* Glyderin; Kali bich.; Menthol; Nux v.; Strych.; *Sul.;* Ver. v.

Drawing—Bism.; *Bry.; Caps.;* Carbo v.; Caul.; *Caust.; Cham.;* Kali c.; Nux v.

Excruciating, violent—Agar.; Amyl; *Anac.;* Arg. n.; Aur.; *Bell.;* Bry.; *Cim.; Cinch.; Glon.;* Kali iod.; Meli.; Oreodaph.; Plat. mur.; *Sang.;* Scutel.; Sil.; *Spig.;* Strych.; Zinc. v.

Heaviness—*Acon.; Aloe;* Arg. n.; *Bapt.;* Bar. m.; Bell.; *Bry.;* Cact.; Calc. c.; Carbo v.; *Cocc.; Gels.; Glon.;* Glycerin; Hydr.; Hyper.; *Ign.;* Iris; *Lach.;* Lil. t.; Meli.; *Menyanth.;* Merc.; *Nux v.;* Onosm.; *Op.;* Oreodaph.; Petrol.; *Phell.; Phos. ac.;* Phos.; Picr. ac.; Plat.; Puls.; Rhus t.; *Sep.; Sul.;* Ther.

Periodical, intermittent—Acon.; Am. picr.; Arg. n.; *Ars.; Bell.;* Cact.; *Ced.;* Chel.; *Cinch.;* Eup. perf.; Gels.; Ign.; Kali cy.; Mag. m.; Niccol.; Niccol. s.; *Sang.;* Sep.; *Spig.;* Tab.; Tela ar.; Zinc. v.

Periodical, intermittent, alternate days—*Anhal.; Cinch.*

Periodical, intermittent, every third day—seventh day—Eup. perf.

Periodical, intermittent, every seventh day—Calc. ars.; Sabad.; *Sang.;* Sil.; Sul.

Periodical, intermittent, every eighth day—Iris.

Periodical, intermittent, every week or two—Sul.

Periodical, intermittent, every two-three weeks—Ferr. m.

Periodical, intermittent, every six weeks—Mag. m.

Periodical, intermittent, lasting several days—Tab.

Periodical, with increase and decrease of sun—Glon.; Kal.; Nat. c.; *Nat. m.; Sang.; Spig.;* Tab.

Piercing, as from nail—*Agar.;* Ananth.; Aquil.; *Coff.; Hep.; Ign.;* Mag. pol. am.; *Nux v.;* Paraf.; Ruta; Sil.; *Thuya;* Zinc v.

Pressing—*Acon.; Aloe; Anac.; Bell.; Bry.;* Cact.; *Caps.; Carb. ac.; Cham.; Chel.;* Chionanth.; Cim.; Epiph.; *Eup. perf.;* Ferr.; *Glon.;* Hydroc. ac.; *Ign.;* Kali c.; Lach.; Meli.; *Menyanth.; Nux v.;* Onosm.; Op.; Oreodaph.; Petrol.; *Phos. ac.; Plat.;* Pod.; Puls.; Rhus t.; Sang.; Sep.; Stann.; Sticta; *Sul.;* Sul. ac.; Thasp.; Ver. a.; *Zinc. m.*

Pressing, as from pincers, or vise—Act. spic.; Bism.; *Cact.;* Cham.; Lyc.; Menisp.; *Menyanth.;* Phos. ac.; *Plat.;* Puls.; *Verbasc.;* Viola tr.

Pressing asunder—Arg. n.; *Asaf.;* Aur.; *Bry.;* Carbo an.; *Cim.;* Cinch.; Coral.; Eriod.; *Fagop.; Menisp.;* Prun. sp.; *Ptel.;* Stront.

Pressing, dull as from weight—Aloe; Alumen; *Anac.; Cact.;* Carbo v.; *Cim.;* Eup. perf.; Hyper.; *Lach.;* Menyanth.; *Naja; Nux v.;* Op.; Petrol.; *Phell.; Phos. ac.;* Puls.; *Sep.; Sul.;* Ther.

Pressing, in small spots—Arg. n.; *Ign.; Kali bich.;* Plat.; Poth.; Thuya.

Shifting, shooting, stinging, tearing—Acon.; Æsc.; Apis; Arn.; Ars.; *Bell.; Caps.; Ced.;* Cim.; *Cinch.;* Col; Ign.; *Iris;* Kali bich.; Kali c.; Lac c.; *Prun. sp.;* Puls.; Sang.; Sil.; Spig.; Vinca.

Shock (electric) like stabbing—Apis; *Aster.; Bell.;* Can. ind.; Cic.; Cocc.; *Glon.;* Rhodium; *Sang.; Sep.;* Tab.; Zinc. v.

Stitching, sticking—Acon.; Æsc.; Arn.; Ars.; Bell.; *Bry.;* Can. ind.; *Caps.;* Cycl.; *Kali c.;* Niccol.; Puls.; Tar. h.

Stupefying—Arg. n.; *Bell.;* Bry.; Gels.; *Glon.;* Senec.; Staph.; Syph.

Throbbing, beating, hammering, pulsating—*Acon.;* Act. spic.; Amyl; Arg. n.; Ars.; *Bell.;* Bry.; Cact.; Can. ind.; *Caps.;* Chin. ars.; Chin. s.; Cim.; *Cinch.;* Croc.; Eup. perf.; *Ferr. m.;* Ferr. p.; Gels.; *Glon.;* Glycerin; Hyper.; *Iris; Lac d.;* Lach.; Lyc.; *Meli.; Nat. m.;* Nux v.; Paul.; Psor.; Puls.; Sang.; Sep.; Sil.; *Spig.; Sul.;* Tongo; Ver. v.

CONCOMITANTS—Anguish, anxiety—Acon.; Ars.; Plat.

Arterial excitement, tension—Acon.; *Bell.; Glon.;* Glycerin; Meli.; Poth.; Usnea; *Ver. v.*

Burning along spine—Picr. ac.

Chilliness—*Arg. n.;* Camph.; Lact. v.; Mang. m.; *Puls.; Sang.;* Sil.

Coldness in back and occiput—Berb. v.

Coldness in head—Calc. ac.; Calc. c.; Sep.; Ver. a.

Coldness of hands and feet—Bell.; *Calc. c.;* Ferr. m.; Lach.; Meli.; *Menyanth.;* Naja; Sep.; Sul.; Ver. a.

Colic—Aloe; Cocc.

Constipation—Aloe; Alum.; *Bry.;* Euonym.; *Hydr.;* Lac d.; Niccol.; *Nux v.;* Op.; Plumb. m.

Coryza—Agar.; Camph.; Cepa.

Cough—Arn.; Caps.; Lyc.

Delirium—Agar.; Bell.; Syph.; Ver. a.

Diarrhoea—Aloe; Cham.; Pod.; Ver. a.

Drowsiness—*Ail.;* Ant. t.; Branca; Chel.; Dub.; *Gels.; Indium;* Lept.;
Myr.; Stellar.

Ears, burning—Rhus t.

Ears, deafness—Chin. s.; Verbasc.

Ears, roaring—Aur.; *Chin. s.; Cinch.;* Ferr. m.; Sang.; Sulphon.

Ears, stitching—Caps.

Empty feeling in stomach—*Ign.;* Kali p.; *Sep.*

Excitement, emotional—Can. ind.; Pall.

Excitement, sexual—Apis; Plat. mur.

Exhaustion, asthenia—*Ars.;* Aur. br.; *Cinch.; Gels.;* Ign.; Indium; Lac
d.; Lob. infl.; *Picr. ac.;* Sang.; Sul.

Eyes: blindness, or visual disturbances, precede or attend—Anhal.; Bell.;
Cycl.; Epiph.; *Gels.;* Ign.; *Iris; Kali bich.;* Kali c.; Lac c.; *Lac d.;*
Nat. m.; Niccol.; Nux v.; Picr. ac.; Pod.; Psor.; *Sang.;* Sil.; Spig.;
Ther.; Zinc. s.

Eyes, enlarged feeling—Arg. n.

Eyes, heaviness—Aloe.

Eyes, heaviness of, and lids—Bell.; Gels.

Eyes, injection—*Bell.;* Meli.; Nux v.

Eyes, lachrymation—Chel.; Phell.; Rhus t.; Spig.; Taxus.

Eyes, soreness, pain—Aloe; Ced.; *Cim.; Eup. perf.; Gels.;* Homarus;
Menthol; Myr.; Nat. m.; Phell.; *Scutel.;* Sil.; *Spig.*

Eyes, vision returns as headache comes on—*Iris;* Lac d.; Nat. m.

Face, flushed, hot—*Acon.;* Amyl; *Bell.;* Cham.; Ferr. p.; Gels.; *Glon.;*
Mag. p.; *Meli.;* Naja; Nat. m.; Nux v.; Pod.; *Sang.;* Sep.

Face, pale—Acon.; *Calc. c.;* Cinch.; Ign.; *Lach.;* Lob. infl.; Meli.; Nat.
m.; Sil.; Spig.; Tab.; *Ver. a.*

Faintness—Nux v.; Ver. a.

Fever—Acon.; Ars.; *Bell.;* Ferr. p.

Flatulence—Asclep. t.; Calc. ac.; Calc. p.; Can. ind.; *Carbo v.;* Xanth.

Gastralgia, attending or following—Bism.

Gastro-intestinal derangements—Agar.; Aloe; Arg n.; Ars.; *Bry.;* Can.
ind.; *Carbo v.; Cinch.;* Iris; *Nux v.;* Pod.; *Puls.*

Hair, falling out—Ant. c.; Nit. ac.; Sil.

Head nodding—Lamium; Sep.

Head retracted—Bell.; Cocc.; *Gossyp.*

Heart's action labored—Lycopus.

Haemorrhoids—Nux v.

Hunger—Anac.; Cact.; *Epiph.;* Ign.; *Lyc.; Psor.*

Hypochondrium, right, stitches—Æsc.

Irritability—Anac.; *Bry.; Cham.;* Ign.; *Nux v.*

Liver disturbance—Chel.; Jugl. c.; *Lept.;* Nux v.

Loquacity—Can. ind.

Lumbago, alternating—Aloe.

Mental depression, despondency—Aloe; *Arg. n.;* Aur.; *Ign.;* Indol; Iris;
Lac d.; Naja; Picr. ac.; Plumb. m.; *Puls.; Sars.;* Sep.; Zinc. m.

Mental weakness—Arg. n.; Nux v.; Sil.

Muscular soreness—Gels.; Rhus t.

Nausea—Aloe; *Ant. c.;* Ars.; *Bry.; Cocc.;* Ferr. m.; Gels.; Indol; *Ipec.; Iris;* Lac c.; Lac d.; Lob. infl.; Lob. purp.; Naja; Nat. m.; *Nux v.;* Paul.; Petrol.; *Puls.; Sang.; Sep.;* Sil.; *Tab.*

Nodules, gouty of scalp—Sil.

Nosebleed—Agar.; Amyl; Ant. c.; Ham.; *Meli.*

Nose, dry, neuralgia—Dulc.

Numbness, tingling, of lips, tongue, nose—Nat. m.

Numbness—Chel.; Indol; Plat.

Occipital soreness—Cim.; Sil.

Oversensitiveness—Ars.; *Bell.; Cham.;* Cinch.; Coff.; *Ign.; Nux v.; Sil.;* Spig.; Tela ar.

Pains in abdomen—Cina; Col.; Ver. a.

Pains in limbs—Sang.

Pains in lumbar region—Radium.

Palpitation—Cact.; Spig.

Polyuria—Asclep. s.; *Gels.; Ign.;* Lac d.; *Sang.;* Scutel.; Sil.

Ptyalism—Fagus; Iris.

Respiratory affections—Lact. v.

Restlessness—*Ars.;* Helleb.; Ign.; Pyr.; Spig.

Scalp, bruised feeling—Æsc.; *Cinch.;* Col.; Sil.

Scotoma—Aspar.

Sleeplessness—*Coff.;* Indium; Syph.; Zinc. v.

Spasmodic symptoms—Ign.

Sweat profuse—Lob. infl.; Tab.

Temporal veins engorged—Carls.; Gels.

Thirst—Pulex.

Tongue coated, fetor oris, etc.—Calc. ac.; Card. m.; Euonym.; Gymnocl.; *Puls.*

Toothache—Sang.

Trembling all over—*Arg. n.;* Bor.; *Gels.*

Vertigo—Acon.; Agrost.; Bry.; Chin. s.; *Cinch.; Cocc.; Eup. purp.; Gels.;* Glon.; Ign.; Lept.; Lob. purp.; *Nux v.;* Pod.; Sep.; Xanth.

Vomiting—Arg. n.; *Ars.; Bry.;* Calc. ac.; Cham.; Cinch.; Cocc.; Glon.; *Ipec.; Iris;* Lac c.; *Lac d.;* Lob. infl.; Meli.; Nat. m.; *Nux v.;* Puls.; Robin.; *Sang.;* Sep.; Sil.; Tab.; Ver. a.; Zinc. s.

Yawning—Kali c.; Staph.

MODALITIES—Aggravation: After drugging: Nux v.

After midnight—Ferr. m.

Afternoon—Ananth.; Bad.; *Bell.;* Cycl.; Eup. purp.; Indol; Lob. infl.; Meli.; Selen.

Air, open—*Ars.;* Bcv.; Branca; *Cinch.;* Cocc.; Coff.; Mag. m.; *Nux v.;* Sep.

Anger—Nux v.

Ascending—Ant. c.; Bell.; But. ac.; *Calc. c.;* Conv.; *Menyanth.*

Attention, close—Ign.

Awaking from sleep—Lach.

Beating time—Anhal.

Bending head backward—Glon.

Bending head forward—Bell.; Cob.

Closing teeth—Am. c.

Cold, draft of air—*Ars.;* Bell.; *Cinch.;* Eup. purp.; Ferr. p.; Ichth.; Ign.; Iris; Nux v.; Rhod.; Rhus t.; Sil.

Contact, touch—*Bell.; Cinch.;* Ferr. p.; Rhus t.; *Tar. h.*

Coughing—Acon.; Arn.; *Bell.; Bry.; Caps.;* Carbo v.; Iris; Kali c.; *Nat. m.; Nux v.;* Petrol.; Phos.; Sep.; Sul.

Dinking coffee—Act. spic.; Ign.; Nux v.

Drinking milk—Brom.

Eating—Am. c.; Arn.; *Ars.;* Atrop.; *Bry.;* Cact.; Cocc.; Coff.; Gels.; Ign.; Lach.; *Lyc.; Nux v.*

Evening—Aur.; Caust.; *Cepa;* Cycl.; Eup. purp.; Indol; Kali s.; *Puls.;* Thlaspi.

Exertion, mental or physical—Aloe; *Anac.; Arg. n.;* Cocc.; *Epiph.;* Gels.; Nat. c.; *Nux v.;* Phos. ac.; Phos.; *Picr. ac.;* Sep.; Sil.; Tub.

Gradually: crescendo, decrescendo—Plat.; Stann.

Hawking—Conv.

Jar, misstep, etc.—Aloe; *Bell.;* Bry.; Cinch.; Crot.; Ferr. p.; *Glon.;* Lach.; Lyc.; Menyanth.; Rhus t.; Sil.; *Spig.; Ther.*

Left side—Anac.; Ars. m.; *Brom.;* Chin. s.; *Cycl.;* Epiph.; Eup. purp.; *Lach.;* Niccol.; Oreodaph.; Paraf.; Sapon.; *Senec.;* Sep.; *Spig.;* Thuya.

Light—*Bell.;* Ferr.; Lac d.; Lyssin; *Ign.;* Kali bich.; Kali c.; *Nux v.;* Oreodaph.; Phell.; Sang.; Scutel.; Sil.; Tar. h.

Lying down—Ars. m.; *Bell.;* Bov.; Cinch.; Col.; Eup. perf.; Gels.; *Glon.;* Lach.; Lyc.; Rhus. t.; Sang.; Ther.

Lying on back of head—Cocc.; Col.

Lying on painful side—Sep.

Menses—Croc.; Lac d.; *Nat. m.;* Sep.

Morning—Æsc.; Alum.; *Am. m.;* Aspar.; Cycl.; Hep.; Lac d.; Myr.; *Nat. m.;* Niccol.; *Nux v.;* Phos. ac.; Pod.; Sang.; Spig.; Stellar.; Sul.

Morning on awaking, opening eyes—Bov.; *Bry.;* Graph.; *Nat. m.; Nux v.;* Onosm.; Strych.; Tab.

Motion—Acon.; Anac.; *Apis; Bell.; Bry.;* But. ac.; Cinch.; Cocc.; *Gels.; Glon.;* Glycerin; Ign.; Iris; Lach.; Mag. m.; Menthol; Nat. m.; *Nux v.; Phos. ac. ;* Ptel.; Rhus t.; Sep.; *Sil.; Spig.;* Stann.; Ther.

Motion of eyes—Bell.; *Bry.;* Cim.; Col.; Cupr. m.; Gels.; Ichth.; Ign.; Nux v.; *Physost.;* Puls.; Rhus t.; Spig.

Muscular strain—Calc. c.

Narcotics—Coff.

Night—Ars.; *Aur.;* Bov.; Merc. d.; Ptel.; *Puls.;* Strych.; Sul.; Syph.; Tar. h.

Noises—Acon.; Ars.; *Bell.;* Coff.; Ferr. p.; *Ign.;* Lac d.; Lachnanth.; Nit. ac.; *Nux v.;* Phell.; *Phos. ac.;* Ptel.; Sang.; Scutel.; *Sil.;* Spig.; Tab.; *Tar. h.*

Noon—Chin. s.; Sang.; Tab.

Nosebleed—Amyl; Ant. c.

Objects, bright—*Bell.;* Oreodaph.; Phos. ac.; *Sil.;* Spig.

Odors—Coff.; Ign.; Scutel.; *Selen.*

Overheating—Carbo v.; Sil.; Thuya.

Pressure—Diosc.; Hep.; Lach.; Nat. ars.; Ptel.; Sil.

Riding in cars—Cocc.; Kali c.; Petrol.

Right side—*Bell.;* Bry.; *Cact.;* Carb. ac.; *Chel.;* Crot.; Hep.; Iris; *Lyc.;* Mez.; *Sang.;* Taxus.

Rising in bed—*Bry.;* Cocc.

Sitting—Cinch.; Rhus t.

Sleep after—Crot. casc.; Ign.; *Lach.*

Stimulants, abuse—Ign.; *Nux v.*

Stool.—Aloe; Ign.; Ox. ac.

Stooping—Acon.; Ars. m.; *Bell.; Bry.;* Glon.; *Ign.;* Lach.; *Nux v.;* Puls.; Rhus v.; Sep.; Sil.; *Spig.;* Sul.

Sun—*Bell.;* Gels.; *Glon.;* Kali bich.; Lach.; *Nat. c.;* Nux v.; *Sang.; Selen.;* Spig.

Talking—Cact.; Coff.; Ign.; Mez.

Tobacco—Carb. ac.; Gels.; Hep.; *Ign.;* Lob. infl.; Nat. ars.

Warmth in general—Aloe; Bry.; *Cepa;* Euphras.; *Glon.;* Hyper.; *Led.;* Niccol.; Phos.; *Puls.;* Sep.

Water, sight of—Lyssin.

Weather changes—*Calc. p.;* Dulc.; Guaiac.; *Phyt.;* Psor.; Rhod.; Spig.

Wine—Nux v.; Rhod.; Zinc.

Winter—Aloe; Bism.; Carbo v.; Nux v.; Sabad.; Sul.

Working in black—Ced.

AMELIORATION—**After rising:** Kali p.

Bending head backward—*Bell.;* Murex.

Bending head forward—Cim.; Hyos.; Ign.

Closing eyes—Ant. t.; Bell.

Cold in general—Aloe; Alumen; Ars.; Bism.; *Cepa;* Cycl.; Ferr p.; Lyc.; Phos.; Poth.; *Puls.;* Spig.; *Tab.*

Conversation—Dulc.

Dark room—Sang.; Sil.

Eating—Alum.; *Anac.;* Apium gr.; Carls.; *Chel.;* Coca; Kali p.; *Lith. c.; Psor.*

Holding hands near head—Carbo an.; Glon.; Petrol.; Sul. ac.

Lying—Anac.; *Bry.; Cinch.;* Ferr.; Gels.; Ign.; Lach.; Mag. m.; Nux v.; Phos. ac.; *Sang.; Sil.;* Ther.

Lying on painful side—Calc. ars.; Ign.

Lying on painful side with head high—*Bell.;* Gels.

Lying on painful side with head low—Absinth.; Æth.

Menses, during—Bell.; Cepa; Glycerin; Jonosia; Lach.; *Meli.;* Zinc. m.

Mental exertion—*Helon.;* Picr. ac.

Motion, gentle—Cinch.; Glon.; Helon.; Iris; Kali p.; *Puls.*

Motion, hard, continued—Indigo; Rhus t.; Sep.

Nosebleed—Bry.; Bufo; Ferr. p.; Mag. s.; *Meli.;* Psor.; Rhus t.

Open air—Acon.; Act. spic.; *Cepa; Coca;* Indol; Jonosia; *Puls.;* Radium; Sep.; Thuya.

Partially closing eyes—*Aloe;* Coccinel.; Oreodaph.

Polyuria—Acon.; *Gels.; Ign.; Phos. ac.;* Sang.; Sil.; Ver. a.

Pressure—*Apis; Arg. n.; Bell.;* Bry.; Carbo an.; *Cinch.;* Col.; **Gels.;**

Glon.; Ign.; Indigo; Lac c.: Lac d.; *Mag. m.;* Mag. p.; *Menyanth.;* Nux m.; Nux v.; Paris; *Puls.;* Sang.; Sep.; Sil.; Spig.; Thuya; *Ver. a.*
Raising head—Sulphon.
Rest, quiet—Bell.; *Bry.;* Cocc.; *Gels.;* Lith. c.; Menyanth.; Nux v.; Oreodaph.; Puls.; *Sang.; Sil.;* Spig.
Rubbing—Indigo; Tar. h.
Semierect posture—Bell.
Sleep—Coccinel.; Gels.; Nat. m.; *Sang.;* Scutel.; Sil.
Smoking—Aran.
Stimulants—Gels.
Stool and expelling flatus—Æth.; Sang.
Stooping—Cina; Ign.; Menyanth.
Sweating—Nat. m.
Tea—Carb. ac.
Thinking of pain—Camph.; Helon.; *Ox. ac.*
Turning head forward—Ign.
Uncovering head—Glon.; Lyc.
Warmth in general—Am. c.; Cinch.; Col.; Ichthy.; *Mag. p.;* Nux v.: Phos.; Rhus t.; *Sil.*
Wrapping or bandaging tightly—Agar.; *Apis;* Arg. n.; Bell.; Glon.; Ign.; Lac d.; Mag. m.; *Pier. ac.;* Puls.; *Sil.;* Stront.

HYDROCEPHALUS—(acute and chronic): **hydrocephaloid:** Acon.; *Apis; Apoc.;* Arg. n.; Arn.; Ars.; *Bac.;* Bar. c.; *Bell.; Bry.;* Calc. c.; *Calc. p.;* Canth.; Carb. ac.; Chin. s.; *Cinch.; Cupr. ac.;* Cyprip.; Dig.; Gels.; *Helleb.; Iod.; Iodof.;* Ipec.; Kali br.; Kali iod.; Laburn.; Merc. s.; Œnothera; Op.; Phos.; Pod.; *Sil.;* Solan. n.; *Sul.;* Tub.; Ver. a.; Zinc. br.; *Zinc. m.;* Zinc. mur.

MOTION—POSITION OF HEAD—Boring back into pillow or rolling sideways:—*Apis;* Arum; *Bell.; Helleb.; Pod.;* Zinc. m.
Cannot hold head up, neck so weak—Abrot.; *Æth.;* Cocc.; Nat. m.; Ver. a.
Drawn back, retracted—*Agar.;* Art. v.; *Bell.;* Camph. monobr.; *Cic.;* Cur.; Hydroc. ac.; Iodof.; Morph.; Nat. s.; Sec.; Stram.; Sul.; *Ver. v.*
Motion constant, jerking trembling—*Agar.;* Ant. t.; Ars.; *Bell.;* Can. ind.; Cham.; *Hyos.;* Lamium; Myg.; Nux m.; Op.; *Stram.;* Strych.; Ver. v.; Zinc. m.

SCALP—Dandruff (seborrhoea):—Am. m.; *Ars.;* Bar. c.; Branca; Bry.; Fluor. ac.; *Graph.;* Hep.; Heracl.; Iod.; *Kali s.;* Lyc.; Nat. m.; Phos.; Sanic.; *Sep.;* Sul.; Sul. iod.; Thuya.

ERUPTIONS—Boils: Anac.; *Ant. t.;* Aur.; *Calc. mur.;* Calc. s.; Dulc.; Hep.; Jugl. r.; Scrophul.; *Sil.*
Crusta lactea—Arct. l.; Asatacus; Bar. c.; *Calc. c.;* Calc. iod.; Calc. s.; Cic.; Clem.; *Dulc.;* Graph.; *Hep.;* Kali m.; *Lyc.;* Merc.; *Mez.;* Oleand.; Petrol.; Psor.; Rhus t.; Sars.; Scrophul.; *Sep.;* Sil.; Sul.; *Trifol.; Vinca m.; Viola tr.*
Eczema—*Arct. l.;* Astac.; *Calc. c.;* Clem.; *Graph.;* Hydr.; Lyc.; Mez.; *Oleand.; Petrol.;* Psor.; Selen.; Sul.; Tellur.; Viola od.
Erysipelas—Bell.; Euphorb.; Rhus t.
Favus (porrigo, scald head)—Æthiops; Ars.; Ars. iod.; Calc. c.; Calc. iod.;

Calc. mur.; Calc. s.; *Dulc.;* Ferr. iod.; Graph.; *Hep.;* Jugl. r.; Kali s.: Nit. ac.; Sep.; *Sil.;* Sul.; Viola tr.

Growths, tumors, exostoses—Ananth.; Aur. m.; *Calc. fl.;* Cupr. m.; Fluor. ac.; *Hekla; Kali iod.;* Merc. phos.; Merc.; Sil.; Still.

Herpes—Ananth.; Chrys.; Nat. m.; Oleand.; *Rhus t.*

Itching eruptions—Clem.; *Oleand.;* Sil.; Staph.; *Sul.*

Moist, humid eruptions—*Calc. s.;* Clem.; *Graph.; Hep.;* Lyc.; Merc.; *Mez.; Oleand.; Petrol.;* Psor.; *Rhus t.;* Sep.; *Sil.;* Staph.; *Vinca.*

Moist, humid eruptions, behind ears—*Graph.;* Lyc.; *Oleand.; Petrol.;* Staph.; Thlaspi; Tub.

Moist, humid eruptions, of margin of hair, nape of neck—*Clem.;* Hydr.; Nat. m.; *Oleand.;* Sul.

Plica polonica—Ant. t.; Bar. c.; Bor.; Graph.; *Lyc.;* Nat. m.; Psor.; Sars.; Tub.; *Vinca;* Viola tr.

Pustules—Arundo; Cic.; *Clem.;* Graph.; Iris; Jugl. c. ; Mez.

Ringworm (tinea capitis)—Ars.; *Bac.;* Bar. m.; Calc. c.; Chrys.; Dulc.; *Graph.;* Kali s.; *Mez.;* Petrol.; *Psor.; Sep.;* Sil.; Sul.; *Tellur.;* Tub.; Viola tr. See Skin.

Scabs, crusts—Ant. c.; Ars.; Calc. s.; Cic.; *Dulc.; Graph.;* Hep.; Lyc.; *Mez.;* Sul.; Trifol.

Scales, dry—*Ars.;* Kali s.; Mez.; *Nat. m.;* Phos.; Phyt.; Psor.; Sanic.; Thlaspi.

Spots, red—Tellur.

Wens—*Bar. c.; Benz. ac.;* Graph.; Hep.; *Kali iod.;* Nit. ac.; Phyt.

HAIR—Brittle, harsh, dry: Bad.; Bell.; Bor.; Graph.; *Kali c.;* Plumb. m.; *Psor.;* Sec.; Staph.; Thuya.

Falling out (alopecia)—*Alum.;* Ant. c.; *Ars.;* Arundo; Aur.; Bac.; Bar. c.; Calc. c.; Calc. iod.; Carbo v.; Chrysar.; *Fluor. ac.; Graph.;* Hyper.; Kali c.; Lyc.; Mancin.; Mez.; *Nat. m.; Nit. ac.;* Petrol.; *Phos. ac.; Phos.;* Pix liq.; *Selen.; Sep.;* Sil.; Strych. ars.; *Syph.; Thallium;* Thuya; Thyr.; Sphingur.; *Vinca;* Zinc. m.

Greasy—Benz. nit.; Bry.; Merc.

Gray, premature—Lyc.; *Phos. ac.;* Sec.; Sul. ac.

Tangled, in bunches—*Bor.;* Fluor. ac.; Lyc.; *Psor.;* Tub.; Vinca.

ITCHING of scalp—Alum.; Ant. c.; *Ars.;* Arundo; *Bov.; Calc. c.;* Carbo v.; Clem.; Graph.; Heracl.; Iodof.; Jugl., r.; Mag. c.; Mancin.; Menisp.; Nit. ac.; *Oleand.;* Phos.; Sep.; Sil.; Strych.; *Sul.;* Tellur.; *Vinca.*

Neuralgia—*Acon.; Cim.;* Hydr.; Phyt.

Numbness—*Acon.;* Alum.; Ferr. br.; *Graph.; Petrol.*

Sensitive to touch, combing—*Acon.;* Apis, Arn.; Ars.; Azar.; *Bell.;* Bov.; Bry.; Carbo v.; Caust.; *Cinch.;* Euonym.; *Eup. perf.; Gels.;* Hep.; Kali bich.; Lachnanth.; Meli.; Merc.; Nat. m.; Nit. ac.; Nux m.; *Nux v.;* Oleand.; *Paris;* Rhus t.; Sep.; *Sil.;* Strych.; Sul.

Sweat—*Calc. c.;* Calc. p.; *Cham.;* Graph.; Helleb.; Hep.; Heracl.; Hyper.; Mag. m.; Merc.; Pod.; *Rheum.;* Sanic.; *Sil.*

Tension—*Acon.;* Arn.; Asar.; *Bapt.;* Canchal.; Caust.; Iris; *Merc.; Paris;* Ratanh.; Selen.; Sticta; *Viola.*

712 HEAD

SENSATIONS—As if a ball, firmly lodged in forehead: Staph.

As if brain were frozen—Indigo.

As if brain were loose, in forehead, falling laterally—Bell.; Bry.; Rhus t.; Sul. ac.

As if hair were pulled, on vertex—Acon.; *Arg. n.;* Kali n.; Lachnanth.; Mag. c.; *Phos.*

As if top would fly off—Acon.; *Can. ind.; Cim.* Passif.; Syph.; Visc. a.; Yucca.

Bewildered, confused, stupid, intoxicated feeling—*Absinth.;* Acon.; *Ail.;* Aloe; Anac.; *Apis;* Aran.; Arn.; *Bapt.;* Bell.; *Bry.;* Can. ind.; Carbo v.; Cinch.; *Cocc.; Gels.; Glon.; Helleb.;* Menthol; Nat. c.; Nux m.; *Nux v.; Op.; Phos. ac.; Phos.; Quercus;* Rhus t.; Sep.; *Sul.;* Tanac.; Xerophyl.; Zinc. m.

Bruised, sore feeling, of brain—Arg. m.; *Arn.; Bapt.;* Bell.; *Bellis;* Bov.; *Cinch.;* Eupion; Led.; *Nux v.;* Petrol.; Rhus t.; Ver. a. See Headache.

Burning, head—*Acon.;* Alumen; Apis; Arn.; *Ars.; Aster.;* Bell.; Canth.; Nux v.; *Phos.;* Zinc.

Burning on vertex—Avena; Cupr. s.; Daphne; *Frax. am.; Graph.;* Helon.; *Lach.;* Rhus t.; *Sul.;* Tarax.

Bursting—*Acon.;* Arg. n.; *Bell.; Bry.;* Caps.; Cinch.; Cocaine; Formica; *Gels.; Glon.;* Nat. c.; Nat. m.; Nux m.

Coldness—*Agar.;* Ars.; Bar. c.; *Calc. c.;* Calc. p.; Calc. sil.; Carbo v.; Con.; Helod.; Laur.; Nat. m.; *Sep.;* Sil.; Val.; *Ver. a.*

Coldness in occiput—Berb. v.; Calc. p.; Dulc.; Ferrula; *Helod.; Phos.*

Compressed in vise—*Anac.;* Antipyr.; Arg. n.; *Berb. v.; Cact.;* Can. ind.; *Carb. ac.;* Cim.; Coca; *Eup. perf.;* Franciscea; Gels.; Hyper.; Mag. p.; Nit. ac.; *Plat.;* Stann.; Sul.; Tub. See Headache.

Crawling, formication—*Acon.;* Calc. c.; Petrol.; Ran. b.; Ran. rep.; Sul.

Emptiness, hollowness—*Arg. m.;* Caust.; *Cocc.;* Cupr. ac.; Cupr. m.; Granat.; *Ign.;* Mancin.; *Phos.;* Puls.; Zinc.

Enlarged, full, expanded feeling—Acetan.; *Acon.; Arg. n.; Ars. m.; Bapt.; Bell.;* Bov.; Bry.; Cim.; Cocc.; *Gels.; Glon.;* Jugl. c.; Justicia; Lachnanth.; *Meli.;* Menthol; Nat. c.; *Nux v.;* Oxytr.; Paris; Rhus t.; Usnea; *Ver. v.*

Gnawing in spot—Nat. s.; Ran. s.

Heaviness—*Acon.;* Agar.; *Aloe;* Arn.; Apis; *Bapt.;* Calc. c.; Chel.; Cim.; Cinch.; *Gels.;* Mur. ac.; Op.; Oreodaph.; *Petrol.;* Phos. ac.; Plat.; Rhus t.; Sep. See Headache.

Lightness—Abies c.; Hyos.; *Jugl. c.;* Mancin.; Nat. ars.; Nat. chlor.

Looseness of brain—*Am. c.;* Ars.; Bell.; Bry.; Cinch.; Hyos.; Kali c.; *Rhus t.;* Spig.; Sul. ac.; Sul.

Numbness—Alum.; *Bapt.;* Bufo; Calc. ars.; Cocc.; Con.; Graph.; *Kali br.;* Oleand.; Paris; Petrol.; *Plat.*

Opening and shutting—*Can. ind.; Cim.;* Cocc.; Lac c.

Tired feeling—*Apis;* Arn.; Chin. ars.; Con.; Ferr. p.; *Phos.;* Zinc. v.

Undulating, surging, wavelike—*Acon.;* Aur.; *Bell.;* Canth.; Chin. s.;

Cim.; *Cinch.; Glon.;* Hep.; Hyos.; Ind.; Lach.; Mag. p.; *Meli.;* Nux v.; Pall.; Rhus t.; Senec.; Sul.

Wild, crazy feeling on vertex—Lil. t.

VERTIGO—Dizziness: Remedies in general: *Absinth.; Acon.;* Adren.; Æsc. gl.; *Æth.; Agar.; Alum.;* Ambra; Ant. c.; *Apis;* Apomorph.; *Arg. n.;* Arn.; Ars. iod.; Aur. mur.; Bapt.; *Bell.;* Bism.; Bor.; *Bry., Calc. c.;* Can. ind.; *Carb. ac.; Carbo v.;* Chenop.; *Chin. s.;* Cim.; *Cinch.; Coca; Cocc.; Con.;* Cycl.; Dig.; Eup. perf.; Ferr. m.; Formal.; *Gels.;* Gins.; *Glon.; Granat.; Hydroc. ac.;* Iod.; Kali c.; Laburn.; Lach.; *Lith chlor.;* Lol.; Lupul.; Merc. v.; *Morph.;* Mosch.; Nat. sal.; Nicot.; *Nux v.; Op.;* Ox. ac.; Petrol.; *Phos.; Picr. ac.;* Pod.; *Puls.;* Quercus; Radium; Sal. ac.; Senec.; Sep.; *Sil.;* Spig.; Stront.; Strych.; Sul.; *Tab.;* Tar. h.; *Ther.;* Wyeth.

CAUSE AND TYPE—Anæmia of brain: Arn.; Bar. m.; Calc. c.; Chin s..; *Cinch.;* Con.; Dig.; Ferr. carb.; *Ferr.;* Hydroc. ac.; Nat. m.; Sil.

Cerebral origin—Bell.; *Cocc.;* Gels.; Sulphon.; Tab.

Congestion of brain—*Acon.;* Arn.; *Bell.;* Cinch.; *Cupr. m.; Glon.;* Hydroc. ac.; *Iod.; Nux v.;* Op.; Stram.; *Sul.*

Epileptic—Arg. n.; Calc. c.; *Cupr. m.;* Kal.; Nux v.; *Sil.*

Gastro-enteric derangement—Aloe; *Bry.;* Cinch.; *Cocc.;* Ipec.; Kali c.; *Nux v.; Puls.;* Rham. cal.; *Tab.*

Hysterical—*Asaf.; Ign.;* Val.

Labyrinthic origin (Meniere's disease)—Arn.; Bar. m.; Bry.; Carbon. s.; Caust.; *Chenop.; Chin. sal.; Chin. s.;* Cinch.; Con.; Ferr. p.; Gels.; Hydrobr. ac.; Kali iod.; *Nat. sal.;* Onosm.; Petrol.; Piloc.; Pyrus; *Sal. ac.;* Sil.; Tab.; *Ther.*

Mal-de-mer—Apomorph.; *Cocc.;* Petrol.; Staph.; Tab.

Mental exertion—*Arg. n.;* Nat. c.; *Nux v.*

Nervous origin—Ambra; Arg. n.; Cocc.; Nux v.; *Phos.;* Rhus t.; Ther.

Noises—Nux v.; *Ther.*

Odor of flowers—Nux v.; Phos.

Old age (senile changes)—*Ambra; Ars. iod.;* Bar. m.; Bellis; Con.; Dig.; *Iod.;* Op.; *Phos.;* Rhus t.; Sul.

Open air—Arn.; Calc. ac.; Canth.; Cycl.; *Nux v.*

Optical disturbances—Con.; *Gels.;* Piloc.

Pelvic troubles—Aloe; Con.

Sunlight—Agar.; Nat. c.

Worms—Cina; Spig.

OCCURRENCE—Alternates with colic: Col.; Mag. c.; Spig.

Beginning in nape of neck, or occiput—*Gels.;* Iberis; Petrol.; *Sil.*

When ascending stairs—Ars. hydr.; *Calc. c.*

When closing eyes—Apis; Arn.; *Lach.;* Mag. p.; *Ther.;* Thuya.

When coughing—Ant. t.

When descending stairs—*Bor.;* Con.; Ferr.; Meph.; *Sanic.*

When eating—Am. c.; Cocc.; Mag. m.; *Nux v.;* Puls.

When entering warm room—Ars.; *Iod.;* Plat.; Tab.

When frightened—Op.

When in high-ceilinged room—Cupr. ac.

When looking at colored light—Art. v.

When looking at running water—Arg. m.; Brom.; *Ferr. m.; Ver. a.*

When looking down—*Bor.;* Oleand.; Kal.; *Spig.*

When looking fixedly—Caust.; Con.; Lach.; Oleand.

When looking up—Calc. c.; Chin. ars.; *Granat.;* Kali p.; Petrol.; *Puls.,* *Sil.;* Tab.

When lying down—Adon. v.; Apis; Calad.; *Con.;* Lach.; Nat. m.; Nux v.; Rhod.; Rhus t.; Sil.; Staph.; *Ther.;* Thuya.

When opening eyes—Lach.; *Tab.*

When reading—Am. c.; Arn.; Cupr. m.; Nat. m.

When riding in carriage—*Cocc.;* Hep.; Lac d.; Petrol.

When rising from bed or chair—Acon.; Adon. v.; Bell.; *Bry.;* Can. ind.; *Cocc.;* Con.; Ferr. m.; *Nat. sal.; Nux v.;* Oleand.; Op.; Petrol.; Phos.; Rhus t.; Sul.

When rising in morning—*Alum.; Bry.;* Jacar.; *Lach.;* Lyc.; *Nux v.;* Op.; Phos.; Pod.; Puls.

When shaking or turning head—*Acon.;* Calc. c.; *Con.;* Hep.; Kali c.; *Morph.;* Nat. ars.

When standing with eyes closed—Arg. n.; Lathyr.

When stooping—*Acon.;* Bar. c.; Bell.; Bry.; Glon.; Iod.; *Kal.;* Nux v.; Oreodaph.; *Puls.; Sul.;* Ther.

When turning eyes—Con.

When turning head—Bry.; Calc. c.; Col.; *Con.;* Kali c.; Menthol; *Morph.;* Nat. ars.

When turning head to left—*Col.;* Con.

When turning in bed—Bell.; *Con.*

When walking—Acon.; Agar.; *Bell.; Caust.;* Cinch.; Dig.; *Gels.;* Kali c.; Lach.; Mag. p.; Nit. ac.; Nux m.; *Oreodaph.;* Petrol.; *Phos. ac.;* Rhus t.; *Ther.*

When walking in dark—Stram.

When walking in open air—Agar.; Arn.; *Cycl.;* Dros.; *Nux v.;* Sep.; *Sul.*

When walking over bridge or water—Ferr.; Lyssin.

CONCOMITANTS—**Buzzing, tinnitus:** Arg. n.; Bell.; Carbo v.; Chenop.; *Chin. s.; Gels.;* Picr. ac.; *Strych.;* Val.

Deathly pallor—*Dub.;* Puls.; *Tab.*

Debility, prostration—Ambra; *Arg. n.;* Bapt.; Cinch.; Con.; Echin.; Gels.; *Tab.;* Ver. a.

Dim vision, diplopia, etc.—Arg. n.; Bell.; *Gels.;* Glon.; Nux v.; Val.; Vinca.

Drowsiness, hot head—Æth.

Fainting, unconscious—Acon.; Alet.; Berb. v.; *Bry.;* Camph.; *Carbo v.;* Glon.; *Nux v.;* Phos.; Sabad.; Tab.

Gastralgia, spasms—Cic.

Head feels elongated, urging to urinate—Hyper.

Headache—Acon.; Agrost.; Apis; Cocc.; *Nux v.*

Intoxicated feeling—Abies c.; Arg. m.; Bell.; Cinch.; *Cocc.;* Con.; **Gels.;** *Nux v.;* Op.; Oxytr.; Petrol.

Liver disturbances—Bry.; Card. m.; Chel.

Nausea, vomiting—Acon.; *Bry.*; *Cocc.*; Euonym.; *Kali bich.*; *Nux v.*; *Petrol.*; Piloc.; *Pod.*; Puls.; Stront.; *Tab.*; Ther.

Nervous phenomena—Ambra; Cocc.; *Gels.*; *Ign.*; Phos.

Nosebleed—Bell.; Bry.; Carbo an.

Opisthotonos—Cic.

Palpitation, heart symptoms—Æth.; Bell.; *Cact.*; Dig.; Spig.

Pressure at root of nose—Bapt.

Relief from closing eyes—Aloe; Lol.

Relief from food—Alum.

Relief from holding head perfectly still—Con.

Relief from lying down—Apis; Antham.; Aur.; Bry.; Cinch.; *Cocc.*; Nit. ac.; Puls.

Relief from nosebleed—Brom.

Relief from rest—Arn.; Colch.; Cycl.; Spig.

Relief from vomiting—Tab.

Relief from walking in open air—Am. m.; Kali c.; Mag. p.; *Puls.*; *Rhus t.*; Tab.

Relief from warmth—Mang. m.; Sil.; Stront.

With balancing sensation—Ferr. m.

With staggering, trembling, weakness—*Arg. n.*; Crot.; *Gels.*; Nux v.; Phos. ac.; Phos.; Stram.

With tendency to fall backward—*Absinth.*; Bell.; Bry.; Kali n.; Nux v.

With tendency to fall forward—Alum.; *Bry.*; Card. m.; Caust.; Chel.; Elaps.; Guarea; Mag. p.; Petrol.; *Pod.*; Spig.; Stram.; Urt.; Vib. op.

With tendency to fall to left—Aur.; Bell.; *Con.*; *Dros.*; Eup. perf.; Iod.; Sal. ac.; Sil.; Stram.; Zinc.

With tendency to fall to right—Helod.; Kali n.

EYES

BROWS—Hair falls out: *Alum.;* Bor.; Merc.; *Nit. ac.;* Plumb. ac.; Sanic.; *Selen.:* Sil.

Pimples on—Fluor. ac.; Sil.; Thuya.

Warty growths on—Ananth.

CANTHI (angles)—Itching, smarting: Alum.; Apium gr.; Ars.; Carbe v.; Fluor. ac.; *Gamb.; Hep.;* Lyc.; Nat. m.; Nux v.; Phos.; Succin. ac.; Sul.; *Zinc. m.*

Sore, raw, fissured—*Ant. c.;* Bor.; *Graph.;* Petrol.; *Sil.;* Staph.; Zinc. m.

Swollen, red—Agar.; *Arg. n.;* Cinnab.; Graph.; Zinc. m.

CATARACT—Am. c.; Arg. iod.; Calc. c.; *Calc. fl.;* Can. s.; *Caust.;* Chimaph.; *Ciner.;* Cochlear; Colch.; *Con.; Euphras.;* Iod.; Kali m.; Led.; Mag. c.; *Naph.;* Nat. m.; *Phos.;* Platan.; Puls.; Quass.; Santon.; Sec.; Senega; Sep.; *Sil.; Sul.;* Tellur.; *Thiosin.;* Zinc.

CHAMBER, anterior, pus in—Hep.; Sil.

Chamber, hemorrhage after iridectomy—Led.

CHOROID—Congestion: Agar.; Phos.; Rhod.; Ruta; *Santon.*

Choroid, Detachment—Acon.; Arn.; Nux v.

Choroid, Extravasation—Ham.

Choroid, Inflammation (choroiditis), Atrophic—Nux v.; Phos.; *Piloc.*

Choroiditis, disseminated and si. ple—Ars.; *Bell.;* Bry.; Ced.; Gels.; Ipec.; *Kali iod.;* Merc.; Merc. i. r.; Naph.; Phos.; *Prun. sp.;* Santon.; Tab.; Tellur.; Thuya.

Choroiditis, suppurative—Hep.; Rhus t.

Choroiditis, suppurative, with iris involvement—Kali iod.; *Prun. s.;* Sil.

Choroiditis, suppurative, with retinal involvement (syphilitic)—Aur.; *Kali iod.;* Kali m.; Merc. c.; *Merc. i. r.*

CILIARY MUSCLE—Accommodation disturbed: Ipec.; Ruta.

Ciliary muscle, paretic condition—*Arg. n.;* Atrop.; Caust.; Dub.; *Gels.;* Paris; Physost.

Ciliary muscle, spasm—*Agar.;* Eser.; Ipec.; Jabor.; Lil. t.; *Physost.;* Piloc.

CILIARY NEURALGIA—Ars.; *Ced.;* Chel.; Chenop.; *Cim.;* Cinch.; *Cinnab.;* Col.; Commocl.; Croc.; Crot. t.; *Gels.;* Lach.; Mez.; Nat. m.; Paris; Phos.; Plant.; *Prun. sp.; Rhod.;* Sapon.; Spig. See Pain.

CONJUNCTIVA—Chemosis: Apis; Guarea; Hep.; *Kali iod.;* Rhus t.; Sul. ac.; *Vespa.*

Discharge, acrid—Ars.; Arum; *Euphras.;* Merc. c.; *Merc.;* Psor.; Rhus t.

Discharge, clear mucus—Ipec.; Kali m.

Discharge, creamy, profuse—*Arg. n.;* Calc. s.; Dulc.; Hep.; *Nat. p.;* Nat. s.; Picr. ac.; *Puls.;* Rhus t.; Syph.

Discharge, ropy—Kali bich.

Ecchymoses and injuries—Acon.; *Arn.; Ham.;* Lach.; Led.; **Nux v.**

Foreign bodies, irritation—*Acon.;* Sul.

Granulations, blisters or wart like—Thuya.

Hyperemia—*Acon.;* Ars.; *Bell.;* Cepa; Ipec.; *Nux v.;* Rhus t.; Sul.; *Thuya.*

Inflammation (conjunctivitis)—Acute and sub-acute catarrhal:—*Acon.;* Apis; *Arg. n.;* Ars.; *Bell.;* Canth.; *Chloral.;* Dub.; Dulc.; *Euphras.;* Ferr. p.; Guarea; *Hep.;* Kali m.; Merc. c.; Merc. per.; *Merc.;* Nat. ars.; Op.; Picr. ac.; *Puls.;* Rhus t.; Sep.; Sticta; Sul.; Upas.

Inflammation, chronic—*Alum.;* Ant. t.; Arg. n.; *Ars.; Aur. mur.;* Bell.; Euphras.; *Kali bich.;* Merc. s.; Picr. ac.; Psor.; *Puls.; Sul.;* Thuya; Zinc. m.

Inflammation, croupous, diphtheritic—Acet. ac.; Apis; Guarea; Iod.; *Kali bich.; Merc. cy.*

Inflammation, follicular (granular)—Apis; Arg. n.; *Ars.;* Aur. m.; *Aur. mur.;* Calc. iod.; Crot. t.; Jequir.; *Kali bich.;* Nat. m.; Phyt.; Puls.; *Thuya;* Zinc. s.

Inflammation, gonorrhoeal—*Acon.;* Ant. t.; Apis; *Arg. n.;* Calc. hypoph.; *Hep.;* Kali bich.; Merc. c.; *Merc.; Puls.;* Rhus t.; Ver. v.

Inflammation, gonorrhoeal, sympathetic form—*Arg. n.;* Euphras.; Merc.; Puls. See Purulent.

Inflammation, phlyctenular—Ant. t.; *Calc. c.; Calc. picr.;* Con.; Euphras.; Graph.; Ign.; Merc. c.; Puls.; *Rhus t.;* Sil.; Sul.

Inflammation, purulent—*Arg. n.;* Calc. hypoph.; Hep.; *Merc. c.;* Merc.; Puls.; *Rhus t.;* Sil.

Inflammation, pustular—*Ant. t.;* Arg. n.; Ars.; Calc. c.; Graph.; *Hep.;* Jequir.; Kali bich.; *Merc. c.;* Merc. nit.; Puls.; Rhus t.

Inflammation, traumatic—*Acon.;* Arn.; Bell.; *Calend.;* Canth.; Euphras.; *Ham.;* Led.; Symphyt.

ORNEA—Abscess of: Calc. s.; *Hep.;* Kali s.; Merc. c.; Sil.; Sul.

Ectasia—Calc. p.

Exudation, serous—Apis.

Foreign bodies—*Acon.;* Calc. hypoph.; Hep.; Rhus t.; Sul.

Inflammation, (keratitis)—Acon.; Apis; Ars.; Ars. iod.; *Aur. mur.;* Bell.; Can. s.; Con.; Euphras.; Hep.; Ilex; *Kali bich.;* Kali m.; *Merc. c.;* Nux v.; Phos.; Sang.; Sul.; Thuya.

Inflammation, arthritic—Clem.; Colch.; Col.

Inflammation, herpetic, vesicular—*Apis; Ars.;* Calc. p.; Euphras.; Ran. b.; Tellur.

Inflammation, interstitial, in persons of hereditary syphilis—Aur. m.; *Aur. mur.;* Can. s.; Merc. c.; Merc. cy.

Inflammation, parenchymatous, syphilitic origin—*Aur. mur.;* Calc. hypoph.; *Kali iod.;* Kali m.; Merc. s.; Sul.

Inflammation, phlyctenular—*Apis;* Bell.; Calc. c.; *Calc. fl.;* Calc. p.; Con.; *Graph.;* Hep.; Ipec.; *Merc. c.;* Puls.; Rhus t.; Syph.; Thuya.

Onyx—Hep.

Opacities—Arg. n.; Aur.; Aur. mur.; Bar. c.; Cadm. s.; Calc. c.; *Calc. fl.;* Calc. hypoph.; Calc. iod.; *Caust.; Can. s.; Ciner.;* Con.; *Euphras.;* Hep.; Kali bich.; Kali m.; Merc. c.; Merc. s.; *Naph.;* Nit .ac.; Phos.; Puls.; Sacchar. of.; Senega; *Sil.;* Sul.; Thiosinam.; Zinc. m.; Zinc. s.

Pustules—*Ant. c.;* Calc. c.; Con.; Crot. t.; Euphras.; *Hep.;* Kali bich.; Kali iod.; Merc. nit.; Nit. ac.

Staphyloma, after suppurative inflammation—*Apis;* Euphras.; Ilex; Physost.

Ulcers—Æthiops antim.; Apis; *Arg. n.;* Ars.; Aur. mur.; *Calc. c.;* Calc. hypoph.; Calc. iod.; Calc. sil.; *Euphras.;* Graph.; *Hep.; Kali bich.;* Kali m.; *Merc. c.;* Merc. i. fl.; Nat. m.; Nit. ac.; Rhus t.; *Sil.;* Sul.; Thuya; Zinc. m.

Ulcers, deep—Ars.; Euphras.; *Kali bich.; Merc. c.;* Merc. i. fl.; Merc. i. r.; Sil.

Ulcers, indolent—Calc. c.; *Kali bich.; Sil.;* Sul.

Ulcers, superficial, flat—Ars.; Asaf.; Euphras.; Kali m.; Merc.; Nit. ac.

Ulcers, vascular—Aur. m.

Wounds, incised, lacerated—Staph.

EYE-BALLS—**Bad effects from exposure to snow:** Acon.; Cic.

Bad effects from electric or artificial light—Glon.; Jabor.

Bad effects from glare of fire—Acon.; Canth.; Glon.; Merc.

Bad effects from operations—*Acon.;* Arn.; Asar.; Bry.; Croc.; Ign.; *Led.;* Rhus t.; Senega; Stront.; Thuya.

Bad effects from sight seeing, moving pictures—Arn.

Burning, smarting—*Acon.;* Ars.; Ars. m.; Aur. mur.; *Bell.;* Calc. c.; Canth.; *Cepa;* Croc.; *Euphras.;* Fagop.; Ferr. p.; Lept.; Lyc.; Mag. p.; *Merc. c.; Nat. ars.; Nat. m.;* Op.; Phyt.; Piloc.; Puls.; Ran. b.; Sang.; *Sul.; Thuya; Zinc. m.*

Coldness—Alum.; Asar.; Con.; Mez.; Nat. m.; Plat.

Coldness, as if wind blowing under lids—*Croc.;* Fluor. ac.; Syph.; Thuya.

Dryness, heat—*Acon.;* Alum.; Ars.; *Bell.;* Berb. v.; Clem.; Croc.; Grat.; *Lyc.; Merc. c.;* Nat. ars.; Nat. c.; Nat. m.; Nat. s.; Nux m.; Op.; Senega; Sep.; Sticta; *Sul.;* Zinc. m.

Edema of ocular conjunctiva, translucent—Apis.

Enlarged, swollen feeling—Acon.; *Bell.;* Ox. ac.; Paris; Phos. ac.; *Rhus t.;* Sarrac.; *Senega; Spig.;* Trill.

Eruptions about—Ant. t.; Crot. t.; Guaiac.

Heat, and flickering, worse in damp weather—Aran.

Heat, and sensitive to air—Clem.; Coral.

Heat—Æsc.; Carbo v.; Indol; Lil. t.; Meph.; Op.; Phos.; *Ruta;* Sapon.; Strych.; *Sul.*

Heaviness—Bapt.; *Gels.;* Meli.; *Onosm.;* Op.; Paris; Parth.; Sep.; Solan. lyc.; Sulphon.

Hemorrhage (inter-ocular)—Arn.; *Ham.;* Lach.; Led.; *Sul. ac.;* Supraren. ext.

Injuries—Acon.; *Arn.;* Calend.; Canth.; Cochlear.; *Ham.;* Led.; Physost.; *Rhus t.;* Sul. ac.; *Symphyt.*

Itching—Agar.; *Agn.;* Ant. c.; Ars. m.; *Aur. mur.;* Calc. c.; Caust.; Cepa; Croc.; *Fagop.;* Gamb.; *Merc.;* Nux v.; Puls.; *Rhus t.;* Scilla; *Sul.;* Zinc. m.

LOOK—**CONDITION**—**Dull:** Ant. c.; *Ant. t.;* Bapt.; Diph.; Merc.; Onosm.; Solan. lyc.

Fixed, staring, distorted—*Bell.;* Can. ind.; *Cic.;* Cupr. m.; Glon.; *Helleb.;* Hyos.; *Morph.;* Œnanthe; Op.; Phos. ac.; Piscidia; *Stram.;* Strych.

Glazed, death-like—*Op.;* Phos. ac.; Zinc. m. See Face.

Glistening, dazzling, brilliant—*Bell.;* Bry.; *Canth.;* Cupr. m.; Hyos.; Merc. c.; *Stram.;* Ver. v.

Looking downwards—*Æth.;* Hyos.

Protruding, bulging (exophthalmus)—Amyl; *Bell.;* Clem.; Commocl.; Ferr. p.; Glon.; Helod.; *Lycop.;* Paris; Sang. tart.; Sapon.; Spong.; Stellar.; *Stram.;* Strych.; *Thyr.*

Red, blood-shot, suffused—*Acon.;* Æsc.; Ail.; *Bell.;* *Cepa;* Cinnab.; Dulc.; *Gels.;* Ham.; Hyos.; *Merc. c.;* Morph.; Op.; Ruta; Sil.; Sulphon.; Sul.; *Thuya;* Ver. v.

Red, inflamed—*Acon.;* Ant. c.; Arg. n.; Ars.; Aur. mur.; *Bell.;* Caust.; Clem.; *Euphras.;* Ferr. p.; Hep.; Indol; Ipec.; Jacor.; Lyc.; Merc. s.; Nat. m.; Rhus t.; Sang. n.

Red, raw—Arg. n.; Crot. t.

Red, with yellow vision—Aloe.

Rolling downwards—*Æth.;* Hyos.

Rolling in vertical axis—*Benz. nit.;* Zinc. m.

Rolling on falling asleep—Æth.

Rolling quickly with closed eyes—Cupr. m.

Rolling upwards—Bell.; *Cic.;* Helleb.; Mur. ac.; Œnanthe.

Sensation as if fat on eyes—Paraf.

Sensation as if sand or sticks in—*Acon.;* Alum.; Ars.; *Caust.;* Coccus c.; Euphras.; Ferr. p.; Graph.; *Nat. m.;* Phos.; Phyt.; *Sul;* Xeroph.

Sensation as if wind blowing in eyes—Fluor. ac.

Squinting to relieve pain in forehead—Aloe.

Stiffness—Asar.; Aur.; *Kal.;* Med.; Nat. ars.; Rhus t.

Sunken, surrounded by blue rings—Acet. ac.; Ant. c.; Apium gr.; *Ars.;* Camph.; *Cinch.;* Cupr. m.; Granat.; Helleb.; Ipec.; Nat. c.; *Phos ac.;* Phos.; Sec.; *Staph.;* Upas; *Ver. a.;* Visc. a. See Face.

Syphilitic diseases—Jacar. g.; Kali iod.; Merc. i. fl.; Nit. ac.; Thuya.

Trembling (nystagmus)—*Agar.;* Benz. nit.; Carbon. hydr.; *Cic.;* Gels.; Iod.; Kali iod.; Mag. p.; Physost.

Unable to keep eyes fixed steadily—Arg. n.; Paris.

Whites of, yellow—Brassica; Cham.; *Chel.;* *Cinch.;* Crot.; Dig.; Euonvm. tarop.; Iod.; Lach.; Merc.; Myr.; Nat. p.; Nat. s.; *Pod.;* Plumb.; Sep. See Face.

EYELIDS AND MARGINS—**Agglutination:** Agar.; Alum.; *Ant. c.;* Apis; Arg. n.; Bor.; Calc. c.; Caust.; Dig.; *Euphras.;* *Graph.;* Kali bich.; Kali c.; Lyc.; *Merc. s.;* Nat. ars.; Nat. m.; Psor.; *Puls.;* Rhus t.; Sep.; *Sul.;* Thuya; Uran.; Zinc. m.

Blueness—Dig.; Morph.

Drooping (ptosis)—Alum.; Caul.; *Caust.;* *Con.;* Dulc.; *Gels.;* Graph.; Hæmat.; Helod.; Kal.; *Morph.;* Naja; Nat. ars.; Nit. ac.; Nux m.; Nux v.; Op.; Phos.; Plumb.; Rhus t.; *Sep.;* Spig.; Stram.; Sulphon.; Syph.; Upas; Ver. a.; *Zinc. m.*

Dryness—*Acon.;* Alum.; Ars.; *Bell.; Graph.;* Lith. c.; Nux v.; Puls.; Senega; Sep.; Sul.; Zinc. m.

Dryness, scaliness—*Ars.;* Bor.; Sep.; Tellur.; Thuya.

Ectropion—Apis; Graph.; Thiosinam.

Entropion—*Bor.;* Graph.; Nat. m.; Tellur.

ERUPTIONS, growths, blisters, vesicles—Canth.; *Nat. s.;* Pall.; *Rhus t.;* Sep.; *Thuya.*

Chalazae, tarsal tumors—Ant. t.; Calc. c.; Caust.; *Con.;* Ferr. pyropn.; *Kali iod.;* Platanus; Sil.; *Staph.; Thuya;* Zinc. m.

Cysts, sebaceous—*Benz. ac.;* Calc. c.; *Calc. fl.;* Iod.; *Kali iod.;* Merc. s.; Platanus; *Staph.*

Eczema, fissures—Bac.; Chrysarob.; *Graph.; Petrol.;* Staph.; Sul.; Tellur.

Granular lids (trachoma)—*Alum.;* Ars.; Aur. mur.; *Calc. c.;* Cinnab.; Dulc.; *Euphras.;* Graph.; Hep.; Jequir.; *Kali bich.;* Kali m.; Merc. per.; Nat. ars.; Nat. s.; Puls.; Sep.; Sul.; *Thuya;* Zinc. s.

Pustules—Ant. c.; Hep.

Scabs, crusts, scurfs—Arg. n ; *Ars.;* Bor.; Calc. c.; *Graph.;* Kali m.; Lyc.; Senega; *Sep.*

Styes (hordeolum)—Agar.; Apis; Aur. m. n.; *Calc. picr.;* Con.; *Graph.; Hep.;* Lyc.; Merc.; *Puls.; Sep.; Sil.; Staph.; Sul.;* Thuya; Uran.

Styes, followed by hard nodosities—Con.; Staph.; Thuya.

Ulcers—Arg. n.; *Ars.; Caust.;* Euphras.; *Graph.;* Hep.; Lappa; Lyc.; *Sul.; Tellur.* See Tissues.

Inflammation (blepharitis)—Acute: *Acon.;* Apis; Arg. n.; *Ars.:* Cham.; Dig.; Dulc.; *Euphras.;* Hep.; Kreos.; Merc. i. fl.; *Merc. pr. rub.; Merc. s.;* Nat. ars.; Petrol.; *Puls.;* Rhus t.; Sul.; Upas; Uran.

Inflammation, chronic—*Alum.;* Ant. c.; *Arg. n.;* Aur.; Bar. c.; *Bor.;* Calc. c.; Clem.; Euphras.; *Graph.;* Hep.; Jugl.; Merc. c.; Merc. pr. r.; Petrol.; Psor.; Sep.; *Sil.; Staph.; Sul.; Tellur.*

Inflammation, erysipelatous—*Apis;* Bell.; *Rhus t.;* Vespa.

Redness—Agar.; Am. br.; *Ant. c.;* Apis; Arg. n.; Ars.; *Bell.;* Cinnab.; Clem.; Dig.; Euphras.; Graph.; Hep.; Lyc.; *Merc. c.;* Merc. s.; Rhus t.; Sabad.; *Sul.* See Inflammation.

SENSATIONS—Burning and smarting:—Agar.; Alum.; Apis; *Ars.;* Arundo; Bell.; Calc. c.; Cepa; Cham.; Croc.; *Euphras.;* Graph.; Kali bich.; Kali iod.; Lyc.; Merc.; Mez.; Nat. m.; Puls.; Sabad.; *Sul.*

Coldness—Croc.; Phos. ac.

Heaviness—Caul.; *Gels.;* Hæmat.; Helod.; Nat. m.; *Sep.* See Drooping.

Itching—Agar.; Alum.; *Ambros.;* Calc. c.; *Gamb.;* Graph.; Lyc.; Mez.; *Morph.; Puls.;* Rhus t.; Staph.; Succin. ac.; *Sul.;* Tellur.; Zinc.

Pulsation of superciliary muscle—Cina.

Rawness and soreness—*Ant. c.;* Arg. n.; Ars.; Bor.; Euphras.; *Graph.;* Hep.; Merc. c.; Petrol.; Sul.; Zinc. See Belpharitis.

Spasms of eyelids, twitching, (blepharospasm, nictitation)—*Agar.;* Ars.; Atrop.; *Bell.;* Calc. c.; Cham.; Cic.; *Cod.;* Croc.; Eser.; Gels.; Guaiac.; *Hyos.;* Ign.; Lob. purp.; Mag. p.; Nat. m.; Nicot.; *Nux v.;* Physost.; *Puls.;* Ruta; Strych.; Sul. ac.

Stiffness—Caust.; Gels.; Kal.; Rhus t.

Swelling (Œdema)—Am. br.; *Apis;* Arg. n.; *Ars.;* Ars. m.; Aur. mur.; Bell.; Calc. c.; Dig.; Euphorb. d.; *Euphras.;* Graph.; Hep.; *Kali c.;* Kali iod.; Merc. c.; Nat. ars.; Nat. c.; Phos.; Puls.; *Rhus t.;* Rhus v.; Sabad.; Sep.

Thickening—*Alum.;* Arg. n.; Calc. c.; *Graph.;* Hep.; Merc.; *Tellur.*

GLAUCOMA—*Acon.;* Atrop.; Aur.; *Bell.;* Bry.; Caust.; Ced.; Cocaine; Col.; Commocl.; Croc.; Eser.; *Gels.;* Mag. c.; Nux v.; Op.; *Osm.;* Phos.; Physost.; Prun. sp.; Rhus t.; *Spig.;* Supraren. ext.

HYPOPION—Crot. t.; *Hep.;* Merc. c.; Merc.; Plumb.; *Sil.*

IRIDO-CHOROIDITIS—Kali. iod.; Prun. sp.; *Sil.*

Irido-cyclitis, traumatic, with infection and sequelæ—Nat. salic.

IRIS—Prolapse: Ant. s. a.; Physost.

IRITIS—Remedies in general: *Acon.;* Ars.; Bell.; Ced.; *Cinnab.; Clem.;* Dub.; *Euphras.;* Ferr. p.; Gels.; Grind.; Hep.; Iod.; Kali bich.; Kali iod.; *Merc. c.;* Merc. s.; Puls.; *Rhus t.;* Spig.; Sul.; Syph.; Tellur.; Tereb.; Thuya.

Plastic—*Acon.;* Bry.; Cinnab.; Hep.; *Merc. c.;* Rhus t.; Thuya.

Rheumatic—Arn.; *Bry.;* Clem.; Colch.; *Euphras.;* Formica; Kali bich.; Kal.; Led.; Merc. c.; *Rhus t.;* Spig.; Tereb.; *Thuya.*

Serous—Apis; *Ars.;* Bry.; Ced.; *Gels.;* Merc. c.; Merc.; Spig.

Syphilitic—Asaf.; *Aur.;* *Cinnab.;* Clem.; Iod.; Kali bich.; *Kali iod.;* Merc. c.; Merc. cy.; Merc. i. fl.; *Nit. ac.;* Sul.; Thuya.

Traumatic—Acon.; Arn.; Bell.; *Ham.;* Led.; Rhus t.

Tuberculous—*Ars.;* Kali bich.; Sul.; Syph.; Tub.

LACHRYMAL SAC—Blemorrhœa: Ant. t.; Calc. c.; Calend.; *Hep.;* Merc. d.; Nat. m.; Petrol.; *Puls.;* Sil.; Stann.

Dacryo-cystitis—Apis; Fluor. ac.; *Hep.; Iod.;* Merc.; Petrol.; *Puls.; Sil.; Stann.*

Duct closed, from cold, exposure—Calc. c.

Duct, stricture—Nat. m.

Duct, swollen—Graph.; Sil.

Epiphora—Calc. c.; Graph.; Hep.; *Merc. per.;* Merc. s.; *Nat. m.;* Scilla; Sil.; Tongo. See Lachrymation.

Fistula lachrymalis—*Calc. c.;* Caust.; *Fluor. ac.;* Lach.; Merc. c.; Nat. m.; Nit. ac.; Petrol.; Phos.; Phyt.; *Sil.;* Stann.; Sul.

LACHRYMATION—Acon.; ˜*Ambros.;* Antipyr.; Apis; *Ars.;* Ars. m.; Aur.; Calc. c.; Caust.; *Cepa;* Con.; Eugen. j.; *Euphras.;* Guarea; Ipec.; *Kali iod.;* Lyc.; *Merc. c.;* Merc. per.; Merc. s.; Nat. ars.; *Nat. m.;* Phos.; Phyt.; *Puls.;* Rhus t.; *Sabad.;* Sang. n.; Scilla; Sil.; Sticta; Succin.; Sul.; Taxus.

Acrid, burning, hot—Apis; *Ars.;* Ced.; Eugen. j.; *Euphras.;* Graph.; *Kali iod.;* Kreos.; *Merc. c.;* Naph.; *Nat. m.; Rhus t.;* Sul.

Bland—Cepa; *Puls.*

MODALITIES—Relief in open air: Cepa.

Worse at night—Apis.

Worse from cold application—Sanic.

Worse from coughing—Euphras.; *Nat. m.*
Worse from eating—Ol. an.
Worse from foreign bodies in eyes, cold wind, reflection from snow—Acon.
Worse in morning early—Calc. c.
Worse in open air—Calc. c.; Colch.; Lyc.; Phos.; Sanic.; Sil.

LAGOPHTHALMOS—Physost.

MEIBOMIAN GLANDS—Swollen: *Æth.;* Bad.; Clem.; Dig.; Graph.; Hep.; Puls.; Rhus t. See Blepharitis.

OCULAR MUSCLES—Contracted spasmodically: *Agar.;* Cic.; Physost.; Strych.
Ocular muscles, pain—Carbo v.; Cim.; *Onosm.* See Pain.
Ocular muscles, paralysis—Arg. n.; Bell.; *Caust.; Con.;* Euphras.; *Gels.;* Hyos.; Lach.; Oxytr.; Phos.; Physost.; *Rhus t.; Ruta;* Santon.; Senega; Syph.
Ocular muscles, paralysis, extrinsic—Gels.; Phos.
Ocular muscles, paralysis, intrinsic—Alum.; Con.; Lach.; Nat. m.; Onosm.; Ruta.
Ocular muscles, paralysis superior rectus—Senega.
Ocular muscles, paralysis, weak—*Gels.;* Lach.; Nat. m.; Physost.; *Ruta;* Tilia.

OCULAR TENSION—Decreased:—Apium v.; Ced.; Eser.; Nat. m.; Osm.; Prun. sp.; Ran. b.; Rhod.
Increased—See Glaucoma.

OPHTHALMIA—Catarrhal: *Acon.;* Am. m.; Apis; Ars.; Bell.; Cham.; Dulc.; *Euphras.;* Gels.; *Kali bich.;* Merc. c.; Merc.; Nux v.; *Puls.;* Sul.
Chronic—*Alum.;* Arg. n.; Ars.; Con.; Euphras.; *Graph.;* Kali bich.; Lyc.; *Psor.;* Sep.; *Sul.;* Zinc. m.
Follicular, granular—Aur. mur.; Euphras.; Jequir.; *Puls.*
Gonorrhoeal (neonatorum)—Acon.; *Arg. n.;* Bell.; Calc. s.; Can. s.; *Hep.;* Kali s.; *Merc. c.; Merc. pr. rub.; Merc.;* Nit. ac.; *Puls.;* Rhus t.: Syph.; Thuya.
Gonorrhoeal, constitutional—Acon.; *Clem.;* Nit. ac.; Puls.
Purulent—Apis; *Arg. n.;* Calend.; Grind.; *Hep.;* Merc. c.; Merc. pr. rub.; Nat. s.; Plumb.; Puls.; *Rhus t.*
Rheumatic—Acon.; Bell.; *Bry.;* Calc. c.; Caust.; Clem.; Colch.; Euphras.; Ilex; *Kali bich.;* Led.; Lith. c.; Lyc.; Merc. c.; Merc.; Nux v.; Phyt.; *Rhus t.;* Sil.; Spig.; Sul.
Scrofulous—*Æthiops; Æthiiops antim.;* Æth.; Apis; Arg. n.; Ars.; Ars. iod.; Aur.; Aur. mur.; Bar. c.; Bar. iod.; Bell.; *Calc. c.; Calc. iod.;* Can. s.; Cist.; Clem.; *Cochlear.;* Colch.; Con.; *Euphras.; Graph.; Hep.;* Iod.; *Kali bich.; Merc. c.;* Merc. d.; Merc. nit.; Merc. pr. rub.; Nat. m.; *Nit. ac.;* Psor.; Puls.; Rhus t.; Scrophul.; Sil.; *Sul.;* Thuya; Viola tr.; Zinc. s.
Senile—Alum.
Sympathetic—*Bell.;* **Bry.;** **Calend.;** Merc.; *Rhus t.;* Sil. See Conjunctivitis.

Syphilitic—Apis; Asaf.; Gels.; Kali iod.; Merc. c.; Nit. ac.

OPTICAL—Hyperæsthesia:—Chrysar.

OPTIC DESKS—Hyperemic, retinal vessels enlarged:—Bell.; Onosm.

Optic disks, pallor, visual field contracted, retinal vessels shrunken—Acetan.

OPTIC NERVE—Atrophy: Agar.; Arg. n.; Atoxyl; Carbon. s.; Iodof.; Nux v.; *Phos.;* Santon.; *Strych. nit.;* Tab.

Inflammation (neuritis)—*Apis;* Ars.; Bell.; Carbon. s.; Kali iod.; *Merc. c.;* Nux v.; Picr. ac.; Plumb. m.; Puls.; Rhus t.; Santon.; Tab.; Thyr.

Neuritis, choked—Bell.; Bry.; Dub.; Gels.; Helleb.; Nux v.; Puls.; Ver. v.

Neuritis, descending—Ars.; Cupr. m.; Merc. c.

Paralysis—Nux v.; Oxytr.; Phos. ac.

ORBITS—Bony tumors: Kali iod.

Cellulitis—*Apis;* Hep.; Kali iod.; Phyt.; *Rhus t.;* Sil.

Injuries—Acon.; *Arn.;* Ham.; Symphyt.

Pain around—Apis; *Asaf.;* Aur. m.; Bell.; *Cinnab.;* Hep.; Hydrocot.; Ilex; Plat.; Plumb. m.; Spig.

Pain, deep|in—*Aloe;* Gels.; Merc. c.; Phos.; Phyt.; Plat.; Ruta; Sarrac.; *Spig.;* Stann.; Upas. See Pain.

Periostitis—Asaf.; *Aur.; Kali iod.;* Merc.; Sil.

PAIN: LOCATION—Ciliary body—Ars.; *Ced.;* Chenop.; Chrom. oxy.; *Cim.; Cinnab.; Commocl.;* Crot. t.; *Gels.;* Paris; Phos.; Plant.; *Prun. sp.;* Rhod.; *Spig.;* Thuya.

Eyeballs—*Acon.;* Alfal.; Am. br.; Asaf.; Aur.; Azar.; Bapt.; *Bell.; Bry.; Ced.;* Chel.; Chimap.; *Cim.;* Cinch.; *Clem.;* Cocc.; Col.; *Commocl.;* Con.; Crot. t.; Eser.; *Eup. perf.; Euphras.; Gels.;* Grind.; Guarea; Hep.; Indol.; Jabor.; Kali iod.; Kal.; *Lycop.;* Menthol; *Merc. c.;* Nat. m.; Niccol. s.; Nit. ac.; Oleand.; Onosm.; Osm.; Paris; Passif.; Phos.; Phos. ac.; Physost.; Plat.; *Prun. sp.;* Puls.; Rhod.; Rhus t.; *Ruta;* Sang.; *Spig.;* Staph.; Symphyt.; Syph.; Tereb.; Ther.; Thuya; Upas; Viola od.

Orbits—*Aloe;* Am. picr.; *Asaf.;* Aur. m.; Chel.; Cim.; Cinnab.; Crot. t.; Gels.; Ilex; *Kali iod.;* Menthol; *Phos.;* Ruta; *Spig.;* Ther.; *Upas.*

Supra-orbital—Asaf.; *Bry.;* Carb. ac.; *Ced.; Chin. s.;* Dub.; *Gels.; Kali bich.;* Mag. p.; Meli.; Menthol; Merc. c.; Plat.; Ruta; *Spig.;* Thuya.

TYPE—Aching, sore: Æsc.; Alfal.; Aloe; Arn.; Arg. n.; Bapt.; *Bry.;* Cim.; *Eup. perf.;* Euphras.; Eser.; Gels.; *Ham.;* Led.; Lept.; Menthol; *Nat. m.;* Niccol. s.; Nit. ac.; Onosm.; Radium; Rhus t.; *Ruta;* Sep.; *Spig.*

Boring—*Asaf.; Aur.; Col.; Crot. t.;* Hep.; Merc. c.

Bruised—*Arn.;* Aur. mur.; Cim.; Cupr. m.; *Gels.;* Hep.; Nat. m.

Burning, smarting—*Acon.;* Am. gummi; *Ars.;* Asaf.; Carbo v.; Cepa; Clem.; Euphras.; Ilex aq.; Indol; Iod.; Jabor.; Lyc.; Merc. c.; *Nat. m.; Phos.;* Ran. b.; *Ruta;* Sil.

Enlarged feeling, bursting—Am. br.; Bry.; *Cim.; Commocl.;* Paris; *Prun. sp.; Spig.*

Neuralgic—*Ars.;* Asaf.; Bell.; *Ced.;* Chin. s.; *Cim.;* Cinch.; *Cinnab.;*

Col.; Commocl.; Crot. t.; *Gels.;* Kali iod.; **Kal.;** **Mag. p.;** **Meli.;**
Mez.; Osm.; Phos.; Physost.; *Prun. sp.;* Rhod.; *Spig.*

Periodically, intermittent—Ars.; Asaf.; *Ced.;* Chin. s.; Cinch.; *Spig.*

Piercing, penetrating—Apis; Aur.; Millef.; Rhus t.

Pressing inwards, as if retracted—Aur. mur.; *Crot. t.;* Hep.; Oleand.;
Paris; Phos. ac.

Pressing outwards—Asar.; *Bry.;* Cim.; *Cocc.;* Col.; Commocl.; Guarea;
Lycop.; Merc. c.; Passif.; *Spig.;* Ther.

Pressive, crushing—*Acon.;* Asaf.; Aur. mur.; Cinch.; Clem.; Crot. t.;
Cupr.; Euphras.; Hep.; Menthol; Nit. ac.; Oleand.; *Paris; Phos. ac.;*
Phos.; *Prun. sp.;* Ran. b.; Rhus t.; *Ruta;* Sang.; Sep.; *Spig.*

Sensitive to touch—*Acon.;* Arn.; Ars.; Aur.; *Bell.; Bry.;* Cim.; Clem.;
Eup. perf.; *Ham.; Hep.;* Lept.; Rhus t.; Sil.; *Spig.;* Thuya. See
Aching.

Shooting, stitching, darting, cutting—Acon.; Asaf.; *Bry.;* Calc. c.; Chimap.;
Cim.; Cinnab.; Clem.; *Col.;* Euphras.; Graph.; Helleb.; Hep.; *Kali
c.;* Kal.; Mag. p.; Merc. c.; *Nit. ac.;* Physost.; Prun. sp.; Rhod.; Rhus
t.; Sil.; *Spig.*

Splinter-like—Apis; Aur.; *Hep.;* Med.; Merc.; *Nit. ac.;* Sul.; Thuya.

Stinging—*Apis;* Euphras.; Hep.; Kali c.; Puls.; Thuya.

Strained, stiff feeling—*Guaiac.;* Jabor.; *Kal.;* Med.; *Nat. m.;* Onosm.;
Rhus t.; *Ruta.*

Tearing—Ars.; Asaf.; *Aur. mur.;* Bell.; Chel.; Colch.; Crot. t.; Guarea;
Merc. c.; *Puls.;* Sil.

Throbbing—Asaf.; *Bell.;* Bry.; Cim.; *Hep.;* Merc.; Ther.

MODALITIES—**Aggravation: At night:** *Ars.;* Asaf.; Cinnab.; Con.; Euphras.; Hep.; *Kali iod.;* Lyc.; Merc. c.; *Merc. s.;* Puls.; Rhus t.;
Sep.; Spig.; *Syph.;* Thuya.

Before a storm—Rhod.

From closing eyes—Sil.

From cold air—*Asar.; Clem.:* Hep.; Mag. p.

From damp, cold, rainy weather—Merc. c.; *Rhus t.; Spig.*

From glare of light—Asar.; Con.; Merc.

From looking down—Nat. m.

From looking up—Chel.

From lying down—Bell.

From motion—Ars.; *Bry.;* Cim.; Crot. t.; Grind.; Indol; Kal.; Rhus t.;
Spig.

From motion, or use of eyes—*Arg. n.;* Arn.; *Bry.;* Cim.; Euphras.; Kal.;
Nat. m.; Onosm.; Physost.; Puls.; Rhus t.; *Ruta; Spig.*

From sunlight—Asar.; Merc.

From sunrise to sunset—Kal.; Nat. m.

From touch—*Bry.; Hep.;* Phos.; Plant.

From warmth—Arg. n.; *Commocl.;* Puls.; Sul.; Thuya.

Worse on left side—Menthol; Onosm.; *Spig.;* Ther.

Worse on right side—*Bell.;* Ced.; *Chel.;* Commocl.; Kal.; *Mag. p.:* Prun.
sp.; Ran. b.; Ruta.

AMELIORATION—Cold air, applications: Arg. n.; *Asar.;* Puls.
Darkness—Con.; Lil. t.
Lying down on back—Puls.
Motion—Kali iod.
Pressure—Arg. n.; Asaf.; Chel.; *Chin. s.; Col.;* Con.; Lil. t.
Rest—Asaf.; Bry.; Cim.
Touch, pressure—Asaf.; Chel.
Warmth—Ars.; *Hep.;* Mag. p.; *Thuya.*

PANNUS—Apis; *Aur. mur.;* Chin. mur.; *Hep.;* Kali bich., Merc. i. r., Nit. ac. See Cornea.

PAN-OPHTHALMITIS—Hep.; Rhus t.

PERCEPTIVE POWER lost—Kali p.

PHOTOPHOBIA—*Acon.;* Agn.; Ail.; Ant. t.; Apis; *Arg. n., Ars.;* Ars. m.; Asar.; Aur. mur.; *Bell.;* Benzol; Calc. c.; Calc. p.; Cepa; Cim.; Clem.; *Con.;* Croc.; Elaps; *Euphras.; Graph.;* Hep.; *Ign.;* Kali c.; Lil. t.; Lyc.; *Merc. c.; Merc. s.;* Nat. s.; Nux m.; *Nux v.;* Op.; Phos. ac.; Phos.; Psor.; *Puls.; Rhus t.;* Scrophul.; Sil.; Spig.; *Sul.;* Ther.; Zinc.

PTERYGIUM—Am. br.; Apis; Calc. c.; *Can. s.;* Guarea; Lach.; *Ratanh.;* Spig.; *Sul.;* Tellur.; *Zinc. m.*

PUPILS—Contracted (myosis): Acon.; Cina; *Eser.;* Gels.; Helleb.; Ign.; Iodof.; Lonic.; Merc. c.; *Morph.;* Op.; Oxytr.; Phos.; *Physost.;* Piloc.; Solan. n.

Dilated (mydriasis)—Acetan.; Agar.; *Agn.; Ail.; Atrop.; Bell.;* Calc. c.; Camph.; *Cic.; Cocaine;* Dig.; *Dub.;* Gels.; Glon.; Helleb.; *Hyos.; Iodof.;* Nit. ac.; *Nux m.;* Œnanthe; Sec.; *Stram.;* Ver. v.; Zinc. m.

Insensible, poor reaction—Bell.; Benzol; Camph.; *Cic.; Gels.;* Helleb.; Hydroc. ac.; Hyos.; Laur.; Nit. ac.; *Op.;* Phos.; Piloc.; Stram.; *Zinc.*

RETINA—Anemia: Lith. c.

Apoplexy (hæmorrhage from, traumatism, cough, etc.)—Acon.; *Arn.;* Bell.; Bothrops; Croc.; *Crot.; Ham.;* Lach.; *Led.;* Nat. sal.; Phos.; Symphyt.

Artery, spasm—Nux v.

Congestion—Acon.; *Aur.; Bell.;* Carbon. s.; *Dub.;* Ferr. p.; Gels.; Phos.; Puls.; *Santon.*

Congestion, from cardiac disease—Cact.

Congestion, from light, artificial, brilliant—Glon.

Congestion, from menstrual suppression—Bell.; Puls.

Congestion, from overuse of eyes—*Ruta;* Santon.

Detachment—*Aur. mur.;* Dig.; *Gels.;* Naph.; Piloc.

Edema—*Apis;* Bell.; Canth.; *Kali iod.;* Phos.

Hyperæsthesia (optical)—*Bell.;* Cim.; Con.; Lil. t.; Macrot.; *Nux v.; Ox. ac.;* Phos.; Strych.

Inflammation (retinitis), albuminuric and chronic—Crot.; Gels.; Kal.; *Merc. c.;* Nat. sal.; Phos.; *Plumb. m.;* Sal. ac.

Inflammation, apoplectic—Glon.; Lach.

Inflammation, leukemic—Nat. s.; Thuya.

Inflammation, pigmentary—Nux v.; Phos.

Inflammation, proliferating—Kali iod.; Thuya.

Inflammation, punctata albescens—Bell.; Kali iod.; Merc. c.; Merc. i. r.; Naph.; Sul.

Inflammation, simple and serous—*Aur.*; Bell.; *Benz. dinit.*; Bry.; *Dub.*; Gels.; *Merc.*; Picr. ac.; Puls.; Santon.

Inflammation, syphilitic—Iod.; *Kali iod.*

Injuries—Acon.; *Arn.*; Bell.; *Ham.*; Lach.; Led.; Phos.

Thrombosis and degeneration—Ham.; Phos.

SCLEROTICA—Degeneration: Aur.; Bar. mur.; Plumb.

Ecchymosis—*Arn.*; Bell.; Cham.; Ham.; Lach.; *Led.*; Nux v.; Senega.

Inflammation, deep (scleritis)—*Acon.*; *Ars.*; Aur. mur.; Eryng. aq.; Hep.; Kal.; *Merc. c.*; Sep.; *Spig.*; Thuya.

Inflammation, superficial (episcleritis)—*Acon.*; Bell.; Bry.; Kali iod.; Merc. c.; Rhus t.; Tereb.; *Thuya.*

STRABISMUS (squinting)—Alumen; Alum.; Apis; Apoc.; *Bell.*; Benz. dinit.; Calc. p.; *Cic.*; Cina; Cupr. ac.; Cycl.; *Gels.*; *Hyos.*; Nux v.; *Santon.*; Sec.; Spig.; *Stram.*; Tab.; *Zinc.*

Convergent—Cycl.; Jabor.

Dependent on convulsions—Bell.; *Cic.*; Hyos.

Dependent on injuries—Cic.

Dependent on worms—Bell.; *Cina;* Cycl.; Hyos.; Merc.; *Santon.*; Spig.

Divergent—Morph.; Nat. sal.

VISION—AMAUROSIS (blindness): Acon.; Apis; *Aur. m.*; Bell.; Calc. c.; Caust.; Chin. s.; Cinch.; *Con.*; Cycl.; Dulc.; *Gels.*; Hep.; Hyos.; Mancin.; *Merc.*; Mormord.; Naph.; Nat. m.; Nux m.; Nux v.; *Phos.*; *Plumb. ac.*; Plumb. m.; Santon.; Sep.; Sil.; Stram.; Strych.; Tab.; Vanad.; Zinc. m.

Colors—*Benz. dinit.*; Carbon. s.; Physost.; *Santon.*

Day—Acon.; *Bothrops;* Castor.; Lyc.; Phos.; Ran. b.; Sil.

Hysterical—Phos.; Plat.; Sep.

Night—*Bell.*; Cadm. s.; Cinch.; Helleb.; Hep.; Hyos.; Lyc.; *Nux v.*; Physost.; Puls.; Strych.

Retro-bulbar neuritis—Iodof.

Tobacco—*Nux v.*; Phos.; Piloc.; Plumb. ac.

AMBLYOPIA—(blurred, weak vision): Acon.; *Agar.*; *Anac.*; Arn.; *Aur.*; Bapt.; *Benz. dinit.*; *Caust.*; Cinch.; *Con.*; Colch.; *Cycl.*; Dig.; Elaps; Eser.; Euphras.; *Gels.*; Hep.; *Jabor.*; *Kali c.*; Kali p.; Lil. t.; *Lith. chlor.*; Lyc.; Mag. p.; Naph.; *Nat. m.*; Nux m.; Nux v.; *Onosm.*; Ox. ac.; Osm.; Phos. ac.; *Phos.*; Physost.; Piloc.; *Puls.*; Ran. b.; Rhus t.; *Ruta;* Santon.; Senega; Sep.; Sil.; Stront.; *Tab.*; Thuya; Titan.; Zinc. m.

Objects appear as looking through mist or veil—Agar.; Calc. c.; *Caust.*; Cina; Croc.; *Cycl.*; *Gels.*; Kali c.; Lil. t.; *Mormord.*; *Nat. m.*; *Phos.*; Physost.; Plumb.; *Puls.*; *Ruta;* Sep.; *Tab.*

Objects appear elongated—Bell.

Objects appear inverted—Bell.; Guarea.

Objects appear too large—Bov.; Hep.; *Hyos.;* Niccol.; Nux m.; *Ox. ae.*

Objects appear too small—Benz. dinit.; Glon.; Nicot.; *Plat.;* Stram.

Retinal images persist—Jabor.

When reading, eyes easily fatigued—Ammon.; Calc. c.; Cina; *Jabor.;* Nat. ars.; Nat. m.; Phos.; *Ruta;* Sep.; Sul.

When reading, eyes feel pressed asunder or outward, relieved by cold bathing—Asar.

When reading, letters appear red—Phos.

When reading, letters disappear—Cic.; Cocc.

When reading, letters run together—*Agar.;* Bell.; *Calc. c.;* Can. ind.; Cina; Cinch.; Con.; Elaps; Ferr.; Hyos.; Lyc.; *Nat. m.;* Sil.

ASTHENOPIA—(eye-strain, with spasm of accommodation): *Agar.;* Alum.; Am. c.; Am. gutti; Apis; Arg. n.; Arn.; Artem.; Bell.; Carbon. s. *Caust.; Cim.;* Cina; Croc.; *Gels.;* Ign.; *Jabor.;* Kali c.; Kal.; *Lac. f.; Macrot.* *Nat. m.;* Niccol. sul.; Nicot.; Nux v.; Onosm.; Paris; *Phos.; Physost.,* Rhod.; *Ruta;* Santon.; Senega; Sep.; Stront.

External recti—Cupr. ac.; Gels.

Internal recti—Jabor.; Muscar.; Nat. m.; Physost.; Piloc.

Myopic—Eser.; Lil. t.

ASTIGMATISM—Gels.; *Lil. t.;* Physost.

DIPLOPIA—(double vision): Agar.; Aur.; *Bell.;* Cic.; Con.; *Cycl.;* Dig.; *Gels.;* Gins.; *Hyos.;* Nat. m.; *Nit. ac.;* Oleand.; Onosm.; Phos.; Physost.; Plumb.; Sec.; Stram.; Sulphon.; Sul.; Syph.; Ver. v.

HEMIOPIA—Calc. s.; Glon.; Hep.; *Lith. c.;* Lyc.; Mur. ac.; Nat. m.; *Titan.;* Ver. v.

Left-half—Calc. c.; Lith. c.; Lyc.

Lower-half—Aur.; Digit.

Vertical—Ferr. p.; *Lith. c.;* Morph.; Mur. ac.; *Titan.*

HYPERMETROPIA—Calc. c.; Con.; *Jabor.;* Nat. m.; Petrol.; Ruta; Sep.; Sil.

MYOPIA—Acon.; *Agar.;* Aur. mur.; Bell.; Carbon. s.; Euphras.; Gels Lil. t.; Nit. ac.; Phos.; *Physost.; Piloc.;* Ruta; Viola od.

OPTICAL ILLUSIONS—(chromopsia, photopsia): **Black before eyes:** Agar.; *Atrop.;* Bell.; *Carbo v.; Carbon. s.;* Cinch.; Cycl.; Dig.; Lach.; Lyc.; Mag. c.; Mag. p.; Merc.; Nat. m.; Phos.; Physost.; Sep.; Stront.; *Tab.;* Zinc.

Blue before eyes—Crot.; Trill. cer.; Trill. p.

Confusion of colors—*Bell.;* Calc. c.; Croc.; Merc.; Puls.; Ruta; Staph.; Stram.

Flashes, flames, flickering—Agar.; Aloe; *Bell.;* Calc. fl.; Caust.; Clem.; *Cycl.;* Glon.; Hep.; Ign.; *Iris;* Lyc.; Phos.; Physost.; Puls.; Senega; Viola od.

Gray—Arg. n.; Conv.; Guarea.

Green—Dig.; *Osm.; Phos.*

Halo around light—Bell.; Chloral; Hyos.; Sul.

Objects appear white—Chloral.

Objects, brilliant, fantastic, colored, fiery—*Anhal.;* Aur.; *Bell.;* Cinch.; *Cycl.;* Nat. m.; Sep.

Red before the eyes—Antipyr.; Apis; *Bell.;* *Dub.;*   Elaps;   Hep.; *Phos.;* Stront.

Sparks, stars—Aur.; *Bell.;* Calc. fl.; Caust.; Croc.; *Cycl.;* Glon.; Lyc.; Naph.; Sil.; Strych.

Spots (muscæ volitantes)—*Agar.;* Anac.; *Atrop.;* Aur.; Carbo v.; Caust.; *Cinch.;* Colch.; Con.; *Cycl.;* Cyprip.; Kali c.; Meli.; *Merc.;* *Nit. ac.;* *Nux v.;* *Phos.;* Physost.; Sep.; Sil.; Sul.; Tab.

Yellow before eyes—*Aloe;* Canth.; Cina; Digitox; *Santon.*

VITREOUS OPACITIES—diffused: Ham.; Hep.; Kali iod.; Merc. c.; Merc i. r.; Thuya.

Turbid—Cholest.; *Kali iod.;* Phos.; Prun. sp.; *Senega;* Solan. n. Su¹

EARS

AUDITORY NERVE—Torpor: *Chenop.*

AURICLE—(external ear): Burning, as if frost-bitten—Agar.; Caust.; Sang.

ERUPTIONS—Remedies in general: *Ant. c.;* Bar. c.; *Calc. c.;* Calc. s.; *Graph.;* Lyc.; *Mez.;* Petrol.; Rhus t.; Tellur.

Acne—Calc. s.

Eczema around—*Ars.;* Arundo; Bov.; Chrysarob.; *Clem.;* Crot. t.; *Graph.;* Hep.; Kali m.; *Mez.;* Oleand.; Petrol.; Psor.; *Rhus t.;* Sanic.; Scrophul.; Tellur.

Erysipelas—*Apis;* Bell.; Rhus t.; Rhus v.

Fissures—Calc. c.; Graph.

Frost-bites—Agar.; *Apis;* Bell.; Rhus t.

Intertrigo—Petrol.

Herpes—Cistus; Graph.; Psor.; Rhus t.; *Sep.;* Tellur.

Moist, oozing—Ant. c.; Calc. c.; *Graph.;* Hep.; *Mez.;* Petrol.; *Psor.;* Sanic.

Pustules—Ars.; *Hep.;* Psor.

Scabs, scurfs—Chrysar.; Hep.; *Psor.*

Glands, swollen, painful, around—*Bar. c.;* Bell.; *Calc. c.;* Caps.; Graph.; Iod.; *Merc.*

Itching—*Agar.;* Ars.; Hep.; Nat. p.; *Sul. iod.;* Tub.

Lobe, eruption on—Bar. c.

Lobe, ulceration of ring hole—Stann.

Numbness—Mag. c.; Plat.; Verbasc.

Pain, tearing, with tophi—Berv. v.

Red, raw, sore—Graph.; Petrol.; Sul.

Red, swollen—*Acon.;* *Agar.;* Anac.; Apis; *Bell.;* Cinch.; Graph.; Hep.; Kali bich.; Medusa; Merc.; Puls.; *Rhus t.;* Scrophul.; Sul.

Sensitive to touch—Arn.; *Bell.;* Bry.; *Caps.;* *Cinch.;* Ferr. p.; *Hep.;* Psor.; Sanic.; Sep.

CERUMEN—Carbo v.; Caust.; *Con.;* Elaps; Graph.; Lach.; Puls.; Sep.; Spong.

DEAFNESS—HARDNESS OF HEARING—Remedies in general: Agar.; *Agraph.;* Ambra; Am. c.; Arn.; Ars. iod.; *Bar. c.;* *Bar. mur.;* Bell.; Calc. c.; Calc. fl.; Calend.; Carbo an.; Carbon. s.; *Caust.;* Cheiranth.; *Chenop.;* *Chin. s.;* *Cinch.;* Con.; Dig.; Dulc.; Elaps; Ferr. p.; Ferr. picr.; *Graph.;* Hep.; Hydr.; Hydrobr. ac.; Iod.; Kali ars.; Kali c.; *Kali m.;* Lob. infl.; *Lyc.;* Mang. ac.; *Merc. d.;* Merc. s.; Mez.; Nat. c.; *Nat. sal.;* *Nit. ac.;* Petrol.; Phos. ac.; *Phos.;* Psor.; Puls.; Rham. c.; Sal. ac.; Sang. n.; Sep.; *Sil.;* Tellur.; *Thiosin.;* *Verbasc.;* Viola od.

CAUSE—Abuse of Mercury: Hep.; Nit. ac.

Adenoids and hypertrophied tonsils—*Agraph.;* Aur.; Bar. c.; Calc. p.; Merc.; Nit. ac.; Staph.

Alternate with sensibility of ear—Sil.

Apoplexy—Arn.; Bell.; Caust.; Hyos.; Rhus t.

Bone conduction, deficient, or absent—Chenop.

Catarrh (eustachian, middle ear)—Ars. iod.; Asar.; *Calcareas;* Caust.; Gels.; Graph.; *Hep.;* Hydr.; *Iod.;* Kali bich.; *Kali m.;* Kali s.; Mang. ac.; Menthol; *Merc. d.;* Merc. s.; Petrol.; *Puls* ; Rosa d.; Sang.; Sep.; Sil.; Thiosin.

Cerebral—Chenop.; Mur. ac.

Cold exposure—Acon.; Kali m.; Visc. a.

Concussion—Arn.; Chin. s.

Damp weather—Mang. ac.

Discharge suppressed or eczema—Lob. infl.

Eruption of scalp, suppressed—Mez.

Human voice, difficult to hear—Calc. c.; *Chenop.;* Ign.; Phos.; Sil.; Sul.

Infectious diseases—Arn.; *Bapt.; Gels.;* Hep.; Lyc.; Petrol.; Phos.; Puls.

Nervous exhaustion, and nervous origin—*Ambra;* Anac.; Aur.; *Bell.;* Caust.; Chin. s.; Cinch.; *Gels.; Ign.; Lach.;* Phos. ac.; Phos.; Plat.; Tab.; *Val.*

Nutritional disturbance, in growing children—Calc. c.; Merc. i. r.

Old age—Kali m.; Merc. d.; Phos.

Rheumatico-gouty diathesis—*Ferr. picr.;* Ham.; Kali iod.; Led.; Sil.; Sul.; Visc. a.

Sclerotic condition of conducting media—Ferr. picr.; Thiosin.

Scrofulous diathesis—*Æthiops;* Calc. c.; Merc.; Mez.; Sil.; *Sul.*

Sounds, low toned—Chenop.

Syphilis—Kreos.

Work'ng in water—Calc. c.

Aggravated before menses—Ferr. picr.; Kreos.

Ameliorated from noise, riding in cars—Calend.; *Graph.;* Nit. ac.

EUSTACHIAN TUBES—(catarrh or closure): Alfal.; Alum.; Bar. m.; *Calcareas;* Caps.; *Caust.;* Ferr. iod.; Ferr. p.; Gels.; *Graph.;* Hep.; Hydr.; *Iod.;* Kali bich.; Kali chlor.; *Kali m.;* Lach.; Lob., cer.; Menthol; *Merc. d.;* Merc.; Nit. ac.; Penthor.; Petrol.; Phyt.; *Puls.;* Rosa d.; Sang. n.; *Sil.;* Visc. a.

Eustachian tube inflamed, sub-acute, great pain—Bell.; Caps.

Eustachian tube, tickling inducing swallowing, cough—Gels.; Nux v.; Sil.

EXTERNAL AUDITORY CANAL—Boils, pimples: Bell.; *Calc. picr.;* Hep.; *Merc. s.; Picr. ac.; Sil.;* Sul.

Burning—Ars.; Arundo; *Caps.;* Sang.; Strych.

Digging and scratching Into—Cina; Psor.

Dryness—Calc. picr.; Carbo v.; Ferr. picr.; *Graph.;* Nux v.; Petrol.; Verbasc.

Exostoses—Calc. fl.; *Hekla;* Kali iod.

Feels, as if distended by air—Mez.; Puls.

Fissures—*Graph.;* Petrol.

Inflammation and pain—*Acon.;* Apis; Ars. iod.; *Bell.;* Bor.; Brachygl.; *Cal. picr.; Cham.; Ferr. p.;* Hep.; Kali bich.; *Kali m.; Merc. s.;* Nit. ac.; Psor.; *Puls.;* Rhus t.; *Tellur.*

Itching—*Alum.;* Anac.; Calc. c.; Caust.; Elaps; Hep.; Kali bich.; Kali c.; Psor.; *Puls.;* Sabad.; *Sep.;* Sil.; *Sul.; Tellur.;* Viola od.

Polypoid excrescenses, granulations—Alum.; Calc. c.; *Calc. iod.;* Calc. p.; Formica; Kali bich.; Kali iod.; *Kali m.;* Merc. s.; *Nit. ac.;* Phos.; *Sang.;* Sil.; Staph.; Teucr.; *Thuya.*

Scales, epithelial, exfoliated, with scurfy accumulation—Calc. picr.

Sensation, as if drop of water in left ear—Acon.

Sensation, as if heat emanated from—*Æth.;* Caust.

Sensation, as if obstructed—Æth.; Anac.; Asar.; Carbon. s.; *Cham.;* Crot.; Glon.; Merc.; Nit. ac.; *Puls.; Verbasc.*

Sensation, as if open too much—Mez.

Sensitive to air, touch—Ars.; Bell.; *Bor.;* Caps.; *Cham.;* Ferr. p.; *Hep.;* Merc.; Mez.; Nux v.; Petrol.; Tellur.

HYPERSENSITIVE—to noises, sounds, voices:—Acon.; Anhal.; *Asar.;* Aur.; *Bell.; Bor.;* Chenop.; Cim.; *Cinch.; Coff.;* Ferr. p.; Ign.; Iod.; Lach.; Mag. m.; *Nat. c.;* Nit. ac.; Nux m.; *Nux v.;* Op.; Petrol.; Phos. ac.; Phos.; Plant.; Puls.; Sang.; Sep.; *Sil.;* Spig.; Tereb.; *Ther.*

LABYRINTH—Bloody, serous effusion, in: Chenop.

Inflamed (otitis interna)—Aur.; Kali iod.; Merc. i. r.

MASTOID PROCESS—Caries: *Aur.;* Caps.; Fluor. ac.; *Nit. ac.;* Sil.

Inflammation (mastoiditis)—*Am. picr.;* Asaf.; *Aur.; Bell.;* Benz. ac.; Canth.; *Caps.;* Hep.; Kali m.; Mag. p.; Menthol; *Onosm.;* Oniscus.; Tellur.

MEMBRANA TYMPANI—Calcareous deposits: Calc. fl.

Inflammation (myringitis)—*Acon.;* Atrop.; Bell.; Bry.; Cinch.; *Hep.* See Otitis.

Perforated—Aur.; Calc. c.; Caps.; Kali bich.; Merc.; *Sil.;* Tellur.; *Tub.*

Thickened—Ars. iod.; Merc. d.; Thiosin.

Thin, white, scaly deposit—Graph.

Ulceration—Kali bich.

OSSICLES—Caries:—Asaf.; *Aur.;* Calc. c.; Caps.; Fluor. ac.; Hep.; Iod.; *Sil.;* Syph.

Petrous bone, tender to touch—*Caps.;* Onosm.

Sclerosis, also petrous portion of temporal bone—Calc. fl.

TYMPANUM (middle ear): Inflammation (otitis):

Catarrhal, acute—*Acon.; Bell.;* Cham.; *Ferr. p.;* Gels.; Hep.; *Kali m.;* Merc.; *Puls.,* Rhus t.; Sil.

Catarrhal, chronic—Agar.; Ars.; *Bar. m.; Calc. c.; Caust.;* Cinch.; Graph.; *Hydr.; Iod.;* Jabor.; Kali bich.; Kali iod.; *Kali m.; Merc. d.;* Nit. ac.; Phos.; Sang.; Teucr. See Eustachian Tubes.

Suppurative, acute (otitis media suppurative, acute)—Acon.; Ars.; Ars. iod.; *Bell.;* Bor.; Bov.; Calc. s.; Caps.; Cham.; *Ferr. p.;* Gels.; Guaiac.; Hep.; Kali bich.; Kali m.; Merc. s.; *Merc. v.;* Myrist.; *Plant.; Puls.;* Sil.; Thiosin.

Suppurative, chronic—*Æthiops;* Alum.; *Ars. iod.;* Aur.; Bar. m.; *Calc. c.;* Calc. fl.; *Calc. iod.;* Caps.; *Caust.;* Chenop.; Elaps; *Hep.;* Hydr.; Iod.; *Kali bich.;* Kali iod.; Kali m.; Kali p.; *Kali s.;* Kino; Lapis alb.;

Lyc.; Merc. s.; *Merc. v.;* Naja; Nit. ac.; *Psor.; Puls.; Sil.; Sul.;* Tellur.; *Thuya;* Viola od.

TYPE OF DISCHARGE—(otorrhœa): Bloody—Ars.; Ferr. p.; Hep.; Kali iod.; Merc. s.; *Merc.;* Psor.; Rhus t.; Shook. ch.

Excoriating, thin—*Alum.;* Ars.; Ars. iod.; Calc. iod.; Calc. p.; Cistus; *Iod.;* Merc.; Syph.; *Tellur.*

Muco-purulent, fetid, acrid or bland—Æthiops; Ars. iod.; Asaf.; Aur.; Bor.; *Calc. c.; Calc. s.;* Caps.; *Carbo v.;* Elaps; Ferr. p.; Graph.; *Hep.;* Hydr.; Kali bich.; *Kali s.;* Kino; Lyc.; Merc. pr. rub.; Merc. s.; *Merc. v.;* Nat. m.; Psor.; *Puls.; Sil.;* Sul.; *Tellur.;* Thuya; Tub.

PAIN (otalgia)—*Acon.;* Antipyr.; Apis; *Bell.;* Bor.; *Caps.; Cham.;* Chin. s.; Coff.; Dulc.; *Ferr. p.;* Gels.; *Hep.;* Iod.; Kali bich.; Kali iod.; Mag. p.; Menthol; *Merc. s.; Merc. v.;* Naja; *Plant.; Puls.;* Sang.; Tereb.; Val.; Viola od.; Visc. a.; *Verbasc.*

TYPE—Aching, constant—Caps.; Guaiac.; Merc.

Boring—Am. picr.; *Asaf.;* Aur.; Bell.; *Caps.;* Kali iod.; Sil.; Spig.

Burning—*Ars.;* Caps.; Kreos.; Sang.; Sul.

Cramp-like, pressing, piercing—*Anac.;* Calc. c.; *Cham.;* Kali bich.; Merc.; *Puls.*

Neuralgic, lancinating, shifting, shooting, paroxysmal—Acon.; *Bell.;* Caps.; Cepa; *Cham.;* Cinch.; Ferr. p.; Kali c.; *Mag. p.;* Nit. ac.; *Puls.;* Sil.; *Spig.;* Viola od.

Pulsating, throbbing—Acon.; *Bell.;* Cact.; Calc. c.; *Ferr. p.; Glon.;* Merc. c.; Merc. s.; Puls.; Rhus t.; Tellur.

Stinging—Acon.; Apis; Caps.

Stitching—Bor.; *Cham.;* Ferr. p.; Hep.; Kali bich.; *Kali c.;* Merc.; Nit. ac.; *Plant.;* Puls.; Viola od.

Tearing—*Bell.;* Caps.; *Cham.;* Kali bich.; Kali iod.; Merc. s.; Plant.; *Puls.*

MODALITIES—Aggravation: At night—*Acon.;* Ars.; Bell.; Calc. p.; *Cham.;* Dulc.; Ferr. p.; Hep.; Kali iod.; *Merc.; Puls.;* Rhus t.

From cold air—Calc. p.; Caps.; *Cham.; Hep.;* Kali m.; Mag. p.; Sang.

Noise—Bell.; Cham.

Pressure, motion—Menthol.

Warmth—Acon.; Bor.; Calc. p.; *Cham.;* Dulc.; *Merc.;* Nux v.; *Puls.*

Washing face and neck with cold water—Mag. p.

AMELIORATION—During day: Acon.

From being carried, motion—Cham.

From cold applications—Puls.

From motion, covering—Aur.

From sipping cold water—Bar. m.

From warmth—*Bell.;* Caps.; Cham.; Dulc.; Hep.; *Mag. p.*

In open air—Acon.; Aur.; Ferr. p.; *Puls.*

TINNITUS AURIUM—(noises in ears): Remedies in general: Adren.; Am. c.; Antipyr.; Ars.; *Bar. c.; Bar. m.;* Bell.; Canchal.; Carbon. s.; *Caust.; Chenop.* gl.; *Chin. sal.; Chin. s.;* Cim.; *Cinch.;* Cistus dec.; Con.; Dig.; Ferr. p.; Ferr. picr.; *Graph.;* Hep.; Hydr.; Jabor.;

Kali c.; Kali iod.; *Kali m.;* Kali p.; Lach.; Lecith.; Lith. chlor.; Merc.; Merc. d.; Nat. m.; *Nat. sal.;* Parth.; Petrol.; Phos.; Piloc.; Plat.; Plumb. m.; *Puls.;* *Sal. ac.;* Sang.; *Sang. n.;* Sil.; Sulphon.; Sul.; *Viola od.*

Buzzing—Am. c.; Anac.; Antipyr.; *Bar. m.;* Calc. c.; Canchal.; Caust.; *Chenop.; Chin. s.;* Cinch.; Dig.; Diosc.; Ferr. p.; Formica; Graph.; Iod.; Iris; Kali p.; Kreos.; Lach.

Cracking, snapping, when blowing nose, chewing, swallowing, sneezing—Ambra; *Bar. c.; Bar. m.;* Calc. c.; Chenop. gl.; Formica; Gels.; *Graph.;* Kali c.; *Kali m.;* Lach.; *Nit. ac.;* Petrol.; Puls.; Sil.; Thuya.

Hissing—Can. ind.; *Chin. s.;* Dig.; *Graph.;* Teucr.

Humming—Alum.; Anac.; Calc. c.; *Caust.;* Cinch.; Ferr. p.; *Kali p.;* Kreos.; *Lyc.;* Petrol.; Puls.; Sang.; Sep.; Tereb.

Intolerance of music—*Acon.;* Ambra; Bufo; Viola od.

Pulsating, throbbing—Calc. c.; Caust.; *Ferr. p.; Glon.;* Hep.; Hydrobr ac.; Lach.; Merc.; *Morph.;* Nit. ac.; *Puls.*

Re-echoing of voice, sounds—Bar. c.; *Bar. m.;* Bell.; *Caust.;* Col.; Lyc.; Phos.; Tereb.

Ringing as of bells—*Bell.;* Calc. fl.; Carbon. s.; Caust.; Cham.; *Chin. s.; Cinch.;* Formica; *Graph.;* Iris; Lach.; Mez.; *Nat. sal.;* Petrol.

Roaring—Aur.; Calc. c.; Caust.; *Chin. s.;* Cinch.; Elaps; Ferr. p.; *Graph.;* Kreos.; *Lyc.;* Merc. d.; Merc.; Nat. m.; Nat. sal.; Nit. ac.; Petrol.; Phos. ac.; *Puls.; Sal. ac.;* Sang.; *Sil.;* Strych.; Viola od.

Roaring, relieved by music—Ign.

Rushing—Ferr. p.; Gels.; Puls.

Singing—*Chin. s.;* Dig.; Graph.; Lach.; Puls.

Whizzing—Bar. m.; Bell.; *Hep.;* Rhod.; Sul.

NOSE

AFFECTIONS, syphilitic—Asaf.; *Aur.;* Aur. mur.; *Cinnab.;* Fluor. ac.; *Kali bich.; Kali iod.;* Merc. c.; Sil.

BONES—Caries: Asaf.; *Aur.;* Aur. mur.; Cadm. s.; Kali bich.; Merc. i. r.; Merc.; *Phos.* See Tissues (Generalities).

Pain—*Asaf.; Aur.;* Cinnab.; *Hep.;* Kali iod.; Lach.; *Merc.;* Puls.; *Sil.*

Periostitis—Asaf.; *Aur.;* Merc.; *Phos.* See Tissues.

Ulceration—Asaf.; *Hekla;* Hep.; Kali bich. See Tissues.

EXTERNAL NOSE—ERUPTIONS, growths—Acne: Ars.; *Ars. br.;* Aster.; Bor.; *Caust.;* Clem.; Elaps; Kali br.; Nat. c.; Sil. ; Zing.

Eczema—Bals. per.; Iris; Sars.

Erysipelas—Bell.; Canth.; Rhus t.

Freckles—Phos.; Sul.

Furuncles—Cadm. s.; Cur.; *Hep.;* Sil.

Herpes—Acon. lyc.; Alum.; Bell.; Mur. ac.; Nat. m.; *Sep.;* Sul.

Lupus—Ars.; Aur. mur.; Kali bich.; Kreos.; Thuya; X-ray.

Pustules—*Hep.;* Petrol.; Psor.; Sil.

Scales—*Caust.*

Warts—Caust.; Thuya. See Skin.

Inflammation—Acon.; Agar.; *Apis; Aur.;* Aur. mur.; *Bell.;* Bor.; Carbo an.; Ferr. iod.; *Ferr. picr.;* Fluor. ac.; Graph.; *Hep.;* Hippoz.; *Kali iod.;* Medusa; Merc. c.; Naph.; Nat. c.; *Nit. ac.;* Sil.; Sul.

Itching—*Agar.; Cina;* Filix m.; *Ign.;* Iod.; Phos. ac.; Pin. syl.; Teucr.; Zing.

Numbness—Nat. m.

Redness—Agar.; Alum.; *Apis;* Ars.; Bell.; *Bor.;* Iod.; *Kali iod.;* Nat. c.; Psor.; Rhus t.; Rhus v.; Yucca; Zinc.

Soreness to touch—Alum.; Aur. m.; Bry.; Calc. c.; *Cinnab.;* Con.; Graph.; *Hep.;* Kali bich.; Lachnanth.; Lith. m.; *Merc.; Nit. ac.;* Rhus t.; Sil.

Varicose veins—Carbo v.

Yellow saddle—Sep.

ALAE—(wings): Burning, hot, biting: Ars.; Chenop. gl.; *Sang. n.;* Senega; Sinap.; Sul.

Dryness—Chlorum; Helleb.; *Sang. n.*

Eczema—*Ant. c.;* Bals. per.; Bar. c.; *Graph.; Petrol.*

Eruptions, growths, cracks, crusts, ulcerations—Alum.; *Ant. c.; Arum;* Aur.; Aur. m. n.; Bov.; *Calc. c.;* Caust.; Condur.; Coral.; *Graph.;* Ign.; *Kali bich.;* Kali c.; Lyc.; Merc.; *Nit. ac.; Petrol.;* Sul.; Tereb.; *Thuya.*

Fanning—*Ant. t.;* Brom.; *Chel.;* Gadus m.; Kali br.; *Lyc.;* Phos.; Pyr.; Sul. ac.

Herpes—Dulc.; Nat. m.; Physost.; Sil.

Itching—Carbo v.; *Cina;* Nat. p.; *Santon.;* Sil.; Sul.

Red, inner angles—Agar.; Merc. s.; Plumb. ac.; Sul.

Soreness to touch—*Alum; Ant. c.;* Ars.; *Arum;* Aur. mur.; Calc. c.; Cop.;

Coral.; Fagop.; *Graph.*; *Hep.*; *Kali bich.*; Merc. c.; Merc.; *Nit. ac.*; Petrol.; Scilla; Uran.

Sooty, dirty nostrils—Helleb.

Throbbing—Acon.; Brom.

TIP—Blueness:—Carbo an.; *Dig.*

Burning—Bell.; Bor.; Ox. ac.; Rhus t.

Cold, pale, pointed—Apis; *Ars.*; Calc. p.; *Camph.*; Carbo v.; *Cinch.*; Helleb.; *Tab.*; *Ver. a.* See Face.

Congestion—Am. c.

ERUPTIONS, growths—Acne: Am. c.; Caust.; Sep.

Cracks—Alum.; *Graph.*; Petrol.

Furuncles—Ananth.; Bor.

Herpes—*Æth.*; Clem.; Conv.; Dulc.; Nat. m.

Knobby—Aur.

Pustules—Kali br.

Scales—Caust.; Nat. c.

Ulcers—Bor.; Rhus t.

Tumors—Ananth.; Carbo an.

Warts—Caust.

Inflammation—Bell.; Bor.; Cistus; Euphorbia; Niccol.; Nit. ac.; Rhus t.; Sep.

Itching—Carbo an.; Caust.; *Cina*; *Morph.*; Petrol.; *Santon.*; Sil.

Redness—Bell.; *Bor.*; Calc. c.; *Caps.*; Kali iod.; Kali n.; Niccol.; Nit. ac.; *Rhus t.*; Salix; *Sil.*; Sul.; Vinca m.

Soreness to touch—Bor.; *Hep.*; *Mentha*; Rhus t.

Tingling—Bell.; *Morph.*

Torpor, as from blow—Viola od.

INTERNAL NOSE—Abscess of septum: Acon.; *Bell.*; Calc. c.; *Hep.*; Sil.

Bleeding (epistaxis): Remedies in general—Abrot.; *Acon.*; Agar.; Ambros.; Am. c.; *Arn.*; Ars.; *Bell.*; *Bry.*; Cact.; Calc. c.; Carbo v.; *Cinch.*; Croc.; Crot. casc.; Elaps; Ferr. ac.; *Ferr. p.*; Ferr. picr.; Ficus; Ham.; *Ipec.*; Kali c.; Kali chlor.; Lach.; *Meli.*; Merc.; *Millef.*; Mur. ac.; Nat. nit.; Nat. sal.; *Nit. ac.*; Nux v.; Oniscus; Osm.; *Phos.*; Puls.; Sec.; Sep.; Sul.; *Thlaspi*; Tilia; *Trill.*; Vipera.

CAUSE—Blowing nose: Agar.; Aur. m.; Bov.; *Carbo v.*; Caust.; Graph.; *Phos.*; *Sec.*; Sep.; Sul.

Cough—Arn.

Eating—Am. c.

Hemophilia—Ars.; Crot.; Ham.; Ipec.; *Lach.*; *Phos.*

Hæmorrhoids, suppressed—Nux v.

Menses, absent (vicarious)—*Bry.*; *Ham.*; Lach.; Nat. s.; *Phos.*; Puls.; Sep.

Motion, noise, light—Bell.

Operations—Thlaspi.

Recurrent cases—Ars.; Ferr. p.; Millef.; Phos.

Stooping—Rhus t.

Straining—Carbo v.

Symptomatic (fevers, purpura)—Arn.; Ham.; Ipec.; Lach.; Phos.; Rhus t.
Traumatism—Acet. ac.; *Arn.;* Ham.; Millef.
Washing—*Am. c.; Ant. s. a.;* Arn.; Kali c.; Mag. c.

OCCURRENCE AND CONCOMITANTS—At night during sleep—*Merc. s.;* Nux v.

In children growing rapidly—Abrot.; Arn.; *Calc. c.;* Croc.; Phos.
In daily attacks—Carbo v.
In morning from washing face—Am. c.; Arn.; *Kali c.;* Oniscus.
In morning on awaking, arising, etc.—Aloe; Ambra; Bov.; *Bry.;* Cinch.; Lach.; *Nux v.*
In old people—Agar.; *Carbo v.*
Persistent, with goose flesh—Camph.
Preceded by heat and pain in head—Nux v.
With biliousness—Chel.
With chest affections—Ham.; Nit. ac.
With chronic vertigo—Sul.
With face congested, red—Bell.; *Meli.;* Nux v.
With face pale—Carbo v.; Ipec.
With prostration—Carbo v.; Cinch.; Diph.
With relief of chest symptoms—Bov.
With relief of headache—Ham.; *Meli.*
With tightness, pressure at root of nose—Ham.

TYPE OF BLOOD—Black, stringy: *Croc.;* Crot.; Merc. s.
Bright red—*Acon.;* Bell.; Bry.; Carbo v.; Erecht.; *Ferr. p.;* Ipec.; *Millef.; Trill.*
Coagulated—Cinch.; Nat. chlor.; Nux v.
Dark, fluid—Arn.; Ham.; Lach.; Mur. ac.; *Sec.*
Non-coagulable, passive, profuse—Bry.; Carbo v.; Crot.; *Ham.; Phos.;* Thlaspi; Trill.

BLOWS NOSE continually—Am. c.; Bor.; Hydr.; Lac c.; Mag. m.; *Sticta;* Tritic.
Boring, digging into—*Arum; Cina;* Helleb.; Phos. ac.; *Santon.;* Teucr.; Zinc. m.
Burning, smarting—Acon.; Æsc.; Am. m.; *Ars.;* Ars. iod.; Arum; Bar. c.; Brom.; Caps.; Cepa; Cop.; Hep.; *Hydr.;* Kaolin; Merc. c.; *Merc. s.;* Penthor.; Sabad.; *Sang.;* Sang. n.; Sinap.
Coldness—*Æsc.; Camph.; Cistus;* Coral.; Hydr.; Lith. c.; Ver. a.
Congestion, violent—Bell.; Cupr. m.; *Meli.*
Dryness—*Acon.;* Æsc.; *Am. c.;* Bell.; Calc. c.; *Camph.;* Con.; Cop.; Glycerin; *Graph.;* Kali bich.; Kali c.; Kali iod.; Lemna; *Lyc.;* Nat. m.; Nit. ac.; Nux m.; *Nux v.;* Onosm.; Petrol.; *Phos.;* Rumex; *Samb.; Sang.;* Sang. n.; Senec.; Sep.; Sil.; Sinap.; *Sticta;* Sul. See Stoppage.

ERUPTIONS, growths—Furuncles, pimples: Sil.; Tub.; Vinca.
Lupus—*Ars.;* Calc. c.; Cic.; Hydr.; *Hydrocot.;* Merc.; Rhus t.; Sul.; Tub.
Nodular swelling—Ars.
Papilloma—Caust.; Nit. ac.; *Thuya.*

Polypi—Cadm. s.; *Calc. c.;* Calc. iod.; Calc. p.; Caust.; *Cepa;* Con.; Formica; Kali bich.; Kali n.; Lemna m.; Merc. i. r.; Nit. ac.; *Phos.;* Psor.; *Sang.; Sang. n.;* Staph.; *Teucr.; Thuya;* Wyeth.

Scabs, crusts, plugs, clinkers—*Alum.;* Ant. c.; *Arum;* Aur., Bor.; Cadm. s.; Calc. fl.; Cop.; Dulc.; Elaps; *Graph.;* Hep.; *Hydr.; Kali bich.;* Lemna m.; *Lyc.;* Nat. ars.; Nat. m.; Nit. ac.; *Puls.;* Sang. n.; *Sep.;* Sil.; Sticta; Sul.; *Teucr.;* Thuya.

Ulcerations, exocriations—Alum.; Ars.; Ars. iod.; Arum; Aur.; Bor.; Cepa; *Graph.;* Hep.; *Hydr.; Kali bich.;* Kali c.; Kreos.; Merc. c.; Merc.; *Nit. ac.;* Ran. s.; *Sil.;* Thuya; *Vinca.*

HARDNESS (rhino-sclerma)—Aur. m. n.; Calc. fl.; Con.

Inflammation (rhinitis): Acute, catarrhal from pollen irritation, HAY FEVER, rose cold, summer catarrh: *Ambros.; Aral.; Ars.; Ars. iod.;* Arum; Arundo; Benz. ac.; Cepa; Chin. ars.; Cocaine; Cupr. ac.; Dulc.; Euphorb. pil.; *Euphras.;* Gels.; Hep.; Ipec.; Kali iod.; Kali s. chrom.; *Lach.;* Linum usit.; Merc. i. fl.; *Naph.;* Nat. iod.; Nat. m.; Nux v.; Pollantin; *Psor.; Ran. b.;* Rosa d.; *Sabad.;* Sang.; *Sang. n.;* Sil.; *Sinap.;* Skook. ch.; Solid.; *Sticta;* Supraren. ext.; Trifol.; Tub.

Inflammation, acute, catarrhal, ordinary cold in head: Acon.; Æsc.; Am. c.; Am. m.; *Ars.; Ars. iod.; Arum;* Avena; Bell.; Brom.; *Bry.; Camph.; Cepa;* Cham.; *Dulc.;* Eup.; perf.; *Euphras.;* Ferr. p.; *Gels.;* Glycerin; Hep.; *Hydr.;* Hydroc. ac.; *Iod.; Justicia; Kali bich.; Kali iod.;* Lach.; Menthol; *Merc. s.; Nat. ars.; Nat. m.; Nux v.;* Phos.; Puls.; *Quill.;* Sabad.; Samb.; Sang.; *Sang. n.;* Solid.; *Sticta;* Tereb.; Ther.; Tromb.

CONCOMITANTS—Aching in limbs: Acon.; Bry.; *Eup. perf.; Gels.*

Chilliness (initial stage)—*Acon.;* Bapt.; *Camph.;* Caps.; Ferr. p.; *Gels.;* Merc. i. r.; *Nat. m.;* Nux v.; Phyt.; *Quill.;* Sapon.

Predisposition to colds—Agraph.; Alum.; Ars.; Bac.; Bar. c.; *Calc. c.;* Calc. iod.; Calc. p.; Calend.; Dulc.; Ferr. p.; Gels.; *Hep.;* Hydr.; Kali c.; Merc.; *Nat. m.;* Nux v.; Phos.; *Psor.;* Sep.; Solid.; *Sul.; Tub*

CORYZA—Dry (stuffy colds, snuffles): Acon.; Ambros.; *Am. c.;* Am. m.; Arum; *Calc. c.;* Camph.; Caust.; *Cham.;* Cistus; Con.; Dulc.; Elaps; Glycerin; Graph.; *Hep.;* Iod.; *Kali bich.; Kali c.;* Lach.; *Lyc.;* Menthol; *Nat. m.;* Nit. ac.; *Nux v.;* Osm.; Puls.; *Samb.;* Sep.; Sil.; Sinap.; *Sticta;* Teucr. See Stoppage.

Alternately dry and fluent—Am. c.; *Ars.; Lac c.;* Lach.; Mag. m.; *Nat. ars.; Nux v.;* Puls.; Quill.; *Sinap.;* Solan. n.; Spong.

Coryza, fluent, watery (running cold)—Æsc.; Agraph.; *Ail.; Ambros.;* Am. m.; Am. phos.; *Aral.; Ars.; Ars. iod.; Arum;* Brom.; *Cepa;* Cycl.; Eucal.; Eup. perf.; *Euphras.; Gels.;* Hydr.; Iod.; Ipec.; *Justicia;* Kali chlor.; *Kali iod.;* Merc. c.; *Merc. s.;* Narcissus; *Nat. ars.; Nat. m.; Quill.;* Sabad.; *Sang. n.;* Scilla; Sil.; Solan. n.; Trifol.

Coryza, periodic—Ars.; Cinch.; Nat. m.; Sang.

Coryza, with chronic tendency—Am. c.; Calc. c.; Calc. iod.; *Con.;* Graph.; Hep.; *Kali bich.;* Kali iod.; *Puls.; Sars.; Sil.;* Sul.;

Coryza, with palpitation, especially in aged—Anac.

Coryza, with thick mucus—*Aur.;* Ferr. iod.; *Hep.;* *Kali bich.;* **Kali s.;** *Merc. s.;* Penthor.; *Puls.;* Sang. n.; Sep.; *Sticta.*

Coryza, worse in evening—Cepa; Glycerin; Puls.

Coryza, worse in newborn—Dulc.

Coryza, worse in warm room, better in open air—Ars.; Cepa; Nux v.

Cough—Alum.; *Bell.;* Bry.; *Cepa;* Dros.; Euphras.; *Justicia;* Lyc.; Nux v.; Sang.; Sinap.; *Sticta.*

Fever, low type, in old people—Bapt.

Headache—Acon.; Ars.; Beil.; *Bry.;* Cepa; Camph.; Cinch.; Eup. perf.; *Gels.;* Kali bich.; *Kali iod.;* Nat. ars.; *Nux v.;* Sabad.; Sang.

Hoarseness, aphonia—Ars.; *Caust.;* Cepa; *Hep.;* Osm.; Phos.; Pop. c.; Tellur.; Verbasc.

Infants, with snuffles—Acon.; *Am. c.;* Bell.; *Cham.;* Dulc.; Elaps; *Hep.;* Merc. i. fl.; *Nux v.;* Samb.; Sticta; Sul.

Insomnia—Ars.; Cham.

Lachrymation, sneezing—Acon.; Ambros.; Am. phos.; Aral.; *Ars.;* Ars. iod.; Camph.; *Cepa;* Cham.; *Cycl.;* Eup. perf.; *Euphras.; Gels.;* Ipec.; *Justicia;* Kali chlor.; *Kali iod.;* Menthol; Merc. s.; Naph.; *Nat. m.; Nux v.;* Quill.; *Sabad.;* Scilla; Sinap.; Solid.; Sticta. See Lachrymation.

Photophobia—Ars.; Bell.; Cepa; *Euphras.*

Prostration, lassitude—Ars.; Ars. iod.; Bapt.; Gels.; Quill.

Respiration, asthmatic—Ant. t.; *Aral.; Ars. iod.;* Bad.; *Ipec.;* Naph.

Inflammation, acute, croupous, fibrinous—*Am. caust.;* Apis; Ars.; Echin.; Hep.; *Kali bich.;* Lach.; Merc. s.; Nit. ac.

Inflammation, chronic atrophic (sicca)—*Alum.;* Am. c.; Aur.; *Calc. fl.;* Cinnab.; Elaps; Fluor. ac.; Graph.; *Hep.; Kali bich.;* Kali iod.; Kali s. chrom.; *Lemna m.; Lyc.;* Merc.; Sabal; *Sep.; Sticta; Sul.;* Teucr.; Wyeth.

Inflammation, chronic catarrhal—*Alum.;* Am. br.; *Am. m.;* Ars. iod.; Aur. mur.; Bals. per.; Brom.; *Calc. c.;* Calc. p.; Cub.; Elaps; *Eucal.; Hep.; Hippoz.; Hydr.; Kali bich.;* Kali c.; Kali iod.; Kreos.; Lemna m.; Med.; Merc. i. r.; *Merc. s.; Nat. c.;* Nat. m.; Nat. s.; Nit. ac.; Phos.; Psor.; *Puls.;* Sabad.; Sang.; Sang. n.; *Sep.;* Sil.; Spig.; Sticta; Teucr.; Ther.; Thuya.

Inflammation, purulent in children—Alum.; Arg. n.; *Calc. c.;* Cycl.; Hep.; Iod.; *Kali bich.; Lyc.;* Nat. c.; Nit. ac.

TYPE OF DISCHARGE IN RHINITIS—**Acrid, watery, fluent, hot, or thin mucus:** *Ambros.;* Am. caust.; *Am. m.; Aral.; Ars.; Ars. iod.;* Arum; Bell.; Carbo v.; *Cepa;* Cham.; Eucal.; *Gels.;* Glycerin; *Iod.; Kali iod.;* Kreos.; Lach.; *Merc. c.;* Merc.; Mur. ac.; Naph.; *Nat. ars.; Nat. m.;* Nit. ac.; *Sabad.;* Sang.; *Sang. n.;* Scilla; Sul.; Trifol.

Albuminous, clear mucus—Æsc.; Calc. c.; Camph.; Graph.; Hydr.; Kali bich.; Kali iod.; *Kali m.;* Lac c.; Menthol; *Nat. m.;* Phos.

Bland mucus—*Euphras.;* Jugl. c.; Kali iod.; *Puls.;* Sep.

Bloody mucus—Ail.; A.g. n.; Ars.; *Arum;* Aur.; Echin.; *Hep.;* Hydr.; Kali bich.; Merc. c.; *Merc. i. r.;* Penthor.; *Phos.;* Sang. n.; Sil.; Thuya.

Green, yellow, fetid (purulent or muco-purulent)—Alum.; Ars.; Ars. iod.;

Arum; Aur.; *Bals. per.; Calc. c.;* Calc. iod.; Calc. s.; *Dulc.;* Eucal.; *Hep., Hydr.; Kali bich.;* Kali iod.; *Kali s.; Lyc.;* Med.; *Merc.;* Nat. c.; *Nat. s.;* Nit. ac.; Penthor.; Phos.; *Puls.;* Sang. n.; *Sep.;* Sil.; Ther.; Thuya; Tub.

Membranous formation—*Am. caust.;* Echin.; Hep.; *Kali bich.* See Croupous Rhinitis.

Offensive, fetid—Ars. iod.; Asaf.; *Aur.;* Bals. per.; *Calc. c.;* Echin.; Elaps; Eucal.; Graph.; *Hep.; Hydr.; Kali bich.;* Kali iod.; Merc. s.; Nat. c.; Nit. ac.; Psor.; *Puls.;* Sang.; Sep.; *Sil.; Sul.;* Ther.; Tub.

Profuse—Ail; Am. m.; Aral.; *Ars.; Ars. iod.;* Arum; Bals. per.; Calc. iod.; *Cepa; Euphras.; Hep.; Hydr.; Kali bich.; Kali iod.; Merc.;* Nux v.; *Puls.;* Sang.; Sang. n.; Sep.; Thuya.

Salty-tasting—Aral.; Tellur.

Scabs, crusts, plugs—*Alum.;* Ant. c.; Aur.; Aur. mur.; Bor.; Calc. fl.; Calc. sil.; Caust.; Elaps; Fagop.; *Graph.;* Hep.; *Hydr.; Kali bich.;* Kaolin; Lemna m.; *Lyc.;* Merc. i. fl.; Nat. ars.; Nit. ac.; Petrol.; Psor.; *Puls.; Sep.;* Sil.; Sticta; *Sul.; Teucr.;* Ther.; Thuya.

Thick—Alum.; Am. brom.; *Calc. c.;* Hep.; Hydr.; *Kali bich.; Merc. c.; Merc. s.;* Nat. c.; Penthor.; *Puls.;* Sep.; Ther.; Thuya.

Unilateral—Calc. s.; Calend.; Phyt.

Viscid, ropy, stringy—*Bov.;* Gall. ac.; *Hydr.; Kali bich.;* Myr.; Sticta; Sumb.

ITCHING in nose—*Agn.;* Am. c.; Ars. iod.; *Arundo;* Aur.; Brom.; Cepa; *Cina;* Fagop.; Glycerin; *Hydr.;* Nat. m.; Ran. b.; Rosa d.; Sabad.; Sang.; *Santon.;* Sep.; Sil.; *Teucr.; Wyeth.*

Nervous disturbance—Agar.

Numbness, tingling—Acon.; Jugl. c.; *Nat. m.;* Plat.; Ran. b.; Sabad.; Sang.; Sil.; *Sticta.*

OZAENA—Odor:—Alum.; Ars. iod.; *Asaf.;* Aur. m.; *Aur. mur.; Cadm. s.;* Calc. c.; Calc. fl.; Carb. ac.; Diph.; Elaps; Ferr. iod.; Graph.; *Hep.;* Hippoz.; *Hydr.;* Hydrast. mur.; *Iod.; Kali bich.;* Kali c.; Kali chrom.; Kali iod.; Kali p.; Kreos.; Lach.; Lemna m.; Merc. i. fl.; Merc. pr. rub.; *Merc. s.; Nit. ac.;* Phos. ac.; Phos.; *Psor.; Puls.; Sep.;* Sil.; Teucr.; Ther.; Thuya; *Triost.*

Syphilitic—Asaf.; *Aur.;* Aur. mur.; Crot.; *Fluor ac.;* **Kali bich.; Kali** iod.; *Nit. ac.;* Syph.

PAIN in—Aching in dorsum, better from pressure—Agn.

Boring, gnawing—Asaf.; *Aur.;* Brom.; Kali iod.; Merc. i. r.

Burning—Æsc.; Ars.; *Ars. iod.;* Arum; Chrom. ac.; *Kali iod.;* **Lach.;** Merc. c.; *Sang.* See Burning.

Cramp-like—Plat.; Sabad.

Pressing at root of nose—*Acon.;* Alum.; Arum; Caps.; *Cepa;* Cinnab.; Gels.; Hep.; Iod.; *Kali bich.;* Kali iod.; Menyanth.; Nat. ars.; ' *Nux v.;* Oniscus; *Paris;* Plat.; Puls.; Ran. b.; Ruta; *Sang. n.; Sep.; Sticta;* Ther.

Pressing in frontal sinuses—Gels.; Ign.; Iod.; Kali bich.; *Kali iod.;* Merc.; Nux v.; Sang.; *Sticta.*

Sharp to ears—Merc. c.

Splinter-like, sticking—*Aur.;* *Hep.:* Kali bich.; *Nit. ac*

String-like to ear—Lemna m.

Throbbing—Bell.; *Hep.;* Kali iod.

Violent shooting, from occiput to root of nose, from suppressed discharge— Kali bich.

POSTERIOR NARES—(naso-pharynx): Inflammation of: Acute: *Acon.;* Camph.; Cistus; Gels.; Kali bich.; Menthol; *Merc. c.;* Nat. ars.; Wyeth. See Rhinitis, Pharyngitis.

Chronic—Aur.; Calc. fl.; Elaps; Fagop.; *Hydr.; Kali bich.;* Kali c.; Merc. c.; Penthor.; Sep.; *Spig.; Sticta;* Sul.; Thuya.

Chronic with dropping of mucus--Remedies in General: *Alum.;* Am. br.; Ant. c.; Ars. iod.; Aur.; Calc. sil.; *Coral.;* Echin.; Glycerin; *Hydr.;* Irid.; *Kali bich.;* Kali m.; *Lemna m.;* Merc. i. r.; Nat. c.; *Penthor.; Phyt.; Sang. n.;* Sinap. n.; *Spig.;* Sticta; Teucr.; Ther.; Wyeth.

Clear, acrid, thin mucus—Ars. iod.

Clear mucus—Cepa; *Kali m.;* Nat. m.; Solan. lyc.

Lumpy—Osm.; Teucr.

Thick, tenacious, yellow, or white mucus—Alum.; Am. br.; Ant. c.; Calc. sil.; Coral.; *Hydr.; Kali bich.;* Lemna m.; Menthol; Merc. i. fl.; Nat. c.; Sang. n.; Sep.; Spig.

Tumors—Chrom. ac.; Osm.

Wet, raw feeling—Penthor.

SENSE OF SMELL—Diminished: *Alum.; Cycl.;* Helleb.; *Hep.;* Kali c.; Menthol; Mez.; Rhod.; Sil.; Tab.

Hypersensitive—*Acon.;* Agar.; Aur.; *Bell.; Carb. ac.;* Carbo v.; *Cham.;* Cinch.; Coff.; *Colch.;* Graph.; Ign.; Lyc.; Mag. m.; *Nux v.; Phos.;* Sang.; Sabad.; *Sep.;* Sul.

Hypersensitive to flowers—Graph.

Hypersensitive to food—Ars.; Colch.; Sep.

Hypersensitive to tobacco—Bell.

Lost (anosmia) or perverted—*Alum.;* Am. m.; amyg. pers.; *Anac.;* Apoc. andr.; Aur.; Bell.; Calc. c.; *Hep.;* Ign.; Iod.; Justicia; *Kali bich.;* Lemna m.; *Mag. m.; Nat. m.;* Nit. ac.; *Puls.;* Sang.; Sep.; Sil.; Sul.; Teucr.; Zinc. mur.

Parosmia (illusions)—Agn.; *Anac.;* Apoc. andr.; Ars.; Aur. ; *Bell.;* Calc. c.; Coral.; Diosc.; Graph.; Ign.; *Kali bich.;* Mag. m.; *Merc.;* Nit. ac.; Nux v.; *Phos.; Puls.;* Sang.; Sul.

SENSITIVENESS of nose to air, touch—*Æsc.;* Alum.; *Ant. c.;* Aral.; Ars.; *Arum;* Aur.; Aur. mur.; Bell.; Calc. c.; Camph.; *Hep.;* Kali bich.; Kaolin; *Merc.;* Nat. m.; Osm.; Sil.

SINUSES—(antrum, frontal, sphenoidal): Affections in general: Ars.; *Asaf.;* Aur. m.; Bell.; Calc. c.; Camph.; Eucal.; *Hep.; Iod.;* Kali bich.; *Kali iod.;* Kali m.; Lyc.; *Merc. i. fl.;* Merc.; Mez.; Phos. ac.; *Phos.; Sil.; Spig.; Sticta;* Teucr.

Catarrh of frontal sinuses—Ammoniacum; Ign.; Iod.; *Kali bich.; Kali iod.;* Lyc.; Menthol; Merc. i. fl.; Nat. m.; Nux v.; Sabad.; Sticta; Thuya.

Pain and swelling of antrum—Phos.; Spig.

Syphilitic affections—Aur.; *Kali iod.;* Nit. ac.

SNEEZING—(sternutation): Acon.; Ambros.; Am. m.; *Aral.; Ars.;* Ars. iod.; Arum; Arundo; Calc. c.; Camph.; *Cepa; Cycl.;* Eup. perf.; Euphorbia; *Euphras.; Gels.;* Ichthy.; Iod.; *Ipec.;* Kali bich.; *Kali iod.;* Lob. cer.; Menthol; Merc.; Naph.; Nat. m.; Nit. ac.; Nux v.; Rosa d.; Rhus t.; *Sabad.;* Succin. ac.; Sang.; *Sang. n.;* Sapon.; Scilla; Senec.; Senega; Sinap.; *Sticta.*

Sneezing, chronic tendency—Sil.

Sneezing, ineffectual—*Ars.;* Carbo v.; Sil.

Sneezing, worse coming into warm room: rising from bed: handling peaches —Cepa.

Sneezing, worse in cool air—Ars.; Hep.; Sabad.

Sneezing, worse in evening—Glycerin.

Sneezing, worse in morning—Camph.; Caust.; *Nux v.;* Sil.

Sneezing, worse immersing hands in water—Lac. d.; Phos.

STOPPAGE—**Stuffiness:** *Acon.;* Ambros.; *Am. c.;* Am. m.; Anac.; Apoc.; Ars.; Ars. iod.; *Arum; Aur.;* Aur. m. n.; *Calc. c.;* Camph.; Caust.; *Cham.;* Con.; Cop.; Elaps; Eucal.; Fluor. ac.; *Formica;* Glycerin; Graph.; Helianth.; *Hep.; Kali bich.;* Kali c.; Kali iod.; Lemna m.; *Lyc.;* Menthol; Nat. ars.; Nat. c.; Nat. m.; Nit. ac.; *Nux v.;* Paris; Penthor.; Petrol.; *Puls.;* Radium; Sabad.; *Samb.; Sang. n.;* Sapon.; Sep.; Sil.; *Sinap.;* Spong.; *Sticta.*

Stoppage, alternating nostrils—Acon.; Am. c.; Bor.; *Lac c.;* Mag. m.; *Nux v.*

Swelling—Antipyr.; Ars.; *Ars. iod.; Aur.;* Aur. s. a.; Bar. c.; Bell.; Calc. c.; Hep.; *Kali bich.; Lemna m.; Merc. c.;* Merc. i. r.; *Nit. ac.;* Sabad.; Sang.; Sep. See Inflammation.

ULCERATION OF SEPTUM—Alum.; Aur.; Brom.; Calc. c.; Carb. ac.; Fluor. ac.; Hippoz.; *Hydr.; Kali bich.;* Kali iod.; Merc. c.; Nit. ac.; *Sil.;* Vinca.

Ulceration, syphilitic—*Aur.;* Aur. mur.; Coral.; Kali bich.; *Kali iod.;* Lach.; Merc. aur.; *Nit. ac.*

Wet feeling not relieved by blowing—Penthor.

FACE

APPEARANCE—CONDITION—Anemic, alabaster-like, waxen: *Acet. ac.;* *Apis; Ars.;* Calc. p.; Ferr. m.; Lach.; Merc. c.; Nat. c.; Sep.; Sil.

Bloated, puffy—Æth.; *Am. benz.; Apis; Ars.;* Bor. ac.; Bothrops; Calc. c.; Ferr. m.; *Kali c.;* Helleb.; Hyos.; Lach.; Medusa; *Merc. c.; Op.; Phos.;* Taxus; Xerophyl.

Bloated about eyes—*Am. benz.;* Ars.; Bor. ac.; Elaps; *Merc. c.;* Nat. c.; *Phos.;* Rhus t.; Thlaspi; Xerophyl.

Bloated about lower eyelids—*Apis;* Xerophyl.

Bloated about upper eyelids—Kali c.

Blue, livid (cyanosis)—Absinth.; Am. c.; Ant. t.; Arg. n.; *Ars.;* Aur.; *Camph.;* Carbo an.; *Carbo v.;* Chlorum; *Cic.;* Cina; Cinnab.; Crot.; *Cupr. ac.;* Cupr. m.; *Dig.;* Ferr.; *Hydroc. ac.; Ipec.;* Lach.; *Laur.; Morph.;* Œnanthe; Op.; Phenac.; Rhus t.; *Samb.;* Sec.; Strych.; *Tab.; Ver. a.* See Circulatory System.

Blue rings around, dull looking eyes—*Abrot.;* Acct. ac.; *Ars.;* Berb .v.; Bism.; Calc. c.; *Camph.; Cina; Cinch.;* Cycl.; Ipec.; Nat. c.; *Œnanthe; Phos. ac.; Phos.; Santon.;* Sec.; Sep.; Spig.; Stann.; *Staph.;* Tab.; *Ver. a.;* Zinc. m.

Blushing—Ambra; *Amyl;* Carbo an.; Carls.; *Coca;* Ferr.; Stram.; Sul.

Bronzed—Ant. c.; Nit. ac.; Sec.; Spig.

Brown spots on—Caul.; Sep.

Coppery look—Alum.; Nit. ac.

Distorted—Absinth.; Art. v.; Bell.; Camph.; *Cic.;* Cupr. ac.; *Cupr. m.;* Crot.; Helleb.; Hyos.; Nux v.; *Op.;* Sec.; *Stram.*

Earthy, dirty, sallow, cachectic—*Acet. ac.; Ars.;* Berb. v.; Calc. p.; Camph.; *Carbo v.; Caust.;* Chel.; *Cinch.;* Ferr.; Glycerin; Hydr.; Iod.; *Lyc.;* Merc. c.; Merc.; *Nat. m.;* Nux v.; Phos. ac.; Phos.; Picr. ac.; *Plumb. m.;* Psor.; *Sanic.; Sec.; Sep.;* Spig.; Staph.; Sul.

Expression anxious, suffering—*Acon.;* Æth.; *Ars.;* Bor.; *Camph.;* Canth.; Cina; Cinch.; Iod.; Kreos.; Merc. c.; Plumb.; *Stram.;* Strych.; *Tab.; Ver. a.*

Expression drowsy, stupid—Ail.; Apis; *Bapt.;* Can. ind.; *Gels.;* Helleb.; *Op.;* Rhus t.

Expression stolid, mask-like—Mang. ac.

Greasy, shiny, oily—*Nat. m.;* Plumb.; Psor.; Sanic.; Selen.; Thuya.

Hippocratic (sickly, sunken, deathly cold)—Acon.; Æth.; *Ant. t.;* Arn.; *Ars.;* Berb. v.; *Camph.; Carbo v.;* Cinch.; Cyprip.; Helleb.; Lach.; Merc. cy.; Plumb. m.; Pyr.; *Sec.; Tab.; Ver. a.;* Zinc. m.

Jaundiced, yellow—*Ars.;* Berb. v.; Blatta am.; Bry.; Calc. c.; Carbo v.; *Chel.; Chionanth.; Cinch.;* Crot.; *Dig.;* Hep.; Hydr.; Iod.; Kali c.; Lach.; Lyc.; Merc.; *Merc. d.;* Myr.; Nat. m.; Nat. p.; Nat. s.; *Nux v.;* Ol. j. as.; Petrol.; Picr. ac.; *Plumb. m.;* Pod.; *Sep.; Tarax.;* Yucca. See Jaundice.

Pale—Abrot.; *Acet. ac.; Ant. t.;* Apis; Arg. n.; *Ars.;* Bell.; Berb. v.; Bor.; Calc. c.; Calc. p.; *Camph.; Carbo v.; Cina;* Cinch.; Cupr. m.;

Cycl.; Dig.; *Ferr. ac.*; *Ferr. m.*; *Ferr. mur.*; Ferr. red.; Glon.; Helleb.;
Ipec.; Kali c.; Lach.; Lecith.; Med.; *Merc. c.*; Merc. d.; *Morph.*;
Nat. c.; Nat. m.; Nit. ac.; Phos. ac.; Phos.; *Plumb. m.*; *Puls.*; Pyr.;
Santon.; *Sec.*; Sep.; Sil.; Spig.; Stann.; Staph.; *Tab.*; *Ver. a.*; Zinc. m.

Parchment-like—Ars.

Red, becomes deathly pale on rising—*Acon.*; Ver. a.

Red, dark, dusky, besotted, bloated—*Ail.*; Apis; Ars. m.; *Bapt.*; Bothrops;
Bry.; Carb. ac.; Diph.; *Gels.*; Hyos.; Lach.; *Morph.*; Nux v.; *Op.*;
Rhus t.; Stram.

Red, distorted—Bell.; *Cic.*; Cupr. ac.; *Cupr. m.*; Crot.; Hyos.; Op.;
Stram.

Red, flushed after eating—Alum.; Carbo an.; Carls.; Coral.; Stront.

Red, flushed, from emotion, pain, exertion—Acon.; *Ferr. m.*; Ign.; Meli.

Red, flushed, hot, florid—Acet. ac.; *Acon.*; Agar.; *Amyl*; *Aster.*; Bapt.;
Bell.; Canth.; Caps.; *Ferr. p.*; Gels.; *Glon.*; Glycerin; Kreos.; *Meli.*;
Myg.; Op.; Quercus; Rhamnus c.; *Sang.*; *Stram.*; Sul.; *Ver. v.*

Red, semi-lateral—Acon.; *Cham.*; *Cina*; Dros.; Ipec.; *Nux v.*

Red, though cold—Asaf.; Caps.

Sensitive, after neuralgia—Cod.

Sweating—*Acet. ac.*; Amyl; *Ant. t.*; Ars.; *Cham.*; Glon.; Samb.; Sil.;
Tab.; *Ver. a.*; Viola tr.

Sweating, cold—*Ant. t.*; *Ars.*; Camph.; *Carbo v.*; Cina; Euphorbia; *Lob.
infl.*; *Tab.*; *Ver. a.*; Zinc. mur.

Sweating, in small spots, while eating—Ign.

Sweating on forehead—Cham.; Euphorbia; Op.; *Ver. a.*

Swelling—*Acon.*; Ant. ars.; Antipyr.; *Apis*; Ars.; Ars. m.; *Bell.*; Cepa;
Colch.; *Helleb.*; Lach.; *Merc. c.*; Œnanthe; Op.; Phos.; *Rhus t.*; Rhus
v.; Ver. a.; Vespa; Vipera.

Swelling from toothache—*Bell.*; Cham.; Coff.; Mag. c.; *Merc.*

Wrinkled, shrivelled, old-looking—Abrot.; *Arg. n.*; *Bar. c.*; Bor.; Calc.
p.; Con.; *Fluor. ac.*; Iod.; Kreos.; Lyc.; *Nat. m.*; Op.; *Psor.*; *Pulex*;
Sanic.; Sars.; Sec.; Sil.; Sul.

BONES—(facial): Caries: Aur. m.; Cistus; Fluor. ac.; Hekla.

Exostoses—Fluor. ac.; Hekla.

Inflammation—Aur. m.

Pains,—Alum.; Arg. n.; Astrag.; *Aur.*; Carbo an.; Caust.; Dulc.; *Hep.*;
Merc.; Nit. sp. d.; *Phos.*; *Sil.*; Zinc.

Sensitive—Aur.; *Hep.*; Kali bich.; Mez. See Jaws.

CHEEKS—Bites when chewing, talking—Caust.; *Ign.*; Ol. an.

Burning—Agar.; Euphorb.; Ferr. p.; Nit. sp. d.; Phos. ac.; Phos.; Sul.
See Sensation.

Eruptions—*Ant. c.*; Dulc.; Graph.; *Led.*; *Mez.* See Eruptions on face.

Lumpy—Antipyr.

Pains—Agar.; August.; Ver. a. See Prosopalgia.

Redness—Brom.; *Caps.*; *Cic.*; Coff.; Colch.; Euphorbia; Euphras.; *Meli.*
See Red Face.

Redness, unilateral—*Acon.*; *Cham.*; Cina; Dros.; Ipec.; *Nux v.*

Spots, circumscribed, red, burning—Benz. ac.; Bry.; *Cina;* Ferr. mur.; Lachnanth.; *Phos.;* Samb.; *Sang.;* Stram.: Sul.

Swelling—*Acon.;* Bell.; Bov.; *Calc. fl.;* Euphorb.; Kali m.; *Plant.;* Plat. See Swelling of Face.

Tingling, numbness—*Acon.;* Plat.

Ulcers, wart-like—Ars.

Yellow saddle in uterine disease—Sep.

CHIN—Eruptions: *Ant. c.;* Aster.; *Cic.;* Dulc.; *Graph.;* *Hep.;* Nat. m.; Phos. ac.; Rhus t.; Sep.; Sil.; *Sul. iod.;* Zinc.

ERUPTIONS ON FACE—**Acne rosacea**—*Ars. br.;* Carbo an.; Chrysar.; *Eug. j.; Kreos.;* Ophor.; Psor.; Sul.; Sulphurous ac.

Acne simplex—Ambra; *Ant. c.; Bell.; Berb. aq.;* Calc. p.; Calc. s.; Carbo v.; Cim.; Clem.; Con.: Crot. t.; *Eug. j.;* Graph.; Ind.; *Jugl. r.;* Kali ars.; Kali br.; Kali c.; *Led.;* Med.; Nat. m.; *Nux v.;* Phos. ac.; *Sul.:* Thuya.

Angioma—Abrot.

Blotches—*Berb. aq.;* Kali c.; Nux v.

Cancer, open, bleeding—Cistus.

Chilblains—Agar.

Comedones—*Abrot.;* Eug. j.; Jugl. r.; Nit. ac.; *Sul.*

Crusta-lactea—Calc. c.; Hep.; Merc. pr. rub.; *Rhus t.;* Sil.; Viola tr. See Scalp.

Eczema—Anac.; *Ant. c.; Ars.;* Calc. c.; Carb. ac.; *Crot. t.;* Dulc.; *Graph.;* Hep.; Led.; Merc. pr. rub.; *Mez.;* Nat. m.; Sep.; Sil.; Sul.; Sul. iod.; *Vinca;* Viola tr.

Epithelioma—Ars.; Kali s.; Lob. erin.

Erysipelas—Anac. oc.; Ananth.; *Apis; Bell.;* Bor.; *Canth.;* Carbo an.; *Euphorb.;* Ferr. mur.; *Graph.;* Gymnocl.; Hep.; *Rhus t.;* Sep.; Solan. c.; Ver. v.

Erythema—Ars. iod.; *Bell.;* Condur.; Echin.; Euphorbia; *Graph.;* Nux v.

Furuncles—Alum.; *Ant. c.;* Calc. p.; *Hep.; Led.;* Med.

Herpes (tetter)—Anac. oc.; Canth.; Clem.; *Dulc.;* Euphorb.; Limulus; Lyc.; *Nat. m.; Rhus t.;* Sep.

Humid, moist—Ant. c.; Cic.; Dulc.; *Graph.;* Hep.; Mez.; Psor.; Rhus t.; Viola tr.

Itching eruption on forehead during menses—Eug. j.; Psor.; Sang.; Sars.

Lentigo (freckles)—Am. c.; Iris germ.; Graph.; Lyc.; *Mur. ac.;* Nat. c.; *Nit. ac.;* Phos.; Sep.; *Sul.;* Tab.; Thuya.

Lupus—Cistus.

Pustules—*Ant. c.;* Bell.; Calc. c.; *Calc. s.; Cic.;* Graph.; *Hep.;* Indium; Merc.; Psor.

Rough, harsh—*Berb. aq.;* Kali c.; *Petrol.;* Sul.

Scabs, crusts, scurfs—Ars.; Cic.; Cistus; Dulc.; Graph.; Hep.; Mez.; Rhus t.

Scales—Ars.; Euphorbia.

Spots, copper-colored—Benz. ac.; *Carbo an.;* Lyc.; Nit. ac.

Spots, red—*Berb. aq.;* Euphorbia; Kali bich.; *Kali c.;* Œnanthe: Petrol.

Spots, yellow—Nat. c.; *Sep.*

SYPHILIDAE—Areolæ, papules:—Kali iod.

Copper spots—Carbo an.; Lyc.; *Nit. ac.*

Crusts, areolæ—Nit. ac.

Pustules—Kali iod.; Nit. ac.

Tubercles—Alum.; Carbo an.; Fluor. ac.

Ulcer, eroding—Con.

Warts—Calc. s.; Castorea; *Caust.;* Kali c.

Whiskers, eruptions—Hep.

Whiskers, falling out—Graph.; Selen. See Scalp.

Whiskers, itching—Calc. c. See Skin.

FOREHEAD feels contracted, wrinkled—Bapt.; Bellis; Grat.; *Helleb.;* Lyc.; Phos.; Primula.

Glabella, swelling—Sil.

JAWS—Cracking when chewing: Am. c.; Granat.; Lac c.; *Nit. ac.; Rhus t.*

Dislocated easy—Ign.; *Petrol.; Rhus t.;* Staph.

Growths, swelling—Amphis.; *Calc. fl.;* Hekla; Plumb.; Thuya.

Pain—Acon.; Agar.; Alum.; Am. m.; Am. picr.; *Amphis.;* August.; Arum; Astrag.; Aur. m.; Bapt. conf.; Calc. caust.; Carbo an.; *Caust.;* Merc.; Phos.; Rhus t.; Sang.; *Sphingur.;* Spig.; Xanth.

Stiffness (trismus, lockjaw)—Absinth.; Acon.; Arn.; Bell.; Carbon. oxy.; Caust.; Cham.; *Cic.; Cupr. ac.; Cupr. m.;* Cur.; Dulc.; Hydroc. ac.; *Hyper.; Ign.;* Merc. c.; *Morph.;* Nerium; Nicot.; *Nux v.;* Œnanthe; Physost.; Solan. n.; Stram.; *Strych.;* Ver. a.

Trembling—Alum.; *Ant. t.;* Cadm. s.; *Gels.*

LOWER JAW—Caries, necrosis:—Amphis.; Angust.; *Phos.;* Sil.

Chewing motion—Acon.; Bell.; Bry.; *Helleb.;* Stram.

Epulis—Plumb. ac.; Thuya.

Hanging down, relaxed—Arn.; Ars.; Gels.; *Helleb.;* Hyos.; Lach.; Lyc.; *Mur. ac.; Op.*

Nodes, painful—Graph.

Pain—Caust.; Chin. s.; Cinch.; Sil.; Spig.; Xanth. See Jaws.

Swelling—Amphis.; Aur. m. n.; Merc.; *Phos.;* Sil.; Symphyt.

UPPER JAW—Affections of Antrum of Highmore: Arn.; Bell.; Chel.; Commocl.; Euphorb. amyg.; Hep.; *Kali iod.;* Kali s.; Mag. c.; Merc. c.; Paris; *Phos.;* Sil.; Tilia.

Pain—Astrag.; Calc. p.; Euphorbia; *Fluor. ac.;* Merc. i. r.; *Phos.;* Polygon.; *Spig.*

Tumor—Hekla.

MUSCLES—(facial) Distortion (risus sardonicus): *Cic.;* Cupr. ac.; Hydroc. ac.; Op.; *Sec.;* Stram.; Strych.; Tellur.

Pain—Anac.; Angust.; Cocc.; Colch.; Oxytr.; Sab. See Prosopalgia.

Paralysis—Bell's palsy: *Acon.;* Alum.; *Am. phos.;* Bell.; Cadm. s.; *Caust.;* Cocc.; Cur.; *Dulc.;* Formica; *Gels.;* Graph.; Hyper.; *Kali chlor.; Kali iod.;* Merc. c. k.; Physal.; *Rhus t.;* Ruta; *Senega;* Zinc. picr.

Left side—Cadm. s.; Senega.

Right side—Bell.; Caust.

Stiffness—Absinth.; Acon.; *Agar.;* Bapt.; *Caust.;* Gels.; Helod.; **Nux v.;** Rhus t. See Trismus.

Twitching, spasmodic—Agar.; Arg. n.; *Bell.;* Caust.; Cham.; *Cic.; Cina; Gels.; Hyos.; Ign.;* Laburn.; Laur.; Menyanth.; *Myg.;* Nux v.; Œ*nanthe;* Op.; Sec.; Stram.; Tellur.; Visc. a.

PROSOPALGIA—Pain (face-ache):

TYPE—Congestive, inflammatory, neuralgic: Acon.; *Agar.;* Aran.; Arg. n.; *Ars.; Bell.;* Cact.; *Caps.;* Caust.; *Ced.;* Cepa; *Cham.;* Chin. ars.; *Chin. s.;* Cim.; *Cinch.* Coff.; *Col.;* Ferr.; *Gels.;* Hekla; *Kali iod.;* Kali p.; Kal.; *Mag. p.;* Menthol; Merc. c.; Merc. s.; *Mez.;* Nit. sp. d.; Phos.; *Plant.; Plat.;* Puls.; Radium; Rhodium; *Rhus t.;* Sang.; Sil.; *Spig.;* Stann.; Sul.; Thuya; Tilia; *Verbasc.;* Zinc. p.; *Zinc. v.*

Reflex, from decayed teeth—Coff. tosta; Hekla; Merc. s.; *Mez.;* Staph.

Rheumatic—*Acon.;* Act. sp.; *Caust.;* Cham.; Colch.; Col.; *Dulc.;* Puls.; *Rhod.; Rhus t.;* Spig.

Syphilitic (mercurial)—*Kali iod.;* Mez.; Nit. ac.

Toxic (malarial, quinine)—Ars.; Cinch.; Ipec.; Nat. m.

LOCATION—Eyes: Ars.; *Cim.;* Clem.; Nux v.; Paris; *Spig.;* Thuya. See Eyes.

Jaw, lower—*Amphis.;* Calc. c.; Lach.; Nit. sp. d.; Plat.; Radium; *Rhod.;* Xanth.; Zinc. v.

Jaw, upper—*Amphis.;* Bism.; Calc. *caust.;* Cham.; Col.; Dulc.; *Euphorb. amyg.;* Graph.; Iris; *Kali cy.; Kali iod.;* Kal.; *Kreos.;* Mez.; Paris; Sang.; Thuya; *Verbasc.*

Jaw, upper, (infra-orbital)—Colch.; Iris; Mag. p.; *Mez.;* Nux v.; *Phos.;* Verbasc.

Jaw, upper, to teeth, temples, ears, eyes, malar bones—*Act. sp.;* Arg. n.; Ars.; Bell.; Bism.; *Cham.;* Clem.; *Coff.; Col.;* Dulc.; *Kali cy.; Mez.;* Phos.; Plant.; Rhod.; Sang.; *Spig.;* Thuya; *Verbasc.*

Malar bones (zygoma)—Angust.; Arg. m.; Aur.; *Calc. caust.;* Caps.; *Cim.;* Col.; Hydrocot.; Lecith.; Menthol; Ol. an.; Mag. c.; Mez.; Paris; *Plat.;* Rhus t.; *Sphingur.; Spig.;* Strych.; Thuya; *Verbasc.;* Zinc. m.

Unilateral, left—*Acon.;* Arg. n.; *Col.;* Coral.; Hydrocot.; *Lach.;* Paris; Plat.; Sapon.; Senec.; *Spig.; Verbasc.;* Zinc. v.

Unilateral, right—Aran.; *Cact.;* Caps.; Ced.; Clem.; Coff.; Colch.; Hyper.; *Kal.; Mag. p.; Mez.; Puls.*

TYPE OF PAIN—Cramp-like drawing, pressing: Angust.; Bism.; Bry.; *Cact.;* Cocc.; Col.; *Mez.; Plat.;* Thuya; Ver. a.; *Verbasc.*

Cutting, tearing, jerking, stitching, rending—Acon.; Amphis.; *Ars.;* Aur.; Caust.; *Cham.;* Cinch.; *Col.;* Dulc.; Hyper.; Mag. p.; Merc.; Mez.; Nux v.; Phos.; *Puls.;* Rhodium; Rhod.; Senec.; Sil.; *Spig.*

Fine line of pain coursing along the nerve—Caps.; Cepa.

Gradual onset and cessation—Plat.; *Stann.*

Gradual onset and sudden cessation—Arg. m.; *Bell.;* Puls.

Hot needles, penetrating—Ars.

Icy needles, penetrating—Agar.

Lancinating, paroxysmal, lightning-like, radiating—Arg. n.; Ars.; *Bell.;*

Cocc.; *Col.;* Gels.; Graph.; Hep.; *Kali iod.;* Kreos.; Mag. p.; *Nux v.;* Phos.; Plant.; *Rhodium;* Sang.; *Spig.;* Strych.; Zinc. m.

Periodical intermittent—Cact.; Ced.; Chin. s.; *Cinch.; Col.;* Graph.; Mag. p.; Plant.; *Spig.;* Ver. a.; Verbasc.

CONCOMITANTS—Acid, sour eructations: Arg. n.; Nux v.; Verbasc.

Canine hunger, preceded by coldness—Dulc.

Catarrh (coryza, lachrymation)—Verbasc.

Cheek, dark red—Spig.

Chilliness—Col.; Dulc.; *Mez.; Puls.;* Rhus t.

Gastralgia, alternating—Bism.

Lachrymation—Bell.; Ipec.; Nux v.; Plant.; *Puls.;* Verbasc.

Mental irritability—Cham.; Coff.; Kreos.; Nux v.

Numbness—*Acon.;* Menthol; Mez.; Plat.; Rhus t.

Photophobia—Nit. sp. d.; Plant.

Ptosis—Gels.

Restlessness, palpitation—Spig.

Salivation, stiff neck—Mez.

Tenderness to touch—Acon.; *Bell.; Cinch.;* Col.; *Hep.;* Mez.; Paris; Spig.; Verbasc.

Twitching about face—Agar.; Bell.; *Colch.;* Kali c.; Nux v.; Thuya; *Zinc. m.*

Vision veiled—Tilia.

MODALITIES—Aggravation: From acids, motion, emotion: Kali c.

From chewing, opening mouth—Angust.; Cocc.; Helleb.; Hep.; Mez.

From cold, dry exposure—*Acon.;* Coff.; Kal.; Mag. c.; Mag. p.; Nit. sp. d.

From cold, wet exposure—Col.; *Dulc.;* Mag. m.; Rhus t.; *Sil.; Spig.;* Thuya.

From contact, touch—*Bell.;* Caps.; *Cinch.;* Col.; *Cupr. m.; Hep.;* Mag. p.; *Mez.;* Paris; *Spig.;* Verbasc.

From eating, drinking—Bism.; Iris; *Mez.*

From eating motion—Col.; Phos.; Verbasc.

From eating, motion, stooping, jar, etc.—*Bell.;* Ferr. p.; *Spig.*

From morning until sunset—Spig.

From motion, noise—Ars.; Chin. s.; Cinch.; *Spig.*

From pressure—Caps.

From rest—Mag. c.; Plat.; Rhus t.

From talking, motion, sitting or lying on unaffected side—Kreos.

From talking, sneezing, change of temperature, pressure of teeth—Verbasc.

From tea—Selen.; Spig.; Thuya.

From thinking of pain—Aur.

From tobacco—Sep.

From warmth—Cham.; Glon.; Kali s.; Merc. s.; Mez.; *Puls.*

In afternoon—Cocc.

In daytime—Ced.; Plant.; Spig.

In evening, night—*Ars.;* Caps.; Mag. c.; Merc. s.; Mez.; *Puls.;* Rhus t.

AMELIORATION—From chewing—Cupr. ac.

From cold applications, cold—Bism.; *Clem.;* Kali p.; Phos.; *Puls.*

From eating—Rhod.

From kneeling, and pressing head firmly against floor—Sang.

From motion, open air—Thuya.

From pressure—Cinch.; *Col.;* Mag. m.; *Rhod.*

From rest—Col.; Nux v.

From rubbing—Acon.; *Plat.*

From warmth—Ars.; Calc. c.; *Col.;* Cupr. ac.; Mag. m.; *Mag. p.;* Mez.; Thuya. See Modalities.

SENSATIONS—Burning heat: *Agar.;* Agrost.; Ant. c.; *Ars.;* Arum; *Canth.; Caps.; Cham.; Euphorbia;* Kali c.; Nat. c.; Sang.; Senega; Sil.; Stront.; *Sul.;* Viola tr.

Cobwebs dried on, as if—Alum.; *Bar. c.; Bor.;* Brom.; Euphorbia; *Graph.;* Phos. ac.; *Ran. s.*

Coldness—Abrot.; *Agar.; Ant. t.; Camph.;* Carbo v.; Dros.; *Helod.;* Phos. ac.; *Plat.; Ver. a.* See Hippocratic Face.

Contracted, wrinkled feeling, in forehead—*Bapt.; Bellis;* Grat.; *Helleb.;* Phos.; Primula.

Formication (numbness, tingling, crawling)—*Acon.;* Agar.; Colch.; Gymnocl.; Helod.; Myr.; Nux v.; *Plat.*

Itching—*Agar.;* Ant. c.; *Mez.;* Myr.; Nat. m.; Rhus t.; Sep.; Stront.

TIC-DOULOUREUX—*Acon.; Aconit.;* Ananth.; Arg. n.; *Ars.; Bell.;* Caps.; Cim.; *Coccinel.; Colch.;* Cupr. m.; *Gels.;* Glon.; Graph.; Kali c.; Kali chlor.; *Kali iod.; Mag. p.; Mez.;* Nat. s.; Nux v.; *Phos.;* Rhus t.; Sep.; Stann.; Staph.; Sul.; *Strych.; Thuya; Verbasc.;* Zinc. m. See Prosopalgia, Trifacial Neuralgia.

MOUTH

BREATH, cold—Ant. t.; Ars.; *Camph.; Carbo v.;* Cistus; Cupr. m.; Euphorb. dath.; *Helod.;* Jatropha; *Tab.;* Tereb.; *Ver. a.*

Breath, offensive (fetor oris)—Abies n.; Alum.; Ambra; Anac.; *Ant. c.; Arn.; Ars.; Aur.; Bapt.;* Bor.; Bry.; Calc. c.; Caps.; *Carb. ac.;* Carbo v.; Chel.; Cinch.; Cistus; Daphne; *Diph.;* Graph.; Helleb.; *Hep.;* Indol; *Iod.;* Kalagua; Kali chlor.; Kali per.; Kali p.; *Kali tell.;* Kreos.; Lach.; Merc. c.; Merc. cy.; Merc. d.; *Merc. s.;* Mur. ac.; *Nat. tell.; Nit. ac.;* Nux v.; *Petrol.;* Phyt.; Psor.; *Puls.; Quercus;* Rheum; *Sep.;* Sinap.; Spig.; Stann.; Sul. ac.; Tereb.

Breath offensive, after meals only—Cham.; *Nux v.;* Sul.

Breath offensive, in evening or night—Puls.; Sul.

Breath offensive, in girls at puberty—Aur. m.

Breath offensive, in morning only—*Arn.;* Bell.; *Nux v.;* Sil.; Sul.

EXTERNAL MOUTH—Commissures (corners): Color: **pearly white about:** Æth.; *Cina;* Santon.

Color, yellow about—Sep.

Cracks, ulcerations—Am. m.; *Ant. c.;* Ars.; *Arum;* Arundo; Bov.; *Condur.;* Echin.; Eup. perf.; *Graph.;* Helleb.; *Hep.;* Nat. m.; *Nit. ac.;* Petrol.; Rhus t.; Sec.

Eruptions around—Ant. c.; *Ars.;* Aster.; Echin.; *Graph.; Hep.;* Naph.; Mez.; Mur. ac.; *Nat. m.;* Petrol.; Senega.

LIPS—Black:—*Ars.;* Bry.; *Merc. c.;* Vipera.

Blue, cyanosed—Ars.; *Camph.;* Carbo an.; Carbo v.: *Cupr. m.;* Cupr. s.; *Dig.;* Hydroc. ac.; Sec.; *Ver. a.; Zinc.* See Face.

Burning, hot, parched—Acon.; Arn.; *Ars.;* Arum; *Bry.;* Caps.; Illic.; Nat. m.; Phos.; Rhus t.; *Sul.;* Thyr.

Cancer—Acet. ac.; *Ars.;* Ars. iod.; Clem.; Commocl.; Condur.; Con.; *Hydr.;* Kreos.; Lyc.; *Sep.;* Tab.; Thuya.

Chewing motion—Acon.; *Bell.; Bry.;* Helleb.; Stram.

Cold sores, herpes, hydroa—Agar.; Ars.; Calc. fl.; *Caps.;* Dulc.; Frax. am.; Hep.; Med.; *Nat. m.; Rhus t.;* Rhus v.; *Sep.;* Sul. iod.; Upas.

Cracks, ulcerations—Ant. c.; *Ars.; Arum;* Bry.; Carbo v.; Carbon. s.; *Clem.; Condur.;* Echin.; Glycerin; *Graph.;* Kali bich.; Merc. pr. rub.; Mur. ac.; Nat. m.; *Nit. ac.;* Phos.; *Rhus t.;* Sil.

Cracks, ulcerations in middle of lower lip—Am. c.; Graph.; *Hep.;* Nat. m.; Puls.; Sep.

Distortion—*Art. v.;* Cadm. s.; *Cic.; Cupr. ac.;* Cur.; Stram.

Dryness—Acon.; Ant. c.; *Bry.;* Chionanth.; Cinch.; Euonym.; Glycerin; Helleb.; Helon.; Mur. ac.; *Nat. m.; Nux m.;* Phos. ac.; Puls.; Rhus t.; Senec.; Sep.; *Sul.; Zinc. m.* See Burning.

Eczema—*Ant. c.;* Aur. mur.; Bov.; Calc. c.; Graph.; Lyc.; Mez.; *Rhus v.*

Eruptions—Acne: Bor.; Psor.; Sars.; *Sul. iod.*

Exfoliation—Con.; Sep.

Foam at the mouth—Absinth.; Cic.; Cupr. ac.; *Cupr. m.; Hydroc. ac.;* Hyos.; Lyssin; *Œnanthe;* Op. See Convulsions (Nervous System).

Glued together—Can. ind.; Helon.

Licks them frequently—Puls.

Numbness, tingling—*Acon.*; Crot.; Echin.; *Nat. m.*

Pain, soreness—*Arum;* ᵗᵒr.; Calc. c.; Illic.; Nat. m.; *Rhus t.; Rhus v.;* Sep.

Picks them until they bleed—*Arum;* Helleb.; Zinc. m.

Red, bleeding—*Arum;* Kreos.

Red, crimson—Aloe; *Sul.;* Tub.

Swelling—Antipyr.; *Apis;* Bov.; Bry.; Caps.; Medusa; Merc. c.; *Rhus v.; Vipera.*

Swelling of lower—Puls.; Sep.

Swelling of upper—Apis; *Bell.;* Calc. c.; *Hep.;* Nat. c.; *Nat. m.;* Psor.; *Rhus t.*

Twitching, spasmodic—*Agar.;* Art. v.; Cim.; *Gels.; Ign.;* Myg.; Niccol.; Op.; Strych.

Ulcer, cancerous—Ars.

INNER MOUTH—(buccal cavity): Bleeding, after tooth extraction: Arn.; Bov.; Cinch.; Ham.

Burning, smarting—Acon.; Aesc.; Apis; *Ars.; Arum;* Bell.; Bor.; Bry.; Caps.; *Canth.;* Carb. ac.; Carbo v.; Colch.; Ferr. p.; *Iris;* Merc. c.; *Sang.;* Sul.; *Tarax.;* Vespa.

Canker-sores—Agave; *Ant. c.; Arg. n.;* Ars.; *Bor.;* Caps.; Carbo v.; Echin.; Hydr.; Kali bich.; *Kali chlor.;* Lach.; Lyc.; *Merc. c.;* Merc.; Mur. ac.; Nat. hypochlor.; *Nat. m.; Nit. ac.;* Phyt.; Sal. ac.; *Sul. ac.;* Sul. See Aphthous Stomatitis.

Coldness—Camph.; *Cistus;* Coccinel.; Sinap. n.; Ver. a.

Dryness—*Acon.;* Aesc.; Alum.; *Apis; Ars.; Bell.;* Bor.; *Bry.;* Cupr.; Dub.; Hyos.; Iris ten.; Kali bich.; Kali p.; Lach.; *Lyc.;* Merc. c.; Merc. per.; *Morph.;* Mur. ac.; Nat. m.; Nat. s.; *Nux m.;* Op.; Phos.; Puls.; *Radium;* Rhus t.; Sang.; Senec.; Sep.; Tereb.

Dryness, with great thirst—Acon.; *Ars.; Bry.;* Rhus t.; Sul.; Ver. a.

Dryness, yet no thirst—*Apis;* Lach.; *Lyc.; Nux m.;* Paris; *Puls.;* Sabad.

Glands, salivary cellular tissue inflamed—Anthrac.; Bry.; *Hep.;* Merc.; Mur. ac.

Inflammation (stomatitis)—in general: Acon.; Alum.; Arg. n.; Arum; *Bapt.;* Bell.; *Bor.;* Caps.; Corn. c.; *Hydr.; Kali chlor.;* Kali m.; *Merc. c.; Merc. s.;* Nat. m.; *Nit. ac.;* Nux v.; Ran. s.; Sep.; Sinap. n.; Sul.; *Sul. ac.;* Vespa.

Inflammation, aphthous (thrush)—Æth.; Ant. t.; Ars.; Bapt.; *Bor.;* Bry.; Carbo v.; Eup. arom.; Hydr.; *Hydrast. m.; Kali chlor.;* Kali m.; *Merc. c.; Merc. s.; Mur. ac.;* Nat. m.; Nit. ac.; Rhus gl.; Sars.; *Semperv. t.; Sul. ac.; Sul.*

Inflammation, follicular, vesicular—Anac.; Ananth.; Canth.; *Caps.;* Kali chlor.; *Hydrast. m.;* Mag. c.; Nat. m.; *Mur. ac.; Rhus t.;* Sul.

Inflammation, gangrenous (noma, cancrum oris)—*Ars.;* Bapt.; Hydr.; *Kali chlor.;* Kali p.; *Kreos.; Lach.; Merc. c.;* Merc. s.; *Mur. ac.;* Sec.; Sul. ac.

Inflammation, mercurial—Bapt.; Carbo v.; Hep.; Hydr.; Mur. ac.; *Nit. ac.*

Inflammation, ulcerative—Agave; Alnus; *Arg. n.;* *Ars.;* Arum; Bapt.; Bor.; Chlor.; *Cinnab.;* Coryd.; *Hep.;* *Hydrast. m.;* Kali bich.; *Kali chlor.;* Kali cy.; Mag. c.; Menthol; *Merc. c.;* *Merc. s.;* *Mur. ac.;* *Nit. ac.;* Nit. mur. ac.; Phos.; *Rhus gl.;* Sul. ac.; Sulphurous ac.; **Tarax.**

Itching—Arundo; Bor.; Kali bich.

Mucous membrane glossy, as if varnished—*Apis;* Nit. ac.; Tereb.

Mucous membrane inflamed from burns—Apis; Canth.

Mucous membrane pallid—Ferr. m.; Morph.

Mucous membrane red, dusky—*Bapt.;* Lach.; Morph.; *Phyt.*

Mucous membrane red, tumid, with gray-based ulcers—Kali chlor. See Stomatitis.

Pain—Apis; *Arum;* Bell.; Bor.; Hep.; *Merc.;* *Nit. ac.;* Upas. See Stomatitis.

Pain from plate of teeth, worse on touch, eating—Alumen; Bor.

PALATE—Aphthæ: Agave.

Blisters—Nat. s.

Coating, creamy—Nat. p.

Constriction, scratching—Acon.

Dryness—Carbo an.

Edema—Apis.

Elongated—Strych. See Uvula.

Itching, tickling—*Arundo;* Gels.; Wyeth

Necrosis, caries—*Aur.;* Merc. cy.

Red, swollen—Acon.; *Apis;* Aur.; Bell.; Fluor. ac.; *Kali iod.;* Merc. c.

Ulceration, rawness—Ant. c.; *Arum; Cinnab.;* Hep.; Merc. c.; Merc. per.; *Nit. ac.;* Sul. ac.; Tarax. See Throat.

Wrinkled; pain on chewing, nursing—Bor.

PTYALISM—Saliva, increased: *Acet. ac.;* Allium s.; Anac.; Ant. c.; *Arum;* Bapt.; Bism.; Bry.; Cham.; Chionanth.; Cinch.; Colch.; Cupr. m.; Daphne; Dig.; Dulc.; *Epiph.; Euphorb.;* Granat.; Hep.; *Iod.; Ipec.; Iris; Jabor.;* Kali chlor.; *Kali iod.;* Kali perm.; Lac c.; Lact. ac.; *Lob. infl.; Merc. c.;* Merc. cy.; Merc. d.; Merc. i. r.; *Merc. s.;* Mez.; Muscar.; Nat. m.; *Nit. ac.;* Nit. mur. ac.; Phos.; *Piloc.;* Pod.; Ptel.; *Puls.;* Rhus t.; Sang.; Sars.; Sep.; Sul.; *Syph.;* Tab.; Trifol.

After eating—Allium s.

During pregnancy—Acet. ac.; *Granat.; Iod.; Jabor.;* Lact. ac.; *Merc.;* Muscar.; Nit. ac.; Piloc.; Sep. See Pregnancy (Female Sexual System).

During sleep—*Cham.;* Coccinel.; Lact. ac.; *Merc.;* Rheum; *Syph.*

From mercurialization—*Hep.;* Iod.; *Iris;* Kali chlor.; Nit. ac.

Saliva acrid, hot—Ars.; *Arum;* Bor.; Daphne; *Kali chlor.;* Kreos.; **Merc.;** *Nit. ac.;* Taxus.

Bitter—*Ars.;* Atham.; Bry.; Kali s.; *Puls.;* Sul.

Bloody—Antipyr.; *Ars.;* Mag. c.; *Merc.;* *Nit. ac.;* Nux v.

FETID, offensive—Ars.; *Iod.;* Kreos.; Mancin.; Merc. d.; **Merc. s.;** *Nit. ac.;* Psor.; Rheum.

Frothy, cotton-like—Alet.; Aqua mar.; *Berb. v.;* Bry.; Canth.; Lyssin; *Nux m.;* Nux v.; Phos. ac.; Sul.

Metallic—Bism.; Cham.; Cocc.; *Cupr. m.; Merc.; Nit. ac.;* Zinc.
Milky—Plumb. oxy.
Mucus—Bell.; Colch.; *Dulc.; Nit. ac.;* Phos. ac.; *Phos.;* Puls.
Ropy, tenacious, slimy, soapy—Am. m.; Ant. c.; Arg. n.; Dulc.; *Epiph.; Hydrast. m.;* Hydr.; Iod.; Iris; *Kali bich.;* Kali chlor.; Lyssin; *Merc. s.; Merc. v.;* Myr.; Nat. m.; Piloc.; *Puls.;* Tarax.
Salty—Ant. c.; *Euphorb.;* Lact. ac.; *Merc. c.; Nat. m.;* Phos.; Sep.; Ver. a.
Sour—*Iris; Nit. ac.;* Nux v.; Paris; Pod.
Sweetish—Cupr. m.; Merc.; Plumb. ac.; *Puls.;* Stann.
Watery—Asar.; Bism.; Iod.; Jabor.; Lob. infl.; *Nat. m.;* Phos.; Trifol.
ULCERATIONS—Soreness of mouth: Alum.; *Arg. n.; Ars.; Arum; Bor.;* Caps.; *Hep.; Hydrast. mur.;* Hydr.; Kali chlor.; *Merc. c.; Merc. s.; Mur. ac.; Nit. ac.;* Nux m.; Phyt.; *Ran. s.; Rhus gl.;* Semperv. t.; Sinap. n.; Sul. ac.; Tarax. See Stomatitis (Ulcerative).
Ulcerations, syphilitic mucous patches—*Cinnab.:* Kali bich.; *Merc. c.;* Merc. nit.; Merc. pr. rub.; Merc. s.; *Nit. ac.;* Still.; *Thuya.* See Male Sexual System.
Varicose veins—Ambra; Thuya.

TONGUE

COATING—COLOR—Blackish—*Ars.;* Bapt.; Camph.; Lach.; Lyc.; Merc. c.; *Merc. cy.;* Merc. d.; Merc. v.; *Op.;* Phos.; Rhus t.; Vipera.

Bluish, livid, pale—Ars.; Cupr. s.; *Dig.;* Gymnocl.; Merc. cy.; *Morph.;* Op.; Mur. ac.; Sec.; Ver. a.; Vipera.

Brownish—Am. c.; Ant. t.; *Ars.;* Bapt.; *Bry.;* Cupr. ars.; Echin.; Hyos.; Med.; *Merc. cy.;* Morph.; Mur. ac.; Nat. s.; Phos.; Sec.; Vipera.

Brown center—*Bapt.;* Phos.; Plumb. m.

Brownish, dry—*Ail.;* Ant. t.; *Ars.;* Bapt.; *Bry.;* Kali p.; *Lach.; Rhus t.;* Spong.; Tart. ac.; Vipera.

Clean—*Ars.; Asar.; Cina;* Cinch.; Coryd.; Dig.; *Ipec.;* Mag. p.; Nit. ac.; *Pyr.; Rhus t.;* Sep.

Clean anteriorly, coated posteriorly—Nux v.

Clean at menstrual nisus, foul after flow ceases—Sep.

Dark streak in center, typhoid tongue—Arn.; Bapt.; Mur. ac.

Flabby, moist, with imprints of teeth—Ars.; Chel.; *Hydr.;* Kali bich.; Merc. c.; *Merc. d.; Merc. s.;* Nat. p.; Pod.; Pyr.; *Rhus t.;* Sanic.; Stram.; Yucca.

Frothy, with bubbles on side—Nat. m.

Furred—Ant. t.; Ars.; *Bapt.;* Canth.; *Card. m.;* Chin. ars.; Coca; Ferr. picr.; Gels.; Guaiac.; Lyc.; Myr.; *Nux v.;* Puls.; Rumex. See White.

Grayish-white base—Kali m.

Greenish—Nat. s.; Plumb. ac.

Mapped—Ant. c.; *Ars.; Kali bich.;* Lach.; Merc. v.; *Nat. m.;* Nit. ac.; Ox. ac.; Phyt.; Ran. s.; Rhus t.; *Tarax.;* Tereb.

Mapped, with red, insular patches—Nat. m.

Red—*Acon.; Apis; Ars.; Bell.;* Bor. ac.; *Canth.;* Crot.; Diph.; Gels.; Hyos.; *Kali bich.;* Lach.; Merc. c.; Mez.; Nux v.; *Pyr.; Rhus t.;* Tereb.

Red, dry, especially center—Ant. t.; Rhus t.

Red edges—Amyg. pers.; Ant. t.; Ars.; Bapt.; *Bell.;* Canth.; Card. m.; *Chel.;* Echin.; Kali bich.; Lac c.; Lach.; Merc. c.; Merc. i. fl.; *Merc.;* Nit. ac.; Pod.; *Rhus t.;* Rhus v.; Sul.; Tarax.

Red edges, white center—Bell.; Rhus t.

Red in center, or streaks—Ant. t.; *Ars.;* Caust.; Crot.; *Ver. v.*

Red, papillæ pale, effaced—Allium s.

Red, papillæ prominent—Ant. t.; *Arg. n.;* Ars.; *Bell.;* Kali bich.; Lyc.; Mez.; Nux m.; *Ptel.; Tereb.*

Red, raw—Ars.; *Arum;* Canth.; Tarax.

Red, shining, glossy, as if varnished—Apis; *Canth.;* Crot.; Jal.; *Kali bich.; Nit. ac.;* Phos.; *Pyr.;* Rhus t.; *Tereb.*

Red spots, sensitive—Ran. s.; *Tarax;* Tereb.

Red tip—Amyg. pers.; *Arg. n.; Ars.;* Cycl.; Merc. i. fl.; Phyt.; *Rhus t.;* Rhus v.; Sul.

Red, wet, central furrow—Nit. ac.

Strawberry—*Bell.;* Fragar.; Sapon.

Unilateral—*Daphne;* Lob. infl.; Rhus t.

White-furred, slimy, pasty—Acon.; Æsc.; *Ant. c.; Ant. t.;* Arg. n.; Arn.; *Bapt.;* Bell.; *Bism.; Bry.;* Calc. c.; Carbo v.; Card. m.; *Chel.;* Cinch.; *Cycl.;* Ferr. ; Glon.; Hedeoma; *Hydr.;* Ipec.; Kali c.; Kali chlor.; Kali m.; Lac c.; Lob. infl.; Lyc.; Merc. c.; *Merc.;* Mez.; Nat. m.; Nux v.; Ox. ac.; Paris; Petrol.; Phos.; *Puls.; Sep.;* Sul.; Tarax.; Ver. v.

Yellow, dirty, thick coating—*Æsc.; Bapt.;* Bry.; Carbo v.; Cham.; *Chel.;* Chionanth.; *Cinch.;* Ferr.; *Hydr.;* Indol; *Kali bich.;* Kali s.; Lept.; Lyc.; *Merc. d.; Merc. i. fl.; Merc.;* Myr.; Nat. p.; *Nat. s.;* Nux v.; *Ostrya;* Pod.; *Puls.;* Sang.; Sul.; *Yucca.*

Yellow patch in center—*Bapt.;* Phyt.

CONDITIONS—**Anæsthesia**—Carbon. s.

Atrophy—Mur. ac.

Biting—Absinth.; Hydr.; Hyos.; *Ign.;* Illic.; Phos. ac.; Sec.

Burning, smarting scalded feeling—*Acon.;* Apis; *Ars.;* Arum; Bapt.; Bell.; Berb. v.; Canth.; Caps.; Carbo an.; Caust.; Col.; *Iris;* Lyc.; Merc. c.; Mez.; *Mur. ac.;* Nat. m.; Phos. ac.; Pod.; *Ran. s.; Sang.;* Sanic.; Sinap.; Sul.

Burning tip—*Ars.;* Bar. c.; Calc. c.; Caps.; *Iris;* Lathyrus; Physost.; *Sang.;* Tereb.

Coldness—Acet. ac.; *Camph.;* Carbo v.; *Cistus; Helod.;* Hydroc. ac.; Sec.; *Ver. a.*

Dryness—*Acon.;* Ail.; Ant. t.; Apis; *Ars.;* Bapt.; *Bell.; Bry.;* Calc. c.; Colch.; Hyos.; Kali bich.; Kali c.; Lach.; Leonur.; Merc. c.; *Merc.; Morph.; Mur. ac.;* Nat. m.; *Nux m.; Paris;* Phos. ac.; Phos.; Puls.; Pyr.; *Rhus t.; Sul.;* Tereb.; *Ver. v.;* Vipera.

ERUPTIONS, growths—**Cancer:** Alumen; Apis; *Ars.; Aur.;* Aur. m. n.; Crot.; Galium; Hoang nan; Kali chlor.; *Kali cy.; Mur. ac.;* Semperv. t.; *Thuya;* Vib. pr.

Cracks, excoriations—Ananth.; *Ars.; Arum;* Arundo; Bapt.; Bell.; Bor. ac.; Bor., Bry.; Cham.; *Kali bich.;* Lach.; Leonur.; Nat. m.; *Nit. ac.;* Phyt.; Plumb. ac.; Pyr.; Ran. s.; *Rhus t.;* Rhus v.; Semperv. t. See Ulcerations.

Epithelioma—Ars.; Carb. ac.; Chrom. ac.; *Hydr.; Kali cy.;* Mur. ac.; *Thuya.*

Furrows lengthwise, in upper part—Merc.

Growths, nodules—Ars. hydr.; *Aur.;* Aur. m. n.; Castor.; *Gall. ap.;* Mur. ac.; Nit. ac.; *Thuya.*

Psoriasis—*Cast. eq.;* Kali bich.; *Mur. ac.*

Ranula—Ambra; *Calc. c.;* Ferr. p.; Fluor. ac.; Merc. s.; Nit. ac.; *Thuya.*

Ring worm—Nat. m.; Sanic. See Red edges.

Ulcerations—Apis; *Arg. n.;* Ars.; Ars. hydr.; Bapt.; Fluor. ac.; Kali bich.; Lyc.; *Merc.;* Mur. ac.; *Nit. ac.; Nit. mur. ac.;* Sang. n.; Semperv. t.; Syph.; Thuya.

Ulcerations, syphilitic—Aur.; *Cinnab.;* Fluor. ac.; *Kali bich.;* Lach.; Merc.; Mez.; *Nit. ac.*

Veins, varicose—Ambra; *Ham.;* Thuya.

Vesicles, blisters—Am. c.; Apis; Berb. v.; Bor.; *Canth.;* Carbo an.; Lacert.; *Lyc.;* Merc. per.; Mur. ac.; *Nat. p.; Nat. m.;* Nit. ac.; Phyt.; *Rhus t.;* Sul. ac.; *Sul.;* Thuya.

Warts—Aur. mur.; Mang. ac.

Hard, induration of—Alumen; Aur. m.; *Calc. fl.;* Mur. ac.; Semperv. t.; *Sil.*

Heaviness—Caust.; Colch.; Gels.; Guaco; Merc. per.; Mur. ac.; Nux v.

Inflammation (glossitis)—*Acon.; Apis;* Ars.; Bell.; Canth.; Crot.; *Lach.; Merc. c.;* Merc.; *Mur. ac.; Ox. ac.;* Phyt.; Ran. s.; *Sul. ac.; Vipera.* See Swelling.

Numbness, tingling—*Acon.;* Con.; Echin.; *Gels.;* Ign.; Lathyrus; Merc. per.; *Nat. m.;* Nux m.; Nux v.; Plat.; Radium; Rheum; Sec.

Pain—Acon.; *Ars.;* Arum; Bell.; Kali ars.; Kali iod.; Merc. v.; *Nit. ac.; Phyt.;* Ruta; Semperv. t.; *Thuya.* See Soreness.

Paralysis—Acon. cam.; Acon.; Anac.; Arn.; Ars.; Bar. c.; *Bell.; Bothrops;* Can. ind.; *Caust.;* Cocc.; *Con.;* Cupr.; *Cur.; Dulc.; Gels.;* Guaco; Hyos.; Lach.; Lob. purp.; *Mur. ac.;* Nux m.; Oleand.; Op.; *Plumb. m.;* Sec.; Stram.; Zinc. s. See Nervous System.

Protrusion, difficult—Anac.; *Apis;* Ars.; Calc. c.; *Caust.;* Crot.; Dulc.; *Guaco; Gels.; Hyos.; Lach.;* Merc.; Mur. ac.; *Myg.;* Nat. m.; Pyr.; Plumb. m.; Stram.; Sulphon; Tereb.

Protrusion, snake-like—Absinth.; Crot.; *Cupr.; Lach.;* Lyc.; *Merc.;* Sanic.; *Vipera.*

Rawness, roughness—Apis; *Ars.; Arum;* Canth.; Dulc.; *Nit. ac.;* Phyt.; *Ran. s.;* Tarax.

Sensation, as if hair on tongue—Allium s.; Kali bich.; Nat. m.; *Sil.*

Sensation, as if swollen, enlarged—Absinth.; Æth.; *Anac.;* Crot.; Nux v.; Ptel.; Puls.

Soreness—*Apis; Arum;* Cistus; Kali c.; Merc. c.; Mur. ac.; *Nit. ac.;* Ox. ac.; Phelland.; Physost.; *Ran. s.; Rhus t.;* Semperv. t.; Sep.; Sil.; *Tereb.;* Thuya.

Spasm—Acon.; Bell.; Ruta; Sec. See Trembling.

Stiffness—Con.; *Dulc.;* Hyos.; Lac c.; Merc. i. r.; Nicol.; Sec.; Stram.

Swelling—*Acon.; Apis;* Ars.; Arum; Aster.; Bapt.; *Bell.;* Bism.; Cajup.; *Canth.; Crot.;* Diph.; Fragar.; Kali tell.; Lach.; Mag. p.; *Merc. c.; Mez.; Mur. ac.;* Œnanthe; Ox. ac.; Pelias; Ruta; Thuya; *Vespa; Vipera.*

Trembling—*Absinth.; Agar.; Agraricin;* Apis; Ars.; Bell.; Camph.; Caust.; Cham.; *Gels.; Lach.; Merc.;* Plumb.; Stram.

TASTE

LOST—*Amyg. per.; Ant. c.;* Bry.; Cycl.; Formal.; Gymnema; **Justicia;** Lyc.; Mag. c.; *Mag. m.; Nat. m.;* Pod.; *Puls.;* Sang.; Sil.; Sul.

PERVERTED—ALTERED—in general: Æsc.; *Alum.;* Ant. t.; *Arg. n.;* Arn.; Ars.; Calc. c.; Camph.; Carbo v.; Chel.; *Cinch.;* Cycl.; Fagop.; *Gymnema; Hydr.;* Kali c.; Lyc.; Mag. c.; Mag. m.; Merc. c.; *Merc. s.; Nat. m.;* Nit. ac.; *Nux v.;* Paris; Pod.; *Puls.;* Rheum; *Sep.; Sul.;* Zinc. mur.

After eating—Ars.; Carbo v.; *Nat. m.;* Nit. ac.; Zinc.

After sleep—Rheum.

Acid, astringent, sour—Aloe; Am. c.; *Calc. c.;* Carbo v.; Cham.; Cinch.; Euphorbia; Hep.; *Hydr.;* Ign.; Iris; Kali c.; Lob. infl.; *Lyc.; Mag. c.;* Nat. p.; Nit. ac.; *Nux v.;* Phos. ac.; Phos.; *Puls.;* Sep.; *Sul.*

Bitter, bilious—*Acon.;* Aloe; Ars.; *Atham.;* Bapt.; *Bry.;* Camph.; *Card. m.; Cham.; Chel.; Cinch.; Col.;* Cupr.; Dig.; *Hydr.;* Ipec.; Kali c.; *Lyc.;* Merc. c.; *Myr.;* Nat. m.; Nat. s.; *Nux v.;* Paris; *Pod.;* Ptel.; *Puls.;* Rhus t.; Sabad.; *Sep.;* Stann.; *Sul.;* Tarax.

Bitter from tobacco—*Asar.;* Euphras.; Puls.

Bloody-like—*Alum.;* Chel.; Kali c.; Mancin.; *Nit. ac.;* Sil.; Sul.; Trifol. Zinc.

Coppery, metallic—*Æsc.;* Arg. n.; Ars.; Bism.; Cocc.; *Cupr. ars.; Cupr m.;* Lact. ac.; *Lob. infl.; Merc. c.;* Nit. mur. **ac.;** Nux v.; *Rhus t.;* Sul.

Delicate, changeable—Coff.; *Puls.*

Disgusting, putrid, foul, slimy—*Arn.;* Aur. mur.; Bor.; Calc. c.; *Carbo v.;* Chel.; Ferr. m.; Graph.; Hep.; Indol; Led.; Lemna m.; Lyc.; Merc. c.; *Merc.;* Nat. m.; Nat. s.; Nux v.; Petrol.; Phos.; Pod.; *Puls.; Pyr.;* Sep.; Yucca.

Flat, insipid, straw-like, pappy—*Ant. c.;* Ant. t.; *Ars.;* Bapt.; Bor.; *Cinch.; Cycl.;* Euphor. amyg.; *Ferr. m.;* Glycerin; Ign.; Kali s.; Nux m.; *Puls.*

Greasy, fatty, pasty—Arn.; Carbo v.; Caust.; Euonym.; Ol. an.; Phos.; *Puls.;* Trill. cer.

Peppery—Hydr.

Perverted in morning—Fagop.; Graph.; Hydr.; *Nux v.;* Puls.

Salty—Ant. c.; Ars.; *Bell.;* Cadm. s.; *Carbo v.;* Cinch.; *Cycl.;* Merc. c.; *Merc.; Puls.; Sep.;* Sul.; Zinc. m.

Sweet—Agar.; *Apoc. andr.;* Bism.; Chel.; Cupr. m.; Dig.; Glycerin; *Merc.; Nit. ac.;* Phelland.; *Plumb.;* Puls.; *Pyr.; Sabad.;* Selen.; Stann.

GUMS

BLEEDING easily—*Agave; Alum.;* Ambra; Ant. c.; *Arg. n.; Arn.; Ars.;* Bapt.; Benz. ac.; Bor.; Calc. c.; *Carbo v.;* Cistus; Crotal.; Echin.; Hep.; *Iod.; Kreos.;* Lach.; Merc. c.; *Merc.; Nit. c.; Phos.;* Plant.; Sep.; Sil.; Staph.; Sul. ac.; Sul.; Zinc.

Bleeding protractedly, after tooth extraction—Ars.; Bov.; *Ham.; Kreos.;* Phos.; Trill.

Blue line along margin—Plumb.

Burning—Antypr. See Pain.

Cold feeling—Coccinel.

Desire to press teeth together—Phyt.; Pod.

Epulis—Calc. c.; Plumb.; *Thuya.*

Inflammation (gumboil)—*Acon.; Bell.;* Bor.; *Calc. fl.;* Calc. s.; Cham.; *Hekla;* Hep.; Kreos.; Merc. c.; *Merc.;* Phos.; Rhus t.; *Sil.* See Pain, Swelling.

Painful after tooth extraction—Arn.; Sep.

Painful, sore, sensitive—Alum.; Am. c.; Arg. n.; *Bapt.;* Bell.; Bor.; Calc. c.; *Carbo v.;* Caust.; *Cham.;* Dolichos; *Hep.; Kreos.; Merc.; Nit. ac.;* Plant.; Rhus t.; *Sil.;* Sul.; Thuya.

Red seam (strophulus)—*Ant. c.;* Apis; *Cham.;* Kali p.; *Puls.;* Rhus t.

Scorbutic (soft, spongy, receding)—*Agave;* Alum.; Ant. c.; Arn.; *Ars.;* Bapt.; *Carbo v.;* Cistus; Echin.; Hep.; *Iod.;* Kali c.; Kali chlor.; Kali p.; *Kreos.; Merc.; Mur. ac.;* Nat. m.; *Nit. ac.; Phos.; Staph.;* Sul.; Thuya.

Swelling—*Apis;* Bell.; Bism.; Calc. c.; Caust.; *Cham.;* Cistus; Graph.; Kreos.; Lach.; Mag. m.; Merc. c.; Merc. d.; *Merc. i. r.; Merc. v.;* Mur. ac.; Nit. ac.; *Phos.;* Plumb.; Rhod.; Sep.; Sil.; Staph.; Sul.; Tereb.

Ulceration (pyorrhœa alveolaris)—Aur.; *Bapt.;* Carbo v.; *Caust.; Cistus;* Emetine; Kali c.; Kreos.; *Merc. c.; Merc.; Nit. ac.;* Phos.; *Plant.; Sep.; Sil.; Staph.;* Sul. ac.; Thuya.

TEETH

ALVEOLAR abscess—Hep.; Merc.; Sil.

Black, dark, crumbling—Ant. c.; *Kreos.*; Merc.; Phos. hydr.; *Staph.*; Syph.; Thuya.

Caries, decay, premature—Calc. c.; Calc. fl.; *Calc. p.*; Cocc.; Fluor. ac.; Hekla; *Kreos.*; Merc.; *Mez.*; Phos.; *Plant.*; Sil.; *Staph.*; Tub.

Caries at crown—Merc.; *Staph.*

Caries at root—*Merc.*; Mez.; Sil.; Syph.; *Thuya.*

Cupped, dwarfed, serrated—Staph.; *Syph.*

DENTITION—(teething difficult, delayed): Acon.; *Bell.*; *Bor.*; *Calc. c.*; *Calc. p.*; Caust.; *Cham.*; Cheiranth.; *Coff.*; *Cupr.*; Gels.; *Hekla*; *Kali br.*; *Kreos.*; Mag. p.; Merc.; Nux v.; Passifl.; Phyt.; *Pod.*; Puls.; *Sil.*; Solan. n.; Staph.; Sul.; *Tereb.*; Zinc. br.; Zinc. m.

With cerebral, nervous symptoms—Acon.; Agar.; *Bell.*; *Cham.*; Cim.; Cyprip.; Dolichos; *Helleb.*; Kali br.; *Pod.*; Solan. n.; Tereb.; *Zinc.*

With compression of gums—Cic.; Phyt.; Pod.

With constipation, general irritation, cachexia—*Kreos.*; Nux v.; Op.

With convulsions—*Bell.*; Calc. c.; *Cham.*; Cic.; Cupr.; Glon.; Kali br.; *Mag. p.*; Solan. n.; Stann.; *Zinc. br.*

With cough—Acon.; Bell.; Ferr. p.; Kreos.

With deafness, otorrhœa, stuffiness of nose—Cheiranth.

With diarrhœa—Æth.; *Calc. c.*; *Calc. p.*; *Cham.*; Ferr. p.; Ipec.; Kreos.; Mag. c.; Merc.; Oleand.; Phos.; *Pod.*; Puls.; Rheum; *Sil.*

With effusion threatened, in brain—*Apis*; Helleb.; Tub.; *Zinc. m.*

With eye symptoms—Bell.; Calc. c.; Puls.

With insomnia—Bell.; Cham.; *Coff.*; *Cyprip.*; Kreos.; Passifl.; Scutel.; Tereb.

With intertrigo—Caust.; Lyc.

With milk indigestion—Æth.; Calc. c.; *Mag. m.*

With salivation—Bor.

With sour smell of body, pale face, irritability—Kreos.

With weakness, pallor, fretfulness, must be carried rapidly—Ars.

With worms—*Cina*; Merc.; Stann.

FEEL cold—*Coccinel.*; Gamb.; Phos. ac.; Rheum.

Feel loose—Alum.; Am. c.; Arn.; Bism.; Calc. fl.; Carbo v.; Hyos.; Lyc.; *Merc. c.*; *Merc.*; *Nit. ac.*; *Plant.*; Rhus t.; Sil.; *Zinc.*

Feel numb—Plat.

Feel sensitive to cold, chewing, touch—*Acon.*; Ars.; Bell.; Carbo v.; Cham.; *Coff.*; *Fluor. ac.*; Gymnocl.; Merc.; Parth.; Plant.; *Staph.*   See Pain.

Feel too long—Bry.; Carbo v.; Caust.; *Cham.*; Clem.; Lyc.; Mag. c.; *Merc.*; *Mez.*; Parth.; Plant.; Ratanh.; Rhus t.

Feel warm—Fluor. ac.

FISTULA DENTALIS—Calc. fl.; Caust.; *Fluor. ac.*; Nat. m.; *Sil.*; Staph.; Sul.

GRINDING—Apis; *Bell.*; Can. ind.; *Cic.*; Cina; Helleb.; Myg.; *Phys.*; Plant.; *Pod.*; *Santon.*; Spig.; Zinc.

ODONTALGIA—Toothache—Remedies in general: *Acon.;* Agar.; Ant. c.; Antipyr.; Apis; *Ars.;* Atrop.; *Bell.; Bry.;* Calc. c.; Carb. ac.; Carbo v.; *Cham; Clem.;* Coccinel.; *Coff.;* Col.; Ferr. m.; Gels.; Glon.; Hekla; Ign.; Kali c.; *Kreos.;* Lach.; *Mag. c.; Mag. p.; Merc.* ; Nux v.; Ox. ac.; Phos.; Phyt.; *Plant.; Puls.;* Sep.; Spig.; *Staph.;* Tab.; Ther.; Thuja.

CAUSE—Coffee: Cham.; Ign.

Cold bathing—Ant. c.

Decayed teeth—Cham.; *Kreos.; Merc.;* Mez.; Staph.

Dental pulp, inflamed—Bell.

Drafts, or cold exposure—*Acon.;* Bell.; Bry.; *Calc. c.;* Cham.; Merc.; *Puls.; Rhod.;* Sil.

Extraction of teeth—Arn.; Staph.

Menses, during—Bar. c.; Cham.; Sep.; *Staph.*

Nursing baby—Cinch.

Pregnancy—Alum.; *Calc. c.;* Cham.; *Mag. c.;* Nux m.; Puls.; Ratanh.; *Sep.;* Tab. See Female Sexual System.

Tea—Thuja.

Tobacco-smoking—*Clem.;* Ign.; Plant.; *Spig.*

Washing clothes—Phos.

LOCATION—Decayed teeth: Ant. c.; *Cham.; Kreos.;* Mag. c.; *Merc.; Mez.;* Nux v.; Staph.; Thuya.

Eye-teeth—Ther.

Lower—Antipyr.; Caust.; Merc.; Staph.; Verbasc.

Molars—Antipyr.; Bry.; Caust.

Roots of teeth—Meph.; *Merc.;* Staph.

Sound teeth—Arg. n.; Caust.; Cham.; Plant.; Spig.; Staph.

Upper teeth—Bell.; Fluor. ac.

TYPE—Neuralgic, congestive: *Acon.;* Aran.; Ars.; *Bell.;* Ced.; *Cham.; Coff.;* Dolichos; Ferr. picr.; *Ign.;* Mag. c.; Mag. p.; Merc. v.; Plant.; *Spig.* See Odontalgia.

Rheumatic—Acon.; *Bry.;* Cham.; Chin. s.; Colch.; Guaiac.; Merc.; *Puls.; Rhod.*

TYPE OF PAIN—Aching: Cham.; Kreos.; Merc.; Mez.; Staph.

Burning—*Ars.;* Bell.; Sil.

Drawing, jerking, tearing—*Bell.;* Cham.; Chimap.; Coff.; Cycl.; Kreos.; Meph.; *Merc.; Nux v.; Prun. sp.;* Puls.; Rhod.; Sep.; Sil.; *Spig.;* Sul.

Gnawing boring—Calc. c.; Carbo v.; Mez.; Nux v.; Plant.; Puls.; Sil.; Staph.

Periodical—Ars.; Chin. s.; Coff.

Shock-like—Am. c.; Aran.; Nux v.

Shooting—Calc. c.; *Cham.;* Kali c.; Mag. c.; *Nux v.;* Phos.; Sep.; Sil.

Stitching—*Bry.;* Cham.; Nit. ac.; Puls.

Throbbing—Acon.; *Bell.;* Coccinel.; Glon.; Kali c.; Mag. c.; *Merc.; Sil.;* See Odontalgia.

CONCOMITANTS—Distraction of the mind: Acon.; Cham.

Heat, thirst, fainting—Cham.

Neuralgia of lids, reflex—Plant.

Rush of blood to head, loose feeling of teeth—Hyos.

Soreness of teeth—Bell.; Merc.; Plant.; Zinc. m.

Swelling about jaws, cheeks—Bell.; Bor.; Cham.; *Hekla*; Hep.; Lyc.; *Merc.*; *Sil.* See Gumboil.

MODALITIES—AGGRAVATION—After midnight: Ars.

At night—Ant. c.; Aran.; *Bell.*; Caust.; *Cham.*; *Clem.*; *Mag. c.*; Mag. p.; *Merc.*; Mez.; *Puls.*; Sep.; Sil.; Sul.

From blowing nose—Culex; Thuya.

From change of weather—Aran.; Merc.; *Rhod.*

From cold foods, drinks—*Calc. c.*; Lach.; Mag. p.; *Merc.*; *Nux v.;* Staph.; Sul.

From cold in general—*Ant. c.; Calc. c.;* Hyos.; Lyc.; Mag. c.; Merc.; *Nux v.;* Plant.; *Sil.;* Spig.; Sul.

From contact, touch—Bell.; Calc. fl.; Caust.; Cinch.; Kali c.; Mag. m.; Mez.; Plant.; *Staph.*

From eating—Ant. c.; Bell.; Bry.; *Calc. c.;* Cham.; Chimap.; *Kali c.;* Mag. p.; Mez.; Nux v.; *Puls.;* Sil.; *Spig.;* Staph.; Zinc.

From exertion of mind or body—Chimap.; Nux v.

From lying down, rest, quiet—*Aran.;* Mag. c.; Nat. s.; *Ratanh.;* Sep.

From shrill sounds—Ther.

From smoking tobacco—Clem.; Ign.; *Spig.*

From warm food—*Bism.;* Bry.; Calc. c.; *Caust.; Clem.; Coff.;* Merc.; *Puls.;* Sil.

In intervals between meals—Ign.

In morning—Hyos.

Warmth in general—*Cham.; Merc.;* Prun. sp.; *Puls.;* Sep.

Windy weather, thunder storms—Rhod.

AMELIORATION—Cold air: Nat. s.; Puls.

Cold drinks—*Bism.; Bry.;* Chimap.; *Coff.;* Ferr. m.; Ferr. p.; Nat. s.; *Puls.*

Eating—Ign.; Plant.; *Spig.*

Hot liquids—*Mag. p.*

Lying down—Spig.

Mouth open, sucking in air—Mez.

Pressure external—Bry.; Cinch.

Pressure of teeth—Cinch.; *Ol. an.;* Staph.

Rubbing cheek—Merc.

Sweat in general—Cham.; *Chenop. gl.*

Walking about—Mag. c.: Ratanh.

Warmth—*Ars.;* Cinch.; Lyc.; *Mag. p.;* Merc.; Nux v.

Wet finger—Cham.

RIGG'S DISEASE—Calc. ren.; Merc.; Sil. mar.

SORDES and deposits—*Ail.;* Alum.; Ars.; *Bapt.; Echin.;* Hyos.; Iod.; Kali p.; Merc. c.; *Mur. ac.;* Phos. ac.; Plant.; *Rhus t.*

THROAT

ADENOID VEGETATIONS—*Agraph.;* Bar. c.; Calc. c.; *Calc. fl.; Calc. iod.; Calc. p.;* Chrom. ac.; Iod.; Kali s.; Lob. syph.; Mez.; Psor.; *Sang. n.;* Sul.; Thuya.

DIPHTHERIA—Remedies in general: Ail.; *Apis;* Ars.; Ars. iod.; Arum; *Bapt.; Bell.; Brom.;* Calc. chlor.; *Canth.;* Carb. ac.; *Crot.; Diph.;* Echin.; Guaiac.; *Kali bich.;* Kali chlor.; *Kali m.; Kali per.;* Lac c.; *Lach.;* Lachnanth.; Led.; Lob. infl.; *Lyc.:* Merc. c.; *Merc. cy.;* Merc. i. fl.; Mer. i. r.; *Mur. ac.;* Naja; *Nit. ac.; Phyt.;* Rhus t.; Sang.; Sul.; Tar. c.; Vinca.; Zinc. m.

TYPE—Ataxic: Ars.; Bell.; Lach.; Mosch.; Phos.

    Laryngeal—Apis; *Brom.;* Canth.; Chlorum; Diph.; *Hep.;* Iod.; *Kali bich.;* Lac c.; *Merc. cy.;* Petrol.; Phos.; Samb.; Spong.

    Malignant—*Ail.;* Apis; Ars.; *Carb. ac.;* Chin. ars.; Crot.; Diph.; *Echin.;* Kali p.; Lac c.; *Lach.; Merc. cy.;* Mur. ac.; Pyr.

    Nasal—*Am. c.;* Am. caust.; *Kali bich.;* Lyc.; Merc. cy.; *Nit. ac.*

CONDITIONS—Extension downwards: Iod.; *Kali bich.;* Lac c.; Merc. cy.

    Extension left to right—Lac c.; *Lach.;* Sabad.

    Extension right to left—Lyc.

    Extension upward—Brom.

    With croup—Acet. ac.; *Brom.;* Hep.; *Iod.; Kali bich.;* Kali m.; Lach.; Merc. cy.; Phos.; Samb.; Spong.

    With drooling—Lac c.; Merc. cy.

    With objective symptoms only: painless type; deficient reaction; sopor, stupor, epistaxis—Diph.

    With post-diphtheritic paralysis—*Arg. n.; Caust.;* Cocc.; Con.; Curare; Diph.; *Gels.;* Kali p.; Lach.; Oleand.; *Phos.; Plumb.;* Rhus t.; Sec.

    With prostration from beginning—Ail.; *Apis; Ars.;* Bapt.; Canth.; *Carb. ac.;* Crot.; *Diph.;* Kali per.; *Lach.; Merc. cy.;* Mur. ac.; Phyt.

    With spasm of glottis—Mosch.; Samb.

    With urine scanty—Apis; Ars.; Canth.; Lac c.; Merc. cy.; Naja.

OESOPHAGUS—Burning, smarting: Acon.; *Am. caust.;* Asaf.; Ars.; *Canth.;* Caps.; Carb. ac.; *Crot. t.;* Gels.; *Iris; Merc. c.;* Mez.; Ox. ac.; *Phos.;* Sang.; Sinap. a.; Strych.

    Constriction—Abies n.; *Alum.;* Am. m.; *Asaf.; Bapt.; Bell.;* Cact.; *Cajup.;* Caps.; *Cic.;* Condur.; Gels.; Hyos.; Ign.; *Lyssin;* Merc. c.; Naja; *Phos.;* Plat.; Plumb.; Rhus t.; Stram.; Ver. v.

    Dryness—*Acon.;* Bell.; Cocc.; *Mez.; Naja.*

    Inflammation (esophagitis)—Acon.; Alum.; Ars.; *Bell.;* Merc. c.; Naja; *Phos.;* Sul. ac.; Ver. a.

    Pain—*Am. caust.;* Cocc.; Gels.; *Phos.*

    Spasm (esophagismus)—Aconitin; Arg. cy.; Asaf.; *Bapt.;* Bar. c.; *Bell.;* Canth.; Cic.; Hyos.; *Ign.;* Lach.; Lyssin; Merc. c.; *Naja;* Stram.; Strych.; *Ver. v.* See Pharynx.

FAUCES—Anesthesia: Kali br.

Burning heat—_Acon.;_ _Æsc.;_ Bell.; _Canth.;_ _Caps.;_ Carb. ac.; Gels.; _Phos.;_ _Phyt.;_ Sinap. n.; Still.

Dryness—Acon.; _Æsc.;_ _Bell.;_ Canth.; Caps.; Gels.; Jugl. c.; _Nux m.;_ Phos.; _Phyt.;_ _Sabad.;_ Senec.

Inflammation—Ail.; Apis; _Bell.;_ Ferr. p.; _Kali bich.;_ Menthol; Merc. i. fl.; Merc. s.

Necrosis—Merc. cy.

Redness—_Bell.;_ Carb. ac.; Ferr. p.; Gymnocl.; Menthol; _Merc. cy.;_ _Merc. i. r.;_ Mez.; Naja; Puls.

Roughness, sensitive—_Æsc.;_ Coccus; Dros.; _Nux v.;_ Phos.; _Phyt._

Tingling—_Acon.;_ Echin.; Phyt.

Ulceration—Coryd.; _Kali bich.;_ Merc. i. r.; _Nit. ac.;_ Sang. See Pharynx

PHARYNX—Abscess (retro-pharyngeal): Antipyr.; Bell.; Bry.; _Hep.;_ Lach.; _Merc.;_ Nit. ac.; Phos.; _Sil._

Abscess, predisposition to—Calc. c.; _Calc. iod.;_ Ferr. p.; _Kali iod.;_ _Sil._

Adherent crusts—Elaps; Kali bich.; Kali m.

Anesthesia—Gels.; _Kali br._

Burning, smarting, scalded feeling—Acon.; _Æsc.;_ _Am. caust.;_ Apis; _Ars.;_ Ars. iod.; _Arum;_ _Aur.;_ Bar. c.; Bell.; Camph.; _Canth.;_ _Caps.;_ Carb. ac.; _Caust.;_ Cocaine; Con.; Glycerin; Guaiac.; Hydr.; _Iris;_ Kali bich.; _Kali per.;_ Kreos.; Lyc.; _Merc. c.;_ Merc. i. fl.; Merc.; _Mez.;_ Nat. ars.; Nit. ac.; _Phos.;_ _Phyt.;_ Pop. c.; _Quill.;_ _Sang.;_ Sang. n.; Senec.; _Sul.;_ Wyeth.

Coldness—Cistus.

Constriction, spasmodic—_Acon.;_ _Æsc.;_ Agar.; Alum.; Apis; _Arg. n.;_ Ars.; Arum; Asaf.; _Bapt.;_ _Bell.;_ Bothrops; Cact.; Calc. c.; Cajup.; _Canth.;_ _Caps.;_ _Cic.;_ Cocaine; Cupr. m.; _Hyos.;_ _Ign.;_ Lach.; _Merc. c.;_ Mez.; Morph.; Nux v.; _Phyt.;_ Plumb. m.; Puls.; Ratanh.; _Sang.;_ _Sang. n.;_ Sarcol. ac.; _Stram.;_ _Strych.;_ Sumb.; Val.

DYSPHAGIA—Deglutition painful, difficult: Remedies in general: Agar.; Ail.; Alum.; Amyg. pers.; Anac.; Apis; Ars.; Atrop.; _Bapt.;_ _Bell.;_ Bothrops; Bry.; _Cajup.;_ _Canth.;_ _Caps.;_ Carb. ac.; _Cic.;_ Cocc.; Con.; Cocaine; Cur.; Dub.; Fluor. ac.; Grat.; Hep.; Hydroc. ac.; _Hyos.;_ _Ign.;_ Iod.; Kali bich.; Kali br.; Kali c.; Kali chlor.; Kali m.; Kali perm.; _Lac c.;_ _Lach.;_ Lyc.; Lyssin; _Merc. c.;_ Merc. cy.; Merc. i. fl.; Merc. i. r.; _Merc. s.;_ _Merc. v.;_ Nat. p.; _Nit. ac.;_ Phos.; _Phyt.;_ Pop. c.; Psor.; Sang.; Sang. n.; Senec.; _Stram.;_ _Strych._

Can swallow only liquids—_Bapt.;_ _Bar. c.;_ Cham.; Nat. m.; Plumb.; _Sil._

Can swallow only solids, liquids descend with difficulty—_Alumen;_ _Bell.;_ Bothrops; Bry.; Cact.; _Canth.;_ _Crot.;_ Gels.; _Hyos.;_ Ign.; Lach.; _Lyssin;_ _Merc. c.;_ Sil.

Choking when eating, drinking—Abies n.; _Anac.;_ Cajup.; _Can. s.;_ Glon.; _Kava;_ _Merc. c.;_ Mur. ac.; Niccol.; Nit. ac.; _Phyt.;_ Santon.; Sumb.

Food descends "wrong way"—_Anac.;_ Can. s.; Kali c.; _Meph.;_ Nat. m.

Food regurgitates, per nasum—_Bell.;_ Diph.; Kali perm.; _Lach.;_ Lyc.; _Merc. c.:_ Merc. v.

Liquids descend with gurgling sound—Ars.; *Cupr. ac.;* Hydroc. ac.; *Laur.;* Thuya.

Swallows food and drink hastily—Anac.; *Bell.;* Bry.; Coff.; Helleb.; *Hep.;* Oleand.; Zinc. m.

DEPOSITS—Membranous—*Acet. ac.;* Apis; Brom.; Carb. ac.; *Kali bich.;* Kali m.; Kali perm.; Lach.; Merc. cy.; Mur. ac.; *Nit. ac.;* Phyt. See Diphtheria.

Dryness—*Acon.; Æsc.;* Agar.; *Alum.; Apis; Ars.;* Asaf.; *Atrop.; Bell.; Bry.;* Canth.; *Caps.;* Caust.; Cistus; Cocaine; Cocc.; Dros.; *Dub.;* Ferr. p.; *Guaiac.;* Hep.; Hyos.; Justicia; Kali bich.; Kali c.; Kali chlor.; *Lach.;* Lemna m.; *Lyc.;* Merc. c.; Merc. per.; Merc.; Mez.; *Morph.;* Nat. m.; Nat. s.; Nit. ac.; *Nux m.;* Onosm.; *Phos.; Phyt.;* Puls.; Quill.; Rhus t.; *Sabad.; Sang.;* Sang. n.; Sarcol. ac.; Sep.; *Spong.;* Strych.; Sul.; *Wyeth.*

Edema—Ail.; *Apis;* Ars.; Kali perm.; Lach.; Mag. p.; Mur. ac.; *Nat. ars.;* Phos.; Phyt.; Rhus t.

Erysipelas—*Apis;* Bell.; *Canth.;* Euphorb. of.; Lach.; *Rhus t.*

Globus hystericus—*Ambra; Aquil.; Asaf.;* Bell.; Gels.; Hyos.; *Ign.;* Kali p.; Lach.; Lob. infl.; Mag. m.; Mancin.; *Mosch.; Nux m.;* Plat.; Raph.; *Val.* See Hysteria.

HAWKING—Hemming (clearing throat):—*Æsc.; Alum.;* Am. m.; *Arg. m.; Arg. n.; Arum;* Bry.; Calc. c.; Canth.; Carbo v.; *Caust.;* Cistus; Cocc.; *Coccus;* Con.; *Coral.;* Eucal.; Guaiac.; Gymnocl.; *Hep.;* Hepat.; *Hydr.;* Iberis; Justicia; *Kali bich.;* Kali c.; *Kali m.;* Lach.; *Lyc.;* Merc. i. fl.; *Merc. i. r.; Nat. c.; Nat. m.;* Nit. ac.; *Nux v.; Phos.; Phyt.;* Psor.; *Selen.;* Sep.; Silph s.; Spong.; *Stann.;* Sul.; *Tab.;* Trifrol. pr.; Vinca m.; Viola tr.; *Wyeth.* See Chronic Pharyngitis.

Hawking with cheesy, fetid, lumps—*Agar.;* Kali bich.; Kali m.; Mag. c.; Merc. i. r.; *Psor.;* Sec.; Sil. See Follicular Pharyngitis.

Hawking, with fetid pus—Antipyr.; *Hep.;* Lyc.; Sil.

Hawking, with gelatinous, viscid, gluey mucus; difficult raising—*Æsc.;* Aloe; *Alum.;* Am. br.; Am. m.; *Arg. n.; Arum; Canth.;* Carbo v.; *Caust.;* Cistus; Coca; *Coccus;* Euphras.; *Hydr.;* Iberis; *Kali bich.;* Kali c.; Lach.; *Merc. i. fl.; Merc. i. r.;* Myr.; Nat. c.; Nat. m.; Nat. s.; Nux v.; Petrol.; Phos. ac.; Phos.; *Phyt.;* Psor.; *Rumex;* Sang.; *Selen.;* Sep.; Silph. s.; *Stann.*

Hollow feeling, as if pharynx had disappeared—Lach.; Phyt.

Inclination to swallow constantly—Æsc.; Asaf.; *Bell.;* Caust.; Lac c.; *Lach.;* Lact. ac.; Lyssin; *Merc. i. fl.; Merc.;* Myr.; Phyt.; Sumb.; Wyeth.

INFLAMMATION-(Pharyngitis): Atrophic (sicca): Æsc.; *Alum.;* Dub.; Arg. n.; Ars. iod.; Kali bich.; Nux v.; Sabal.

Inflammation, catarrhal, acute—Acon.; *Æsc.;* Apis; Arg. n.; *Bell.;* Bry.; Canth.; *Caps.;* Caust.; Cistus; Eucal.; Ferr. p.; *Gels.;* Glycerin; *Guaiac.;* Gymnocl.; *Hep.;* Iod.; *Justicia; Kali bich.;* Kali c.; Kali m.; Lach.; Lachnanth.; Led.; Menthol; Merc. c.; Mer. i. fl.; Merc. i. r.; *Merc.;* Naja; Nat. ars.; Nat. iod.; Nux v.; *Phyt.;* Quill.; Sal. ac.; *Sang.; Sang. n.;* Scilla; *Wyeth.*

Inflammation, catarrhal, acute, predisposition to—Alumen; *Bar. c.;* Graph.; Lach.; Sul.

Inflammation, catarrhal, chronic—*Æsc.;* *Alum.;* Am. br.; *Am. caust.;* Arg. iod.; *Arg. m.; Arg. n.;* Ars.; Arum; Aur.; Bar. c.; Brom.; Calc. p.; Can. ind.; Carbo v.; Caust.; Cinnab.; Cistus; *Coccus;* Cub.; Elaps; Ferr. p.; Graph.; *Hep.; Hydr.; Iod.; Kali bich.;* Kali c.; Kali chlor.; Lach.; *Lyc.;* Med.; Merc. c.; Merc. i. fl.; *Merc.; Nat. c.;* Nat. m.; *Nux v.;* Ox. ac.; Penthor.; Petrol.; Phos.; Puls.; *Rumex;* Sabad.; Sabal; *Sang.;* Sec.; Senega; *Sep.;* Stann.; Sumb.; Tab.; *Wyeth.*

Inflammation, follicular, acute—*Æsc.;* Apis; Bell.; Caps.; *Ferr. p.;* Iod.; Kali bich.; *Kali m.;* Merc.; *Phyt.;* Sang. n.; Wyeth.

Inflammation, follicular, chronic (clergymen's sore throat)—*Æsc.; Alum.;* Am. br.; *Arg. n.;* Arn.; Ars. iod.; *Arum;* Calc. fl.; Calc. p.; Caps.; Caust.; Cinnab.; Cistus; Dros.; *Hep.; Hydr.;* Ign.; *Kali bich.;* Kali m.; *Lach.;* Merc. cy.; *Merc. i. r.;* Nat. m.; Nux v.; Phos.; *Phyt.; Sang. n.;* Sticta; Still.; Sul.; *Wyeth.*

Inflammation, herpetic—*Apis;* Ars.; Bor.; Hydr.; Jacar.; *Kali bich.;* Kali chlor.; Lach.; Merc. i. fl.; Nat. s.; *Phyt.;* Sal. ac.

Inflammation, rheumatic—Acon.; Bry.; Colch.; Guaiac.; Phyt.; Rhus t.

Inflammation, septic—Am. c.; *Hep.;* Mur. ac.; *Sil.*

Inflammation, tubercular—Merc. i. r.

AGGRAVATIONS—From cold—*Cistus;* Fluor. ac.; Hep.; *Lyc.*

From drinks, warm or hot—*Lach.;* Merc. i. fl.; Phyt.

From menses—Lac c.

From pressure—Lach.; Merc. c.

From sleep—*Lach.;* Lyc.

From suppressed foot sweat—*Bar. c.;* Psor.; Sil.

From swallowing, empty—Antipyr.; *Bar. c.;* Crotal.; Dolichos; *Hep.; Justicia;* Lac c.; *Lach.;* Merc. i. fl.; Merc. i. r.; *Merc.;* Phyt.; Sabad.

From swallowing liquids—Bell.; Bry.; Ign.; *Lach.*

From swallowing solids—Bapt.; Merc. s.; Morph. See Deglutition.

From swallowing sweet things—Spong.

From warmth—Coccus; Iod.; Lach.; *Merc.*

In afternoon—Lach.

In bed—Merc. i. fl.; *Merc.*

In intervals of swallowing—Caps.; Ign.

On left side—*Lach.; Merc. i. r.;* Sabad.

On lef. to right—Lac c.; *Lach.;* Sabad.

On right side—Bar. c.; *Bell.;* Guaiac.; *Lyc.;* Mag. p.; *Merc. i. fl.;* Merc.; Niccol.; Phyt.; Pod.; *Sang.;* Sul.

AMELIORATIONS—From inspiring cold air:—Sang.

From swallowing—Gels.; *Ign.*

From swallowing liquids—Cistus.

From swallowing liquids, warm—*Alum.;* Ars.; Calc. fl.; Lyc.; Morph.; Sabad.

From swallowing solids—*Ign.;* Lach.

PAPULES—Hippoz.; Iod. See Follicular Pharyngitis.

Paralysis, neuroses—*Alum.;* Bar. m.; *Bell.; Caust.;* Cocc.; *Con.;* Cur.;

Gels.; Hep.; *Hyos.;* *Ign.;* *Lach.;* Lob. infl.; Lyc.; Merc.; Morph.; Nit. ac.; *Nux m.;* Plumb. m.; *Pop. c.;* Rhus t.; *Sil.;* Stram.; Sul.

Peristalsis reversed—Ambra; Asaf.

Plug or lump sensation—Alum.; Bar. c.; *Bell.;* Carbo v.; Graph.; *Hep.;* *Ign.;* *Lach.;* Lob. infl.; Merc. i. fl.; Nat. m.; *Nux v.;* Plumb. ac.; Phyt.; Puls.; Rumex; Sul.; Wyeth.

Pustules—Æth. See Ulceration.

Rawness, roughness, scraping—Acon.; *Æsc.;* *Alum.;* Am. c.; *Am. caust.;* Am. m.; *Arg. m.;* *Arg. n.;* *Arum;* Bar. c.; Bell.; *Bry.;* Brom.; *Carbo v.;* *Caust.;* Coccus; Con.; Cub.; *Dros.;* Fagop.; Gels.; *Hep.;* *Hepat.;* Homar.; Hydr.; *Iod.;* *Kali bich.;* Kali c.; Lact. ac.; Merc. cy.; Merc.; Nit. ac.; *Nux v.;* Onosm.; Penthor.; *Phos.;* *Phyt.;* *Pop. o.;* Puls.; *Rumex;* *Sang.;* Sang. n.; Sep.; Sticta; Sul.

Redness—Acon.; Æsc.; *Bell.;* Ferr. p.; Gins.; Merc. i. fl.; Merc. i. r.; Merc. nit.; Merc.; Sal. ac.; *Sul.*

Redness, dark, livid—Ail.; Alum.; *Am. c.;* Am. caust.; Amygd. pers.; *Apis;* Arag.; *Arg. n.;* Ars.; *Bapt.;* Bell.; Canth.; Caps.; Crot.; Diph.; *Gymnocl.;* *Lach.;* Merc. c.; Mur. ac.; *Naja;* Nat. ars.; Penthor.; *Phyt.;* Puls.; Wyeth.; Zinc. carb.

Redness, glossy, as if varnished—Alum.; *Apis;* Arag.; Bell.; Cistus; Hydr.; Kali bich.; *Lac c.;* Phos.

Relaxation—Æsc.; Alumen; *Alum.;* Am. m.; Bar. c.; *Calc. p.;* Eucal.; Penthor.

Sensitive, sore, tender—Acon.; Æsc.; Ail.; *Apis;* Arg. m.; *Arg. n.;* Arn.; *Arum;* Atrop.; Bar. c.; *Bell.;* Brom.; Bry.; Calc. p.; *Canth.;* Caps.; Carb. ac.; *Caust.;* Dolichos; Fagop.; Ferr. p.; Fluor. ac.; Graph.; Gymnocl.; *Hep.;* Homar.; Hydr.; Ign.; *Kali bich.;* Kali c.; Kali iod.; *Kali per.;* Lac c.; *Lach.;* Lachnanth.; Led.; Lyc.; Menthol; *Merc. c.;* *Merc. cy.;* Merc. i. fl.; *Merc. i. r.;* *Merc.;* Mur. ac.; Naja; Nit. ac.; *Nux v.;* Ox. ac.; Petrol.; Phos.; *Phyt.;* Pop. c.; Quill.; Rhus t.; Sabad.; *Sang.;* Sang. n.; Spong.; Sul.; Trifol.; Verbasc.; Wyeth.

Sore, irritable of smokers—Æsc.; Arg. n.; Caps.; Nat. m.; Nux v.

Spasm—Bell.; Canth.; *Sumb.* See Constriction.

Sticking, pricking, splinter-like pains, extending to ears, worse swallowing, yawning, etc.—Agar.; Alum.; *Arg. n.;* Dolichos; Ferr. iod.; Gels.; Guaiac.; *Hep.;* *Kali bich.;* *Kali c.;* Lac c.; *Nit. ac.;* *Phyt.;* Psor.; Sil.; Staph.

Stiffness—Æsc.; Kali m.; Mag. p.; Mez.; Nux m.; Phyt.; *Rhus t.* See Constriction.

Swelling—Acon.; Æsc.; Ail.; *Apis;* Arg. n.; Arum; Bapt.; *Bar. c.;* *Bell.;* Canth.; *Caps.;* Crot.; Gymnocl.; *Hep.;* Kali bich.; Kali m.; *Kali per.;* Lac c.; *Lach.;* Merc. c.; *Merc. cy.;* *Merc. i. fl.;* *Merc. i. r.;* *Merc.;* Naja; Nat. ars.; *Phyt.;* Sabad.; Sang.; Vespa; Wyeth. See Inflammation.

Syphilis—Aur.; Bell.; Cinnab.; Fluor. ac.; Hydr.; *Kali bich.;* Kali iod.; Merc. c.; *Merc. i. fl.;* *Merc. i. r.;* Merc. nit.; Mez.; *Nit. ac.;* *Phyt.;* Sul.

Tickling, as from hair—Æsc. gl.; Allium s.; Ambra; *Arg. n.;* Caust.; Dros.;

Hepat.; *Kali bich.;* Lach.; Nat. m.; Nit. ac.; Nux v.; Pulex; *Sabad.;* Sang.; Sul.; *Val.;* Yucca.

Ulceration—Ail.; Am. c.; *Apis;* Aral.; Bapt.; *Cinnab.;* Hydr.; *Hydrast. mur.; Kali bich.;* Kali m.; *Lach.; Merc. c.;* Merc. cy.; Merc. i. fl.; Merc. i. r.; Merc.; Mur. ac.; *Nit. ac.; Phyt.;* Sang.; Vinca m.

Ulceration, aphthous—*Canth.;* Eucal.; *Hydrast. mur.;* Nit. ac.

Ulceration, gangrenous—Ail.; Am. c.; *Ars.;* Bapt.; Crot.; Echin.; Kali chlor.; Kali perm.; Kali n.; *Lach.; Merc. cy.;* Merc.; Mur. ac.; Sil.

Ulceration, mercurial—Hep.; Hydr.; Lyc.; Nit. ac.

Ulceration, syphilitic—Aur. m.; Calc. fl.; *Fluor. ac.;* Hippoz.; Jacor. gual.; *Kali bich.;* Kali iod.; Lach.; Lyc.; *Merc. c.;* Merc. i. fl.; Merc. i. r.; Merc.; *Nit. ac.;* Phyt.: Still.

Veins, varicose—*Æsc.;* Aloe; *Bar. m.;* Ham.; Phyt.; Puls.

TONSILS—**Abscess (peritonsillar):** Calc. s.

DEPOSITS ON—**Creamy, extends over tonsils, uvula, soft palate:**—Nat. p.
Dark, dry, wrinkled—Ars.
Dark, gangrenous—Bapt.
Grayish, dirty, like macerated skin, covering tonsils, uvula pharynx—Phyt.
Grayish, dirty, thick, with fiery red margins—Apis.
Grayish, extends to posterior nares, air passages, later purplish black— Echin.
Grayish patch on tonsils—Kali m.
Grayish, thick; shred-like borders, adherent or free—Merc. v.
Grayish-white, in crypts—Ign.
Grayish-yellow, slight; easily detached; worse on left—Merc. i. r.
Patchy on right tonsil and inflamed fauces, easily detached—Merc. i. fl.
Plugs of mucus constantly form in crypts—Calc. fl.
Shining, glazed white or yellow patch—Lac c.
Thick, brownish-yellow like wash leather, or firm, fibrinous, pearly, extends over tonsils, soft palate—Kali bich.
Thick, dark gray, or brownish black—Diph.
Thin, false; on yellowish red tonsils and fauces—Merc. s.
Thin, then dark, gangrenous—Merc. cy.

HYPERTROPHY—**Induration:** Alumen; Ars. iod.; Aur.; Bac.; *Bar. c.; Bar. iod.;* Bar. m.; Brom.; Calc. c.; Calc. fl.; *Calc. iod.; Calc. p.;* Ferr. p.; Hep.; *Iod.; Kali bich.;* Kali m.; Merc. i. fl.; *Merc. i. r.;* Plumb. iod.; Phyt.; Sil.; Sul. iod.; Thuya.

Hypertrophy, with hardness of hearing—*Bar. c.;* Calc. p.; *Hep.;* Lyc.; Plumb.; Psor.

Inflammation (tonsillitis): Acute Catarrhal and Follicular: *Acon.; Ail.;* Am. m.; Amyg. pers.; *Apis; Bapt.;* Bar. ac.; *Bar. c.;* Bar. m.; *Bell.;* Brom.; Caps.; Dulc.; Eucal.; Ferr. p.; Gels.; Gins.; *Guaiac.; Gymnocl.;* Hep.; *Ign.;* Iod.; Kali bich.; *Kali m.;* Lac c.; *Lach.;* Lyc.; *Merc. i. fl.; Mers. i. r.; Merc. s.;* Naja; Nat. s.; *Phyt.;* Rhus t.; Sabad.; *Sang., Sil.;* Sul.

Inflammation, acute phlegmonous (quinsy): Acon.; Apis; *Bar. c.;* Bar. iod.; *Bell.;* Caps.; Cinnab.; Guaiac.; *Hep.;* Lac c.; Lach.; Lyc.;

Merc. i. fl.; Merc. i. r.; *Merc. s.; Merc. v.; Phyt.; Psor.;* Sang.; Sang. n.; Sil.; *Tar. c.;* Vespa.

Inflammation, chronic tendency—*Bar. c.;* Calc. p.; Fucus; Hep.; Lach.; Lyc.; Psor.; *Sil.*

Redness, dark—Ail.; Amyg. am.; *Bapt.;* Brom.; Caps.; Diph.; Gymnocl.; *Lach.;* Merc.; *Phyt.*

Swelling—*Acon.;* Am. m.; *Apis;* Ars. iod.; Bar. ac.; *Bar. c.; Bell.;* Brom.; Calc. c.; Calc. p.; Caps.; Cinnab.; Cistus; Diph.; Ferr. p.; Gels.; Guaiac.; *Hep.;* Ign.; Iod.; Kali bich.; Kali m.; *Lach.;* Lyc.; Merc. c.; *Merc. i. fl.; Merc. i. r.; Merc.; Phyt.;* Psor.; *Sang. n.* See Tonsillitis.

Ulceration—*Ars.;* Bar. c.; Echin.; *Hep.;* Ign.; *Kali bich.;* Lach.; Lyc.; Merc. c.; Merc. i. fl.; Merc. i. r.; Merc. per.; Merc. s.; Nat. s.; Nit. ac.; Phyt.; *Sil.* See Follicular Tonsillitis.

Ulceration, gangrenous—Am. c.; Ars.; Bapt.; Crot.; *Lach.; Merc. cy.;* Mur. ac.

UVULA—Constricted feeling—Acon.

Edematous, sac-like—*Apis;* Ars.; Caps.; *Kali bich.;* Mur. ac.; *Nat. ars.;* Phos.; Phyt.; Rhus t.

Elongation, relaxation—*Alumen;* Alum.; Bar. c.; Bell.; Calc. fl.; Canth.; *Caps.;* Coccinel.; *Coccus;* Croc.; Fagop.; Hep.; *Hyos.; Kali bich.; Merc. c.;* Merc.; Nat. m.; Nux v.; *Phos.; Phyt.;* Rumex ac.; Sabad.; Wyeth.

Inflammation (uvulitis)—*Acon.;* Amygd. pers.; *Bell.;* Caps.; Cistus; Iod.; *Kali bich.; Kali per.; Merc. c.;* Merc.; Nat. s.; Nux v.; Puls.; Sul. iod.

Pain—Trifol.; Tussil.

Sore spot behind, better by eating—Am. m.

Ulceration—Indium; *Kali bich.;* Merc. c.

Whitened, shrivelled—Carb. ac.

White, tenacious, mucus—Am. caust.

STOMACH

APPETITE—Defective, lost (anorexia)—*Abies n.;* Alet.; Alfal.; Am. c.;
Ant. c.; Arn.; *Ars.; Bapt.;* Bism.; But. ac.; Calc. c.; Calc. p.; Caps.;
Carb. ac.; Carbo v.; Card. m.; *Chel.; Chin. ars.;* Chionanth.; *Cinch.;*
Coca; Cocc.; Coff.; Colch.; Cycl.; Dig.; *Ferr. m.; Gent.;* Glycerin;
Helon.; Hydr.; *Ign.; Ipec.;* Iris; Kali bich.; *Lecith.; Lyc.;* Merc. d.;
Myr.; Niccol.; *Nux v.;* Phos. ac.; Phos.; Plat.; Prun. sp.; Prun. v.;
Puls.; Raph.; *Rhus t.;* Sep.; Stront.; Strych. ars.; *Strych. p.;* Sul.;
Symphor.; Tarax.

Appetite, increased, ravenous (bulimy)—Abies c.; *Abrot.;* Agar.; *Alfal.;*
Allium s.; *Anac.;* Ars.; Ars. br.; Bell.; Brassica; Bry.; Cact.; *Calc. c.;*
Calend.; Chel.; Cim.; *Cina;* Cinch.; Ferr. m.; Glycerin; Granat.;
Graph.; Hep.; Ichth.; Ign.; *Iod.;* Kali c.; Lact. ac.; Lap. alb.; Lob.
infl.; *Lyc.;* Merc.; Nat. c.; *Nat. m.; Nux v.;* Oleand.; Op.; *Petrol.;*
Petros.; *Phos.; Psor.;* Rhus t.; Sec.; Stann.; *Sul.; Thyr.; Uran. n.;*
Zinc. m.

Appetite, increased, hungry at night—Abies. n.; *Cina;* Cinch.; Ign.; **Lyc.;**
Nat. c.; Petrol.; *Phos.; Psor.;* Selen.; *Sul.*

Appetite, increased, hungry before noon—Hep.; *Sul.;* Zinc. m.

Appetite, increased, hungry, even after a meal—*Alfal.;* Calc. c.; Casc.;
Cina; Iod.; Indol; Lac c.; *Lyc.;* Med.; *Phos.;* Phyt.; *Psor.;* Staph.;
Stront.; Sul.; Zinc.

Appetite, increased, yet loses flesh—Abrot.; Acet. ac.; *Iod.; Nat. m.;*
Sanic.; Tub.; Uran. n.

Appetite, increased, yet quickly satiated—Am. c.; Arn.; Ars.; Bar. c.;
Carbo v.; *Cinch.; Cycl.;* Ferr.; Lith. c.; *Lyc.;* Nat. m.; Nux v.; Petros.;
Pod.; Prun. sp.; *Sep.; Sul.*

APPETITE PERVERTED—AVERSIONS: Alcoholic beverages:—Ign.; Sil.

Beer—Asaf.; Bell.; Cinch.; Nux v.; Puls.

Boiled food—Calc. c.

Brandy—Ign.; Lob. erin.

Bread—Chenop. gl.; Cycl.; Ign.; *Lyc.; Nat. m.;* Puls.; Sul.

Butter—Cycl.; Hep.; *Puls.;* Sang.

Coffee—*Cham.;* Fluor. ac.; *Nux v.;* Sul. ac.

Drinks in general—Bell.; *Canth.;* Cocc.; Ign.; Kali bich.; Lyssin; Nux
v.; Stram. See Hydrophobia.

Drinks, warm and hot—Cham.; Kali s.; *Puls.*

Eggs—Ferr. m.

Fats—*Calc. c.;* Carbo an.; *Carbo v.; Cycl.;* Hep.; Nat. m.; Petrol.; *Puls.;*
Sep.

Food cooked—Graph.; Sil.

Food in general—*Ant. c.;* Ars.; Canth.; Cocc.; *Colch.;* Dulc.; Ferr. m.;
Ign.; *Ipec.; Kali bich.;* Kali c.; *Nux v.;* Pod.; Puls.; Rheum; Rhus t.;
Sabad.; Yerba. See Anorexia.

Food, smell, sight of—Ant. c.; *Ars.;* Cocc.; *Colch.;* Dig.; *Nux v.; Sep.;* Sil.; Stann.; Symphor.

Food, warm, hot—Calc. c.; Ign.; Lyc.; Petrol.; *Puls.;* Sil.; Ver. **a.**

Meat—Aloe; *Alum.; Arn.;* Bell.; *Calc. c.; Carbo v.;* Card. m.; Chenop. gl.; Cinch.; Colch.; Crotal.; *Cycl.;* Ferr. p.; *Graph.;* Lyc.; Morph.; *Mur. ac.; Nit. ac.;* Petrol.; *Puls.; Sep.;* Sil.; Stront.; Sul.; Thuya.

Milk—Arn.; Bell.; *Carbo v.;* Ferr. p.; *Guaiac.;* Nat. c.; Pastin.; Puls.; Sep.; Sil.; *Sul.*

Potatoes—Alum.; Thuya.

Salt food—Graph.; Selen.

Sour things—Dros.; Ferr. m.; Sul.

Sweets—Bar. c.; Caust.; *Graph.;* Radium; Sul.

Tobacco—Arn.; Calc. c.; Canth.; Cocc.; *Lob. infl.;* Nat. m.; *Nux v.;* Plant.

Tobacco, odor of—Cascar.; *Ign.;* Lob. infl.

Wine—Sul.

APPETITE—PERVERTED CRAVINGS (pica): Acids, pickles, sour things: *Abies c.;* Alum.; Am. m.; *Ant. c.;* Ant. t.; Arn.; *Ars.;* Arundo; Calc. c.; Carbo an.; Chel.; *Cinch.;* Cod.; *Hep.;* Ign.; Jonosia; Kali bich.; Lact. v.; *Mag. c.;* Myr.; Nat. m.; *Phos ac.; Puls.;* Sec.; *Sep.;* Thea; *Ver. a.*

Alcoholic beverages—*Ars.; Asar.;* Calc. ars.; *Caps.; Carb. ac.;* Carbo v.; Cinch.; *Coca;* Cocc.; Ferr. p.; *Kali bich.;* Lach.; Lecith.; Med.; Mosch.; *Nux v.;* Phos.; Psor.; Puls.; *Selen.;* Staph.; Stront.; *Sul.; Sul. ac.; Syph.;* Tub.

Apples—Aloe; *Ant. t.;* Guaiac.; Tellur.

Beer, bitter—Aloe; Cocc.; *Kali bich.;* Nat. m.; Nux v.; Puls.

Bread—Ferr. m.; Stront.

Butter—Ferr. m.

Buttermilk—Elaps.

Charcoal coal, chalk, etc.—*Alum.;* Calc. c.; Cic.; Ign.; Nit. ac.; *Psor.*

Cheese—Arg. n.; Cistus.

Coffee—*Angust.;* Ars.; Con.; Lecith.; Mosch.

Drinks, cold—*Acon.; Ant. t.;* Asim.; *Ars.;* Bell.; *Bry.;* Calc. c.; Cocc.; *Cupr. m.;* Dulc.; *Merc.;* Nat. s.; Onosm.; Phos.; Rhus t.; *Ver. a.* See Thirst.

Drinks, hot—Angust.; Cascar.; Castan.; *Chel.; Lyc.;* Med.; Sabad.; Spig.

Effervescent beverages—Colch.

Eggs—Calc. c.

Farinaceous food—Calc. p.; Sabad.

Fats—Mez.; Nit. ac.; Nux v.; Sul.

Food, coarse, raw—*Abies c.;* Sil.

Food, cold—Bry.; *Phos.; Puls.;* Sil.

Food, fish—Sul. ac.

Food, warm, hot—Chel.; Cupr. m.; Sabad.

Fruits, juicy things—Aloe; *Ant. t.;* Cinch.; Mag. c.; Med.; *Phos. ac.;* Phos.; Ver. a.

Ham rind—Calc. p.
Lemonade—Am. m.; Cycl.; Puls.; Sab.; Sec.
Meat—*Abies c.; Calc. p.; Lil. t.; Mag. c.;* Menyanth.
Meat, salt, smoked—Calc. p.
Milk—Apis; Ars.; *Phos. ac.; Rhus t.;* Sabal; Sul.
Oysters—Lach.
Salt—Calc. c.; Carbo v.; *Caust.;* Con.; Med.; Nat. m.; Nit. ac.; *Phos.:* Sul.; Ver. a
Spices—Alum.; *Cinch.;* Fluor. ac.; *Hep.;* Nux m.; *Nux v.;* Phos.; Sang.; Staph.
Sweets, candy—Alfal.; Am. c.; *Arg. n.;* Calc. c.; *Cina;* Coca; *Cocaine;* Crot.; Jonosia; *Kali c.; Lyc.;* Mag. m.; Med.; Sabad.; *Sul.*
Tea—Alum.; Hep.
Tobacco—*Asar.; Carb. ac.;* Carbo v.; Coca; Daphne; *Staph.*
Tonics—Puls.
Various things—Bry.; Cham.; *Cina; Cinch.;* Fluor. ac.; Rheum; Sang.
Vegetables—Abies c.; Mag. c.
Water, cold—*Acon.;* Agar. emet.; *Ant. t.;* Apoc.; *Ars.;* Asim.; Bell.; *Bry.; Colc. c.; Eup. perf.;* Onosm.; Op.; *Phos.;* Ver. a. See Thirst.
APPETITE—THINGS THAT DISAGREE—Beer:—Ferr. m.; *Kali bich.*
Bread—Ant. c.; *Hydr.;* Lyc.; *Nat. m.;* Nit. ac.; Puls.
Butter—Carbo an.; *Carbo v.;* Nat. m.; Puls.
Cabbage—*Bry.;* Carbo v.; Kali c.; Lyc.; Petrol.
Cheese—Col.
Coffee—Carbo v.; Lyc.; *Nux v.*
Drinks, cold—*Ars.;* Calad.; Dig.; Elaps; Kali iod.; *Ver. a.*
Drinks, warm, hot—Bry.; Graph.; *Phos.;* Puls.; Pyr.
Eggs—Colch.
Fats—Ant. c.; Calc. c.; Carbo v.; *Cycl.;* Lyc.; *Puls.;* Thuya.
Fish—Carbo v.
Food, cold—Kali iod.
Food of any kind—Alet.; Amyg. pers.; *Carbo v.;* Lach.; Mosch.; Nat. c.
Food, warm—Puls.
Meat—Ars.; Bor.; *Bry.;* Carbo v.; *Cinch.;* Mag. m.; Nat. m.; *Puls.;* Selen.; Sil.; Ver. a.
Meat in excess—Allium s.
Fruits—*Ars.;* Carbo v.; *Caust.;* Ferr. m.; Kali bich.; *Rumex.*
Melons—Zing.
Milk—*Æth.;* Calc. c.; *Carbo v.;* Cinch.; Kali iod.; Lact. v.; Mag. c.; *Mag. m.;* Niccol.; Ol. j. as.; Pod.; Rheum; Sep.; *Sul.*
Mushrooms, poisonous—Camph.
Odor of food nauseates—*Ars.;* Cocc.; *Colch.;* Dig.; *Sep.*
Onions—Brom.; Lyc.; Thuya.
Oysters—Carbo v.; Lyc.
Pastry—Ant. c.; Lyc.; *Puls.*
Pork—Ant. c.; Carbo v.; Cycl.; *Puls.*
Potatoes—*Alum.;* Sep.
Salt food—Carbo v.

Sausage—Acet. ac.; Ars.; Puls.
Soup—Kali c.
Sour foods, drinks—*Ant. c.;* Carbo v.; Dros.; Nat. m.; Phos. ac.
Starchy food—*Carbo v.;* Cinch.; Lyc.; *Nat. c.;* Nat. s.; Sul.
Strawberries—Ox. ac.
Sweets—*Arg. n.;* Ipec.; Lyc.; Sul.; Zinc.
Tea—*Cinch.;* Diosc.; Ferr. m.; Kali hypoph.; *Selen.;* Thuya.
Tobacco—*Ign.;* Kali bich.; Lob. infl.; Lyc.; Phos.; *Selen.;* Tab.
Vegetables—Hydr.
Vinegar—Ant. c.; Carbo v.
Water—*Ars.;* Chin. ars.
Water, impure—Zing.
Wine—Ant. c.; *Zinc. m.*

ATONY—(myasthenia): Bell.; Ign.; Podophylin; *Strych. p.*

BILIOUSNESS—*Æsc.;* Aloe; Aqua mar.; *Bapt.;* Berb. v.; *Bry.;* Card. m.; Cham.; *Chel.;* Chionanth.; *Cinch.;* Crot.; Diosc.; *Euonym.;* Eup. perf.; Ferr. m.; Gent.; *Hydr.; Iris;* Kali c.; *Lept.;* Lyc.; Mag. m.; *Merc.;* Myr.; *Nat. s.;* Nitro-mur. ac.; *Nux v.;* Pod.; Ptel.; *Puls.;* Sep.; Sul.; *Tarax.; Triost.;* Yucca. See Liver.

CANCER—Acet. ac.; Am. m.; Arg. n.; Ars.; *Bell.;* Bar. c.; Bism.; Cadm. s.; Calc. fl.; *Condur.;* Con.; Carbo v.; Graph.; *Hydr.; Kali bich.;* Kali c.; *Kreos.;* Mag. p.; Nux v.; *Ornithog.;* Phos.; Plumb. m.; Sec. See Generalities.

CARDIAC ORIFICE—Contraction: Alum.; *Bar. m.;* Bry.; Datura; *Phos.;* Plumb. m.

Pain (cardialgia)—*Agar.;* Arg. n.; Asaf.; Bar. c.; Bism.; Can. ind.; *Carbo v.;* Caul.; *Cupr. m.; Ferr. cy.;* Ferr. tart.; Formica; Ign.; Mag. m.; Nat. m.; Nit. ac.; *Nux v.; Oniscus;* Stront. c.; Thea. See Pain.

Spasmodic contraction, painful, cardio-spasm—Æth.; *Agar.;* Am. c.; *Arg. n.;* Ars.; *Bell.;* Calc. c.; Caul.; *Con.;* Hyos.; *Ign.;* Nat. m.; *Nux v.;* Phos.; Puls.; Rhus t.; Sep.; Sil.

Dilatation (gastroptosis)—Bism.; Graph.; *Hydrast. mur.;* Kali bich.; *Nux v.;* Phos.; Puls.; Xanthor.

GASTRALGIA—See Pain.

GASTRIC AFFECTIONS, better in open air—Adon.

GASTRIC AFFECTIONS, of cigar-makers—Ign.

HEMORRHAGE (hemetemesis): Acet. ac.; Acon.; *Arn.; Ars.;* Bothrops; *Cact.;* Canth.; Carbo v.; *Cinch.; Cocaine;* Crot.; Cupr. m.; Erig.; Ferr. p.; Ficcus; *Geran.; Ham.;* Hyos.; *Ipec.;* Kreos.; Mangif. ind.; *Millef.;* Nit. ac.; Nux v.; *Phos.; Sec.;* Trill.; Zinc. m.

HICCOUGH—(singultus): Æth.; Agar.; Amyl; Ars.; Bell.; *Cajup.;* Caps.; Carbo an.; Carbo v.; *Cic.;* Cocaine; Cocc.; *Cupr. m.; Cycl.;* Diosc.; Eup. perf.; *Gins.;* Hep.; Hydroc. ac.; Hyos.; *Ign.;* Kali br.; Mag. p.; *Morph.; Mosch.;* Nat. m.; Niccol.; Nicot.; Nux m.; *Nux v.;* Ol. succin.; Ran. b.; Stram.; *Sul. ac.;* Tab.; Ver. a.; Ver. v.; Zinc. oxy.; *Zinc. v.*

Hiccough, after smoking—Ign.; Selen.

Hiccough, followed by spasm—Cupr. m.

Hiccough, with belching—Ant. c.; *Cajup.;* Cic.; Cinch.; *Diosc.; Nux v.;* Wyeth.

Hiccough, with hysterical, nervous symptoms—Gels.; *Ign.; Mosch.;* Nux m.; Zinc. v.

Hiccough, with pains in back, after eating, nursing—Teucr.

Hiccough, with retching, vomiting—Jatropha; Mag. p.; Merc.; *Nux v.*

Hiccough, with spasm of esophagus—Ver. v.

Hiccough, with yawning—Amyl; Carls.; *Cocc.*

HYPER-ACIDITY (hyperchlorhydria): Acet. ac.; Anac.; Ant. c.; *Arg. n.; Atrop.;* Bism.; Caffeine; *Calc. c.;* Calc. p.; *Carbo v.;* Cham.; Chin. ars.; Cinch.; Con.; Grind.; Hydr.; Ign.; *Iris;* Lob. infl.; Lyc.; Mag. c.; Mur. ac.; *Nat. c.;* Nat. p.; *Nux v.; Orexine tan.;* Petrol.; Phos.; Prun. v.; *Puls.;* Robin.; Sul.; *Sul. ac.*

Hyperæsthesia—*Arg. n.;* Ars.; Bism.; Chin. ars

Hyperperistalsis—Ars.; Fel. tauri; Hyos.; *Ign.;* Phos.

INDIGESTION—DYSPEPSIA—Remedies in general: *Abies c.; Abies n.;* Abrot.; Acet. ac.; *Æsc.;* Æth.; Agar.; Alet.; Alfal.; Allium s.; Alnus; Aloe; Alum.; *Anac.; Ant. c.;* Ant. t.; Apoc.; *Arg. n.;* Aristol.; *Arn.; Ars.;* Atrop.; Bapt.; Bar. c.; Bell.; *Bism.;* Brom.; *Bry.;* Calc. c.; Calc. chlor.; Caps.; *Carb. ac.; Carbo v.; Card. m.;* Cascara sag.; *Cham.; Chel.;* Cina; *Cinch.; Coca;* Cochlear.; *Colch.;* Col.; Corn. fl.; Cupr. ac.; *Cycl.; Diosc.;* Fel tauri; Ferr. m.; Gent.; *Graph.;* Hep.; *Homar.; Hydr.; Ign.;* Iod.; *Ipec.;* Iris; *Kali bich.; Kali c.;* Kali m.; *Lach.;* Lept.; *Lob. infl.; Lyc.;* Merc.; *Nat. c.;* Nat. m.; Nat. s.; Nit. ac.; *Nux m.; Nux v.;* Op.; Petrol.; Phos. ac.; *Phos.;* Picr. ac.; Pod.; Pop. tr.; Prun. sp.; Prun. v.; Ptel.; *Puls.; Robin.;* Sal. ac.; Sang.; *Sep.;* Stann.; *Strych. ferr. cit.; Sul.;* Sul. ac.; Uran. n.; Xerophyl.

CAUSE—Abuse of drugs—Nux v.

Acids—*Ant. c.;* Ars.; Cinch.; Nat. m.

Aged, debilitated—Abies n.; Ars.; Bar. c.; *Carbo v.;* Cinch.; Fluor. ac.; *Hydr.;* Kali c.

Beer—Ant. t.; Bapt.; Bry.; *Kali bich.;* Lyc.; *Nux v.*

Bread—Ant. c.; Bry.; Lyc.; Nat. m.

Bright's disease—Apoc. See Urinary System.

Buckwheat cakes—Puls.

Cheese—Ars.; Carbo v.; Col.; Nux v.

Coffee—Cham.; Kali c.; Lyc.; *Nux v.*

Cold bathing—Ant. c.

Debauchery in general—Ant. t.; *Carbo v.; Cinch.;* Nat. s.; *Nux v.*

Decayed meat, fish—Ars.; Carbo v.

Dietetic indiscretions—Allium s.; *Ant. c.;* Bry.; *Carbo v.;* Cinch.; Coff.; *Ipec.;* Lyc.; Nat. c.; *Nux v.; Puls.;* Xanth.

Egg albumen—Nux v.

Excesses—Carbo v.; *Cinch.;* Kali c.; *Nux v.*

Fat food—Ant. c.; *Calc. c.;* Carbo v.; *Cycl.;* Ipec.; *Kali m.; Puls.;* Thuya.

Fatigue, brain fag, in children—Calc. fl.

Fevers, acute, after—Cinch.; Quass.

Flatulent food—Cinch.; Lyc.; Puls.

Fruits—Ars.; *Cinch.;* Elaps; *Puls.;* Ver. a.

Gastric juice, scanty—Alnus; *Alum.;* Lyc.

Gout—Ant. t.; Cinch.; *Colch.;* Nux m.; Thuya.

Hasty eating, drinking—Anac.; Coff.; *Oleand.*

Hot weather—Ant. c.; *Bry.*

Ice water, ices—*Ars.;* Carbo v.; Elaps; Ipec.; Kali c.; Nat. c.; *Puls.*

Lactation—*Cinch.;* Sinap. a.

Meats—*Caust.;* Ipec.; Puls.; Sil.

Melons—Ars.; Zing.

Menstruation—Arg. n.; Cop.; Sep. See Female Sexual System.

Milk—*Æth.;* Calc. c.; Carbo v.; Mag. c.; Mag. m.; Nit. ac.; Sul. ac.; Sul.

Nervous, from unpleasant emotions—Cham.; Nux m.; Nux v.

Night watching—Nux v.

Pastry—Ant. c.; Carbo v.; Ipec.; Kali m.; Lyc.; *Puls.*

Pork sausage—Cinch.; Puls.

Pregnancy—Sabad.; *Sinap a.;* Thea.

Salt, abuse of—Phos.

Sedentary life—Nux v.

Sweets—Ant. c.; *Arg. n.;* Ipec.; *Lyc.;* Zinc. m.

Tea—Abies n.; *Cinch.;* Diosc.; Puls.; Thea; Thuya.

Tobacco—Abies n.; *Nux v.;* Sep.

Urticaria—Cop.

Vegetables, tobacco—Ars.; Asclep t.; Nat. c.; Nux v.; *Sep.*

Water—Ars.

Wines, liquors—*Ant. c.;* Caps.; Carbo v.; Coff.; Nat. s.; *Nux v.;* Sul.; Sul. ac.; Zinc. m.

TYPE—**Atonic, nervous, acid**—Alet.; *Alfal.;* Alston.; *Anac.;* Angust.; *Arg. n.;* Calc. c.; Caps.; Carb. ac.; *Carbo v.; Cinch.;* Ferr.; Grind.; Hep.; *Ign.;* Jugl. c.; *Kali p.;* Lob. infl.; *Lyc.;* Mag. c.; Nat. c.; *Nux v.; Phos.; Ptel.;* Quass.; Ratanh.; Robin.; Sul. ac.; Sul.; Val.

Catarrhal—Abies c.; Abies n.; *Ant. c.; Arg. n.;* Bals. per.; Calc. c.; Carb. ac.; Carbo v.; Cinch.; Collins.; Coryd.; Geran.; *Hydr.;* Hydroc. ac.; Illic.; *Ipec.; Kali bich.;* Lyc.; Nux v.; Ox. ac.; *Puls.;* Sul. See Chronic Catarrhal Gastritis.

Latent or masked—Cact.; Carbo v.; Cinch.; Hydroc. ac.; *Nat. m.; Sep.;* Spig.; Tab.

SYMPTOMS AND CONDITIONS—**Acidity:** Arg. n.; *Calc. c.;* Carbo v.; Ign.; Lob. infl.; Lyc.; Nat. c.; *Nux v.;* Puls.; *Robin.;* Sul. See Hyperchlorhydria.

Cough—Lob. syph.; Taxus. See Respiratory System.

Digestion, weak. slow (bradypepsia)—Alston.; *Anac.; Ant. c.; Arg. n.;* Ars.; Asaf.; Bism.; *Bry.;* Caps.; *Carbo an.; Carbo v.; Cinch.;* Cochlear.; Coff.; Colch.; *Cycl.; Diosc.;* Eucal.; Granat.; *Graph.; Hydr.;* Ipec.;

Kali bich.; *Lyc.;* Merc.; *Nat. c.;* Nat. m.; *Nux v.;* Prun. v.; *Puls.;* Zing. See Indigestion.

Distress from simplest food—Alet.; Amyg. pers.; *Ant. c.;* Carbo an.; *Carbo v.; Cinch.;* Dig.; *Hep.; Kali c.;* Lach.; *Nat. c.; Nux v.;* Puls.

Drowsiness, sleepiness—Æth.; Ant. c.; Bism.; *Carbo v.; Cinch.; Epiph.; Fel tauri;* Graph.; Grat.; Kali c.; *Lyc.; Nat. chlor.; Nat. m.; Nux m.;* Nux v.; Phos. ac.; Phos.; Sarrac.; Staph.; Sul.

Eructations, belching—*Abies n.;* Acet. ac.; Agar.; Alum.; *Anac.; Ant. c.; Arg. n.;* Arn.; *Asaf.;* Bism.; *Bry.; Cajup.; Calc. c.;* Calc. p.; Caps.; Carb. ac.; Carbo an.; *Carbo v.;* Cham.; *Cinch.; Cycl.; Diosc.;* Fagop.; Ferr. m.; Ferr. p.; Glycerin; *Graph.;* Grat.; *Hep.;* Hydr.; Ind.; *Iod.;* Ipec.; Jugl. c.; Kali bich.; *Kali c.;* Lob. infl.; *Lyc.;* Mag. c.; *Mosch.; Nat. c.;* Nat. p.; Nat. m.; Nit. ac.; *Nux m.; Nux v.;* Petrol.; *Phos.;* Pod.; *Puls.; Robin.;* Rumex; Sal. ac.; Sang.; *Sep.;* Sil.; *Sul.;* Sul. ac.; Uran. n.; Val.

Eructations, odorless, tasteless, empty—*Agar.;* Aloe; *Ambra;* Am. m.; Anac.; Asar.; Bism.; Calad.; Calc. iod.; Coca; Cocc.; Hep.; Ign.; *Iod.; Oleand.;* Plat.

Eructations, rancid, putrid, foul—*Arn.;* Asaf.; Bism.; Calc. iod.; *Carbo v.; Cham.;* Cycl.; Diosc.; *Graph.;* Hydr.; *Kali c.;* Mag. m.; *Mag. s.;* Ornithog.; Plumb.; Psor.; *Puls.;* Raph.; Sang.; *Sep.;* Sul.; Thuya; Val.; Xerophyl.

Eructations, relieve temporarily—*Arg. n.;* Asaf.; Bar. c.; Bry.; Calc. p.; *Carbo v.;* Kali c.; Lach.; Mosch.; *Nux m.;* Nux v.; Ol. an.; Ox. ac.; Puls.

Eructations, sour, burning, acid, bitter—Acet. ac.; Ant. c.; Arg. n.; Bry.; *Calc. c.;* Calc. iod.; Calc. p.; Carb. ac.; Carbo an.; *Carbo v.;* Cham.; Cinch.; *Diosc.;* Ferr. p.; Fluor. ac.; Graph.; Ipec.; Hep.; *Hydr.; Kali c.; Lact. ac.;* Lact. v.; *Lyc.;* Mag. c.; *Nat. c.;* Nat. m.; Nat. nit.; *Nat. p.;* Nit. ac.; Nit. mur. ac.; *Nux v.;* Ox. ac.; Petrol.; Phos. ac.; *Phos.;* Pod.; *Puls.;* Raph.; *Robin.;* Sabal; Sal. ac.; Senec.; *Sep.;* Sil.; Sinap. n.; *Sul. ac.; Sul.;* Xerophyl.

Eructations, tasting of ingesta—*Ant. c.; Carbo v.;* Cinch.; Cycl.; *Ferr.;* Graph.; *Puls.; Sep.;* Sil.; Sul.

Fainting—Ars.; Cinch.; Mosch.; Nux m.; Nux v.; Phos. ac.

Flatulent distention of stomach drumlike—*Abies c.;* Agar.; Ant. c.; Apoc.; *Arg. n.; Asaf.;* Bry.; But. ac.; *Cajup.; Calc. c.;* Calc. fl.; Caps.; Carb. ac.; *Carbo v.; Cinch.; Colch.;* Cycl.; Diosc.; Ferr. magnet.; *Graph.;* Grat.; Hydr.; *Ign.;* Indol; Iod.; Jugl. c.; Kali bich.; *Kali c.; Lach.; Lyc.;* Mosch.; *Nux m.; Nux v.;* Ox. ac.; Phos. ac.; Phos.; Pop. tr.; *Puls.;* Sil.; Sul.; Thuya. See Sensation.

Headache—Arg. n.; *Bry.;* Carbo v.; Cinch.; Cycl.; Kali c.; Lach.; Lept.; *Ign.;* Nat. m.; Nux m.; *Nux v.;* Puls.; Robin.; *Sang.;* Tarax. See Head.

Heartburn, pyrosis—Am. c.; Ant. c.; Apomorph.; *Arg. n.;* Ars.; Bism.; *Bry.;* Cajup.; *Calc. c.;* Calend.; Caps.; Carb. ac.; *Carbo v.;* Chin. s.; Datura; *Diosc.;* Fagop.; Gall. ac.; Graph.; Iod.; Kali c.; Lach.; Lob. infl.; *Lyc.;* Mag. c.; Phos. ac.; Mag. m.; *Nat. m.;* Nit. ac.; *Nux v.;*

Nux m.; Ox. ac.; *Puls.;* Robin.; Sang.; Sinap.; Sinap. n.; *Sul. ac.;* Tab.

Hiccough—Bry.; Hyos.; Ign.; *Nux v.;* Paris; Sep.

Lassitude, weakness—Act. sp.; Ant. t.; *Ars.;* Can. s.; Caps.; Carbo an.; *Carbo v.;* Cinch.; Graph.; Grat.; Hydr.; *Lyc.; Nux v.;* Phos.; Puls.; Sep.

Mental depression, dullness—Anac.; Cinch.; Cycl.; Hydr.; Lyc.; Nat. c.; Nit. ac.; *Nux v.;* Puls.; Sep.; Tab. See Mind.

Nausea, vomiting—Æth.; *Ant. c.;* Ant. t.; *Arg. n.; Ars.;* Atrop.; Bism.; *Bry.; Carb. ac.;* Carbo v.; Cham.; Cocc.; *Ferr. m.;* Graph.; Ign.; *Ipec.; Kali bich.; Kreos.;* Lept.; Lob. infl.; Lyc.; Nat. c.; *Nux v.;* Petrol.; Phos.; *Puls.;* Rhus t.; *Sang.;* Sep.; Sil. See Vomiting.

Pain—*Abies n.;* Æsc.; Anis.; *Arg. n.;* Arn.; *Ars.; Bry.;* Calc. iod.; Calc. mur.; Carbo v.; Cinch.; Col.; Cupressus; Diosc.; Gamb.; *Hedeoma;* Homar.; Ipec.; Kali m.; Nat. m.; *Nux v.;* Paraf.; *Phos.;* Puls.; Scutel.; Sep.; *Stann.;* Thuya. See Pain.

Pain immediately after eating—*Abies n.;* Arn.; Ars.; Calc. c.; *Carbo v.;* Cinch.; Cocc.; *Kali bich.; Kali c.; Lyc.; Nux m.;* Physost.

Pain several hours after eating—Æsc.; *Agar.;* Anac.; Bry.; Calc. hypoph.; Con.; *Nux v.;* Ox. ac.; *Puls.*

Palpitation of the heart—Abies c.; *Arg. n.; Cact.; Carbo v.;* Hydroc. ac.; Lyc.; *Nat. m.; Nux v.; Puls.;* Sep.; *Spig.;* Tab. See Circulatory System.

Pressure as from a stone—*Abies n.;* Acon.; Æsc.; Anac.; *Arg. n.;* Arn.; *Ars.; Bry.; Calc. c.;* Carbo v.; Cham.; Cinch.; Dig.; Ferr. m.; Graph.; Hep.; *Kali bich.;* Lob. infl.; *Lyc.; Nux v.;* Phos. ac.; *Phos.; Puls.;* Rhus t.; Rumex; Scilla; Sep.; Sul.

Pulsation in epigastrium—*Asaf.;* Eucal.; *Hydr.;* Nat. m.; *Puls.;* Selen.; *Sep.*

Pulsation in rectum—Aloe.

Regurgitation of food—Æth.; *Alum.;* Am. m.; *Ant. c.;* Asaf.; *Carbo v.;* Cham.; Cinch.; Ferr. iod.; Ferr.; Graph.; Ign.; *Ipec.;* Merc.; Nat. p.; *Nux v.; Phos.; Puls.;* Quass.; *Sul.*

Salivation—Cycl.; Lob. infl.; *Merc.;* Nat. m.; Puls.; Sang. See Mouth.

Sweating—Carbo v.; Nat. m.; Nit. ac.; Sep.

Toothache—Cham.; Kali c.; Lyc.; Nat. c.; Nit. ac.

Vertigo—Bry.; Carbo v.; Cinch.; Cycl.; *Grat.;* Ign.; *Nux v.;* Puls.; Rhus t. See Head.

Waterbrash—*Abies n.;* Acet. ac.; *Ant. c.;* Ars.; Bism.; *Bry.;* Calc. c.; *Carbo v.;* Diosc.; Fagop.; Graph.; Hep.; Hydr.; Kali c.; Lact. ac.; *Lyc.;* Mag. m.; Nat. m.; Nit. ac.; *Nux v.;* Pod.; *Puls.;* Sep.; Sul.; Symphor.; Ver. a.

INFLAMMATION (gastritis): acute: Acon.; Agar. emet.; *Ant. t.; Ars.; Bell.;* Bism.; Bry.; Canth.; Ferr. p.; Hedeoma; *Hydr.;* Hyos.; *Ipec.;* Iris; *Kali bich.;* Kali chlor.; Merc. c.; *Nux v.;* Ox. ac.; *Phos.;* Puls.; Santon.; Sinap. a.; *Ver. a.;* Zinc.

Inflammation, acute, from alcoholic abuse—Arg. n.; *Ars.;* Bism.; Crot.; *Cupr.; Gaulth.;* Lach.; *Nux v.;* Phos.

Inflammation, acute, with intestinal involvement (gastro-enteritis): Alumen; *Arg. n.; Ars.; Bapt.;* Bism.; Bry.; *Cupr.;* Merc. c.; Merc.; *Rhus t.;* Santon.; Zinc.

Inflammation, chronic (catarrh of stomach)—Alum.; *Ant. c.; Ant. t.; Arg. n.;* Arn.; Ars.; *Bism.;* Calc. c.; Calc. chlor.; Caps.; Carb. ac.; *Carbo v.;* Cinch.; *Colch.;* Dig.; *Graph.; Hydr.;* Hydroc. ac.; Illic.; Iod.; Ipec.; *Kali bich.;* Kali c.; Lyc.; *Merc. c.; Nux v.;* Op.; Ox. ac.; *Phos.;* Pod.; *Puls.;* Rumex; Sang.; Sep.; Sil.; Sul.; Ver. a.; Zinc.

NAUSEA—(qualmishness): *Ant. c.; Ant. t.; Apoc.; Apomorph.; Arg. n.;* Arn.; Ars.; Asar.; Bell.; Berb. v.; Bism.; *Bry.; Cadm. s.;* Carb. ac.; *Carbo v.;* Card. m.; Cascar.; Cham.; Chel.; Chionanth.; *Cocc.; Colch.; Cupr. m.; Cycl.;* Dig.; Eug. j.; Fagop.; *Ferr. m.;* Glon.; Hedeoma; Hyper.; Ichth.; *Ipec.; Iris; Kali bich.; Kali c.;* Kal.; Kreos.; Lach.; Lact. ac.; *Lob. infl.;* Merc. c.; Merc. s.; *Morph.;* Nat. c.; Nat. m.; *Nux v.;* Ostrya; *Petrol.;* Pod.; *Puls.;* Sabad.; Sang.; Sarcol.; ac.; *Sep.;* Spig.; *Strych.; Symphor.; Tab.;* Ther.; *Ver. a.;* Ver. v.

Nausea after abdominal operations—Staph.

Nausea after eating—Am. c.; Asar.; Cycl.; Graph.; Nux v.; Puls.; Sil.

Nausea before breakfast—Berb. v.; Gossyp.; Nux v.; *Sep.*

Nausea from beer—Kali bich.

Nausea from closing eyes—Lach.; *Ther.;* Thuya.

Nausea from coffee—Cham.

Nausea from fat—Nit. ac.

Nausea from ices, cold—Ars.

Nausea from pessaries—Nux m.

Nausea from looking at moving objects—Asar.; Cocc.; Ipec.; Jabor.

Nausea from immersing hands in warm water—Phos.

Nausea from nervousness, emotional excitement—Menthol.

Nausea from pregnancy—Cocc.; Con.; *Lact. ac.;* Lac. v. c.; Lob. infl.; Mag. c.; *Mag. m.;* Phos. ac.; Piloc.; Sep.; *Staph.;* Strych.; Sul. See Female Sexual System.

Nausea from riding in cars, boat—Arn.; *Cocc.; Lac d.; Nux m.;* Nux v.; *Petrol.;* Sanic.; Ther.

Nausea from smell or sight of food—Æth.; Ars.; Cocc.; *Colch.;* Nux v.; Puls.; *Sep.;* Stann.; Symphor.

Nausea from smoking—Euphras.; Ign.; *Ipec.;* Nux v.; *Phos.;* Tab.

Nausea from sweets—Graph.

Nausea from water—Apoc.; Ars.; Ver. a.

Nausea from water, aerated, champagne—Digitox.

With cramps—Triost.

With desire for stool—Dulc.

With diarrhoea, anxiety—Ant. t.

With drowsiness—Apoc.

With faintness—*Bry.; Cocc.;* Colch.; Hep.; Nux v.; Plat.; *Puls.;* Tab.; Val.

With headache—*Aloe;* Formica; Puls.

With hunger—*Berb. aq.;* Cocc.; Ign.; Val.

With menses—*Cocc.;* Crot.; Symphor.

With pain, coldness—Cadm. s.; Hep.

With pale, twitching face, no relief from vomiting—Ipec.

With pressure downward, in intestines—Agn.

With relief from eating—*Lact. ac.;* Mez.; Santon.; *Sep.;* Vip. op.

With relief from lemonade—Cycl.; Puls.

With relief from lying down—Echin.; *Kali c.;* Puls.

With relief from smoking—Eug. j.

With relief from swallow of cold water—Cupr. m.

With relief from uncovering abdomen; in open air—Tab.

With salivation—*Ipec.;* Petrol.; Sang.

With vertigo—*Cocc.;* Hyos.; Lach.; Puls.; Tab.; *Ther.*

With vision dim—Myg.

With weakness, anxiety, recurs periodically—Ars.

Worse after eating—Asar.; Bcrb. aq.; Dig.; *Ipec.; Nux v.;* Puls.

Worse from least sound or noise—Ther.

Worse from motion, rising—Ars.; *Bry.;* Cocc.; Symphor.; *Tab.;* Triost.; Ver. a.

Worse in morning—Anac.; Calc. c.; Fagop.; Carbo v.; *Graph.;* Lact. ac.; Nat. c.; *Nux v.;* Phos.; Puls.; *Sep.;* Sil.; Sul.

NERVOUS DISORDERS—*Agar.;* Bell.; Col.; *Mag. p.;* Nux v.; Sang. See Pain.

PAIN (gastrodynia): Type: Aching:—Æsc.; Anac.; *Hydr.;* Ruta.

Burning, as from ulcer—*Acct. ac.;* Agar. emet.; *Arg. n.;* Arn.; *Ars.;* Asaf.; Bism.; Cadm. br.; Canth.; *Carbo v.; Chin. ars.;* Colch.; *Condur.;* Con.; Datura; Formica; Graph.; *Iod.;* Iris; Kali iod.; Laburn.; Lact. ac.; Lapis alb.; Mancin.; Nat. m.; *Nux v.; Ox. ac.; Phos.;* Robin.; Sep.; *Sul.;* Uran. See Sensations.

Crampy, contractive, colicky, drawing—*Abies n.;* Act. sp.; *Agar. ph.; Arg. n.;* Bapt.; *Bell.; Bism.;* But. ac.; Cact.; Calc. c.; Calc. iod.; *Carbo v.; Cham.;* Cocaine; *Cocc.; Col.;* Con.; Cupr. m.; Datura; Granat.; *Graph.; Ign.;* Ipec.; Jatropha; Kali c.; Lob. infl.; *Mag. p.; Nux v.;* Petrol.; Phos.; Plat.; Ptel.; Sep.; Ver. v. See Sensations.

Cutting, lancinating, stitching, spasmodic, paroxysmal, darting, tearing, shooting—Acon.; Act. sp.; *Arg. n.; Atrop.; Bell.;* Bism.; *Bry.;* Carbo v.; Card. m.; Caust.; *Chin. ars.; Col.;* Con.; *Cupressus; Cupr. ac.;* Cupr. m.; *Diosc.;* Hydr.; Ign.; Iris; Kali c.; *Mag. p.; Nux v.;* Ox. ac.; Ratanh.; Sep.; Sul.; Thall.

Epigastric (pit of stomach)—*Abies c.; Abies n.;* Act. sp.; Æsc.; Aloe; Am. m.; Anac.; *Arg. n.;* Arn.; Ars.; Bar. m.; *Bell.;* Bism.; *Bry.;* Calc. c.; Calc. iod.; Carb. ac.; Carbo v.; Cina; Col.; Cupr. ; *Diosc.;* Graph.; *Hydr.;* Jatropha; Kali bich.; Kali c.; Kal.; Lob. infl.; Lyc.; Nat. m.; *Nux v.;* Ox. ac.; Paraf.; *Phos.; Sep.;* Sang.; Ver. a.

Gnawing, hungry-like—*Abies c.;* Abrot.; Æsc.; *Agar.;* Am. m.; *Anac.; Arg. n.;* Asar.; *Cina;* Ign.; *Iod.;* Lach.; Phos.; *Puls.;* Ruta; Sep.; *Uran.* See Sensations.

Neuralgic (gastralgia)—Abies n.; Acet. ac.; Æsc.; Alum.; Anac.; *Arg. n.;* Ars.; Atrop. · Bell.; Bism.; *Bry.; Carbo v.;* Chel.; Cham.; *Chin. ars.;*

Cina; *Cocc.*; Cod.; Colch.; *Col.*; Condur.; *Cupr. ars.*; Dig.; *Diosc.*;
Ferr. m.; Gels.; Glon.; *Graph.*; *Hydroc. ac.*; Ign.; *Ipec.*; Kali c.; Lob.
infl.; *Mag. p.*; Menthol; Niccol.; Nux m.; *Nux v.*; *Ox. ac.*; Petrol.;
Plumb.; Ptel.; Puls.; Quass.; Rham. c.; Ruta; Spig.; Stann.; *Strych.*;
Sul. ac.; Tab.; *Ver. a.*; Zinc.

Concomitants to gastralgia—With anemia—*Ferr.*; Glon.; Graph.

With backache, anxiety, despondency, sallow face—Nit. ac.

With chronic gastritis—Alum.; Atrop.; Bism.; Lyc.

With chronic ulcer—Arg. n.

With constipation—Bry.; Graph.; Nux v.; Physost.; *Plumb.*

With extension to sides, then to back—Cochlear.

With extension to shoulders—Niccol.

With gout—Colch.; Urt.

With hysteria—Asaf.; Ign.; Plat.

With lactation—Carbo v.; Cinch.

With menses—Arg. n.; Cocc.

With nervous depression—Arg. n.; Gaulth.; *Nux v.*

With pain in throat and spine alternately—Paraf.

With pregnancy—Petrol.

With recurrence—Graph.

With uterine disorder—Bor.

Sickening pain—Ostrya.

MODALITIES TO PAIN—Aggravation: At night: Anac.; Arg. n.; Ars.;
Cham.; Cocc.; Ign.; Kali bich.

From beer—Bapt.; *Kali bich.*

From bending forward—Kal.

From coffee—Canth.; Cham.; Nux v.; Ox. ac.

From empty stomach—*Anac.*; Cina; Hydroc. ac.; *Petrol.*

From food—*Arg. n.*; Bell.; *Bry.*; Ign.; Kali bich.; *Nux v.*

From food, warm—Bar. c.

From jar—Aloe; *Bell.*; Bry.

From nursing—Æth.

From pressure—Arg. n.; Calc. c.; Cochlear.; Ign.

From touch—Bell.; Ign.; Nux v.; *Ox. ac.*

From walking, descending stairs—Bry.

From water, cold—Calc. c.

From worms—*Cina;* Granat.

AMELIORATION—From bending backward, standing erect: Bell.; *Diosc.*

From drinks, cold—Bism.

From drinks, warm—Graph.; Ver. v.

From eating—*Anac.*; Brom.; Calc. p.; *Chel.*; Graph.; *Hep.*; Homar.;
Hydroc. ac.; Ign.; *Iod.*; Kreos.; Lach.; Nat. m.; *Petrol.*; Puls.; Sep.

From ice cream—Phos.

From pressure—Bry.; Fluor ac.; *Plumb.*

From sitting erect—Kal.

From vomiting—Hyos.; Plumb. m.

PYLORUS—Constriction—Can. ind.; *Cinch.*; Hep.; *Nux v.*; *Phos.*; Ornithog.; Sil.

Induration—Bism.; *Condur.;* Graph.; *Phos.;* Sep.; *Strych. p.*

Pain—Canth.; Cepa; *Hep.;* Lyc.; Merc.; *Ornithog.;* Tussil.; *Uran.* See Constriction.

SENSATION—**Anxiety:** Ars.; Kali c.; Nit. ac.; Phos.; Ver. a.

As if stomach were full of dry food—Calad.

As if stomach were pressed against spine—Arn.

As if stomach were swimming in water—Abrot.

Burning heat—Abies c.; Acet. ac.; *Acon.; Agar.;* Arg. n.; *Ars.;* Bism.; Calopt.; *Canth.;* Carb. ac.; *Carbo v.;* Caust.; Colch.; Col.; Ferr. m.; Glycerin; Graph.; Hep.; *Iris; Lact. ac.;* Merc. c.; Nat. m.; *Phos.;* Sang.; Sep.; *Sul.;* Tereb.

Coldness—Abrot.; Bov.; Calc. c.; Calc. sil.; *Camph.;* Cinch.; *Colch.;* Elaps; Hippom.; Kali c.; Kreos.; *Menyanth.;* Ol. an.; Ox. ac.; Pyrus; Sabad.; *Sul. ac.;* Tab.; *Ver. a.*

Distended, drumlike, tightness, clothing intolerable—*Abies c.;* Absinth.; Agar.; *Ambra; Anac.;* Ant. c.; *Apoc.;* Arg. n.; Ars.; Asaf.; But. ac.; *Cajup.; Calc. c.;* Calc. fl.; Calc. iod.; Calc. p.; Caps.; *Carb. ac.; Carbo v.;* Cham.; *Chel.; Cinch.;* Cocc.; *Colch.; Diosc.;* Euonym.; Fel tauri; Ferr. m.; *Graph.;* Grat.; Ign.; *Kali c.; Lach.;* Lecith.; Lob. infl.; *Lyc.;* Merc. c.; Mosch.; Nat. cholein; Nat. m.; Nit. ac.; *Nux m.; Nux v.;* Ornithog.; Pop. tr.; *Puls.;* Sul.

Empty, faint, sinking, "all gone" feeling—*Abies c.;* Anac.; Apoc.; Asaf.; Bapt.; *Bar. mur.;* Caps.; Carbo an.; *Carbo v.; Cim.;* Cocc.; *Dig.; Diosc.;* Gels.; Graph.; *Hydr.;* Hydroc. ac.; *Ign.;* Kali c.; Kali p.; Lac c.; Latrod.; *Lob. infl.;* Lyc.; *Merc. s.;* Morph.; *Murex;* Ornithog.; Petrol.; *Phos.;* Ptel.; *Puls.;* Radium; Sang.; Sep.; Stann.; *Sul.; Tab.;* Tellur.; Thea; Thuya; Trill.; Vib. op.

Empty feeling, aggravated 11 a. m., unable to wait for lunch—*Sul.;* Zinc. m.

Empty feeling, relieved by eating—*Anac.; Chel.;* Iod.; Nat. c.; Mur.; Phos.; *Sep.;* Sul.

Empty feeling, relieved by lying down, wine—Sep.

Heaviness, pressure, as from stone or lump—*Abies n.;* Acon.; *Arg. n.;* Arn.; *Ars.;* Bism.; *Bry.; Calc. c.; Carbo v.;* Cham.; *Cinch.;* Colch.; Dig.; Ferr. m.; *Graph.; Kali bich.;* Kali c.; Lob. infl.; *Lyc.; Nux v.;* Passifl.; *Phos.;* Piloc.; *Puls.;* Robin.; Sang.; Sep.; Spig.; *Sul.;* Xerophyl.; Zing.

Pulsations, throbbing—*Arg. n.;* Asaf.; *Cact.;* Cic.; *Crot.;* Eucal.; *Hydr.;* Iod.; *Kali c.;* Kali iod.; Lach.; *Nat. m.;* Oleand.; *Puls.;* Rheum.

Relaxed, hanging down feeling—Agar.; *Hydr.;* Ign.; *Ipec.; Staph.;* Sul. ac.; *Tab.*

Tenderness, to contact, pressure, jars—*Apis;* Arg. n.; Ars.; Bell.; Bov.; *Bry.; Calc. c.;* Calc. iod.; Canth.; Carbo v.; Card. m.; *Cinch.;* Colch.; Dig.; *Kali bich.;* Kali c.; *Lach.;* Lecith.; Lyc.; *Merc. c.; Merc. s.;* Nat. c.; Nat. m.; Nux m.; *Nux v.;* Phos.; Puls.; Sang.; Sil.; Spig.; Stann.; Sul.

Trembling—Arg. n.; Crot.

Softening (gastro-malacia)—Calc. c.; Kreos.; Merc. d.

THIRST—*Acet. ac.; Acon.;* Alfal.; Ant. c.; Ant. t.; Apoc.; Arn.; *Ars.;* Ars. iod.; Bell.; Berb. v.; Bism.; *Bry.;* Camph.; *Canth.; Caps.; Cham.;* Chin. ars.; Cinch.; Cocc.; *Colch.;* Crot.; Cupr. ars.; Dulc.; *Eup. perf.;* Helleb.; Helon.; Ichth.; Indol; Iod.; Kali br.; Lact. ac.; Laur.; Lecith.; Mag. c.; Mag. p.; Med.; Merc. c.; *Mcrc.;* Morph.; *Nat. m.;* Nux v.; Op.; Petros.; Phos. ac.; *Phos.;* Pod.; Rhus ar.; *Rhus t.;* Sang.; Scilla; Sec.; Sep.; Stram.; *Sul.;* Tereb.; Thuya; Uran. n.; *Ver. a.; Ver. v.*

Constant sipping of cold water—*Acon.;* Ant. t.; *Ars.;* Hyos.; Onosm.; Sanic.

Drinks seldom, but much--*Bry.;* Helleb.; Pod.; *Sul.;* Ver. a.

Thirstlessness—*Æth.;* Ant. t.; *Apis;* Berb. v.; Cinch.; Coff.; Cycl.; *Gels.;* Helleb.; Menyanth.; Nux m.; *Puls.; Sabad.; Sars.*

ULCER OF STOMACH—*Arg. n.; Ars.; Atrop.;* Bell.; Bism.; Calc. ars.; Condur.; Crot.; Ferr. acet.; *Geran.;* Graph.; Grind.; Ham.; *Hydr.;* Iod.; Ipec.; *Kali bich.;* Kali iod.; Kreos.; Lyc.; *Merc. c.;* Merc.; Op.; *Ornithog.;* Petrol.; *Phos.;* Plumb. ac.; Ratanh.; Sinap. a.; Symphyt.; *Uran.*

VOMITING, retching—Remedies, in general: Abrot.; Acon.; *Æth.;* Agar. phal.; Alumen; Amyg. pers.; *Ant. c.; Ant. t.;* Apoc.; *Apomorph.; Arg. n.; Ars.;* Atrop.; *Bell.; Bism.;* Bor.; *Bry.;* Cadm. s.; Calc. c.; Calc. m.; Camph. monobr.; Can. ind.; Canth.; Caps.; *Carb. ac.;* Card. m.; Cascarilla; *Cerium;* Cham.; Chel.; Cinch.; *Cocc.; Colch.; Cupr. ac.; Cupr. ars.;* Cupr. m.; Dros.; Eup. perf.; *Ferr. m.;* Ferr. mur.; Ferr. p.; Gaulth.; Geran.; Granat.; Graph.; Iod.; *Ipec.; Iris;* Jatropha; *Kali bich.;* Kali ox.; *Kreos.;* Lach.; Lact. ac.; *Lob. infl.; Mag. c.;* Merc. c.; *Morph.;* Nat. m.; Nat. p.; *Nux v.; Op.;* Petrol.; *Phos.;* Pix l.; Plumb.; *Puls.;* Ricin. com.; Sang.; Sarcol. ac.; *Sep.;* Stann.; Strych. et. ferr. cit.; *Symphor.; Tab.;* Uran.; Val.; *Ver. a.;* Xerophyl.; Zinc.

CAUSE—Anger in nursing mother, affecting milk—Val.

Anger, with indignation—Cham.; Col.; Staph.

Beer—Cupr.; Ipec.; *Kali bich.*

Bowels impacted-Op.; Plumb.; Pyr.

Cancer (hepatic, gastric, uterine)—Carb. ac.; Kreos.

Cerebral—Apomorph.; Bell.; Glon.; Plumb. m.

Clearing throat of mucus in morning—Bry.; Euphras.

Climacteric—Aquil.

Closing eyes—Ther.

Cyclic, in infants—Cupr. ars.; Ingluv.; Iris; Kreos.; Merc. d.

Drinks, cold, can only retain hot drinks—Apoc.; *Ars.;* Ars. iod.; Calad.; Cascar.; *Chel.;* Ver. a.

Drinks of any kind—Acon.; Apoc.; Ant. t.; *Ars.; Bism.; Canth.;* Dulc.; *Eup. perf.;* Ipec.; Sanic.; Sil.; *Ver. a.*

Drinks, warm—*Bry.; Phos.; Puls.;* Pyr.; Sanic.

Drunkards in morning—Ant. t.; Ars.; Carb. ac.; *Cupr. ars;* Cupr m.; Ipec.; Lob. infl.; *Nux v.*

Eating, drinking—*Acet. ac.; Ant. c.;* Ant. t.; *Ars.;* Bism.; *Bry.;* Calc.

mur.; Cina; Colch.; Crot.; *Ferr. m.;* Ferr. p.; Hyos.; Iod.; *Ipec.;* Lyc.; Nux v.; *Phos.; Puls.;* Sil.; *Ver. a.;* Ver. v.

Eruptions repercussed—Cupr. m.

Gastric irritation—Ant. c.; *Ars.;* Bism.; Ferr. m.; Ipec.; Nux v.; Phos.; Puls.; Ver. a.

Hysterical—*Aquil.;* Ign.; *Kreos.;* Plat.; Val.

Lying on any side, except right—Ant. t.

Lying on right side or back—Crot.

Menses, after—Crot. See Female Sexual System.

Milk—*Æth.;* Ars.; Calc. c.; Ferr.; Kreos.; Mag. c.; Mag. m.; Merc. d.; Merc. s.

Motion—*Bry.; Cocc.; Colch.;* Dig.; Nux v.; *Tab.;* Ther.; *Ver. a.*

Phthisis—Kali br.; Kreos.

Post-operative (laparotomy)—Æth.; *Bism.; Cepa; Nux v.;* Phos.; Staph.; *Strych.*

Pregnancy—Acet. ac.; Alet.; *Amyg. pers.;* Ant. t.; *Apomorph.;* Ars ; Bism.; Carb. ac.; *Cerium;* Cocaine; *Cocc.; Cod.;* Cucurb.; *Cupr. ac.;* Ferr. m.; Gossyp.; Graph.; Ign.; Ingluv.; *Ipec.;* Iris; *Kreos.;* Lac d.; *Lact. ac.;* Lob. infl.; *Mag. c.; Nux v.;* Petrol.; Phos.; Psor.; Puls.; *Sep.;* Stront. br.; Strych.; Symphor.; *Tab.*

Pressure on spine and cervical region—Cim.

Raising head—Apomorph.; *Bry.;* Stram.

Reflex—Apomorph.; Cerium; Cocc.; *Ipec.;* Kreos.; *Val.*

Renal origin—Kreos.; Nux v.

Riding in cars—Arn.; *Cocc.;* Ipec.; Kreos.; Nux v.; Petrol.; Sanic.; Sil.

Scarlet fever—Ail.; *Bell.*

Sea-sickness; car sickness—*Apomorph.;* Ars.; Bor.; Carb. ac.; Cerium; Cocc.: Coff.; Glon.; Ipec.; *Kreos.;* Nicot.; *Nux v.;* Op.; *Petrol.;* Sep.: *Staph.;* Tab.; Ther.

Water, sight of, must close eyes while bathing—Lyssin; Phos.

TYPE—Acid, sour: Ant c.; Ars.; Bry.; Calad.; *Calc. c.;* Card. m.; *Cham.;* *Ferr. m.;* Ferr. p.; Iod.; *Iris;* Kali c.; Lac d.; Lact. ac.; *Lyc.;* Mag. c.; *Nat. p.; Nat. s.; Nux v.;* Puls.; *Robin.;* Sul.; Sul. ac.

Bilious (green, yellow)—*Acon.;* Æth.; Ant. c.: Ant. t.; Ars.; Bell.; *Bry.;* Carb. ac.; *Card. m.; Cham.; Chel.;* Crot.; Eup. arom.; *Eup. perf.;* Grat.; Ipec.; *Iris;* Kali c.; Lept.; Nux v.; Nyctanth.; Petrol.; *Pod.;* Puls.; Robin.; *Sang.;* Sep.; Tart. ac.

Black—*Ars.; Cadm. s.; Crot.;* Mancin; Pix l.

Bloody—*Acon.;* Arg. n.; *Ars.;* Bothrops; Cadm. s.; *Canth.;* Crot.; Ferr. m.; *Ferr. p.;* Ficcus; *Geran.; Ham.; Ipec.;* Iris; Mez.; *Phos.; Sec.* See Hemetemesis.

Coffee-grounds, like—*Ars.;* Cadm. s.; *Crot.;* Lach.; *Merc. c.;* Ornithog.; Pyr.; Sec.

Fecal—Op.; Plumb.; Pyr.; Raph.

Food, undigested—*Ant. c.;* Apoc.; Atrop.; Bals. per.; Bism.; *Bry.;* Cerium; *Cinch.;* Colch.; Cupr.; *Ferr. m.;* Ferr. mur.; Ferr. p.; Graph.; *Ipec.;* Iris; Kreos.; Lac c.; Nux v.; Petrol.; Phos.; *Puls.;* Sang.; Strych. ferr. cit.; Ver. a.

Milk, coagula—*Æth.;* Ant. c.; *Calc. c.;* Ipec.; *Mag. c.;* Mag. m.; Merc. d.; Merc.; Pod.; Sanic.; *Val.*

Mucus slimy—Æth.; Ant. c.; *Ant. t.;* *Arg. n.;* Ars.; Bals. per.; Cadm. s.; Carbo v.; Colch.; *Ipec.;* Iris; Jatropha; *Kali bich.;* Kali m.; Kreos ; Merc. c.; Nux v.; Ox. ac.; Petrol.; *Puls.;* Ver. a.; Zinc.

Watery—Abrot.; *Ars.;* Bism.; Bry.; *Euphorbia;* Euphorb. cor.; Iod.; Iris; *Kreos.;* Lac c.; *Mag. c.;* Oleand.; Ver. a.

Yeast, like—Nat. c.; Nat. s.

CONCOMITANTS—With abdominal rumbling—Pod.

With appetite—Iod.; Lob. infl.

With bowels obstructed, impacted–Op.; Plumb.; Pyr.

With chilliness—Ars.; Dulc.; Puls.; Tab.

With cholera—*Ars.;* Camph. See Abdomen.

With chronic tendency—Lob. infl.

With clavus, fickle appetite, salivation, copious lemon colored urine—Ign.

With colic, cramps—Bism.; *Cupr. ars.;* *Cupr. m.;* Op.; Plumb.; Pix l.; Sarrac.; *Ver. a.* See Abdomen.

With collapse, weakness—Æth.; *Ant. t.;* Ars.; Cadm. s.; Crotal.; Euphorb. cor.; *Lob. infl.;* *Tab.;* *Ver. a.;* Ver. v.

With constipation—Nux v.; Op.; Plumb.

With depression of spirits—Nux v.

With diarrhoea—Ars.; Bism.; Calc. c.; Cham.; *Cupr. ars.;* Curp. m.; *Ipec.;* Iris; Kreos.; Merc. c.; Phos.; Pulex; Puls.; Resorc.; *Ver. a.* See Abdomen.

With drowsiness—*Æth.;* *Ant. t.;* Ipec.; Mag. c.

With fear, heat, thirst, profuse urine and sweat—Acon.

With fruitless, anxious retching—Ars.; Bism.; Cupr.; Pod.

With headache—Apomorph.; Iris; Petrol. See Head.

With heart, weak—Ars.; Camph.; *Dig.*

With intervals of days between attacks—Bism.

With midnight occurrence; can eat at once after emptying stomach—Ferr. m.

With nausea—Æth.; Amyg. pers.; Ant. t.; Bry.; *Ipec.;* Iris; *Lob. infl.;* *Nux v.;* Petrol.; *Puls.;* Sang.; Symphor.; Ver. a. See Nausea.

With relief of symptoms—Ant. t.; Puls.

With relief from eating, drinking—Anac.; Tab.

With relief from cold drinks—Cupr.; *Phos.;* Puls.

With relief from hot drinks—Ars.; Chel.

With relief from lying down—Bry.; Colch.; Nux v.; Symphor.

With relief from lying on right side—Ant. t.

With relief from uncovering abdomen; in fresh open air—Tab.

With salivation—Graph.; Ign.; *Ipec.;* Iris; Kreos.; Lact. ac.; *Lob. infl.;* Puls.; Tab.

With spasms—*Cupr. m.;* Hyos.; Op.

With tongue clean—Cina; Dig.; *Ipec.*

With vertigo—Cocc.; Ign.; *Nux v.;* *Tab.*

ABDOMEN

APPENDICITIS. See Typhlitis.

BURNING heat—Abies c.; *Acon.;* *Aloe;* Alston.; Ant. c.; *Apis;* Arg. n.; *Ars.;* *Bell.;* Bry.; Camph.; *Canth.;* Carbo v.; Colch.; Crot.; *Iris;* Kali bich.; *Limul.;* Lyc.; *Merc. c.;* Nat. s.; Nux v.; *Ox. ac.;* Phos. ac.; *Phos.;* Pod.; Rhus t.; Sang.; Sec.; Sep.; Sul.; Ver. a.

CÆCUM, affections of—Ars.; *Lach.;* Rhus v.; Ver. v. See Appendicitis, typhlitis.

COLDNESS—*Æth.;* Ambra; Aur. m.; Cadm. s.; *Calc c.;* Camph.; Caps.; *Cinch;* Colch.; Elaps; Grat.; *Kali br.;* *Kali c.;* Lach.; *Menyanth.;* Phell; Phos.; Sec.; Sep.; *Tab.; Ver. a.*

COLIC—PAIN—Remedies in general: Acon.; Adren.; Aloe; Alum.; *Arg. n.;* Arn.; *Ars.;* Bar. c.; *Bell.;* Bry.; *Cajup.;* *Calc. p.;* Carb. ac.; Carbo v.; *Cham.;* Chin. ars.; Cic.; *Cina;* *Cinch.;* *Cocc.;* Coff.; Collins.; *Colch.;* Col.; Crot. t.; *Cupr. ac.;* *Cupr. m.;* Cycl.; Dig.; *Diosc.; Elat.;* Filix m.; *Gamb.;* Grat.; *Ign.;* Illic.; *Ipec.;* Iris ten.; *Iris; Jal.;* Lept.; *Limul.;* Lyc.; *Mag. c.; Mag. p.;* Mentha; *Merc. c.;* Merc.; *Morph.;* Nat. s.; *Nux v.;* Oniscus; *Op.;* Ox. ac.; Paraf.; *Plat.;* Plumb. ac.; Plumb. chrom.; *Plumb. m.;* Pod.; Polyg.; *Puls.;* Raph.; *Rheum; Rhus t.;* Sab.; Samb.; Sars.; *Senna;* Sep.; *Sil.; Sinap. n.; Stann.;* Staph.; Strych.; Thuya; *Ver. a.; Vib. op.;* Zinc. m.

CAUSE AND NATURE—Alternates with vertigo: Col.; Spig.

Babies' colic—Æth.; Asaf.; Bell.; Calc. p.; Cataria; Cepa; *Cham.; Cina;* Col.; *Illic.;* Jal.; Kali br.; Lyc.; *Mag. p.;* Mentha pip.; Nepeta; Rheum, Senna; Staph.

Biliary, gall-stone colic—Atrop.; Bell.; *Berb. v.;* Bry.; *Calc. c.;* Card. m.; Cham.; Chionanth.; *Cinch.;* Col.; Diosc.; Ipec.; Iris; Lyc.; Mentha; Morph. acet.; Pod.; Ricin.; Tereb.; Triost. See Gall Bladder.

Chronic tendency—Lyc.; Staph.

Flatulent colic—Absinth; Agar.; Alfal.; *Aloe;* Anis.; *Arg. n.;* Asaf.; *Bell.;* But. ac.; *Cajup.;* Calc. p.; Carbon. s.; *Carbo v.;* *Cham.;* Cina; *Cinch.; Cocc.;* Col.; *Diosc.;* Hydroc. ac.; *Illic.;* Ipec.; Iris; *Lyc.,* Mag. p.; Mentha; *Nux v.;* Op.; Plumb. m.; *Polygon.;* Puls.; Radium; Raph.; Robin.; Sang.; *Senna;* Zinc.

From anger—*Cham.;* Col.; Staph.

From carriage riding—Carbo v.; Cocc.

From cold—Acon.; Cepa; *Cham.;* Col.; Nux v.

From eating cheese—Col.

From eating cucumber salad—Cepa.

From gastric disorder—Carbo v.; *Cinch.;* Col.; Diosc.; Ipec.; Lyc.; *Nux v.; Puls.*

From lithotomy, ovariotomy, attending abdominal section—Bism.; Hep.; Nux v.; Raph.; *Staph.*

From uncovering—Nux v.; Rheum.

From wet feet—Cepa; Cham.; Dolichos; Dulc.

From worms—Artem.; Bism.; *Cina*; Filix m.; Granat.; *Indigo;* Merc. s.; Nat. p.; Sabad.; Spig.

Hemorrhoidal—Æsc.; Cepa; Col.; *Nux v.;* Puls.; Sul.

Hysterical—Alet.; *Asaf.;* Cajup.; Cocc.; *Ign.;* Val.

Menstrual—Bell.; Castor.; Cham.; *Cocc.;* Col.; *Puls.* See Female Sexual Organs.

Neuralgic, enteralgie—Alumen; Ant. t.; Ars.; *Atrop.; Bell.;* Cham.; *Cocc.; Col.;* Cupr. ars.; Cupr. m.; *Diosc.;* Euphorb.; Hydroc. ac.; Hyos.; Kali c.; *Mag. p.; Nux v.;* Op.; Plumb. ac.; *Plumb. m.;* Santon.; Tab.; Ver. a.; Zinc. m. See Type of Pain.

Renal—*Berb. v.;* Calc. c.; Diosc.; Eryng.; *Lyc.; Morph. acet.;* Occin.; Sars.; *Tab.; Tereb.* See Urinary System.

Rheumatic—Caust.; Col.; Diosc.; Phyt.; Ver. a.

Toxic (lead, copper)—Alumen; *Alum.;* Bell.; Ferr.; Nat. s.; Nux m.; Nux v.; *Op.;* Plat.; Sul.; Ver. a.

LOCATION—Abdominal muscles—Acon.; *Arn.;* Bell.; *Bellis ; Cupr. m.;* Ham.; Mag. m.; Nat. nit.; Plumb. m.; *Rhus t.;* Strych.; Sul.

Abdominal ring—*Cocc.;* Graph.; Mez.; *Nat. m.;* Nux v.; Stront.

Ascending colon—Rhus t.

Groins—Alum.; Am. m.; Merc. c.; Pod.

Hypochondria—Carbo v.; *Cinch.;* Diosc.; *Nux v.;* Pyrus; Sep. See Type of Pain.

Hypogastrium—*Aloe; Bell.;* Bism.; Cepa; Cocc.; *Diosc.;* Eucal.; Ham.; Kali c.; *Lyc.;* Mag. c.; *Nux v.;* Pall.; Paraf.; Plat.; *Sab.;* Sep.; Sul.; Tromb.; Ver. v. See Sexual System.

Ileo-caecal—Aloe; Bell.; Bry.; Coff.; Ferr. p.; *Gamb.;* Iris ten.; Kali m.; Limul.; Mag. c.; *Merc. c.; Merc. s.;* Plumb.; Radium; Rhus t. See Appendicitis.

Inguinal—Am. m.; Ars.; Calc. c.; Graph.; Sep.

In small spots—Bry.; Col.; *Ox. ac.*

Transverse colon—*Bell.;* Cham.; Colch.; Merc. c.; Raph.

Umbilical (about navel)—*Aloe; Ben . ac.;* Berb. v.; *Bov.; Bry.;* Calc. p.; Carbo v.; *Cham.;* Chel.; *Cina;* Col.; *Diosc.; Dulc.; Gamb.; Granat.;* Hyper.; Indigo; *Kali bich.; Ipec.;* Lept.; Lyc.; *Nux m.;* Nux v.; Pelias; Plat.; *Plumb.;* Puls.; Raph.; *Rheum;* Senec.; *Spig.; Stann.;* Sul.; *Ver. a.;* Verbasc.

TYPE OF PAIN—Bruised: Æth.; Allium s.; *Apis;* Apoc.; *Arn.;* Ars.; *Bellis;* Bry.; Carbo v.; Col.; *Con.;* Eucal.; Ferr. m.; *Ham.; Merc. c.;* Nat. s.; Nit. ac.; *Nux v.;* Phyt.; Puls.; *Sul.*

Colicky, crampy, constricting, cutting, griping, pinching—Acon.; *Æsc.;* Agar.; *Aloe;* Ant. t.; Argem. mex.; Arg. cy.; *Arg. n.;* Arn.; Asaf.; *Bell.;* Bism.; Bry.; *Calc. p.;* Cataria; *Cham.; Cina; Cinch.; Cocc.; Col.; Colch.;* Con.; Crot. t.; *Cupr. ars.;* Cupr. m.; *Diosc.; Dulc.; Elat.;* Eup. perf.; Filix m.; *Gamb.;* Grat.; *Hyper.;* Ign.; Iod.; *Ipec.;* Iris; *Jal.; Jatropha;* Kali bich.; Kali c.; Lach.; Lept.; *Lyc.; Mag. c.; Mag. p.; Merc. c.;* Nat. s.; Niccol.; Nit. ac.; *Nux v.;* Phos.; Phyt.; *Plumb. ac.;* Plumb. chrom.; *Polyg.;* Puls.; Radium; Raph.; *Rheum;* Sab.;

Sec.; *Sep.;* Spig.; *Stann.;* Strych.; Sul ; Tromb.; *Ver. a.;* Vib. op.: Zinc.

Pressing, plug-like—*Aloe;* Alum.; *Anac.; Bell.;* Bry.; *Cocc.;* Hyos.: Kali c ; Mez.; *Nux v.;* Œnoth.; *Plat.;* Plumb. m.; Puls.; Ran s.; Sab ; *Sep.*

Pulsating, bubbling—Æth ; *Aloe;* Bar. m.; *Bell.:* Berb *v.:* Calc. c.; Ign.; Sang ; Selen ; Tarax.

Radiating, shooting, darting, tearing, spasmodic—*Acon.;* Argem. mex.; *Bell.; Bry.;* Calc. c.: *Cham.; Cocc.;* Cochlear ; *Col ;* Cupr. ac.; *Cupr. ars ; Diosc.;* Graph.; Ipec.; Kali c.; *Lyc.; Mag. p.:* Merc.; Morph.; *Nux v.;* Ox. ac.; Paraf ; Plat.; *Plumb.;* Pod.; *Puls.; Sul.* See Enteralgia.

Stitching—Agar.; Apis; Arn.; *Bell.; Bry.:* Chin ars.; Hep.; *Kali c.;* Lach.; Spig.

CONCOMITANTS—Abdomen retracted, as if drawn by string—Chel.; *Plumb. m.;* Pod ; Tab.

Abdomen, retracted, tense, scanty urine, desire to stretch—Plumb. m.

Abdomen swollen, pad-like—*Bell.,* Raph.

Agitation, chill ascending from hypogastrium to cheeks—Col.

Alternates with coryza—Calc. c

Alternates with delirium and pain in atrophied limbs—Plumb. m.

Alternates with vertigo—Col ; Spig.

Backache—Cham.; *Lyc.;* Morph.; Puls.; Samb.

Cheeks red, hot sweat—Cham.

Chilliness—Nux v.; Puls.

Collapse—Æth.; Camph.; Cupr.; *Ver. a.*

Constipation—Allium s.; *Aloe; Alum.;* Cocc.; Collins.; Grat.; Lyc.; *Nux v.;* Op.; *Plumb. ac.;* Sil.

Convulsions—Bell.; Cic.

Cramps in calves—Col.; *Cupr. ac.;* Plumb. m ; Pod.

Delirium alternating—Plumb. m

Diarrhoea—Ars.; Cham.; *Col.;* Mag. c.; Polyg.; Puls., Samb.; Ver. a.

Empty feeling, heat, faintness—*Cocc.;* Hydr.

Hands yellow, blue nails—Sil.

Hiccough, suffocative, in chest and stomach—Ver. a.

Hunger, yet refuses food—Bar. c.

Itching of nose, pale, bluish face—*Cina;* Filix m.

Nausea, frequent, watery, slimy stools—Cham.; Samb.

Pain and aching in thighs—Col.

Painful contraction in limbs following—Abrot.

Periodical recurrence—Aran.; *Cinch.;* Diosc.; Illic.; Kali br.

Pulsation in abdominal aorta, epigastric constriction—Dig.

Red urine—Bov.; *Lyc.*

Restlessness, twitching and turning for relief—Col.

Rumbling of flatus, nausea, liquid feces—Polyg.

Scanty stools, flatus without relief—Cina.

Sour stools—Rheum.

Tenesmus (pelvic)—Staph.

Tossing about, anxiety, no relief from flatus—*Cham.;* Mag. p.

Urging to stool—*Aloe;* Cinch.; Lept.; Nat. s.; *Nux v.;* Op.

Urine suppressed—Acon.; Plumb. ac.

Vomiting—*Bell.;* Cadm. s.; Plumb. ac.

Vomiting, hiccough, belching, screaming—Hyos.

Yawning, spasmodic, drowsiness—Spiranth.

MODALITIES—Aggravation: About 4-5 P. M.: Col.; Kali br.; *Lyc.*

After midnight—*Ars.;* Cocc.

At night, after supper—Grat.

At night—Cham.; Cinch.; Cocc.; Senna; Sul.

From bending, coughing—Ars.; Bell.; *Bry.;* Nat. m.

From bending forward—Ant. t.; *Diosc.;* Sinap. n.

From bending forward, lying down, pressure—Acon.; *Diosc.*

From drinking—Col.; Sul.

From drinking cold water—Cupr. m.

From eating—Bar. c.; *Calc. p.;* Cinch.; *Col.;* Kali bich.; *Nux v.; Psor.;* Zinc.

From jar, pressure—Acon.; Aloe; *Bell.;* Plumb.

From motion, relief from lying on side—Bry.; Cocc.

From smoking—Menyanth.

From sweets—Filix m.

From touch, pressure, motion—Bry.

From uncovering arm, leg; standing—Rheum.

From warmth, at night—Cham.

AMELIORATION—From bending double—Bov.; Cinch.; *Col.; Mag. p.;* Pod.; Sep.; *Stann.;* Sul.; Ver. a.

From eating—Bov.; Homar.

From flatus voided per ano—Aloe; *Carbo v.;* Cinch.; Cocc.; *Col.;* Nat. s.; Sul.

From hot applications or warmth—Ars.; Col.; *Mag. p.;* Pod.; Puls.; Sil.

From lying with knees drawn up—Lach.

From pressure—*Col.; Mag. p.;* Nit. ac.; Plumb.; Rhus t.; *Stann.*

From rubbing—Plumb. m.

From rubbing, warmth—Mag. p.

From sitting erect—Sinap. n.

From sitting, lying down—Nux v.

From stool—Aloe; Col.; Tanac.; Ver. a.

From straightening body backward or moving about—Diosc.

From walking about—Cepa; Diosc.; Mag. p.; Puls.; *Rhus t.;* Ver. a.

From walking bent over—Aloe; *Col.;* Nux v.; Rhus t.

From warm soup—Acon.

FLATULENT—Distention, fulness, heaviness, meteorism, tympanites—*Abies n.; Abrot.;* Absinth.; *Acet. ac.;* Acon.; Agar.; Alfal.; *Aloe;* Ant. c.; Apis; *Arg. n.;* Ars.; *Asaf.;* Bar. c.; *Bell.;* Bov.; *Cajup.; Calc. c.;* Calc. iod.; Carb. ac.; *Carbo v.; Cham.;* Chel.; Cina; *Cinch.; Cocc.; Colch.;* Collins.; *Col.;* Cupr. m.; *Diosc.;* Graph.; Ign.; *Illic.;* Indol; Iris; *Kali c.; Lach.; Limul.; Lyc.; Mag. c.; Mag. p.;* Merc. c.; Merc.; Momord.; Mosch.; Mur. ac.; Naph.; Nat. c.; *Nat. n't.;* Nat. m.; *Nat.*

s.; *Nux m.; Nux v.;* Oniscus; *Op.; Opuntia; Ornithog.; Phos. ac.;* Pod.; *Poth.; Puls.;* Radium; *Raph.;* Rheum; Rhod.; *Rhus gl.;* Rhus t.; Sars.; *Senna; Sep.; Sil.;* Stront. c.; Sul.; Sumb.; *Tarax.; Tereb.;* Thea; *Thuya;* Uran. n.; Val.; Xanth.; Zing.

Flatulence, hysterical—Alet.; *Ambra;* Arg. n.; *Asaf.;* Cajup.; Cham.; Cocc.; *Ign.;* Kali p.; *Nux m.;* Plat.; Poth.; *Sumb.;* Tarax.; Thea; *Val.*

Flatulence, incarcerated in flexures—Am. c.; Aur.; Bell.; Calc. c.; Calc. p.; Carb. ac.; *Carbo v.; Cham.; Cinch.;* Colch.; *Col.; Graph.;* Hep.; Ign ; Kali c.; Limul.; *Lyc.; Momord.;* Nux v.; Pall.; Phos.; Plumb. m.; Puls.; *Raph.;* Rhus gl.; Robin.; Staph.; Sul.; Thuya.

Flatulence, offensive, per ano—*Aloe;* Arn.; Bry.; *Carbo v.;* Ferr. magnet.; Graph ; Oleand.; Sil.

Flatulence, post operative, no relief from passing it—Cinch.

Gurgling, rumbling, borborygmus—*Aloe;* Apoc.; Ars.; Bapt.; Bell.; Carbon. s ; Carbo v.; *Cham.;* Cina; *Cinch.; Colch.;* Col.; Conv.; Cupr. ars.; Crot. t.; *Diosc.; Gamb.;* Glycerin; *Graph.;* Grat.; Hep.; Ipec.; *Jatropha;* Kali c.; *Lyc.;* Merc.; *Nat. s.;* Nux v.; Oleand.; *Phos. ac.;* Pod.; Puls.; Ricin. com.; *Rumex;* Sanic.; Sep.; Sil.; Thea; Xerophyl.

Hardness—Abrot.; Anac.; *Bar. c.; Calc. c.;* Carbo v.; *Cina;* Cinch.; Cupr.; *Graph.; Lyc.;* Nat. c.; Nux v.; Op.; *Plumb. ac.; Raph.; Sil.;* Sul.; Thuya.

Jumping, as of living thing—Arundo; Brachygl.; Branca; *Croc.;* Cycl.; Nux m.; *Op.;* Sabad ; Sul.; *Thuya.*

Large, in girls at puberty—Calc. c.; *Graph.;* Lach.; Sul.

Large, pendulous in women who have borne many children—Aur. m.; Aur. mur.; Bell.; Frax. am.; *Helon.;* Phos.; *Sep.*

Large, pot-bellied, flabby—Am. m.; *Calc. c.; Calc. p.;* Mez.; Pod.; Sanic.; Sars ; *Sep.; Sil.;* Sul.; Thuya.

Large, protrudes here and there—Croc.; Nux m.; Sul.; Thuya.

Retracted, sunken, scow-shaped—*Calc p.;* Euphorb.; Iodof.; Kali bich.; *Kali br.; Plumb. ac.;* Plumb. chrom.; *Plumb. m.;* Pod.; Ptel.; Quass.; *Zinc.*

Sensitive, tender to touch, pressure—Acet. ac.; Acon.; Aloe; *Apis; Arg n.; Arn.;* Ars.; Bapt.; *Bell.; Bov.; Bry.;* Calc. c.; *Carbo v.;* Card. m.; Cinch.; Coff.; Col.; Con ; Cupr. m.; Euonym.; Ferr. m.; Gamb.; *Graph.; Ham.;* Hedeoma; Helleb.; Kali bich.; *Lach.; Lyc.; Merc. c.;* Mur. ac.; Nux v.; Pod.; *Ran. b.;* Rhus t.; *Sep.;* Sil.; *Sumb.;* Sul.; *Tereb.; Ver. a.;* Vib. op.

Spots, brown—Caul.; *Lyc.;* Phos.; *Sep.;* Thuya.

Spots, red—Hyos. See Skin.

Trembling in—Lil. t.

Weak, as if diarrhœa would ensue—*Aloe;* Ant. c.; Apium gr.; Bor.; Crot. t.; Eucal.; Ferr. m.; Formica; Nux v.; *Opuntia;* Ran. s. See Diarrhœa.

Weak, empty, sinking, relaxed feeling—Abrot.; Acet. ac.; *Arn.;* Alston.; Ant. c.; Cham.; *Cocc.;* Euphorb.; Glycerin; *Hydr.; Ign.; Opuntia;* Petrol.; Physost.; *Phos.;* Plumb. ac.; *Pod.;* Quass.; *Sep.; Stann.;* Staph.; Sulphon.; Sul. ac.; *Ver. a.*

ANUS—RECTUM—Abscess (peri-rectal): Calc. s.; Rhus t.; Sil.

Burning, smarting, heat—Abies c.; *Æsc.; Aloe;* Alumen; Alum.; Ambra; Am. m.; Ant. c.; *Ars.;* Bell.; Berb. v.; *Canth.; Caps.; Carbo v.;* Cepa; Chenop. gl.; *Collins.;* Con.; Eucal.; Euonym.; *Gamb.;* Graph.; Ham.; Hydr.; *Iris;* Jugl. c.; Jugl. r.; Kali c.; Merc.; *Nat. m.;* Nit. ac.; *Oleand.;* Pæonia; Prun. sp.; *Ratanh.;* Rheum; Sang. n.; Senna; *Sul.;* Tromb.

Burning before and during stool—Aloe; Am. m.; Ars.; Col.; Con.; *Hydr.; Iris;* Jugl. c.; Merc.; Ol. an.; Rheum.

Burning after stool—Æsc.; Alumen; Am. m.; *Ars.;* Aur.; Berb. v.; *Canth.; Caps.; Carbo v.;* Chenop. gl.; *Gamb.; Nat. m.;* Nit. ac.; Ol. an.; *Pæonia;* Prun. sp.; *Ratanh.;* Sil.; *Stront.; Sul.*

Congestion—*Æsc.; Aloe;* Alum.; *Collins.;* Hyper.; Nat. m.; Nit. ac.; Sab.; *Sep.; Sul.*

ERUPTIONS, growths—Cancer, scirrhus of, also sigmoid; intolerable pains: Alumen; Phyt.; Spig.

Condylomata—Benz. ac.; Kali br.; *Nit. ac.; Thuya.*

Eczema—Berb. v.; Graph.; *Merc. pr. rub.* See Skin.

Eminences, studding interior—Polyg.

Fissures, rhagades, excoriations, ulcerations, soreness, rawness—*Æsc.;* Agn.; *Aloe;* Apis; Arg. n.; *Ars.; Calc. fl.; Carbo ɔ ;* Caust.; Cimex; *Condur.; Graph.;* Ham.; *Hydr.; Ign.;* Iris; Kali iod.; Lach.; Led.; *Merc. d ;* Merc.; Morph.; Mur. ac.; *Nat. m.; Nit. ac.;* Nit. mur. ac.; *Pæonia; Petrol.;* Phos.; Phyt.; Plat.; *Plumb.; Ratanh.;* Rhus t.; Sang. n.; Sanic.; *Sedum;* Sep.; *Sil.;* Sul.; Syph.; *Thuya;* Vib. op.

Fistula in ano—Aur. mur.; Bar. mur.; *Berb. v.; Calc. p.;* Calc. s.; Carbo v.; *Caust.; Fluor. ac.;* Graph.; Hydr.; Lach.; Myrist.; *Nit. ac.;* Nux v.; *Pæonia;* Phos.; Quercus; Ratanh.; *Sil.;* Sul.; Thuya.

Fistula in ano alternates with chest disorders—Berb. v.; Calc. p.; *Sil.*

Pockets—Polygon.

Rash, fiery red in babies—Med.

Hæmorrhage (enterrhagia)—Acal.; Acet. ac.; *Æsc.;* Aloe; *Alumen;* Alum.; Arn.; *Cact.; Carbo v.;* Cascar.; Cinch.; *Cinnam.;* Cob.; Cocaine; Crot.; Erig.; *Ham.;* Ign.; *Ipec.;* Kali c.; *Lach.;* Lycop.; Mangif. ind.; Merc. cy.; *Millef.; Mur. ac.;* Nat. m.; *Nit. ac.;* Phos. ac.; *Phos.;* Sedum; Sep.; Sul. ac.; Sul.; *Tereb.;* Thuya.

Haemorrhage during stool—*Alumen;* Alum.; Carbo v.; Ign.; Iod.; *Ipec.; Kali c.; Phos.;* Psor.; Sep.

Inflammation (proctitis)—*Æsc.; Aloe;* Alum.; Ambra; *Ant. c.;* Colch.; *Collins.;* Merc c.; *Merc.; Nit. ac.;* Pæonia; *Phos.; Pod.;* Ricin.; Sabal; Zing.

Inflammation, syphilitic—Bell.; Merc.; *Nit. ac.;* Sul.

Itching (pruritus)—Acon.; *Æsc.;* Aloe; *Alum.; Ambra; Anac.; Ant. c.; Bar. c.;* Bov.; Cadm. iod.; *Calc. c.;* Carbo v.; Cascar.; *Caust.; Cina; Collins.;* Cop.; *Ferr. iod.;* Ferr. m.; Granat.; Graph.; Homar.; *Ign.; Indigo; Lyc.; Med.; Nit. ac.; Pæonia;* Petrol.; Phos.; Pin. sylv.; Plat.; Polyg.; Radium; Ratanh.; Rumex; Sabad.; *Sacchar. ol.;* Sang. n.; Sep.; *Spig.;* Staph.; *Sul.;* Tellur.; Tereb.; *Teucr.;* Uran.; Zinc.

Moisture—Aloe; Am. m.; *Anac.; Ant. c.;* Bar. c; *Calc. c.; Carbo v.;*
Caust.; Graph.: *Hep.;* Med.; Nit. ac.; Nit. mur. ac.; Pæonia; Phos.;
Ratanh.; *Sep.; Sil ;* Sul. ac.

Operations on, to be given preceding—Collins.

PAIN—Aching—*Æsc.;* Alet ; Alumen; Collins ; Graph.; Lyc.; *Ratanh.*
Bearing down, pressing—*Aloe;* Alum ; Ars.; *Cact.;* Ceanoth.; Chenop.
gl ; Euphras.; Hyper.; Kali c.; Lach.; *Lil. t.;* Med.; Op.; Prun. sp.;
Sep ; Sul ; Sul. ac ; Xerophyl.

Contraction, spasmodic—*Æsc.* gl.; *Æsc.;* Anac.; Arg. n.; *Bell.;* Cact.;
Caust ; Collins; Ferr. m.; Grat.; Hydr.; *Ign.; Lach.;* Lyc.; *Med.;*
Meli.; Merc.; Mez.; *Nat m.; Nit. ac.;* Nit. mur. ac.; *Nux v.; Plumb.
ac.; Ratanh.;* Sanic.; *Sedum,* Sep ; *Syph.;* Tab.; Verbasc.

Lancinating, even after soft stool—*Alumen;* Nat. m.; *Nit. ac.; Ratanh.*

Long lasting, after stool—*Æsc.;* Aloe; Alumen; Am. m.; *Graph.; Hydr.;*
Ign.; Merc. cy.; *Mur. ac.; Nat. m.; Nit. ac.;* Pæonia; *Ratanh.; Sedum;*
Sep.; *Sil.;* Sul.; Thuya; Vib. op.

Neuralgic (proctalgia)—*Atrop.;* Bar. m.; *Bell.;* Colch.; *Crot. t.;* Ign.;
Kali c.; Lach.; Lyc.; Ox. ac.; Phos.; Plumb.; *Strych.;* Tar. h.

Splinter-like, pricking, stinging, stitching, cutting, shooting—Acon.; *Æsc.;*
Alum.; Am. m.; Bell.; Caust.; Cepa; *Collins.; Ign.; Kali c.; Lach.;*
Lyc.; Merc.; Mez ; *Nat. m.; Nit. ac.;* Plat ; *Ratanh.;* Ruta; *Sep.;*
Sil.; *Sul.;* Thuya.

Throbbing, pulsating—Aloe; *Bell.;* Caps.; Ham.; Lach.; *Meli.;* Merc.;
Nat. m.

PARETIC—Condition of rectum and sphincters—*Aloe;* Alum.; *Caust.; Erig.;*
Gels.; Graph.; Hyos.; Mur. ac.; Op.; Oxytr.; Phos. ac.; *Phos.;* Plumb.
m.; Sil.; Sulphon.; Tab.

Paretic condition of rectum, feels plugged—*Aloe; Anac.;* Can. ind.; Kali
bich.; Med.; Plat.; Plumb. m.; *Sep.;* Sul ac.

Paretic condition of rectum, with sense of insecurity of sphincters—*Aloe;*
Alum.; Apoc.; Erig.; Ferr. m.; *Nux v.;* Sanic.; Sec.

Patulous anus—*Apis; Phos.;* Sec.; Solan. t.

PROLAPSUS ANI—*Æsc. gl.; Æsc.; Aloe;* Ant. c.; Aral.; *Arn.; Bell.;*
Carbo v.; Caust.; Colch.; *Ferr. m.; Ferr. p.;* Gamb.; Ham.; Hydr.;
Ign.; Kali c.; Mag. p.; *Mur. ac.;* Nux v.; *Phos.;* Plumb.; *Pod.;* Poly-
por.; *Ruta; Sep.;* Solan. tub.; *Sul.;* Tab.; Tromb.

Prolapsus after confinement, stooping—Pod.; Ruta.

Prolapsus from debility—Pod.

Prolapsus from sneezing—Pod.

Prolapsus from straining, overlifting—Ign.; Nit. ac.; Pod.; Ruta.

Prolapsus from urinating—Mur. ac.

Prolapsus in children—Bell.; Ferr. m.; *Ferr. p.;* Ign.; Mur. ac.; Nux v ;
Pod.

Prolapsus, with diarrhæa, stool—*Æsc.; Aloe;* Carbo v.; Colch.; Crot. t.;
Fluor. ac.; *Gamb.;* Ham.; *Ign.;* Kali c.; Mur. ac.; *Pod.;* Phos.; *Ruta;*
Sul.

Prolapsus with piles, in alcoholics, leading sedentary life—Æsc. gl.

Prolapsus with stool, rectal spasm—Ign.

REDNESS—around—*Cham.;* Merc. cy.; Pæonia; *Sul.;* Zing. See Fissures. Proctitis.

Stricture—*Bell.;* Coff.; Hydr.; Ign.; *Nit. ac.;* Phos.; *Sil.;* Tab.; Thiosin. See Pain.

Torn, bleeding, after stool—Lac d.; *Nat. m.; Nit. ac.* See Fissures.

CATARRH—**Gastro-duodenal:** Card. m.; *Cinch.;* Hydr.; Sang. See Stomach.

CHOLERA—ASIATICA: *Acon.;* Agar. phal.; *Ars.;* Bell.; Bry.; *Camph.; Canth.; Carbo v.;* Chin. s.; Cic.; Colch.; *Cupr. ac.; Cupr. ars.; Cupr. m.;* Dig.; Euphorb. cor.; Guaco; *Hydroc. ac.; Ipec.;* Jatropha; Kali bich.; Lach.; Merc. c.; Naja; Nux v.; Op.; *Phos. ac.;* Phos.; Quass.; Rhus t.; *Sec.;* Sul.; Tab.; Tereb.; *Ver. a.;* Zinc. m.

CHOLERA INFANTUM—Summer complaint: *Acon.; Æth.;* Ant. t.; *Apis;* Arg. n.; *Ars.;* Bell.; *Bism.;* Bry.; Cadm. s.; Calc. ac.; *Calc. c.; Calc. p.;* Camph.; Camph. monobr.; Canth.; Cham.; Cinch.; Col.; Crot. t.; *Cuphea;* Cupr. ac.; *Cupr. ars.;* Cupr. m.; Elat.; *Euphorb. cor.;* Ferr. p.; Graph.; Hydroc. ac.; Indol; *Iodof.; Ipec.;* Iris; *Kali br.; Kreos.; Laur.;* Merc.; Nat. m.; Ox. ac.; Passifl.; Phos.; Phyt.; *Pod.;* Psor.; Resorc.; Sec.; Sep.; *Sil.;* Sul.; Tab.; *Ver. a.; Zinc. m.*

CHOLERA MORBUS—*Ant. t.; Ars.;* Bism.; Camph.; Chloral.; Colch.; Col.; *Crot. t.; Cupr. ars.;* Cupr. m.; Elat.; Grat.; Hydroc. ac.; *Ipec.;* Iris; Operc.; Op.; *Pod.;* Sec.; *Ver. a.*

CHOLERINE—Ant. c.; Ars.; *Crot. t.; Cupr. ars.;* Diosc.; Elat.; Euphorb. cor.; *Grat.; Ipec.;* Iris; *Jatropha;* Nuphar; *Phos. ac.;* Sec.; *Ver. a.*

CONSTIPATION—Remedies in general: *Abies n.;* Acon.; *Æsc. gl.; Æsc.;* Agar.; Alet.; *Aloe; Alumen; Alum.;* Am. c.; *Am. m.;* Anac.; Apis; *Arn.;* Asar.; Berb. v.; *Bry.; Calc. c.;* Calc. fl.; Carb. ac.; *Casc. sag.; Caust.;* Chel.; Chionanth.; Cinch.; Coca; *Collins.;* Croc.; *Dolichos;* Eug. j.; Euonym.; *Euphras.;* Fel tauri; Ferr. m.; Gels.; *Glycerin;* Graph.; *Grat.;* Guaiac.; Hep.; *Hydr.;* Ign.; *Iris; Kali bich.; Kali c.;* Kali m.; Lac d.; Lach.; Lact. ac.; *Lyc.; Mag. m.;* Mez.; Morph.; Nabalus; *Nat. m.; Nit. ac.;* Nit. mur. ac.; *Nux v.;* Nyctanth.; *Op.; Paraf.; Phos.;* Physost.; Phyt.; *Plat.; Plumb. ac.;* Plumb. m.; *Pod.; Psor.;* Pyr.; Ratanh.; Rham. c.; Sanic.; *Selen.;* Senna; *Sep.; Sil.;* Sil. mar.; Spig.; *Staph.;* Strych.; *Sul.; Symphor.; Syph.;* Tab.; Tan. ac.; Tub.; *Ver. a.; Zinc. m.;* Zinc. mur.

CAUSE AND TYPE—Abuse of enemas—*Op.*

After confinement, hepatic and uterine inertia—Mez.

Alternating, with diarrhæa—Abrot.; Am. m.; *Ant. c.;* Bry.; Calc. chlor.; Card. m.; Cascar.; *Chel.; Collins.;* Ferr. cy.; *Hydr.;* Iod.; *Nux v.; Pod.;* Ptel.; Radium; Ruta; *Sul.;* Ver. a.

From abuse of purgatives—Aloe; *Hydr.; Nux v.;* Sul.

From cheese—Col.

From gastric derangements—*Bry.;* Hydr.; *Nux v.;* Puls.

From going to sea—Bry.; Lyc.

From gouty acidity—Grat.

From haemorrhoids—*Æsc. gl.; Æsc.;* Caust.; *Collins.;* Hydr.; Nat. m.; *Nux v.;* Pod.; *Sul.* See Piles.

From impaction—Plumb. m ; Pyr.: Selen.

From lead poisoning—Op.; Plat.

From mechanical injuries—Arn.; Ruta.

From mental shock, nervous strain—Mag. c.

From peristaltic irregularity—Anac.; *Nux v.*

From travelling; in emigrants—Plat.

From torpor of rectum—Aloe; *Alum.; Anac.;* Caust.; Cinch.; Lach.; Lyc.; Nat. m.; *Op.;* Psor.; Selen.; *Sep.; Sil.;* Ver. a.

From torpor, inertia, dryness of intestines—*Æsc.;* Æth.; Alet.; Alumen; *Alum.; Bry.;* Caffeine; *Collins.;* Ferr. m.; Hydr.; *Lyc.;* Meli.; Mez.; *Nat. m.;* Nux v.; *Op.;* Physost.; *Plat.; Plumb. ac.;* Pyr.; Ruta; Sanic.; Selen.; *Sul.;* Ver. a.

Infants, bottle fed; artificial food—Alum.; Nux v.; Op.

Infants, children—*Æsc.; Alum.;* Apis; Bell.; *Bry.;* Calc. c.; Caust.; *Collins.;* Croc.; Hydr.; *Lyc.; Mag. m.; Nux v.;* Nyct. arb. tr.; *Paraf.;* Pod.; Psor.; Sanic.; *Sep.; Sil.;* Sul.; *Ver. a.*

In old people—*Alum.;* Ant. c.; Hydr.; Lyc.; *Op.;* Phyt.; *Selen.;* Sul.

In rheumatic subjects, flatulence, indigestion—Mag. p.

In women—*Æsc.;* Alet.; *Alum.;* Ambra; Anac.; Arn.; *Asaf.;* Bry.; Calc. c.; *Collins.;* Con.; *Graph.; Hydr.;* Ign.; Lach.; Lyc.; Mez.; *Nat. m.;* Nux v.; Op.; *Plat.; Plumb.;* Pod.: Puls.; *Sep.;* Sil.; Sul.

TYPE OF STOOL—Dry, crumbling at verge of anus: Am. m.; *Mag. m.; Nat. m.;* Sanic.; Zinc.

Dry, difficult, scanty, knotty, ball or dung-like—Æsc. gl.; Æsc.; *Alumen; Alum.;* Aster.; Bar. c.; *Card. m.;* Caust.; *Chel.;* Collins.; Glycerin; Graph.; Indol; *Lyc.; Mag. m.;* Morph.; Nit. ac.; *Nux v.; Op.;* Petrol.; *Plat.; Plumb.;* Pyr.; Sanic.; *Sep.; Sul.;* Thuya; Ver. a.; Verbasc.; Xerophyl.; Zinc.

Dry, large, painful—*Æsc.;* Alet.; Aloe; *Alum.; Bry.;* Calc. c.; Caust.; Glycerin; *Graph.; Kali c.;* Lac d.; Meli.; Nat. m.; Nux v.; *Op.;* Pyr.; Sanic.; *Selen.;* Sep.; *Sul.; Ver. a.;* Vib. op.

Dry, must be mechanically removed—Aloe; Alum.; Bry.; Calc. c.; Indol; *Op.; Plumb.;* Ruta; Sanic.; *Selen.;* Sep.; *Sil.;* Ver. a.

Dry, with frequent urging—Alumen; *Anac.;* Aster.; Carbo v.; *Caust.;* Con.; Ferr. m.; Glycerin; Granat.; *Ign.;* Iod.; Lac d.; *Lyc.;* Nit. ac.; Nit. mur. ac.; *Nux v.;* Paraf.; *Plat.; Phos.;* Pod.; Robin; Ruta; *Sil.; Sep.;* Spig.; *Sul.*

Dry, with partial expulsion and receding—Op.; Sanic.; Sil.; *Thuya.*

Frequent, ineffectual urging—Ambra; Anac.; Caust.; Ferr. m.; Graph.; Lyc.; Nat. m.; *Nux v.;* Plat.; Sul.

Hard—*Æsc.;* Aloe; *Am. m.;* Ant. c.; Bar. c.; *Bry.;* Calc. c.; *Chel.;* Con.; Glycerin; Indol; Iod.; Lac d.; *Lyc.; Mag. m.; Nat. m.; Op.;* Phos.; *Plumb.;* Ratanh.; Sanic.; Selen.; *Sul.*

Hard, covered with mucus—Alum.; Am. m.; Cascar.; *Caust.; Collins.;* Cop.; *Graph.; Hydr.;* Nux v.; Sep.

Hard, then pasty liquid—Calc. c.; Lyc.

Large, black, carrion like—Pyr.

Light colored, grayish, chalky—Acon.; Alumen; *Calc. c.; Chel.;* Chionanth.;

Cinch.; Collins.; *Dig.;* Dolichos; *Hep.;* Hydr.; Iberis; Indol; **Kali** m.; *Merc. d.; Pod.;* Sanic.; Stellar.

No desire or urging—*Alum.; Bry.;* Graph.; Hydr.; *Op.*

Pasty, tenacious, adhering to anus—Alum.; Chel.; Chionanth.; *Plat.*

Slender, quill-like—Arn.; *Caust.; Phos.;* Staph.

Soft stool even passed with difficulty—Agn.; Alum.; Anac.; Chel.; Chionanth.; *Plat.;* Ratanh.; Sil.

CONCOMITANTS—Abdominal weakness, shuddering: Plat.

Anus very sore—Graph.; Nat. m.; Nit. ac.; Sil.

Backache—*Æsc.;* Euonym.; *Ferr.;* Kali bich.; Sul. See Back.

Bleeding—Alum.; Am. m.; Anac.; Calc. p.; *Collins.;* Lac d.; Lamium; Morph.; Nat. m.; *Nit. ac.; Nux v.;* Phos.; Psor.; Sep.; Vib. op.

Colic, cramps—Collins.; *Cupr.;* Glon.; Op.;⁴ *Plumb. ac.*

Contraction, spasmodic of anus—Caust.; *Lach.; Lyc.; Nat. m.;* Nit. ac.; Plumb. ac.; Plumb. m.; Sil. See Rectum.

Enuresis—Caust.

Fainting—Ver. a.

Fetor oris—*Carb. ac.;* Op.; Psor.

Gall-stones, jaundice—Chionanth. See Gall Bladder.

Headache—Bry.; Gels.; *Hydr.;* Iris; Nux v.; Sep.; Ver. a. See Headache.

Heart weak—Phyt.; Spig.

Hernia, umbilical—Cocc.; Nux v.

Nervous, from presence of others, even nurse—Ambra.

Pain, compels child to desist from effort—Ign.; Lyc.; *Sul.;* Thuya.

Passes better leaning far back—Med.

Passes better standing—Caust.

Piles—*Æsc.; Aloe;* Alumen; *Calc. fl.;* Caust.; *Collins.;* Euonym.; Glon., Graph.; Kali s.; Lyc.; Nit. ac.; *Nux v.;* Paraf.; *Ratanh.;* Sil.; *Sul.;* Wyeth. See Hæmorrhoids.

Prolapsus—*Æsc.;* Alum.; Ferr. m.; *Ign.;* Lyc.; Med.; *Pod.;* Ruta; Sep.; Sul. See Rectum.

Prolapsus uteri—Stann.

Prostate enlarged—Arn.; Sil. See Male Sexual System.

Prostatic fluid—Alum.; Hep.

Rectal pain, persistent—*Æsc.;* Aloe; Alumen; Caust.; Hydr.; *Ign.;* Lyc.; Mur. ac.; *Nat. m.; Nit. ac.;* Ratanh.; Sep.; Sul.; Thuya. See Rectum.

Sensation of lightheadedness—Indol.

Sensation of something remaining behind—Aloe; Alum.; Lyc.; Nat. m.; *Nux v.;* Sep.; Sil.; Sul.

Urging absent, no desire—*Alum.; Bry.;* Graph.; Hydr.; Indol; *Op.;* Sanic.; Sul.; Ver. a.

Urging felt in lower abdomen—Aloe. See Frequent Urging.

Urging felt in upper abdomen—Anac.; *Ign.;* Ver. a.

DIAPHRAGM—Inflammation (diaphragmitis): Atrop.; Bell.; Bism.; *Bry.; Cact.; Cupr.;* Hep.; Hyos.; Ign.; *Nux v.;* Ran. b.; Stram.; Ver. v.

Pain—Asaf.; Bism.; *Bry.;* Cact.; *Cim.;* Nat. m.; Nux v.; Sec.; Spig.; *Stann.;* Sticta; *Strych.;* Ver. a.; Zinc. ox.

Rheumatism—*Bry.;* Cact.; *Cim.;* Spig.; Sticta.

DIARRHOEA—Enteritis: Acute: Acal.; Acet. ac.; *Acon.; Æth.;* Agar. phal.; *Aloe; Alston.;* Andros.; *Ant. c.;* Ant. t.; *Apis;* Apoc.; *Arg. n.; Arn.; Ars.;* Ars. iod.; *Asaf.; Bapt.; Bell.;* Benz. ac.; *Bism.;* Bov.; *Bry.;* Cadm. s.; Calc. ac.; *Calc. c.; Calc. p.; Camph.; Canth.; Caps.; Carb. ac.; Carbo v.; Cham.; Chel.; Chin. ars.;* Cina; *Cinch.;* Colch.; Collins.; *Col.; Corn. c.; Crot. t.;* Cuphea; Cupr. ac.; *Cupr. ars.; Cycl.; Dulc.;* Echin.; *Elat.;* Epilop.; *Eucal.; Euphorb. cor.;* Ferr. m.; Ferr. p.; Fluor. ac.; Formica; *Gamb.; Gels.; Grat.;* Helleb.; Hep.; Hyos.; Iod.; *Ipec.; Iris;* Jal.; *Jatropha; Kali bich.;* Kali chlor.; Kali p.; Lept.; *Mag. c.; Merc. d.; Merc. s.; Merc. v.;* Morph.; Mur. ac.; Nat. m.; *Nat. s.;* Nit. ac.; *Nuphar; Nux v.;* Oleand.; *Op.;* Opuntia; Oreodaph.; Pæonia; Petrol.; *Phos. ac.; Phos.;* Physost.; *Pod.;* Polyg.; *Prun. sp.;* Psor.; *Puls.; Rheum; Rhus t.;* Rhus v.; Ricin. com.; *Rumex;* Santon.; *Sec.; Sep.; Sil.; Sul.;* Sul. ac.; Tab.; Tereb.; *Thuya;* Val.; *Ver. a.;* Zinc.; Zing.

Chronic—Acet. ac.; Allium s.; Aloe; Angust.; Ant. c.; *Arg. n.;* Arn.; *Ars.;* Ars. iod.; Bapt.; *Calc. c.;* Calc. p.; Cetraria; *Chaparro; Cinch.; Coto;* Crot. t.; *Cupr. ars.;* Elaps; *Ferr. m.;* Gamb.; *Graph.;* Hep.; *Iod.;* Iodof.; Ipec.; *Kali bich.;* Lach.; Lact. ac.; *Liatris;* Lyc.; Mag. m.; Merc. d.; *Merc.;* Nabalus; *Nat. s.;* Nit. ac.; Oleand.; *Phos. ac., Phos.; Pod.;* Psor.; Puls.; Rhus ar.; Rhus t.; Rumex; Strych. ars.; *Sul.; Thuya;* Tub.; Urt.

CAUSE—OCCURRENCE—Alternates with headache: Aloe; Pod.

From acids—Aloe; *Ant. c.;* Phos. ac.; Sul.

From acute diseases—Carbo v.; Cinch.; Psor. See Typhoid Fever.

From alcoholic abuse—Ars.; Lach.; Nux v.

From anger—*Cham.;* Col.; Staph.

From bathing—*Ant. c.;* Pod.

From beer, ale—Aloe; Cinch.; Ipec.; *Kali bich.;* Mur. ac.; *Sul.*

From cabbage; saurkraut—Bry.; Petrol.

From camping—*Alston.;* Jugl. c.; Pod.

From catarrh, bronchial, suppressed—Sang.

From change of weather, draughts—*Acon.; Bry.;* Calc. s.; *Caps.;* Colch.: *Dulc.;* Ipec.; *Merc.; Nat. s.;* Psor.; Rhus t.; Sil.

From chilling cold drinks, ices—*Acon.;* Agraph.; *Ars.;* Bell.; *Bry.;* Camph.; Carbo v.; Caust.; Cham.; Grat.; Nux m.; *Puls.;* Staph.

From coffee—Cistus; *Cycl.;* Ox. ac.; Thuya.

From coryza ceasing—Sang.

From disorganization—Ars.

From eggs—Chin ars.

From emotional excitement, fright—*Acon.; Arg. n.; Gels.;* Hyos.; *Ign.;* Kali p.; *Op.; Phos. ac.;* Puls.; Ver. a.; Zinc.

From eruptions repelled—Ant. t.; Apis; *Bry.;* Dulc.; Petrol.; Psor.; *Sul.*

From fats—Cycl.; Kali m.; *Puls.;* Thuya.

From food, crude—Cham.

From fruits—*Ars.; Bry.;* Calc. p.; *Cinch.;* Cistus; Col.; Crot. t.; Ipec.; Pod.; *Puls.;* Ver. a.; Zing.

From gastric derangements—*Ant. c.;* Bry.; Cinch.; Col.; Ipec.; Lyc.; *Nux v.; Puls.*

From high game—Crot.; Pyr.

From hot weather—Acon.; Aloe; Ambros.; *Ant. c.;* Ars.; *Bry.;* Camph.; Caps.; *Cham.; Cinch.;* Crot. t.; *Cuphea;* Ferr. p.; Gamb.; *Ipec.;* Iris; Merc.; Nux m.; *Pod.;* Sil.; Ver. a.

From hydrocephalus acute—Helleb.

From hyperacidity—Cham.; Rheum; Robin.

From intestinal atony, debility—*Arg. n.;* Caps.; *Cinch.;* Ferr.; Œnanthe; Oreodaph.; *Sec.*

From jaundice—*Chionanth.;* Dig.; Nux v.

From meat putrescent—Ars.; Crot.

From milk—*Æth.;* Calc. c.; Cinch.; Lyc.; *Mag. c.;* *Mag. m.;* Nat. c.; Niccol.; *Sep.;* Sul.; Val.

From milk boiled—Nux m.

From motion—Apis; *Bry.;* Cinch.; Colch.; Nat. s.

From motion downward—Bor.; Cham.; Sanic.

From nephritis—Tereb.

From noxious effluvia—Bapt.; Carb. ac.; *Crot.*

From onions—Thuya.

From oysters—*Brom.;* Lyc.; Sul. ac.

From perspiration checked—*Acon.;* Cham.; Ferr. p.

From pork—Acon. lyc.; *Puls.*

From sweets—*Arg. n.;* Calc. s.; Crot .t.; *Gamb.;* Merc. v.

From tobacco—Cham.; Tab.

From tuberculosis—Acet. ac.; Arg. n.; *Arn.;* Ars.; *Ars. iod.; Bapt.;* Bism.; *Cinch.;* Coto; *Cupr. ars.;* Elaps; Ferr. m.; Iod.; Iodof.; Phos. ac.; *Phos.;* Puls.; Rumex. See Tuberculosis.

From typhoid fever—*Ars.; Bapt.;* Echin.; *Epilob.;* Eucal.; *Hyos.;* Lach.; *Mur. ac.;* Nuphar; Op.; Phos. ac.; *Rhus t.;* Stram. See Typhoid Fever.

From ulceration of intestines—Kali bich.; Merc. c.

From urination—Aloe; Alum.; Apis.

From vaccination—*Sil.;* Thuya.

From veal—Kali n.

From vegetables, melons—*Ars.; Bry.;* Petrol.; Zing.

From water polluted—*Alston.;* Camph.; Zing.

In infants, children—*Acon.; Æth.;* Apis; *Arg. n.;* Ars.; Arundo; Bapt.; *Bell.;* Benz. ac.; Bism.; *Bor.;* Calc. ac.; *Calc. c.; Calc. p.;* Camph.; *Cham.;* Cinch.; Cina; *Col.;* Colost.; *Crot. t.;* Dulc.; Ferr.; Grat.; *Helleb.;* Hep.; *Ipec.;* Jal.; Kali br.; *Kreos.;* Laur.; Lyc.; Lyssin; *Mag. c.; Merc. c.; Merc. d.;* Merc.; Nit. ac.; *Nux v.;* Paul.; *Phos. ac.;* Phos.; *Pod.; Psor.; Rheum;* Sabad.; Sep.; *Sil.; Sul.;* Val.; *Ver. a.*

Infants (dentition)—Acet. ac.; *Acon.; Æth.;* Arundo; *Bell.;* Benz. ac.; Bor.; Calc. ac.; *Calc. c.; Calc. p.; Cham.;* Ipec.; Jal.; *Kreos.; Mag. c.;* Merc. v.; Nux m.; Oleand.; Phyt.; *Pod.;* Psor.; Rheum; *Sil.*

In old people—*Ant. c.;* Bov.; *Carbo v.; Cinch.;* Gamb.; Op.; Phos.; *Sul.*

In women, before and during menses—Am. c.; *Am. m.;* Bov.; Ver. a. See Female Sexual System.

In women, lying-in period—*Cham.; Hyos.;* Psor.; *Sec.;* Stram.

TYPE OF STOOL—**Acrid, excoriating, burning:** *Ars.;* Bry.; Carbo v.; *Cham.;*

Cuphea; *Graph.*; Iris; Kreos.; *Merc. c.*; Merc. d.; Merc. sul.; Merc. v.; Pod.; *Sul.*; Tereb.

Bilious—Ant. t.; *Bry.*; Card. m.; *Cham.*; Cinch.; *Corn. c.*; Crot. t.; Fluor. ac.; Gamb.; *Ipec.*; *Iris*; Jugl. c.; *Lept.*; Lyc.; *Merc. d.*; Merc.; Nat. s.; Nyctanth.; *Pod.*; Puls.; Sang.; Tarax.; Yucca.

Black—*Ars.*; Brom.; Camph.; *Caps.*; *Carb. ac.*; Cinch.; *Crot.*; Echin.; *Lept.*; Morph.; *Op.*; Psor.; Pyr.; *Scilla*; Stram.; Sul. ac.; Ver. a.

Blood-streaked slime—Agar.; *Aloe*; Arg. n.; *Arn.*; Bell.; *Canth.*; Caps.; Col.; *Cupr. ars.*; Euphorbia; *Ipec.*; Lil. t.; Kreos.; Mag. c.; *Merc. c.*; Merc. d.; *Merc. v.*; *Nux v.*; Pod.; *Psor.*; *Rhus t.*; Sul.; Trill. See Dysentery.

Bloody—Æth.; Ail.; Aloe; Am. m.; *Arg. n.*; Arn.; Ars.; Bapt.; Bothrops; Cadm. s.; *Canth.*; Caps.; Carb. ac.; *Colch.*; Col.; Crot.; Cupr. ars.; Dulc.; Ferr. p.; Ham.; *Ipec.*; Kali bich.; Kreos.; Lach.; *Merc. c.*; *Merc. d.*; *Merc. v.*; *Nux v.*; Phos.; Pod.; *Sec.*; Senec.; *Sul.*; Tereb.; Tromb.; Val.

Brown, dark—Apis; Arn.; *Ars.*; Asaf.; *Bapt.*; *Bry.*; Cinch.; Col.; Corn. c.; Cupr. ac.; Cupr. ars.; Ferr. mur.; *Graph.*; Kali bich.; Kreos.; *Lept.*; Mur. ac.; Nux v.; Pod.; *Psor.*; Pyr.; *Raph.*; Rheum; Rumex; *Scilla*; *Sec.*; *Senec.*; Sul.; Tub.

Changeable—Am. m.; *Cham.*; Euonym.; Merc. v.; *Pod.*; *Puls.*; Sanic.; Sil.; *Sul.*

Clay-colored, chalk-like, light-colored—Aloe; *Bell.*; Benz. ac.; Berb. v.; *Calc. c.*; Chel.; *Dig.*; Euphorbia; Gels.; *Hep.*; Kali c.; *Merc. d.*; Merc. v.; Myr.; *Phos. ac.*; Phos.; Pod.; Sep.

Coffee-ground-like, mealy—Crotal.; Dig.; *Lach.*; *Pod.*; Tart. ac.

Colliquative (debilitating)—Acet. ac.; Angoph.; Arist.; *Ars.*; Cinch.; *Colch.*; Coto; *Cupr. ars.*; Diosc.; Elaps; Kali p.; Phell.; *Phos.*; *Sec.*; Sep.; *Tab.*; Tart. ac.; Upas; *Ver. a.*

Fatty, oily—Caust.; *Iod.*; Iris; *Phos.*

Fermented, flatulent, noisy, spluttering expulsion—*Acal.*; Agar.; Alfal.; *Aloe*; Apoc.; *Arg. n.*; Arn.; Benz. ac.; Bor.; *Calc .p.*; Cham.; *Cinch.*; Col.; Corn. c.; *Crot. t.*; *Elat.*; Gamb.; Graph.; *Grat.*; Gummi; Iod.; *Ipec.*; *Jatropha*; Kali bich.; *Mag. c.*; *Nat. sulphuros.*; *Nat. s.*; Op.; *Phos. ac.*; Phos.; *Pod.*; Puls.; Rheum; Rhus t.; Sanic.; Sec.; Sticta; *Sul.*; *Thuya*; Triost.; *Ver. a.*; Yucca.

Frequent—Acet. ac.; *Acon.*; Aloe; *Ars.*; Calc. ac.; Caps.; *Carbo v.*; *Cham.*; *Cinch.*; Crot. t.; Cuphea; *Cupr. ars.*; Elat.; Ipec.; Mag. c.; *Merc. c.*; *Merc. v.*; Nit. ac.; Nux v.; *Phos. ac.*; *Pod.*; Rheum; Rhus t.; Sil.; Sul.; Tereb.; *Ver. a.*

Frog spawn or scum-like—Helleb.; Mag. c.; *Phos.*; Sanic.

Gelatinous, jelly-like—*Aloe*; Cadm. s.; *Colch.*; *Col.*; Euphorbia; *Helleb.*; *Kali bich.*; Oxytr.; Phos.; Pod.; *Rhus t.*

Green—*Acon.*; Æth.; Ant. t.; *Apis*; *Arg. n.*; Ars.; *Bell.*; *Bor.*; Bry.; Calc. ac.; Calc. c.; *Calc. p.*; *Cham.*; Col.; Crot. t.; *Dulc.*; Elat.; Gamb.; *Gels.*; Grat.; Gummi; *Hep.*; Iodof.; *Ipec.*; Iris; Kreos.; Laur.; *Mag. c.*; Merc. c.; *Merc. d.*; *Merc. v.*; *Mez.*; Paul; Phos.; *Pod.*; *Puls.*; Sal. ac.; Sanic.; *Sec.*; Sul.; Tab.; Val.; Ver. a.

Green, turning to blue—Calc. p.; Phos.

Gurgling, gushing—Aloe; Apis; *Crot. t.; Elat.: Gamb.;* Grat.; Gummi; *Jatropha;* Kali bich.; Merc. s.; Nat. s.; *Petrol.; Phos.; Pod.;* Sang.; Sec.; *Thuya;* Tub.; Ver. a. See Fermented.

Hot—*Calc. p.; Cham.;* Diosc.; Ferr.; Merc. c.; Merc. sul.; Pod.; *Sul.* See Acrid.

Involuntary—*Aloe; Apis;* Apoc.; *Arn.;* Ars.; *Bapt.;* Camph.; Carb. ac.; *Carbo v.; Gels.;* Helleb.; *Hyos.;* Op.; *Phos. ac.; Phos.;* Pod.; Psor.; Pyr.; Rhus t.; *Sec.;* Strych.; Sul.; *Ver. a.;* Zinc.

Involuntary, as if anus were wide open—*Apis;* Apoc.; *Phos.;* Sec.; Tromb.

Involuntary, when passing flatus—*Aloe;* Calc. c.; Iod.; *Mur. ac.;* Nat. m.; Nat. s.; *Oleand.; Phos. ac.; Pod.;* Pyr.; Sanic.

Involuntary, when passing urine—*Aloe; Alum.;* A♦pis; Cic.; Hyos.; *Mur. ac.; Scilla;* Sul.; Ver. a.

Lumpy, hard—Aloe; *Ant. c.;* Bar. c.; Bell.; *Bry.;* Cham.; Cina; Con.; Cub.; Glon.; *Graph.; Mag. c.;* Petrol.; Phos.; *Pod.;* Senec.; Tromb.

Mucous, slimy—*Aloe;* Am. m.; *Ant. c.;* Apis; *Arg. n.; Arn.; Ars.; Bell.;* Bor.; Calc. ac.; *Calc. p.; Canth.; Caps.;* Carb. ac.; *Carbo v.; Cham.;* Cina; Cinch.; Cocc.; *Colch.; Col.; Cop.; Dulc.;* Ferr.; Graph.; Gummi; Helleb.; Hep.; *Ipec.;* Kali m.; Laur.; *Mag. c.; Merc. c.;* Merc. d.; *Merc. s.; Merc. v.;* Nit. ac.; *Nux v.;* Phos.; Pod.; Prun. sp.: *Puls.;* Rheum; Ricin. com.; Rhus t.; Ruta; Sep.; Spig.; *Sul.;* Tab.; Tereb.; Urt. See Dysentery.

Non-debilitating—Calc. c.; Graph.; *Phos. ac.;* Puls.

Offensive, cadaverous—Ail.; Ant. c.; Arg. n.; *Arn.; Ars.; Asaf.;* Asclep. t.; *Bapt.; Benz. ac.;* Bism.; *Bor.; Bry.;* Calc. c.; Calc. p.; Carb. ac.; *Carbo v.; Cham.;* Cinch.; Col.; Corn. c.; Crotal.; *Graph.; Hep.; Kali p.; Kreos.;* Lach.; *Lept.; Merc. c.;* Merc. d.; Merc. v.; Mur. ac.; Nit. ac.; Nux m.; Op.; *Petrol.;* Phos. ac.; *Phos.; Pod.; Psor.;* Pulex; Pyr.; *Rheum;* Rhus t.; Rumex; Sanic.; *Scilla; Sec.;* Sil.; Stram.; Sul. ac.; *Sul.; Tereb.;* Tub.

Painless—Alfal.; *Alston.;* Amanita; *Apis;* Ars.; *Bapt.;* Bellis; Bism.; Bor.; Chaparro; *Cinch.;* Colch.; Crot. t.; Dulc.; *Ferr. m.; Gels.; Graph.; Grat.;* Hep.; *Hyos.;* Ipec.; Nit. ac.; *Phos. ac.; Phos.; Pod.;* Psor.; *Puls.;* Pyr.; Rhus t.; Ricin.; Rumex; Scilla; Sec.; Sil.; *Sul.*

Papescent—*Æsc.;* Alfal.; Aloe; Ars.; Bism.; *Bor.; Bry.;* Chel.; *Cinch.;* Col.; *Cycl.;* Gamb.; Gels.; *Graph.; Lept.;* Mag. c.; *Merc. d.;* Merc.; Nit. ac.; Pæonia; *Pod.;* Rheum; Sep.; Sil.; *Sul.;* Val.; Zinc.

Profuse—Acet. ac.; Ant. c.; *Asaf.; Benz. ac.;* Bism.; Bry.; Calc. ac.; Calc. c.; Chel.; Cinch.; Coto; *Crot. t.; Elat.; Euonym.;* Euphor. c.; *Gamb.; Jatropha;* Lept.; Merc.; Nat. nit.; Operc.; Paul.; *Phos.; Pod.;* Psor.; Rhus t.; *Sec.;* Sticta; *Tereb.; Thuya; Ver. a.*

Purulent—Apis; Arn.; Calc. s.; *Hep.; Merc.;* Phos.; Sil.

Rice-water—*Ars.;* Camph.; *Jatropha;* Kali p.; Merc. s.; Ricin. com.; Ver. a.

Sago or tallow particles, like—Phos.

Scanty—*Acon.; Aloe; Ars.; Bell.;* Camph.; Canth.; Caps.; *Colch.;* Col.; *Merc. c.;* Merc. d.; *Merc. v.;* Nit. ac.; *Nux v.;* Oleand.; Sul. See Dysentery.

Shreddy, stringy, membranous, like scrapings of intestines—Aloe; *Arg. n.;* Ars.; Asar.; Bolet.; *Canth.; Carb. ac.; Colch.;* Kali bich.; Kali n.; *Merc. c.;* Merc.; Mur. ac.; *Nit. ac.;* Pod.; Puls.; Sul. ac.

Sour—Calc. ac.; *Calc. c.;* Colch.; Col.; *Colost.;* Graph.; *Hep.;* Jal.; *Mag. c.;* Merc. v.; Nit. ac.; *Pod.; Rheum;* Robin.; Sul.

Spinach chopped, like—Acon.; Arg. n.; Cham.

Sudden, imperative, cannot wait—*Aloe;* Cinch.; Cistus; *Crot. t.; Gamb.; Lil. t.;* Nat. c.; Pæonia; Pod.; *Psor.; Rumex; Sul.;* Tab.; Tromb.; Tub.; *Ver. a.*

Tenacious, glairy—*Asar.;* Caps.; Crot. t.; Helleb.; *Kali bich.* See Mucous.

Undigested, lienteric—Abrot.; Æth.; *Ant. c.;* Arg. n.; Ars.; *Asar.;* Bry.; *Calc. c.; Calc. p.;* Cham.; Cinch.; Crot. t.; Ferr. ac.; *Ferr. m.;* Ferr. p.; *Graph.;* Hep.; Iodof.; *Mag. c.;* Nit. ac.; Nux m.; Nux v.; *Oleand.; Phos. ac.; Phos.; Pod.;* Psor.; *Puls.;* Sul.; Val.

Watery, like washing of meat—*Canth.;* Phos.; Rhus t.

Watery, thin—Acet. ac.; Acon.; Æth.; Aloe; *Alston.; Ant. c.;* Ant. t.; *Apis; Apoc.; Ars.;* Asaf.; *Bapt.; Benz. ac.;* Bism.; *Bor.; Bry.;* Calc. ac.; Calc. c.; *Calc. p.;* Carbo v.; *Cham.;* Chel.; *Cinch.;* Colch.; *Col.;* Crotal.; *Crot. t.;* Cuphea; *Cupr. ars.;* Cycl.; *Elat.;* Ferr. m.; *Gamb.;* Graph.; *Grat.;* Hep.; Hyos.; Iod.; Iodof.; Ipec.; *Iris;* Jal.; *Jatropha;* Kali bich.; Kali n.; Laur.; *Mag. c.;* Mur. ac.; Nat. s.; Oleand.; Operc.; Petrol.; *Phos. ac.;* Phos.; *Pod.; Psor.;* Puls.; *Rheum;* Rhus t.; Rumex; *Sec.; Senec.; Sul.;* Tab.; Tereb.; Thuya; Tromb.; Tub.; *Ver. a.;* Zinc.

White—Acon.; Ant. c.; *Bell.; Benz. ac.; Calc. c.;* Caust.; Cham.; Chel.; Cina; Cocc.; *Colch.;* Crot.; Cub.; *Dig.;* Dulc.; *Helleb.; Hep.;* Iod.; Ipec.; Kali m.; Mag. c.; *Merc. d.;* Merc.; Mez.; Nux m.; *Phos. ac.;* Phos.; Pod.; Puls.; Tromb.

Yellow—Æth.; Agar.; Alfal.; Aloe; *Apis; Ars.;* Asar.; *Bor.; Calc. c.;* Card. m.; Cham.; *Chel.; Cinch.;* Col.; *Crot. t.;* Cycl.; Dulc.; *Gamb.;* Gels.; Grat.; Gummi; *Hep.;* Hyos.; Ipec.; Merc.; *Nat. c.;* Nat. s.; *Nuphar;* Nux m.; Petrol.; Phos. ac.; *Pod.;* Puls.; Rheum; Rhus t.; Senna; Sep.; Sul.; Tab.; Thuya.

CONCOMITANTS—BEFORE STOOL: Chilliness: Ars.; Camph.; Elat.; *Merc. v.;* Phos.; Ver. a.

Colic, cramps—Æth.; *Aloe;* Alston.; *Bell.;* Bor.; Cascar.; *Cham.;* Cina; *Cinch.; Col.;* Crot. t.; *Cupr. ars.; Diosc.;* Dulc.; Elat.; Gamb.; Gummi; *Ipec.;* Iris; Lept.; *Mag. c.; Merc. c.;* Merc. d.; Merc.; Nux v.; *Rheum;* Senna; Sul.; Tromb.; *Ver. a.* See Colic.

Flatulent rumbling—*Aloe;* Asaf.; Carbo v.; *Colch.;* Col.; *Gamb.;* Kali c.; *Nat. s.;* Oleand.; *Pod.;* Puls.

Nausea—*Bry.;* Chrom. ac.; *Colch.; Ipec.;* Merc. v.; Rhus t.; Sep.

Urging, painful—*Aloe; Ars.; Bell.;* Camph.; Cistus; *Col.;* Con.; *Crot. t.;* Formica; Gamb.; Grat.; Hep.; *Ign.;* Kali bich.; Lept.; *Merc. c.; Merc. d.;* Merc. v.; Nat. s.; *Nux v.:* Oleand.; Phos.; Pod.; Rheum; Sil.; *Stront.; Sul.; Ver. a.*

DURING STOOL—Backache: *Æsc.;* Caps.; Colch.; *Nux v.;* Puls.

Burning in anus—*Aloe;* Ars.; *Canth.:* Carbo v.; Chenop. gl.; Con.; *Iris;*

Jugl. c.; *Merc. d.; Mur. ac.;* Pod.; Prun. sp.; *Ratanh.;* Rheum; Tereb.; Tromb.; Ver. a. See Anus.

Chilliness—*Ars.;* Bell.; *Colch.;* Ipec.; *Jatropha; Merc. v.;* Rheum; Ricin. com.; *Sec.;* Tromb.; *Ver. a.*

Colic, cramps—*Aloe;* Alston.; *Ars.;* Bry.; Camph.; *Canth.;* Caps.; Ceanoth.; *Cham.; Cinch.; Col.;* Crot. t.; *Cupr. ars.; Cupr. m.;* Dulc.; *Elat.;* Gamb.; *Ipec.;* Iris; *Jatropha;* Lept.; *Merc. c.;* Merc. d.; *Merc. v.;* Pod.; Rheum; Ricin. com.; Sec.; Sil.; Sul.; Triost.; *Tromb.; Ver. a.;* Zing. See Colic.

Fainting—Aloe; *Ars.;* Crot.; *Merc. v.; Nux m.;* Sul.

Flatus, fetid, expelled—Agar.; *Aloe; Arg. n.; Calc. p.; Carbo v.;* Cinch.; Ign.; Jatropha; *Nat. s.;* Phos. ac.; Pod.; Thuya.

Hunger—Aloe; Ferr. m.; Sec.

Nausea, vomiting—Æth.; *Ant. t.; Ars.; Bism.;* Camph.; Carb. ac.; Chrom. ac.; *Colch.;* Crot t.; Cupr.; Filix m.; *Ipec.; Iris; Jatropha;* Merc.; Opuntia; Phos.; *Pod.;* Tab.; Triost.; *Ver. a.*

Pain tearing down posterior limbs—Rhus t.

Stinging pains—Caps.

Tenesmus of bladder—Canth.; Lil. t.; *Merc. c.*

Tenesmus, relieved by stool—Nux v.

Tenesmus, urging painful—*Acon.; Aloe;* Angoph.; Arn.; *Ars.; Bell.;* Calc. c.; *Canth.;* Caps.; Carb. ac.; *Colch.; Col.;* Crot. t.; Cuphea; Cupr. ac.; *Cupr. ars.;* Hep.; *Ign.; Ipec.; Kali bich.;* Kali n.; Liatris; Mag. c.; *Merc. c.;* Merc. d.; *Merc. s.; Merc. v.;* Morph.; Nat. s.; Nit. ac.; *Nux v.;* Op.; Phos.; Plumb. ac.; *Pod.;* Rheum; Rhus t.; *Senec.;* Sil.; *Sul.;* Tab.; Tromb.; Ver. a.

Vomiting, hiccough, suffocative, in stomach and chest—Ver. a.

AFTER STOOL—Anus burning: Aloe; Apoc.; *Ars.;* Bry.; *Canth.; Caps.;* Carbo v.; Col.; *Gamb.;* Grat.; *Iris;* Kali c.; Merc. c.; Merc. s.; Merc. v.; Nit. ac.; Oleand.; Prun. sp.; *Ratanh.;* Sul.; Tromb.; Ver. a. See Anus.

Coldness—Aloe; *Ars.;* Camph.; *Canth.;* Caps.; Carbo v.; Formica; Ipec.; Merc. v.; *Sec.;* Tab.; *Ver. a.*

Debility, exhaustion—Acet. ac.; Æth.; *Ail.;* Aloe; Amanita; *Arg. n.;* Arn.; *Ars.; Bism.; Camph.; Cinch.; Colch.; Con.;* Crot. t.; Cupr. m.; Elat.; Ferr. m.; Iris; Jatropha; *Kali p.;* Mag. c.; Nit. ac.; *Phos.; Pod.; Rhus t.; Sec.;* Sep.; Sul. ac.; *Tab.; Tereb.;* Tromb.; Tub.; Upas; *Ver. a.*

Fainting—*Aloe;* Ars.; Con.; Crot. t.; *Merc.; Nux m.;* Pæonia; Sars.; *Tereb.;* Ver. a.

Hæmorrhoids—*Aloe;* Ham.; Mur. ac.; Sul. See Hæmorrhoids.

Pains persist in abdomen—Aloe; *Col.;* Crot. t.; Diosc.; *Gamb.;* Grat.; *Merc. c.;* Merc. v.; Rheum; Tromb.; Ver. a.

Palpitation, trembling in limbs—Ars.

Prolapsus ani—*Aloe;* Alum.; Calc. ac.; Carbo v.; Ham.; *Ign.;* Merc. v.; Nit. ac.; *Pod.;* Sul.; Tromb. See Rectum.

Sleep, as soon as tenesmus ceases—Colch.; *Sul.*

Stool natural in evening—Aloe; Pod.

Sweat—Acet. ac.; Aloe; Ant. t.; Ars.; Phos. ac.; Tab.; Tub.; *Ver. a.*

Tenesmus (never-get-done feeling)—Æth.; Aloe; Ars.; *Bell.; Canth.; Caps.;* Colch.; *Gamb.;* Ign.; Ipec.; Kali bich.; Mag. c.; *Merc. c.; Merc. d.; Merc. s.; Merc. v.;* Nit. ac.; Nux v.; *Pod.;* Rheum; Senna; Sil.; *Sul.;* Tromb.

Thirst—Acet. ac.; *Caps.;* Dulc.

Vomiting—Arg. n.; Colch.; Cup-.; *Ipec.; Iris; Nux v.;* Ver. a.

Weakness in abdomen and rectum—Pod.

MODALITIES—Aggravations: From eating, drinking: *Aloe; Alston.; Apis;* Apoc.; *Arg. n.; Ars.;* Bry.; Canth.; *Cinch.; Col.; Crot. t.; Ferr. m.;* Kali p.; Lyc.; Nux v.; *Phos.; Pod.;* Puls.; Rheum; Sanic.; Sul.; Tanac.; Thuya; *Tromb.; Ver. a.*

From motion—Aloe; Apis; *Bry.;* Cinch.; *Colch.;* Crot. t.; *Nat. s.;* Rheum; Ver. a.

From sundown to sunrise—Colch.

In afternoon—Bell.; Calc. c.; *Cinch.;* Corn. c.; *Lyc.*

In autumn—Cinch.; *Colch.; Merc.;* Nux m.; Ver. a.

In daytime only—Hep.; *Petrol.;* Piloc.

In evening, night—*Ars.;* Bellis; Bov.; Calc. c.; Chel.; *Cinch.;* Dulc.; Ferr. m.; Iris; *Merc.;* Nat. nit.; Nux m.; Pod.; *Puls.;* Psor.; *Rhus t.;* Stront.; Sul.; Wyeth.

In morning, early—Acet. ac.; *Aloe;* Ichthy.; Iris; Lil. t.; Med.; *Nat. s.;* Nit. ac.; *Nuphar; Nux v.;* Petrol.; Phos.; *Pod.; Psor.;* Rhus v.; *Rumex;* Sticta; *Sul.;* Thuya; Tromb.; Tub.

In morning—*Aloe; Apis;* Bov.; *Bry.;* Cact.; Cistus; Crot. t.; Ferr. m.; Graph.; *Kali bich.;* Lil. t.; Lyc.; Nux v.

In periodical attacks—Apis; Ars.; *Cinch.;* Euphorb. cor.; *Kali bich.;* Iris; Mag. c.; Thuya.

DUODENUM—Catarrhal inflammation (duodenitis): *Ars.;* Aur.; Berb. v.; Cham.; Chel.; *Cinch.; Hydr.; Kali bich.;* Lyc.; Merc. d.; Merc. s.; Nat. s.; Nux v.; *Pod.;* Ricin. com.; Sang.

Ulceration— *Kali bich.;* Symphyt.; Uran.

DYSENTERY—*Acon.; Aloe;* Alston.; Ambros.; Ant. t.; Apis; *Arg. n.;* Arn.; *Ars.;* Asclep. t.; *Bapt.;* Bell.; Calc. c.; *Canth.; Caps.;* Carb. ac.; Carbo v.; Chaparro; *Cinch.; Colch.;* Collins.; *Col.;* Cuphea; *Cupr. ars.;* Dulc.; Emetine; *Erig.; Eucal.;* Ferr. p.; Gamb.; Ham.; Hep.; *Ipec.;* Iris; *Kali bich.; Kali chlor.;* Kali m.; Kali p.; Lach.; Leonur.; Lept.; Lil. t.; Lyc.; *Mag. c.; Merc. c.;* Merc. d.; Merc. s.; *Merc. v.;* Nit. ac.; *Nux v.;* Operc.; Op.; Phos. ac.; *Phos.;* Plumb. ac.; *Pod ;* Puls.; Rheum; *Rhus t.;* Sec.; *Silph.; Sul.; Tanac.;* Trill.; *Tromb.;* Xanth.; Vaccin.; Ver. a.; Zinc. s.

Abuse of local treatment; diphtheritic form—Nit. ac.

Chronic, intractable cases—Aloe; Arg. n.; *Ars.;* Cinch.; Cop.; *Dulc.;* Hep.; *Merc. c.; Nit. ac.; Nux v.;* Phos. ac.; Pod.; Rhus ars.; *Sul.*

Hemorrhoidal form—Aloe; Collins.; Ham.

In old people—Bapt.

In plethoric, nervous, climacteric females—Lil. t.

With nausea from straining pain; little thirst—Ipec.

With long intervals between—*Arn.;* Cinch.

With periodical recurrence in spring or early summer—Kali bich.

With rheumatic pains all over—Asclep. t.

With tearing down thighs—Rhus t.

Worse in autumn—Acon.; *Colch.;* Dulc.; *Ipec.;* Merc. c.; *Merc. v.;* Sul.
See Diarrhœa.

ENTERITIS—See Diarrhœa.

ENTERO-COLITIS—See Diarrhœa.

GALL-BLADDER—BILIARY CALCULI (cholelithiasis)—Aur.; Bapt.; *Berb. v.;* Boldo; Bry.; *Calc. c.; Card. m.;* Chel.; *Chionanth.;* Cholest.; *Cinch ; Diosc.;* Fel tauri; Ferr. s.; Gels.; *Hydr.;* Jugl. c.; Lach.; Lept.; Myr.; *Nux v.;* Pichi; Pod.; Ptel.; Tarax.

Biliary colic—Ars.; Atrop. sul.; *Bell.; Berb. v.; Calc. c.; Card. m.;* Cham.; Chel.; Chionanth.; *Cinch.; Col.;* Dig.; *Diosc.;* Gels.; *Hydr.;* Ipec.; Lyc.; Morph. acet.; *Nux v.;* Op.; Tereb.

HÆMORRHOIDS—(piles): Remedies in general: Abrot.; *Acon.; Æsc. gl.; Æsc; Aloe; Am. c.;* Am. m.; Apis; *Ars.;* Aur. m.; Bar. c.; *Bell.;* Brom.; *Calc. fl.; Caps.;* Carbo an.; *Carbo v.;* Card. m.; Caust.; Cham.; Chrom. ac.; *Collins.;* Cop.; Diosc.; Ferr. p.; *Fluor. ac.;* Grat.; Ham.; Hep.; Hydr.; *Hyper.;* Ign.; *Kali m.;* Kali s.; *Lach.; Lyc.;* Mag. m.; *Millef.; Mucuna;* Mur. ac.; Negundo; *Nit. ac.; Nux v.; Pæonia;* Pinus sylv.; *Pod.; Polyg.;* Puls.; Radium; *Ratanh.;* Sab.; Scrophul.; Sedum; Sep.; *Semperv. t.; Sul.;* Sul. ac.; Thuya; Verbasc.; *Wyeth.;* Zing.

Bleeding—*Acon.; Æsc.; Aloe; Am. c.;* Bell.; Calc. fl.; *Caps.;* Card. m ; Chrom. ac.; *Collins.;* Erig.; Ferr. p.; *Ficcus; Ham.;* Hydr.; Hyper.; Kali m.; Lept.; Lycop.; *Millef.;* Mur. ac.; Nit. ac.; *Nux v.;* Operc.; *Phos.;* Sab.; Scrophul.; Sep.; *Sul.;* Thlaspi.

Bleeding, dark, venous blood—Aloe; *Ham.;* Hydr., Kali m.; *Sul.*

Blind—*Æsc :* Calc. fl.; Collins.; *Ign.;* Mucuna; *Nux v.;* Puls.; *Sul.;* Wyeth.

Bluish, purplish—*Æsc. gl.; Æsc.; Aloe;* Ars.; Caps.; Carbo v.; Ham.; Lach.; Lyc.; *Mur. ac.*

Burning, smarting—*Æsc.;* Aloe; Am. m.; *Ars.;* Calc. c.; *Caps.;* Carbo an ; Carbo v.; Caust.; *Fluor. ac.;* Graph ; *Ign.;* Mag. m.; *Mucuna:* Negundo; *Nux v.;* Psor.; *Ratanh.; Sul.;* Sul. ac.

Inflamed—*Acon.;* Æsc.; Aloe; Bell.; Caust.; Cop.; Ferr. p.; Mur. ac.; Verbasc. See Sensitive.

Itching—*Æsc.: Aloe; Caps.;* Carbo v.; Caust.; Cop.; Glon.; *Ham.,* Mur. ac.; Nit. ac.; *Nux v.; Petros.;* Puls.; *Sul.*

Mucous piles, continually oozing—*Aloe;* Am. m.; *Ant. c.;* Caps.; Carbo v.; Caust.; Puls.; Sep ; Sul. ac.; Sul.

Protruding, grape-like, swollen—Æsc.; *Aloe; Am. c.;* Caps.; *Carbo v.;* Caust.; *Collins.; Diosc.;* Graph.; Ham.; Kali c.; Lach.; *Mur. ac.;* Nux m.; *Nux v.;* Ratanh.; Scrophul.; Sep.; Sul ; Thuya.

Protruding when urinating—Bar. c.; *Mur. ac.*

Sensitive, exquisitely painful—Æsc. gl.; *Æsc.; Aloe;* Ars.; *Bell.;* Cact.; *Caps.:* Carbo v ; *Caust.; Cham.; Collins.;* Ferr. p.; Graph.; Ham.;

Hyper.; Kali c.; *Lach.; Lyc.;* Mag. m.; *Mur. ac.;* Nat. m.; Nit. ac.; *Nux v.;* Plant.; Puls.; *Ratanh.; Scrophul.; Sedum;* Sep.; *Sil.;* Sul.; Thuya; Verbasc.; Zing.

White piles—Carbo v.

CONCOMITANTS—With abdominal plethora—Æsc.; *Aloe;* Collins.; Ham.; Negundo; Nux v.; Sep.; *Sul.*

With backache—Æsc. gl.; *Æsc.; Bell.;* Calc. fl.; Chrom. ac.; Euonym.; Ham.; Ign.; *Nux v.;* Sul. See Back.

With constipation—Æsc. gl.; *Æsc.;* Am. m.; Anac.; *Collins.;* Euonym.; Kali s.; *Nux v.;* Paraf.; Sil.; *Sul.;* Verbasc.

With debility—Ars.; Cinch.; Ham.; Hydr.; Mur. ac.

With epistaxis—Carbo v.

With fissures, soreness of anus—Caps.; Cham.; *Nit. ac.;* Ratanh.; *Sedum.*

With heart disease—Cact.; Collins.; Dig.

With hypochondriasis—Æsc.; Grat.; *Nux v.*

With pelvic congestion—*Aloe; Collins.;* Ham.; Hep.; Mucuna; *Pod.;* Nux v.; Sep.; *Sul.*

With prolapsus ani et uteri—Pod.

With spasm of sphincter—Lach.; Sil.

With stitches in rectum during cough—Ign.; *Kali c.;* Lach.; Nit. ac.

With sudden development in marantic children—Mur. ac.

With tenesmus, anal and visceral, diarrhoea—Caps.

With tenesmus, constriction, lancinating pains—Nux v.

With tenesmus, dysenteric stools—Aloe; Sul.

With tenesmus, in pregnant females—Collins.

With vicarious bleeding—Ham.; Millef.

AGGRAVATIONS—After confinement: Aloe; Apis. See Female Sexual System.

After stool for hours—Æsc.; Am. m.; Ign.; Ratanh.; Sul.

As rheumatic symptoms abate—Abrot.

During climacteric—Æsc.; Lach. See Female Sexual System.

During menses—Am. c.; Lach.

During sitting—Graph.; Ign.; *Thuya.*

From alcoholic abuse, in sedentary persons—Æsc. gl.; Nux v.

From coughing, sneezing—Caust.; *Kali c.;* Lach.

From leucorrhœa suppressed—Am. m.

From talking, thinking of them—Caust.

From walking—Caust.; Sep.

AMELIORATIONS—From cold water: *Aloe;* Nux v.; Ratanh.

From hot water—*Ars.;* Mur. ac.

From lying down—Am. c.

From walking—Ign.

HERNIA—Æsc.; Alum.; Am. c.; Aur.; Calc. c.; Calc. p.; *Cocc.;* Col.; Iris fact.; *Lyc.;* Mag. c.; *Nux v.;* Ox. ac.; Petrol.; Phos.; Picrot.; *Sil.; Sul. ac.;* Ver. a.; Zinc.

Incarcerated—Lob. infl.; *Millef.;* Nux v.; *Op.;* Plumb.

In children—*Calc. c.;* Lyc.; Nit. ac.; *Nux v.;* Sil.; Sul.

Scrotal, congenital—Mag. m.

Strangulated—Acon.; *Bell.;* Lyc.; Nux v.; *Op.;* Plumb.
Umbilical—Calc. c.; Cocc.; *Nux v.;* Plumb. m.

INTESTINES—Intussusception, obstruction: Acon.; Atrop.; *Bell.;* Colch.;
Col.; *Merc. c.; Nux v.; Op.; Plumb.;* Thuya; Ver. a.
Obstruction, post-operative—Acon.; *Arn.;* Bell.; Merc. c.
Paralysis—Eser. sal.; Plumb. ac.
Ulceration—Arg. n.; Cupr.; *Kali bich.;* Merc. c.; Sul. ac.; Sul.; Tereb.;
Uran.

JAUNDICE (icterus)—*Acon.;* Aloe; Am. m.; Arg. n.; Astacus; Ars.; *Aur.
m. n.;* Aur.; *Berb. v.; Bry.; Card. m.;* Cascara sag.; *Ceanoth.; Cham.;
Chel.;* Chelone; *Chionanth.;* Cholest.; *Cinch.;* Corn. c.; Crot.; *Dig.;*
Dolichos; Eup. perf.; Hep.; *Hydr.;* Iod.; Jugl. c.; Kali bich.; Kali c.;
Kali picr.; Lach.; *Lept.; Lyc.;* Merc. c.; *Merc. d.; Merc. s.; Myr.;* Nat.
m.; *Nat. p.;* Nat. s.; Nit. ac.; *Nux v.;* Ostrya; *Phos.;* Picr. ac.; Plumb.;
Pod.; Ptel.; Rumex; Ruta; Sep.; Still.; Sul.; *Tarax.; Yucca;* Veron.;
Vipera.
Anemia; brain disease; pregnancy—Phos.
Chronic—Aur.; Chel.; *Con.;* Iod.; *Phos.*
Extension of catarrhal process—Am. m.; *Chel.;* Chionanth.; *Cinch.;* Dig.;
Hydr.; Lob. infl.; *Merc.;* Nux v.; Pod.
From mental emotion—Bry.; *Cham.;* Lach.; Nux v.; Vipera.
Infantile—Cham.; *Lupul.;* Merc. d.; Merc. s.; Myr.
Malignant—Acon.; *Ars.;* Crot.; Lach.; Merc.; *Phos.*

HYPOCHONDRIA—Pain in left side: *Alum.;* Am. m.; Arg. n.; *Bapt.
conf.;* Carbo v.; *Ceanoth.; Cim.;* Con.; Dig.; Grind.; Kali c.; Lyc.;
Nat. c.; Nat. m.; Nit. ac.; *Ox. ac.;* Parth.; Polymn.; *Puls.;* Quercus;
Scilla; Sep.; Urt. See Spleen.
Pain in right side—*Æsc.; Aloe;* Aur.; Bapt.; *Berb. v.;* Bolet.; *Bry.;* Calc.
c.; Carbo v.; *Chel.; Cinch.;* Con.; *Diosc.;* Gins.; Jacar.; Jatropha;
Kali bich.; Kali c.; Limul.; *Lyc.;* Merc.; *Nat. s.;* Nux v.; Ol. j. as.;
Phyt.; *Pod.; Ptel.;* Quass.; Ran. s.; Sul.; Wyeth. See Liver.

LIVER—Abscess:—Ars.; *Bell.;* Boldo; Bry.; Chin. ars.; *Hep.;* Lach.;
Merc.; Phos.; Raph.; Rhus t.; *Sil.;* Vipera.
Affections in general—Abies c.; *Æsc.; Aloe;* Am. m.; Ars. iod.; *Astacus;*
Aur. m.; *Aur. m. n.; Berb. v.;* Brassica; *Bry.;* Calc. c.; *Card. m.;
Ceanoth.; Cham.; Chel.;* Chelone; Chenop.; *Chionanth.;* Cholest.; *Cinch.;*
Cob.; Con.; Corn. c.; Croc.; Crot.; Diosc.; Dolichos; *Eup. perf.;*
Euonym.; *Ferr. picr.; Hep.;* Hydr.; Iod.; Iodof.; *Iris; Kali c.;* Kali
iod.; Lach.; *Lept.; Lyc.; Mag. m.;* Mang. s.; Marrub.; *Merc. s.;
Myr.; Nat. s.; Nux v.; Phos.;* Pichi; Plumb.; *Pod.; Ptel.;* Puls.;
Querc.; Raph.; Selen.; *Sep.;* Stellar.; *Sul.; Tarax.;* Thlaspi; Uran.;
Vanad.; Veron.
Atrophy, acute, yellow—Dig.; *Phos.;* Pod.
Atrophy (cirrhosis)—Abies c.; Apoc.; Ars.; *Ars. iod.;* Aur. m.; *Aur. mur.;*
Calc. ars.; *Card. m.;* Cascara sag.; *Cinch.;* Fel tauri; Fluor. ac.; Graph.;
Hydr.; *Iod.;* Kali bich.; Kali iod.; *Lyc.;* Merc. d.; *Merc.; Nasturt.
ag.;* Nat. chlor.; Nit. ac.; Nit. mur. ac.; Nux v.; *Phos.;* Plumb.; Pod.;
Quass.; Senec.

Cancer—Ars.; Chel.; *Cholest.;* Con.; Hydr.; Lach.; Nit. ac.; Phos.

CONGESTION (hyperemia, fullness, torpidity)—Abies c.; Æsc. gl.; *Æsc.;*
Agar.; *Aloe;* Ars.; Berb. aq.; *Berb. v.;* Brassica; *Bry.; Card. m.;*
Cham.; *Chel.;* Chelone; Chin. s.; *Cinch.;* Croc.; Dig.; Eup. perf.; Euo-
nym.; *Hep.; Hydr.; Iris;* Kali bich.· *Kali m.; Lach.; Lept.; Lyc.;*
Mag. m.; Merc. d.; Merc.; Mucuna; Nat. s.; Nit. ac.; Nit. mur. ac.;
Nux v.; Phos.; Picr. ac.; *Pod.;* Quass.; Senna; *Sep.;* Stellar.; Still.;
Sul.; Tromb.; *Vipera.*

Congestion, chronic—Am. m.; *Chel.; Cholest.;* Cinch.; Con.; *Hep.;* Hydr.;
Iod.; *Kali c.;* Lept.; *Lyc.;* Mag. m.; Merc. d.; Merc. s.; Nat. s.; *Pod.;*
Selen.; *Sep.; Sul.;* Vipera.

Enlargement (hypertrophy)—Æsc.; Agar.; *Ars.;* Calc. ars.; Card. m.;
Chel.; Chin. ars.; *Chionanth.; Cinch.;* Col.; Con.; *Dig.;* Ferr. ars.;
Ferr. iod.; Glycerin; Graph.; Iod.; Kali c.; Mag. m.; Mang. ac.; *Merc.*
d.; Merc.; Nat. s.; *Nux v.;* Pod.; Sec.; *Selen.;* Stellar.; *Tarax.;* Vipera; Zinc. See Congestion.

Enlargements in drunkards—Absinth.; Am. m.; Ars.; Fluor. ac.; Lach.;
Nux v.; Sul.

Fatty degeneration—Aur. m.; Chel.; Kali bich.; Phlorid.; *Phos.; Picr.*
ac.; Vanad.

Induration—Abies c.; Ars.; Aur.; Cinch.; *Con.; Fluor. ac.; Graph.;* Lyc.;
Mag. m.; Merc.; Nux v.; Sil.; *Tarax.;* Zinc. See Cirrhosis.

Inflammation (perihepatitis, hepatitis)—Acon.; Act. sp.; Ars.; Aur.; *Bry.;*
Cham.; *Chel.;* Corn. c.; *Hep.;* Iod.; Kali iod.; *Lach.;* Merc. d.; *Merc.;*
Nat. s.; *Phos.;* Psor.; Sil.; Stellar.; Sul.

Pain (hepatalgia)—Acon.; *Æsc.;* Aloe; Am. c.; Am. m.; Ars.; Bell.; Berb.
v.; Boldo; *Bry.;* Calc. s.; Carbo v.; *Card. m.; Ceanoth.; Chel.;* Chelone;
Cholest.; *Cinch.;* Cob.; Con.; Crot.; *Dig.; Diosc.;* Jatropha; Kali c.;
Lach.; *Lept.; Lyc.; Mag. m.; Merc.; Merc. d.; Myr.; Nux v.;* Ol.
j. as.; Parth.; *Pod.; Ptel.;* Ran. b.; *Ran. s.;* Sang.; Selen.; *Sep.;*
Stann.; Sul.; Tarax.; Yucca.

Pain dragging, on turning on left side—Bry.; Ptel.

Pain, pressive—Anac.; Carbo an.; Cinch.; *Kali c.;* Lyc.; Mag. m.; Merc.

Pain, stitching—*Acon.; Agar.;* Am. m.; Bell.; Benz. ac.; *Berb. v.; Bry.;*
Carbo v.; *Chel.;* Cinch.; Diosc.; Hep.; Jugl. c.; Kali bich.; *Kali c.;*
Merc. c.; Merc.; Nat. m.; Nat. s.; *Nux v.;* Ox. ac.; Quass.; Ran. b.;
Sep.; Stellar.; Sul.

Pain, relieved lying on painful side—Bry.; Ptel.; Sep.

Pain, relieved rubbing and shaking liver region—Pod.

Pains worse lying on left side—*Bry.;* Nat. s.; *Ptel.*

Pain worse lying on right side—Chel.; Diosc.; Kali c.; *Mag. m.; Merc.*

Pigmentary degeneration—Arg. n.

Sensitiveness to touch, pressure—*Æsc.; Aloe;* Bapt.; *Bell.; Berb. v.;*
Bry.; Calc. c.; *Card. m.:* Chaparro; *Chel.;* Chelone; *Chionanth.; Cinch.;*
Dig.; Eup. perf.; Fluor. ac.; Graph.; Hydr.; Iod.; *Iris; Kali c.; Lach.;*
Lept.; *Lyc.; Mag. m.; Merc. d.;* Merc.; Nat. s.; *Nux v.;* Nyctanth.;
Phos.; *Pod.; Ptel.; Ran. b.;* Sanic.; Senna; *Sep.;* Stellar.; Sul.; Tarax.;
Zinc.

Syphilis—Aur. mur.; Kali iod.; Merc. i. r. See Male Sexual System.

Waxy liver—Calc. c.; *Kali iod.;* Phos.; Sil.

PANCREAS—Affections: Ars.; *Atrop.;* Bar. m.; Bell.; Calc. ars.; Carbo
an.; Carbo v.; Chionanth.; *Iod.; Iris;* Jabor.; Kali iod.; *Merc.;* Nux
v.; Pancreat.; *Phos.;* Piloc.; Puls.

PERINEUM—Ars.; Asaf.; Bell.; Bov.; Can. ind.; Carbo v.; *Chimaph.;*
Cycl.; Kali bich.; Lyc.; Melastoma; Merc.; *Ol. an.; Pæonia; Sanic.;*
Santal; Selen.; Tellur.

PERITONITIS—*Acon.; Apis;* Arn.; Ars.; Atrop.; *Bell.; Bry.;* Calc. c.;
Canth.; Carbo v.; Cham.; Cim.; *Cinch.; Col.; Crot.;* Ferr. p.; Hep.;
Ipec.; Kali chlor.; *Lach.;* Lyc.; *Merc. c.;* Merc. d.; *Merc.; Rhus t.;*
Sang. n.; *Sinap. n.;* Solan. n.; Sul.; Tereb.; Ver. v.; *Wyeth.*

Chronic—Apis; *Lyc.;* Merc. d.; Sul.

Pseudo-peritonitis, hysterical—Bell.; Col.; Ver. a.

Tubercular—*Abrot.;* Ars.; Ars. iod.; Calc. c.; Carbo v.; *Cinch.;* Iod.; Psor.;
Sul.; *Tub.*

PERITYPHLITIS—*Ars.;* Bell.; *Iris min.;* Iris ten.; *Lach.;* Merc. c.; Rhus t.

SPLEEN—Atrophy, induration:—Agn.; Eucal.; *Iod.;* Phos.

Diseases, epidemic, in domestic animals—Anthrac.

Enlargement—Agar.; Agn.; Aran.; *Ars.;* Ars. iod.; Aur. mur.; Bellis;
Calc. ars.; Caps.; Card. m.; *Ceanoth.;* Ced.; Chionanth.; *Chin. s.;*
Cinch.; Ferr. ac.; *Ferr. ars.;* Ferr. iod.; Grind.; *Helianth.;* Iod.; Mag.
m.; Malar.; Merc. i. r.; *Nat. m.;* Persicaria; Phos. ac.; Phos.; *Polym.;*
Querc.; Succin.; Sul. ac.; Urt.

Inflammation (splenitis)—Aran.; Arn.; Iod.; *Ceanoth.; Chin. s.; Cinch.;*
Ferr. p.; Iod.; Plumb. iod.; *Polym.;* Succin.; Ver. v. See Enlargement.

Pain—*Agar.;* Agn.; Am. m.; Arn.; *Ars.;* Ars. m.; Caps.; *Ceanoth.;*
Cim.; Cinch.; Cobalt.; *Diosc.;* Grind.; *Helianth.; Helon.;* Ilex; Iod.;
Kali iod.; Lob. cer.; Nat. m.; Parth.; Plumb.; *Polym. noed.;* Ptel.;
Quass.; Querc.; Ran. b.; Rhus t.; Scilla; Sul.; Urt.

Pain, stitching—Agar.; Alston.; Am. m.; *Bellis;* Berb. v.; Carbo v.;
Ceanoth.; Chel.; Cinch.; Con.; Kali bich.; Nat. m.; Ran. b.; Rhod.;
Sul.; Tarax.; *Ther.*

TYPHLITIS, APPENDICITIS—Acon.; Arn.; *Ars.;* Bapt.; *Bell.; Bry.;*
Canth.; Card. m.; Colch.; Collins.; *Col.;* Crot.; *Diosc.; Echin.;* Ferr.
p.; Gins.; Hep.; Iris ten.; Kali m.; *Lach.;* Lyc.; *Merc. c.;* Merc.;
Nux v.; Op.; Plumb.; Rhamnus; *Rhus t.;* Sil.; Sul.; Ver. a.

UMBILICUS, Navel—Bleeding from, in newborn: Abrot.; *Calc. p.*

Bubbling sensation—Berb. v.

Burning—Acon.; Ars.

Eczema—Merc. pr. rub.

Pain, soreness about—Æsc.; *Aloe;* Anac.; Benz. ac.; Bov.; Bry.; *Calc.
p.;* Carbo v.; Caust.; *Cham.;* Chel.; Chionanth.; *Cina;* Cocc.; Col.;
Con.; Crot. t.; *Dulc.;* Euonym.; *Gamb.; Granat.;* Hyper.; *Ipec.;* Lept.;
Lyc.; *Nux m.*, Nux v.; Oleand.; Ox. ac.; Paraf.; *Phos. ac.;* Plat.;
Plumb. m.; Ran. sc.; Raph.; *Rheum;* Senec.; Sil.; *Spig.; Stann.;* Sul.;
Taxus; Verbasc.; *Ver. a.;* Zinc. m.

Retraction—Calc. p.; *Plumb.;* Pod.

Ulcer, above—Ars.

Urine, oozing from—Hyos.

WORMS—Remedies in general: *Æsc.; Ambros.;* Apoc. andr.; *Ars.;* Bapt.; Bell.; Calad.; *Calc. c.; Chelone;* Cic.; *Cina;* Cupr. ac.; Cupr. oxy.; *Ferr. mur.;* Ferr. s.; *Filix m.; Granat.;* Ign.; Indigo; Ipec.; Kali m.; Kuosso; Lyc.; Merc. c.; *Naph.; Nat. p.;* Passifl.; Puls.; Quass.; *Ratanh.; Sabad.; Santon.;* Sil.; *Spig.; Stann.;* Sul.; Sumb.; Tereb.; *Teucr.;* Ver. a.; *Viola od.*

Ascaris lumbricoides—*Abrot.; Æsc.;* Ant. c.; Calc. c.; *Chelone; Cina;* Ferr. m.; Granat.; Helmintoch.; Ign.; Indigo; Kali chlor.; Lyc.; Merc. d.; Naph.; Pin. sylv.; *Sabad.; Santon.; Spig.;* Stann.; Sul.; Tereb.; *Teucr.;* Urt.

Oxyuris vermicularis—Ars.; Bapt.; *Chelone; Cina;* Ign.; Indigo; Lyc.; *Merc. d.; Merc. s.;* Nat. p.; Ratanh.; *Santon.;* Sil.; Sinap. n.; Spig.; Teucr.; Val.

Taenia—Argem. mex.; Carbo v.; Cucur.; Cupr. ac.; Cupr. oxy.; *Filix m.; Granat.;* Graph.; Kali iod.; Kamala; *Kuosso;* Mag. m.; Merc.; Pelletierine; Phos.; Puls.; Sabad.; Sab.; Santon.; Stann.; Sul ; Tereb.; Val.

Trichinæ—Ars.; Bapt.; Cupr. oxy.

URINARY SYSTEM

AFFECTIONS, in old men—Alfal.; Aloe; Cop.; Hep.; Phos.; *Pop. tr.;* Staph.; Sul. See Weakness.

BLADDER—**Atony:** *Ars.;* Dulc.; Hep.; Op.; *Plumb.;* Rhus ar.; Rhus t.; Scilla; Tereb. See Paralysis.
Cystocele—Staph.

ENURESIS—**Incontinence: Remedies in general:** Acon.; Agar.; Apis; *Arg. n.;* Arn.; Ars.; Atrop.; *Bell.; Benz. ac.;* Calc. c.; Canth.; *Caust.;* Cic.; Cim.; *Cina;* Con.; *Dulc.; Equis.;* Eryng. aq.; Eup. perf.; *Eup. purp.;* Ferr. m.; *Ferr. p.; Gels.;* Hydrang.; Hyos.; *Kali br.;* Kali n.; Kali p.; *Kreos.;* Linar.; *Lupul.;* Lyc.; Mag. p.; Med.; *Nux v.;* Op.; Petrol.; Phos. ac.; Physal.; Plant.; *Puls ; Rhus ars.;* Rhus t.; *Sabal;* Sanic.; *Santon.;* Sec.; Senega; *Sep.;* Sil.; Stram.; *Sul.;* Tereb.; *Thyr.;* Thuya; Tritic.; Tub.; *Uran.; Verbasc.;* Zinc. m. See Flow.

TYPE—OCCURRENCE—**Diurnal:** Arg. n.; Bell.; Caust.; Equis.; *Ferr. m.; Ferr. p.;* Sec.

In old people—Aloe; Ammon. benz.; *Arg. n.; Benz. ac.;* Canth.; Equis.; *Gels.;* Nit. ac.; *Rhus ar.;* Sec.; Senega; *Turnera.*

Nocturnal—Am. c.; Arg. n.; Arn.; Ars.; *Bell.;* Benz. ac.; Calc. c.; *Caust.;* Cina; Coca; *Equis.;* Eup. purp.; Ferr. iod.; Ferr. p.; Gels.; Hep.; Ign.; Kali br.; Mag. p.; *Med.;* Physal.; *Plant.; Puls.;* Quass.; *Rhus ar.;* Santon ; Sec.; *Sil.; Sul.;* Thuya; *Thyr.;* Uran.; Verbasc.

CAUSE—**Catheterization, after:** Mag. p.
Digestive disturbances—Benz. ac.; *Nux v.;* Puls.
During first sleep; child aroused with difficulty—Caust.; Kreos.; *Sep.*
During full moon; intractable cases; eczematous history—Psor.
Habit the only ascertainable cause—Equis.
History of sycosis—Med.
Hysteria—Ign.; Val m.
Weak or paretic sphincter vesicae—Apoc.; *Bell.; Caust.;* Con.; Ferr. p.; *Gels.;* Nux v.; Rhus ar.; *Sabal;* Sec.; *Strych.* See Paralysis.
Worms—Cina; *Santon.;* Sul.

FEELING—**As if ball or plug, in bladder**—Anac.; Kali br.; Lach.; Santal.
Feeling, as if chill rising from, to back—Sars.
Feeling, as if distended—Anthem.; *Apoc.;* Ars.; Berb. v.; *Con.;* Conv.; Dig.; *Equis.;* Eup. perf.; Gels ; *Hyos.;* Mel cum sale; Pareira;, *Puls.;* Ruta: Santon.; *Sars.;* Sep.; Staph.; *Sul.;* Uva.
Hæmorrhage—*Amyg. pers.;* Cact.; Carbo v.; Erig.; *Ham.;* Millef.; *Nit. ac.;* Rhus ar.; *Sec.; Thlaspi.* See Hæmaturia.
Hypertrophy, concentric—Pichi.

INFLAMMATION (cystitis)—**Acute:** Acon.; Ant. t.; Apis; Ars.; Aspar.; *Bell.;* Benz. ac.; Berb. v.; *Camph.;* Camphor. ac.; *Can. s.;* Canth.; Caps.; Chimaph ; Con.; *Cop.;* Cub.; Dig.; *Dulc.;* Elat.; *Equis.;* Erig.; *Eucal.; Eup. purp.;* Ferr. ac.; *Ferr. p.; Gels.;* Helleb.; Hydrang.; Hyos.; Lach.; *Merc. c.;* Methyl. bl.; Nit. ac.; Nux v.; *Ol. sant.; Pareira;*

URINARY SYSTEM   **807**

Petros.; Pichi; Pip. m.; *Pop. tr.*; Prun. sp.; *Puls.*; Sabal; *Sab.*; Sars.; *Saurur.*; Sep.; *Stigm.*; Sul.; *Tereb.*; Tritic.; Uva; Vesic.

From abuse of cantharis—Apis; Camph.

From gonorrhoea—Bell.; Benz. ac.; *Canth.*; *Cop.*; Cub.; Merc. c.; Puls.; Sabal.

From operations, and in pregnancy—Pop. tr.

With fever, strangury—*Acon.*; Bell.; *Canth.*; Gels.; Hydrang.; Stigm.

Inflammation, chronic—*Ars.*; Bals. per.; Baros.; *Benz. ac.*; Berb. v.; *Bu-chu; Can. s.; Canth.*; Carbo v.; *Caust.*; *Chimaph.*; Coccus; Col.; *Cop.*; Cub.; *Dulc.*; *Epig.*; Eryng. aq.; Eucal.; *Eup. purp.*; Fabiana; Grind.; *Hydr.*; Iod.; Junip.; Kava; Lith. c.; Lyc.; *Merc. c.*; Nit. ac.; *Pareira;* Pichi; Pip. m.; *Pop. tr.*; Prun. sp.; *Puls.*; Rhus ar.; *Sabal;* Santon.; Senega; *Sep.*; Silph.; *Stigm.*; *Tereb.*; Thlaspi; Thuya; Tritic.; Tub.; *Uva;* Vesic.; Zea.

IRRITABILITY—**Bladder and neck**: Acon.; Alfal.; Aloe; *Apis;* Baros.; *Bell.*; *Benz. ac.*; *Berb. v.*; Buchu; Calc. c.; *Camph.*; Can. s.; *Canth.*; Caps.; Caust.; *Cop.*; Cub.; Dig.; *Equis.*; Erig.; Eryng. aq.; *Eup. purp.*; Ferr. ac.; Ferr. m.; *Ferr. p.*; Guaiac.; Hyos.; Kali br.; Mitchella; Nit. mur. ac.; *Nux v.*; Oxytr.; Pareira; Petros.; Prun. sp.; Rhus ar.; *Sabal; Senec.*; Senega; *Sep.*; *Staph.*; *Stigm.*; *Tereb.*; Thuya; *Tritic.;* Vesic.

Irritability in women—Berb. v.; Cop.; Cub.; *Eup. purp.*; Gels.; Hedeoma; Kreos.; Senec.; *Sep.*; Staph.

PAIN—*Acon.*; Ambra; *Bell.*; *Berb. v.*; Camph.; *Canth.*; Carbo v.; Caul.; *Caust.*; Coccus; Cop.; Dig.; *Dulc.*; *Equis.*; Erig.; *Eryng.*; Ign.; Lach.; Lyc.; Naph.; Nit. ac.; Op.; *Pareira.*; Pichi; Piloc.; *Pop. tr.*; Prun. sp.; Pulex; *Puls.*; *Rhus ar.*; *Staph.*; Stigm.; Strych.; *Tereb.*; Thuya; Tritic.; Uran. n.; *Uva.* See Cystitis.

TYPE—**Aching**—Berb. v.; Conv.; *Equis.*; Eup. purp.; *Pop. tr.*; Sep.; Stic-ta; Tereb.

Burning—*Acon.*; Ars.; Baros.; *Berb. v.*; Camph.; *Canth.*; Cop.; Ferr. picr.; Staph.; *Tereb.*; Thuya; *Uva.*

Cramp-like, constricting—Bell.; Berb. v.; Cact.; Can. s.; Canth.; Caps.; Lyc.; Op.; *Polyg.*; Prun. sp.; *Sars.*; Tereb.

Cutting, stitching—Acon.; Æth.; Bell.; *Berb. v.*; Canth.; Coccus; Con.; Lyc.; Tereb.

Neuralgic, spasmodic—Bell.; *Berb. v.*; Canth.; Caul.; Lith. c.; *Lyc.*; Merc. c.; *Pareira;* Puls.; *Staph.*; Uva.

Pressing—Aloe; Brachygl.; *Cact.*; Carbo v.; Coccus; *Con.*; Dig.; *Dulc.*; *Equis.*; Lach.; Lil. t.; Lyc.; Mel cum sale; *Pop. tr.*; Pulex; *Puls.*; Ruta; *Sep.*; *Staph.*; Sul.; Tereb.; Verbasc.

Radiating to spermatic cord—Clem.; Lith. c.; Puls.; Spong.

MODALITIES—**AGGRAVATIONS: After urination:**—*Canth.*; Caust.; Epig.; *Equis.*; Pichi; Ruta. See Urination.

From drinking water—Canth.

From lithotomy—Staph.

From walking—Con.; Prun. sp.

AMELIORATIONS—From rest:—Con.
From urination—Coccus.; Hedeoma.
From walking—Ign.; Tereb.

PARALYSIS—Alum.; Apoc.; *Arn.; Ars.;* Aur.; Cact.; Camph.; Can. ind.; *Canth.; Caust.;* Con.; Dig.; Dulc.; Eucal.; *Equis.;* Ferr. m.; Ferr. p.; *Gels.;* Helleb.; *Hyos.;* Lach.; Morph.; *Nux v.; Op.; Plumb. m.;* Psor.: Puls.; *Sec.;* Strych.; Thuya.

Paralysis of sphincter—Ars.; *Bell.; Caust.;* Cic.; *Dulc.; Hyos.;* Ign.: Lach.; Laur.; Nat. m.; Op.; Sul.; Thuya; *Zinc.*

POLYPI—Papilloma:—Ars.; *Calc. c.;* Thuya.

Prolapsus—Hyos.; Pyrus; Staph.

Sensitiveness, tenderness of vesical region—*Acon.; Bell.;* Berb. v.; *Canth.;* Coccus; *Equis.;* Eup. purp.; Merc. c.; Sars.; Sticta; *Tereb.* See Pain.

Spasm (cystopasm)—Canth.; Gels.; *Hyos.;* Nux v.; Puls.

Spasm following operations on orifice—*Bell.;* Col.; *Hyper.*

TENESMUS VESICAE—*Acon.: Apis;* Arn.; *Bell.;* Benz. ac.; Camph.; Can. s.; *Canth.; Caps.;* Cham.; Chimaph.; Coccus; *Col.;* Cop.; Cub.; Epig.; *Equis.;* Eryng.; *Eup. purp.;* Ferr. p.; Hydrang.; Hyos.; Ipec.; *Lil. t.;* Lith. c.; Lyc.; Med.; *Merc. c.;* Nit. ac.; *Nux v.; Oniscus;* Pichi; *Plumb. m ;* Pop. tr.; Prun. sp.; *Puls.;* Rham. c.; Rhus t.; *Sabal;* Sars.; *Senec.;* Staph.; *Stigm.; Tereb.;* Vesic.

WEAKNESS—Inability to retain urine, dribbing—Aloe; Ananth.; *Apoc.; Bell.; Benz. ac.,* Brachygl.; Camph., *Can. ind.; Caust.;* Clem.; *Con., Equis.;* Erig.; Euphras.; *Gels.*. Hep.; *Nux v.·* Petrol.; Picr. ac.; Pulex; Puls.; *Rhus ar.;* Santon.; Sabal; *Sars.;* Selen.; Solan. lyc.; *Staph.;* Tereb.; Thymol; Tribul.; Uva; *Verbasc.;* Vesic.; Xerophyl.

Weakness in old men—Alum.; *Benz. ac.;* Carb. ac.; Clem.; Con.; *Pop. tr.*. Selen.; *Staph.* See Paralysis.

KIDNEYS—Abscess (perinephritic):—Arn.; Bell.; *Hep.;* Merc.; Ver. v.

CALCULI—GRAVEL (nephrolithiasis)—COLIC:—*Arg. n.; Bell.;* Benz. ac.. *Berb. v.;* Buchu; Calc. c.; Calc. ren.; *Canth.;* Cham.; Chin. s.; *Coccus:* Col.; *Diosc.; Epig.;* Erig.; Eryng.; *Eup. purp.;* Hedeoma; Hep.; Hydrang.; Ipomœa; *Lyc.;* Med.; *Nit. ac.; Nux v.; Ocimum;* Oniscus; Op.; Oxyden.; *Pareira; Pichi;* Piperaz.; Polygon.; *Sars.;* Sep.; *Solid.; Stigm.; Tab.;* Thlaspi; Urt.; Uva; Vesic.

Colic, worse left side—*Berb. v.;* Canth.; Tab.

Colic, worse right side—*Lyc.;* Nux v.; Ocimum; Sars.

Inter-paroxysmal treatment—*Berb. v.; Calc. c.;* Chin. s.; Hydrang.; *Lyc.*. Nux v.; *Sep.;* Urt.

CONGESTION, acute—*Acon.;* Arg. n.; Arn.; Aur.; *Bell.;* Benz. ac.; *Berb v.;* Bry.; Camph.; *Canth.;* Dig.; *Dulc.;* Eucal.; Eryng. aq.; *Helleb.; Helon.;* Hydroc. ac.; *Junip.;* Kali bich.; Merc. c.; *Ol. sant.;* Op.; Rhus t.; Senec.; Solid.; *Tereb.;* Ver. v. See Nephritis.

Congestion, chronic (passive, from heart or kidney disease)—Acon.; Arn.; Bell.; *Caffeine; Conv.; Dig.;* Glon.; Phos.; *Stroph.;* Strych.; Ver. v. See Heart.

DEGENERATION, acute, amyloid, fatty—Apis; *Ars.; Aur. mur.;* Bell.:

Cic.; *Cupr. ac.;* Ferr. mur.; Hydroc. ac.; *Kali iod.;* Lyc.; *Nit. ac.;* *Phos. ac.; Phos.;* Rhus t.; Tereb. See Nephritis.

FLOATING KIDNEY (nephroptosis) reflex symptoms:—*Bell.;* Cham.; Col.; Gels.; *Ign.;* Lach.; Puls.; *Strych. ars.;* Sul.; Zinc.

INFLAMMATION (nepritis)—Bright's disease:

ACUTE AND SUBACUTE PARENCHYMATOUS NEPHRITIS—*Acon.;* Ant. t.; *Apis;* Apoc.; *Ars.; Aur. mur.; Bell.;* Berb. v.; *Can. s.; Canth.;* Chel.; *Chimaph.; Chin. s.;* Colch.; Conv.; *Cupr. ars.;* Dig.; Dulc.; Eucal.; Eup. perf.; Ferr. iod.; Fuschina; Glon.; *Helleb.;* Helon.; *Hep.;* Hydrocot.; Irid.; Junip.; Kali bich.; *Kali chlor.;* Kali citr.; **Kal.**; *Koch's lymph;* Lach.; *Merc. s.; Methyl. bl.;* Nit. ac.; *Ol. Sant.;* Phos. ac.; *Phos.; Pichi;* Picr. ac.; Plumb. ac.; Ploygon.; Rhus t.; *Sab.; Samb.; Scilla;* Sec.; Senec.; Serum ang.; *Tereb.; Ver. a.; Ver. v.;* Zing.

CAUSE—**From cold, or wet exposure**—*Acon.;* Ant. t.; *Apis;* Canth.; *Dulc.;* Rhus t.; Tereb.

From influenza—Eucal.

From malaria—*Ars.;* Eup. perf.; Tereb.

From pregnancy—Apis; Apoc.; *Cupr. ars.;* Helon.; Kal.; *Merc. c.;* Sab. See Female Sexual System.

From scarlet fever, diphtheria—Acon.; *Apis; Ars.;* Bell.; *Canth.;* Conv.; Cop.; Dig.; Ferr. iod.; *Helleb.; Hep.;* Kal.; Lach.; *Merc. c.;* Methyl. bl.; Nat. s.; Nit. sp. d.; *Rhus t.;* Sec.; *Tereb.*

From suppurations—Apoc.; Chin. s.; *Hep.;* Phos.; Plumb. c.; *Sil.;* Tereb.

CONCOMITANTS—**Dropsy:**—Acon.; Adon. v.; Ant. t.; *Apis; Apoc.; Ars.;* Aur. mur.; Canth.; Colch.; Cop.; *Dig.; Helleb.;* Merc. c.; Piloc.; *Samb.; Scilla;* Senec.; Tereb. See Dropsy (Generalities).

Heart failure—Adon. v.; Ars.; *Caffeine; Dig.;* Glon.; *Spart.;* Stroph.; Ver. v.

Pneumonia—Chel.; Phos.

Uraemic symptoms—Æth.; Am. c.; Ars.; Bell.; Can. ind.; *Carb. ac.;* Cic.; *Cupr. ars.;* Helleb.; Hyos.; *Morph.; Op.;* Piloc.; Stram.; Urea.

ACUTE, SUPPURATIVE NEPHRITIS—Acon.; Arn.; Bell.; Camph.; Calc. s.; *Can. s.;* Canth.; *Chin. s.;* Eucal.; Hekla; *Hep.;* Kali n.; *Merc. c.;* Naph.; Sil.; Ver. v.

CHRONIC, INTERSTITIAL NEPHRITIS—Apis; *Ars.; Aur. mur.;* Aur. m. n.; Cact.; *Chin. s.; Colch.;* Conv.; *Dig.;* Ferr. m.; *Ferr. mur.; Glon.; Iod.;* Kali c.; *Kali iod.;* Koch's lymph; Lith. ac.; Lith. benz.; Lith. c.; *Merc. c;* Merc. d.; *Nat. iod.; Nit ac.;* Nux v.; Op.; Phos. ac.; Phos.; *Plumb. c.; Plumb. iod.; Plumb. m.;* Sang.; Zinc. picr. See Arteriosclerosis (Circulatory System).

CHRONIC, PARENCHYMATOUS NEPHRITIS—Am. benz.; *Apis; Ars.; Aur. mur.;* Aur. m. n.; Benz. ac.; Berb v.; *Brachygl.;* Calc. ars.; Calc. p.; Can. ind.; *Canth.;* Chin. ars ; Conv.; Dig.; Eup. purp.; *Euonym.; Ferr. ars.;* Ferr. cit.; *Ferr. mur.;* Ferr. p.; Form. ac.; Glon.; *Helon.;* Hydroc. ac.; Junip.; Kali ars.; *Kali chlor.;* Kali cit.; *Kali iod.; Kali m.;* Kal.; Koch's lymph; Lonic.; *Lyc.;* Merc. c.; Nat. chlor.; *Nit. ac.; Piloc.; Plumb.;* Senec.; Solania; Solid.; Spart.; *Tereb.;* Urea; *Vesic.*

SYMPTOMS—URAEMIA: In general:—*Am. c.;* Apis; Apoc.; Ars.; Asclep. c.; *Bell.;* Can. ind.; *Canth.;* *Carb. ac.;* Cic.; Cupr. ac.; *Cupr. ars.;* *Glon.;* *Helleb.;* Hydroc. ac.; Hyos.; Kali br.; *Morph.;* *Op.;* Phos.; *Pier. ac.;* Piloc.; Quebracho; Serum ang.; Stram.; *Tereb.;* Urea; Urt.; *Ver. v.*

  Coma—*Am. c.;* Bell.; Bry.; *Carb. ac.;* Cupr. ars.; *Helleb.;* Merc. c.; *Morph.;* *Op.;* Ver. v.

  Convulsions—Bell.; Carb. ac.; Chloral.; *Cic.;* Cupr. ac.; *Cupr. ars.;* Glon.; *Hydroc. ac.;* Kali br.; Merc. c.; Op.; Piloc.; Plumb.; Ver. v.   See Convulsions (Nervous System).

  Headache—Arn.; Can. ind.; Carb. ac.; Cupr. ars.; *Glon.;* Hyper.; *Sang.;* Zinc. picr. See Head.

  Vomiting—*Ars.;* Iod.; Kreos.; Nux v. See Stomach.

PAIN IN RENAL REGION—Burning:—*Acon.;* Ars.; Aur.; *Berb. v.;* But. ac.; *Canth.;* Hedeoma; *Helon.;* Kali iod.; Lach.; *Lyc.;* Merc. c.; *Phos.;* Sab.; *Sul.;* *Tereb.* See Back.

  Cutting, digging, boring—Arn.; *Berb. v.;* *Canth.;* Eup. purp.; Ipec.; *Lyc.;* Rhus t.; Tereb.

  Drawing, tensive—*Berb. v.;* Can. s.; *Canth.;* Chel.; Coccus; *Colch.;* Dulc.; Lach.; *Lyc.;* Nit. ac.; Solid.; *Tereb.*

  Neuralgic, radiating (nephralgia), tearing, lancinating—*Arg. n.;* Arn.; *Bell.;* *Berb. v.;* Calc. c.; *Canth.;* Chel.; Chin. s.; *Coccinel; Coccus;* Diosc.; Eryng. aq.; Ferr. mur.; *Hedeoma;* *Hydrang.;* Lach.; *Lyc.;* Kali iod.; Nit. ac.; *Nux v.;* *Ocimum;* Oxytr.; Pareira; Phos.; Sab.; *Sars.;* Scrophul.; *Solid.;* *Tab.;* Tereb.; Thlaspi; Vespa. See Nephrolithiasis.

  Pressing—Arg. n.; *Arn.;* Aur. mur.; *Berb. v.;* *Canth.;* Chin. s.; *Lyc.;* Nit. ac.; *Ocimum;* Petrol.; *Phos. ae.;* *Sep.;* *Tereb.;* Uva; Xerophyl.

  Stitching—*Berb. v.;* *Canth.;* Colch.; *Kali c.;* Pareira.

  Throbbing—Act. sp.; *Berb. v.;* Chimaph.; *Med.;* *Sab.*

  Weariness, aching, lameness—*Acon.;* Alum.; Am. br.; Apis; *Arg. n.;* *Benz. ac.;* *Berb. v.;* Can. ind.; *Canth.;* Chel.; Cina; Conv.; Cop.; *Eup. purp.;* *Hedeoma;* *Helon.;* Hydrang.; Junip.; Kali bich.; Lyc.; Nat. chlor.; *Nux v.;* *Ol. sant.;* *Phyt.;* *Picr. ac.;* Pin. sylv.; *Sab.;* Sep.; Solid.; Stellar.; Tereb.; Ustil.; *Uva;* Vespa. See Back.

MODALITIES—AGGRAVATIONS: At 2 P. M.: Kal.

  From lifting, sudden effort—Calc. p.

  From lying down—Conv.

  From motion—*Berb. v.;* *Canth.;* Chel.; Kali iod.

  From pressure—*Berb. v.;* Canth.; Colch.; *Solid.*

  From sitting—*Berb. v.;* Ferr. mur.

  From stooping, lying down—Berb. v.

  From stretching legs—Colch.

  From wine—Benz. ac.

  On left side—Æsc.; Berb. v.; *Hedeoma;* Hydrang.; Tab.; Uva.

  On right side—Am. benz.; Can. ind.; *Chel.;* Equis.; Lith. c.; *Lyc.;* Ocimum; Phyt.; Picr. ac.; *Sars.;* *Tereb.*

AMELIORATIONS—From lying on back: Cahinca.

  From lying on back, legs drawn up—Colch.

From standing—Berb. v.
From urination—Lyc.; Med.
From walking—Ferr. mur.

PERI-NEPHRITIS—Acon.; Bry.; Chin. s.; Hep.; Merc.; Sil.

PYELITIS—Inflammation of pelvis: Acute: Acon.; *Ars.*; Aur.; *Bell.*; *Benz. ac.*; Berb. v.; Bry.; *Can. s.*; *Canth.*; Cinch.; *Cop.*; *Cupr. ars.*; Epig.; *Ferr. mur.*; Hekla; Hep.; Kali bich.; *Merc. c.*; Nit. ac.; *Puls.*; *Rhus t.*; Stigm.; *Tereb.*; Thuya; *Tritic.*; *Uva*; *Ver. v.*

Calculous—Hep.; *Hydrang.*; Lyc.; *Piparaz.*; Sil.; Uva. See Nephrolithiasis.

Chronic—Ars.; *Benz. ac.*; Berb. v.; *Buchu*; *Chimaph.*; Chin. s.; Cinch.; *Cop.*; Hep.; Hydrast. mur.; Hydrast. s.; *Junip.*; *Kali bich.*; *Ol. sant.*; Pareira; Puls.; Sep.; Sil.; Sul.; Stigm.; *Uva*.

SENSITIVENESS, tenderness—*Acon.*; Apis; *Berb. v.*; Calc. ars.; Can. s.; *Canth.*; Equis.; *Helon.*; Phyt.; *Solid.*; *Tereb.* See Pain.

SYPHILIS—Aur.; Kali iod.; Merc. c. See Male Sexual System.
Traumatisms—Acon.; *Arn.*; Bell.; Ver. v.

TUBERCULOSIS—*Ars. iod.*; Bac.; Calc. c.; Calc. hypoph.; *Calc. iod.*; *Chin. ars.*; Chin. s.; Hekla; Kali iod.; Kreos. See Tuberculosis (Respiratory System).

URETHRA—Burning, smarting, heat—*Acon.*; Apis; *Arg. n.*; *Berb. v.*; Cahinca; Calc. c.; *Can. ind.*; *Can. s.*; *Canth.*; *Caps.*; Chimaph.; *Clem.*; Con.; Cop.; Dig.; Gels.; *Hydrang.*; *Merc. c.*; *Merc.*; Mez.; Nat. c.; Nit. mur. ac.; Oniscus; Petrol.; *Petros.*; Phos.; Selen.; Staph.; *Sul.*; Tereb.; *Thuya*; *Uran.*; Zing.

Burning between acts of urination—Berb. v.; Can. s.; Staph.

Caruncle—Can. s.; *Eucal.*; Teucr.; *Thuya*.

Discharge, mucous—Hep.; Merc. c.; Nat. m.

Hæmorrhage—Calc. c.; Lyc.

Inflammation (urethritis)—*Acon.*; Apis; *Arg. n.*; Camph.; *Can. s.*; *Canth.*; Caps.; Caust.; *Cop.*; *Cub.*; *Doryph.*; *Gels.*; Kali bich.; Kali iod.; Merc. c.; Nux v.; Petrol.; Sab.; Sul.; *Thuya*; Yohimb. See Male Sexual System.

Itching—Acon.; Alum.; Ambra; *Arg. n.*; Canth.; Caust.; Col.; *Ferr. iod.*; Ferr. m.; Gins.; Lyc.; *Merc.*; Mez.; *Nit. ac.*; Ol. an.; Pareira; Petrol.; *Petros.*; Staph.; *Sul.*; Thuya; Tussil.

MEATUS—Burning: *Acon.*; Ambra; Bor.; Can. s.; *Canth.*; *Caps.*; Clem.; Gels.; Menthol; *Petros.*; Selen.; *Sul.*; Zing.

Eruptions around—Caps.

Itching—Alum.; *Ambra*; Caust.; Col.; Gins.; *Petros.*

Ulcers around—Eucal.

Swelling—Acon.; Arg. n.; *Can. s.*; *Canth.*; Cop.; Gels.; *Merc.*; *Ol. sant.*; Sul. See Urethritis.

Membranous-prostatic involvement—Sabal.

PAIN IN URETHRA—Constricting: *Arg. n.*; *Can. s.*; Caps.; *Clem.*; Ferr. iod.; Ol. sant.; *Petros.*

Cutting—Alum.; Ant. c.; *Berb. v.*; *Canth.*; Nat. m.; Oniscus; *Petros.*

Soreness, tenderness irritation—Agn.; Anag.; *Arg. n.; Berb. v.;* Brachygl.; *Can. s.; Canth.;* Caust.; Clem.; *Cop.;* Cub.; Ferr. picr.; Gels.; Kali iod.; Tussil.

Stitching, stinging—Agar.; *Apis; Arg. n.;* Aspar.; *Berb. v.;* Can. ind.; *Can. s.;* Caps.; Carbo v.; *Clem.;* Merc. c.; Merc.; Nit. ac.; Petros.; *Thuya.*

SENSIBILITY—Diminished—Kali br.

STRICTURE, organic—Acon.; Arg. n.; Arn.; Calc. iod.; *Canth.; Clem.;* Eucal.; Lob. infl.; Phos.; Puls.; *Sil.; Sul. iod.*

Stricture, spasmodic—*Acon.;* Bell.; *Camph.;* Canth.; Eryng.; Hydrang.; Nux v.; Petros.

URINARY FLOW—DESIRE—Constant desire: Absinth.; *Acon.;* Ananth.; *Bell.;* Berb. v.; Cact.; *Can. s.; Canth.;* Carbo v.; Caust.; Ceanoth.; Coccus; *Cop.;* Dig.; Dulc.; Equis.; *Eup. purp.;* Ferr. mur.; Gels.; Guaiac.; Kreos.; *Lil. t.;* Lyssin; *Murex;* Op.; *Pareira;* Ruta; *Sabal; Senec.;* Sep.; *Staph.;* Sulphon.; *Sul.; Thuya; Tritic.;* Zing. See Cystitis.
Constant after labor—Op.; *Staph.*
Constant at night—Dig.; *Sabal.*
Constant from prolapsus uteri—Lil. t.
Constant, on seeing running water—Canth.; *Lyssin;* Sul.

DIABETES INSIPIDUS—Copious, profuse; polyuria; diuresis: *Acet. ac.;* Acon.; *Alfal.;* Am. acet.; Apoc.; *Arg. m.;* Arg. mur.; Ars.; *Aur. mur.; Bell.;* Bry.; Cahinca; *Can. ind.;* Caust.; Cepa; Chin. s.; Chionanth.; Cina; *Cod.;* Conv.; Dulc.; *Equis.; Eup. purp.; Ferr. mur.;* Ferr. n.; *Gels.;* Glycerin; *Glon.;* Gnaph.; Guaco; *Helleb.; Helon.; Ign.;* Indol; *Kali c.;* Kali iod.; *Kali n.; Kreos.;* Lact. ac.; Led.; *Lil. t.; Lith. c.; Lyc.;* Mag. p.; Merc. c.; Mosch.; *Murex; Nat. m.;* Niccol. s.; *Nit. ac.;* Nux v.; *Ol. an.; Oxytr.; Phos. ac.;* Phos.; Physal.; Picr. ac.; Plat. m. n.; Puls.; Quass.; *Rhus ar.; Samb.;* Sang.; Santon.; Sars.; *Scilla; Sinap. n.;* Spart.; Staph.; *Stroph.; Sul.;* Tarax.; Tereb.; Thymol; Thyr.; *Uran.;* Verbasc.; Ver. v. See Diabetes.
Copious at night—Ambra; Kali iod.; *Lyc.; Murex;* Petrol.; *Phos. ac.;* Quass.; *Scilla.*

DYSURIA—Difficult, slow, painful: *Acon.; Alum.;* Ant. t.; *Apis;* Apoc.; *Arg. n.;* Arn.; Ars.; Bell.; *Lenz. ac.;* Camph.; Can. ind.; *Can. s.; Canth.;* Caps.; Cascara; *Caust.;* Chimaph.; *Clem.;* Coccus; *Con.;* Cop.; Cucurb. cit.; Dig.; Dulc.; *Epig.;* Equis.; *Eup. purp.; Fabiana;* Ferr. p.; *Hep.;* Hydrang.; Hyper.; Hyos.; Kreos.; Lith. c.; *Lyc.;* Med.; Merc. c.; *Morph.;* Mur. ac.; *Nat. m.;* Nit. ac.; Nux v.; Ocimum; *Ol. sant.; Op.; Pareira;* Petros.; Pichi; *Plumb.;* Pop. tr.; Puls.; Rhus t.; Ruta; *Sabal; Santon.; Sars.;* Selen.; *Sep.; Solid.;* Staph.; Stigm.; Taxus; Thlaspi; *Tritic.; Uva;* Verbasc.; Vib. op.; Zinc. See Scanty.
Difficult, in pregnancy. and afer confinement—Equis.
Difficult, in presence of others—Ambra; Hep.; Mur. ac.; *Nat. m.*
Difficult, in young, married women—Staph.
Difficult, must lie down—Kreos.
Difficult, must sit bent backwards—Zinc.

Difficult, must stand with feet wide apart, body inclined forward—Chimaph.

Difficult, must strain—*Acon.; Alum.;* Can. ind.; *Chimaph.;* Equis.; *Hyos.;* Kali c.; *Kreos.;* Lyc.; *Mag. m.;* Nux v.; Op.; Papaya; *Pareira; Prun. s.; Sabal;* Zinc. See Bladder.

Difficult, with prolapsus ani—Mur. ac.

Difficult, with prostatic or uterine diseases—Con.; Staph.

Divided stream—Anag.; Arg. n.; Can. s.; Canth.

Feeble stream—Cham.; Clem.; Helleb.; Hep.; Merc.; Sars.

FREQUENT desire—*Acon.;* Agar.; Agn.; Alfal.; Aloe; *Alum.;* Ant. c.; *Apis;* Arg. n.; *Aspar.; Aur. mur.;* Bar. c.; *Bell.;* Benz. ac.; *Berb. v.;* Bor. ac.; Calc. ars.; Calc. c.; *Can. s.; Canth.;* Caps.; Carls.; *Caust.; Chimaph.;* Clem.; Coccus; *Colch.;* Col.; Conv.; Cub.; Dig.; *Equis.;* Ferr. p.; *Fer. picr.;* Formica; *Gels.;* Glycerin; Helleb.; *Helon.;* Hydrang.; Ign.; Indol; Jatropha; *Kali c.;* Kal.; *Kreos.;* Lact. ac.; *Lil. t.;* Lith. benz.; *Lith. c.; Lyc.;* Merc. c.; Merc. v.; Nat. c.; Nit. ac.; *Nux v.;* Ocimum; *Ol. sant.;* Ox. ac.; *Phos. ac.;* Piloc.; Plumb.; *Prun. sp.;* Pulex; *Puls.;* Sabal; Sab.; *Samb.;* Santon.; *Sars.; Scilla;* Sec.; *Sep.;* Sil.; *Staph.; Sul.;* Tritic.; *Uva; Vespa;* Zing.

Frequent desire at night—Alum.; *Aur. mur.;* Bor.; Calc. c.; Carb. ac.; *Caust.;* Coccus; *Con.;* Ferr.; *Ferr. picr.;* Glycerin; *Graph.; Kali c.; Kreos.;* Murex; Nat. m.; *Phos. ac.;* Physal.; Picr. ac.; *Puls.;* Sang.; Sars.; Scilla; Sep.; Solan. lyc.; *Sul.;* Tereb.; Thuya; Xerophyl.

Imperative, irresistible, sudden desire—Acon.; Agar.; Aloe; *Apis;* Arg. n.; Bor.; Can. s.; *Canth.;* Carls.; Equis.; Hedeoma; Ign.; *Kreos.;* Lathyr.; *Merc. c.;* Merc.; Murex; Naph.; Ol. an.; *Pareira; Petros.; Pop. tr.;* Prun. sp.; Puls.; Quass.; Ruta; Santon.; Scutel.; *Sul.;* Thuya.

Intermittent, interrupted flow—Agar.; Can. ind.; Caps.; *Clem.; Con.;* Gels.; *Hep.;* Mag. s.; Pulex; Puls.; *Sabal;* Sars.; Sedum; Thuya; Zinc. m.

INVOLUNTARY—Alum.; *Arg. n.;* Arn.; Ars.; *Bell.;* Calc. c.; *Caust.; Cina; Dulc.;* Echin.; *Equis.;* Ferr. m.; *Gels.; Hyos.;* Kali br.; *Kreos.;* Op.; Petrol.; *Puls.; Rhus ar.;* Rhus t.; Ruta; *Sabal;* Saponin; Sars.; *Selen.;* Senega; *Sil.;* Solan. lyc.; Sul.; *Uva;* Xerophyl. See Bladder.

Involuntary, at night—Ars.; *Bell.;* Calc. c.; *Caust.; Cina;* Kali br.; *Kreos.;* Plant.; *Puls.;* Rhus t.; Senega; *Sep.;* Sil.; *Sul.;* Uva. See Enuresis.

Involuntary, during first sleep—Kreos.; Sep.

Involuntary, when coughing, sneezing, walking, laughing—Bell.; Calc. c.; Canth.; Caps.; *Caust.;* Ferr. m.; Ferr. mur.; *Ferr. p.;* Ign.; Kali c.; Nat. m.; *Puls.; Scilla;* Selen.; Sul.; Vib. op.; Xerophyl.; *Zinc.*

Involuntary, when dreaming of act—Equis.; Kreos.

Involuntary, without consciousness of—Apoc.; *Arg. n.; Caust.;* Sars.

RETENTION (ischuria)—*Acon.;* Apis; Apium gr.; *Arn.; Ars.; Bell.; Camph.;* Can. ind.; Can. s.; *Canth.; Caust.;* Chimaph.; Cic.; Cup.; Dulc.; *Equis.; Eup. purp.; Hyos.;* Ign.; Lyc.; Merc. c.; *Morph.; Nux v.; Op.; Plumb. m.;* Puls.; Rhus t.; Sars.; *Stigm.;* Strych.; Sul.; *Tereb.;* Zinc. m.

From atony of fundus—Tereb.

From cold or wet exposure—*Acon.; Dulc.;* Gels.; Rhus t.

From fever, acute illness—Ferr. p.; Op.

From fright—*Acon.;* Op.

From hysteria—Ign.; Zinc.

From inflammation—*Acon.;* Can. ind.; *Canth.;* Nux v.; Puls.

From overexertion—Arn.

From paralysis—*Caust.;* Dulc.; Hyos.; Nux v.; *Op.; Plumb. m.;* Strych.

From post partum—Hyos.; Op.

From prostatic hypertrophy—Chimaph.; Dig.; Morph.; Zinc. See Male Sexual System.

From spasmodic constriction of neck of bladder—*Bell.;* Cact.; Camph.; Canth.; *Hyos.;* Lyc.; *Nux v.;* Op.; Puls.; Rhus t.; Stram.; Thlaspi.

From suppressed discharges or eruptions—Camph.

From surgical operations—Caust.

SCANTY FLOW—*Acon.;* Adon. v.; *Alfal.;* Apis; Apoc.; *Arg. n.; Ars.;* Aur. mur.; *Bell.; Benz. ac.; Berb. v.;* Bry.; Camph.; Can. s.; *Canth.:* Carb. ac.; Carbo v.; *Chimaph.;* Clem.; *Colch.;* Col.; Conv.; Cupr. ars.; *Dig.;* Dulc.; Equis.; Eup. purp.; Fluor. ac.; Graph.; *Helleb.; Junip.;* Kali bich.; Kali chlor.; Kali iod.; Kreos.; Lach.; Lecith.; Lil. t.; Lith. c.; Lyc.; Lyssin; Menthol; *Merc. c.;* Merc. cy.; *Nit. ac.; Nux v.;* Op.; Phos.; Picr. ac.; *Piloc.; Plumb.;* Prun. sp.; Pulex; Puls.; Ruta; Sab.; Sars.; Scilla; Selen.; Senec.; Senega; Sep.; Serum ang.; Solid.; Stroph.; Sul.; Sul. ac.; Sulphon.; *Tereb.; Uva;* Zing.

Scanty, drop by drop—*Acon.;* Æsc.; *Apis;* Arn.; *Bell.;* Bor.; *Canth.;* Caps.; Caust.; Clem.; Colch.; *Cop.;* Dig.; Equis.; Inula; *Lyc.; Merc. c.;* Merc.; Nux v.; Plumb.; *Puls.;* Rhus t.; *Sabal;* Staph.; Sul.

STRANGURY—*Acon.;* Ant. t.; *Apis;* Apoc.; *Ars.; Bell.; Camph.; Can. s.; Canth.; Caps.;* Col.; Con.; *Cop.; Dulc.;* Eryng.; *Eup. purp.;* Hydrang.; Juncus; Junip.; Junip. v.; Lyc.; *Merc. c.;* Morph.; Nux m.; *Nux v.; Pareira; Petros;* Prun. sp.; Puls.; Sab.; Sars.; Senna; Stigm.; *Tereb.;* Thlaspi; *Tritic.; Urt.;* Verbasc.; Zing.

In children—*Bor.;* Lyc.; Sars.

In females—Apis; Caps.; *Cop.;* Dig.; *Eup. purp.;* Lil. t.; *Sab.;* Staph.; Ver. v.; Vib. op.

Nervous type—Apis; *Bell.;* Caps.; *Eryng.;* Morph.; Petros.

SUPPRESSION (anuria)—*Acon.;* Agar. ph.; Alfal.; *Apis;* Apoc.; *Ars.;* Ars. hyd.; *Bell.;* Bry.; *Camph.; Canth.;* Coff.; *Colch.; Cupr. ac.; Dig.;* Formal.; *Helleb.;* Junip.; *Kali bich.; Kali chlor.; Lyc.; Merc. c.;* Merc. cy.; Nit. ac.; *Op.; Oxyden.;* Petrol.; Phyt.; Picr. ac.; Puls.; Sec.; *Solid.;* Stigm.; *Stram.; Tereb.;* Ver. a.; Zing.

URINATION—COMPLAINTS BEFORE ACT: Anxiety, agony: *Acon.;* Bor.; *Canth.;* Phos. ac.

Burning—Ars.; *Berb. v.; Camph.; Can. s.; Canth.;* Cochlear.; Cop. See Urethra.

Leucorrhœa, yellow—Kreos.

Pain—*Acon.; Berb. v.; Bor.; Canth.;* Can. s.; Erig.; Kali c.; Lith. c.; *Lyc.;* Piloc.; *Rhus ar.;* Sanic.; *Sars.;* Senega; Sep. See Pain (bladder, kidneys, urethra).

COMPLAINTS DURING ACT—Burning, smarting: *Acon.;* Ambra; Anac.; Anag.; *Apis;* Apoc.; *Arg. n.; Ars.; Berb. v.;* Bor. ac.; *Bor.;* Camph.

Can. ind.; *Can. s.; Canth.;* Caps.; Carbo v.; Cepa; Chimaph.; *Cop.;* Cub.; Dig.; Epig.; *Equis.;* Erig.; Eryng. aq.; *Eup. purp.;* Gels.; Glycerin; Helleb.; *Kreos.; Lyc.; Merc. c.;* Merc. s.; Nit. ac.; Nux v.; Ocimum; *Ol. sant.;* Ox. ac.; *Pareira;* Phos.; Puls.; Rhus ar.; *Sep.;* Staph.; *Sul.; Tereb.;* Thuya; Uva; Verbasc.; *Vespa.*

Chill—*Acon.;* Sars.; Sep.

Meatus, agglutination—Anag.; Can. s.

Meatus, burning (also prepuce)—Calad.; Calc. c.; *Can. s.;* Gels.; Menthol; *Merc. c.;* Puls.

Meatus, itching—Ambra; Cop.; Lyc.; Nux v.

PAINS IN GENERAL—*Acon.;* Apis; *Arg. n.;* Berb. aq.; *Berb. v.;* Blatta am.; Bor. ac.; Camph.; *Can. s.; Canth.;* Caps.; *Chimaph.;* Col.; Dig.; Doryph.; *Equis.;* Erig.; Graph.; Hedeoma; *Lith. c.; Lyc.;* Merc.; Nit. ac.; *Nux v.; Pareira; Petrol.;* Phos.; Puls.; *Rhus ar.;* Sabal; *Sars.; Sep.*

Cutting, stinging, stitching—*Acon.;* Ant. c.; Apis; Berb. aq.; *Berb. v.;* Bor.; Camph.; *Can. s.; Canth.;* Cochlear.; Col.; Con.; Hydrang.; Nux v.; *Pareira; Puls.*

Drawing, radiating to labia—Eupion.

Drawing, radiating to chest and shoulders—Glycerin.

Drawing, radiating to perineum—Lyc.; Sep.

Drawing, radiating to sacrum, coccyx—Graph.

Drawing, radiating to testicles—*Berb. v.;* Cahinca; Erig.

Drawing, radiating to thighs—Berb. v.; Pareira.

Pressive—Camph.; Cop.; Lyc.; *Sep.*

Pressive in heart—Lith. c.

Spasmodic, toward end of act—*Arg. n.;* Bor. ac.; Puls.

Stool, involuntary—Sul.

Sweating—Merc. c.

COMPLAINTS AFTER ACT—Burning, smarting: *Acon.;* Anac.; Apis; *Arg. n.;* Bell.; *Berb. v.;* Camph.; *Can. s.; Canth.; Caps.;* Chimaph.; Cochlear.; Cub.; *Kreos.;* Lyc.; Mag. s.; *Merc. c.;* Nat. c.; *Nat. m.;* Phos. ac.; *Pichi;* Puls.; Rhus t.; Senega; Staph.; *Sul.; Thuya; Uva.*

Dribbling—*Arg. n.;* Benz. ac.; Calc. c.; Camph.; Can. ind.; Caust.; *Clem.;* Con.; Lyc.; *Pareira; Selen.;* Thuya; Zing. See Bladder.

Emission, seminal—Calad.; Hep.; Phos. ac.

Exhaustion—Ars.; Berb. v.

Hæmorrhoids—Bar. c.

Meatus, and urethra, tingling—Clem.; Thuya.

Meatus, burning—Caps.; Puls.

PAINS—Aching, bruised: *Berb. v.;* Equis.; Sul.

Cutting, tearing, stitching—*Berb. v.;* Bov.; Camph.; *Can. s.; Canth.; Caps.;* Cochlear.; *Cub.;* Guaiac.; Mag. s.; Merc. acet.; *Nat. m.;* Nux v.; Petros.; Prun. sp.; *Sars.; Thuya;* Uva.

Pressive, in perineum—Am. m.; Lyc.

Sensation as if urine remained behind—Alum.; *Berb. v.;* Dig.; Eup. purp.; Eryng. aq.; Gels.; *Hep.; Kali bich.;* Ruta; Sec.; Sil.; Staph.; *Thuya.*

Severe, at close, and after act—Apis; *Berb. v.; Canth.;* Echin.; *Equis.;*

Lith. c.; Med.; Merc. acet.; *Nat. m.;* Petros.; Puls.; Ruta; *Sars.;* Staph.; *Thuya.*

Spasmodic—*Nat. m.;* Nux v.; Puls.

Perspiration—Merc. c.

Tenesmus, urging, straining—Arg. n.; *Camph.; Canth.;* Chimaph.; Epig.; *Equis.;* Eryng. aq.; Lith. c.; Nit. ac.; Pichi; *Pop. tr.; Puls.;* Ruta; Sabal; Sars.; *Staph.;* Stigm.; Sul.

URINE—TYPE: Acid: Acon.; *Benz. ac.;* Canth.; Chin. s.; Euonym.; Lith. c.; *Lyc.; Merc. c.;* Mur. ac.; *Nit. ac.;* Nit. mur. ac.; Nux v.; Ocimum; Puls.; *Sars.;* Sep.; *Sul.; Uva.* See Burning.

ALBUMINURIA—Albuminous: Acetan.; Adon. v.; *Am. benz.;* Ant. t.; *Apis; Ars.;* Aur. mur.; Bell.; *Berb. v.; Calc. ars.;* Can. s.; *Canth.;* Carb. ac.; Chin. s.; *Colch.;* Conv.; Cop.; Cupr. ac.; Cupr. ars.; *Dig.;* Equis.; *Euonym.; Eup. purp.;* Ferr. ars.; *Ferr. mur.;* Ferr. picr.; Formica; Fuschina; Glon.; *Helleb.;* Helon.; Kali chlor.; *Kal.;* Lach.; Lecith.; Lith. c.; Lyc.; *Merc. c.;* Merc. cy.; Methyl. bl.; Mur. ac.; Nit. ac.; Ocimum; Ol. sant.; *Osm.;* Phos. ac.; *Phos.; Plumb. c.;* Plumb. m.; Radium; Sab.; Scilla; *Sec.;* Sil.; *Solid.; Stroph.; Tereb.;* Thyr.; Uran. n.; Viscum a.

Alkaline—Am. c.; Benz. ac.; *Kali acet.;* Mag. p.; Med.; *Phos. ac.* See Nephritis.

BLOODY (hæmaturia)—*Acon.;* Ant. t.; Apis; *Arn.;* Ars.; Ars. hydrog.; Bell.; *Berb. v.;* Cact.; Camph.; *Can. s.; Canth.;* Carb. ac.; Chin. s.; Cina; Cinch.; *Coccus; Colch.; Cop.; Crot.;* Dulc.; Epig.; *Equis.; Erig.;* Eucal.; Ferr. p.; Ficcus; Gall. ac.; Geran.; *Ham.;* Hep.; *Ipec.;* Kali chlor.; Kreos.; *Lach.; Lyc.;* Mangif. ind.; Merc. c.; Merc.; *Millef.; Nit. ac.; Nux v.;* Ocimum; Ol. sant.; *Pareira; Phos.;* Pichi; Picr. ac.; Plumb.; *Rhus ar.;* Sab.; Santon.; *Sars.;* Scilla; Sec.; *Senec.; Solid.;* Stigm.; *Tereb.; Thlaspi; Uva.*

Burning, scalding, hot—*Acon.;* Apis; Bell.; Benz. ac.; *Bor.;* Camph.; *Can. s.; Canth.;* Coccus; Conv.; Hep.; Kali bich.; Kal.; *Lyc.; Merc. c.;* Nit. ac.; Phos.; Pichi; Pop. tr.; *Sars.; Sul.* See Acid.

Cold feeling—Nit. ac.

Heavy feeling—Thlaspi.

Oily pellicle—Adon. v.; *Crot. t.;* Hep.; Lyc.; *Iod.;* Petrol.; *Phos.;* Sumbul.

Viscid, gluey—*Col.;* Pareira; *Phos. ac.* See Deposit.

COLOR—APPEARANCE—Black, inky: *Apis;* Arn.; *Benz. din.; Benz. ac.;* Canth.; *Carb. ac.; Colch.;* Dig.; *Helleb.;* Kreos.; Lach.; Merc. c.; Naph.; Nit. ac.; Pareira; *Tereb.*

Brown, dark—*Apis;* Apoc.; Arg. n.; Arn.; Ars.; *Bell.; Benz. ac.; Bry.; Canth.;* Carb. ac.; Carbo v.; *Chel.;* Chin. s.; Coccus; *Colch.;* Crot.; *Dig.;* Fluor. ac.; Helleb.; Kali c.; Kali chlor.; Lach.; *Lyc.;* Merc. c.; Myr.; Nat. c.; Nat. chlor.; *Nit. ac.; Nux v.;* Phos. ac.; Phos.; Phyt.; Picr. ac.; Plumb.; Prun. sp.; *Rhus t.; Sep.;* Solid.; Staph.; Sulphon.; *Tereb.*

Cloudy, turbid—*Ambra;* Am. c.; Apoc.; *Arg. m.;* Ars.; *Aur. mur.; Bell.; Benz. ac.; Berb. v.;* Camph.; *Can. s.; Canth.;* Card. m.: Caust.; Chel.;

Chimaph.; Chin. s.; Cina; Colch.; Col.; Con.; *Cop.;* Crot. t.; Daphne; *Dig.;* Dulc.; Graph.; Helleb.; Helon.; *Hep.;* Kali c.; Kreos.; Lith. c.; *Lyc.;* Lyssin; Nit. ac.; Nit. mur. ac.; *Ocimum;* Petrol.; *Phos. ac.; Phos.; Plumb.; Puls.;* Raph.; Rhus t.; *Sars.; Sep.;* Solid.; Sul.; *Tereb.;* Thuya; Zing.

Deep—*Bell.;* Calc. c.; Dig.; Helleb.; Lach.; *Lyc.;* Merc.; Nit. ac.; *Sep.*

Frothy—Apis; *Berb. v.;* Cop.; Crot. t.; Cub.; *Lach.;* Myr.; Raph.; Sars.

Greenish—Ars.; *Berb. v.;* Camph.; Can. ind.; *Carb. ac.; Ceanoth.;* Chimaph.; Cop.; Laburn.; Mag. s.; Ol. an.; Ruta; *Santon.;* Uva.

Milky—Chel.; *Cina;* Col.; Con.; Dulc.; Eup. purp.; Iod.; Lil. t.; Merc.; *Phos. ac.;* Phos.; Raph.; Still.; Uva; *Viola od.*

Pale, clear, limpid—*Acet. ac.;* Berb. v.; Caust.; Crot. t.; Equis.; *Gels.;* Helon.; *Ign.;* Kreos.; Lycop.; Mag. m.; Mosch.; *Nat. m.;* Nit. ac.; Nux v.; *Phos. ac.; Phos.;* Puls.; Staph.; *Sul.* See Polyuria.

Pink—Sulphon.

Red, dark—*Acon.; Apis;* Bell.; Benz. ac.; *Bry.;* Canth.; Carbo v.; Coccus; Cupr. ac.; *Dig.;* Hep.; *Kali bich.;* Lob. infl.; Merc. c.; Merc. d.; Nux v.; Petrol.; Phyt.; Scilla; Selen.; Solid.

Red, fiery, high colored—*Acon.;* Ant. c.; *Apis;* Apoc.; Arg. n.; Ars.; *Bell.; Benz. ac.; Berb. v.; Bry.;* Camph.; Can. s.; *Canth.;* Carb. ac.; Cepa; Chel.; Chimaph.; Cupr. ac.; *Equis.;* Euonym.; Glon.; *Helleb.; Hep.;* Kali bich.; *Lith. c.; Lyc.;* Merc. d.; *Myr.;* Nit .ac.; Ocimum; Phyt.; Picr. ac.; Puls.; Rheum; *Rhus t.;* Sab.; Sars.; Selen.; Senec.; Sul.; *Tereb.;* Thuya; Uva; Ver. v.

Smoky—Am. benz.; *Benz. ac.;* Helleb.; *Tereb.* See Bloody.

Thick—Ammon. benz.; Ananth.; *Benz. ac.;* Camph.; Cina; Coccus; *Col.;* Con.; Daphne; Dig.; *Dulc.; Hep.;* Iod.; *Merc. c.;* Ocimum; *Phos.;* Still.; Sep.; Zing.

Yellow—Absinth.; Bell.; Berb. v.; *Card. m.;* Ceanoth.; Cinch.; Dahpne; Hydr.; Ign.; Kal.; Lact. ac.; Ocimum; Op.; Plumb. m.; Solid.; Uva.

Yellow, dark—Bov.; Bry.; Camph.; *Chel.;* Chenop.; Crot. t.; *Iod.;* Kali p.; Myr.; Petrol.; *Picr. ac.;* Pod.

ODOR—Fetid, foul: Am. benz.; Am. c.; Apis; Ars.; *Aspar.; Bapt.; Benz. ac.;* Berb. v.; *Calc. c.;* Camph.; Carbo an.; *Chimaph.;* Col.; Conv.; Cupr. ars.; Daphne; *Dulc.; Graph.;* Hydr.; Indium; Kali bich.; Kreos.; Lach.; *Lyc.;* Merc.; Naph.; *Nit ac.;* Ocimum; Petrol.; *Phos.;* Physal.; Pulex; *Sep.; Solid.;* Stront. br.; Sul.; Tropæol.; Uran. n.

Fish-like—Uran. n.

Garlicky—Cupr. ars.

Musk-like—Ocimum.

Pungent, ammoniacal—*Bor.;* Cahinca; Cop.; Dig.; Naph.; *Nit. ac.; Pareira;* Petrol.; Solid.; Stigm.

Sharp, intensely strong—*Absinth.;* Am. benz.; Arg. n.; *Benz. ac.; Bor.; Calc. c.;* Carbo v.; *Chin. s.;* Erig.; *Lyc.;* Picr. ac.; Pin. sylv.; *Sul.;* Viola od.; Zing.

Sharp, like cat's urine—Cajup.; Viola tr.

Sharp, like horse's urine—Benz. ac.; *Nit. ac.*

Sour—Calc. c.; *Graph.;* Nat. c.; Petrol.; Sep.; Solid.

Sweet, violaceous—Arg. m.; *Cop.;* Cub.; Eucal.; Ferr. iod.; Inula; *Junip.;* Phos.; Primula; Salol; *Tereb.;* Thyr.

Valerian, like—Murex.

SEDIMENT—TYPE: Aceton (azoturia): Ars.; Aur. mur.; *Calc. mur.;* Carb. ac.; *Caust.;* Colch.; Cupr. ars.; *Euonym.;* Nat. sal.; Phos.; *Senna.*

Bile—Ceanoth.; Chionanth.; *Chel.;* Kali chlor.; Myr.; Nat. s.; Sep. See Liver.

Blood—Ars.; *Berb. v.;* Cact.; *Can. s.; Canth.; Carb. ac.;* Colch.; Dulc.; *Ham.;* Hep.; Lyc.; *Nit. ac.;* Pareira; *Phos.;* Tereb. See Bloody.

Casts—*Apis;* Ars.; Aur. mur.; Brachygl.; *Canth.; Carb. ac.;* Chel.; Crot.; Kali chlor.; Merc. c.; Nat. chlor.; *Phos.;* Picr. ac.; Pichi; *Plumb.;* Radium; Sulphon.; Tereb. See Nephritis.

Cells, debris—Arg. n.; *Ars.; Berb. v.;* Brachygl.; Cact.; *Canth.; Carb. ac.;* Chel.; Crot.; Hep.; Kali bich.; *Merc. c.; Phos.;* Picr. ac.; Solid.; Tereb. See Nephritis.

Chlorides, diminished—Bar. m.; Chel.; Col.

Chlorides, increased—Chin. s.; Radium; Senna.

Chyluria—Col.; Iod.; *Kali bich.; Phos. ac.;* Uva. See Milky Urine.

Coffee-ground like—Dig.; *Helleb.;* Tereb.

Flocculent, flaky—*Berb. v.;* Caust.; Phos.; *Sars.*

Gelatinous, gluey, viscid—Berb. v.; *Cina; Col.; Ocimum; Phos. ac.;* Puls. See Mucous.

Grayish-white, granular—Berb. v.; Calc. c.; Canth.; *Graph.;* Sars.; Sep.

Hæmatoporphyrinuria—*Sulphon.;* Trion.

Hæmoglobinuria—*Ars. hydrog.;* Carb. ac.; Chin. ars.; Chin. s.; Ferr. p.; Kali bich.; *Kali chlor.;* Nat. nit.; Phos.; Picr. ac.; Santon.

Indican—Alfal.; Indol; Nux m.; Picr. ac.

Lithic acid, uric acid, gravel, brick dust—Arg. n.; Arn.; *Aspar.;* Baros.; *Bar. m.;* Bell.; *Benz. ac.; Berb. v.; Calc. c.;* Calc. ren.; Can. s.; *Canth.;* Caust.; Chel.; *Chin. s.; Cinch.;* Coccin. sept.; Cochlear.; *Coccus;* Colch.; Col.; Dig.; Diosc.; *Epig.; Eup. ar.; Eup. purp.;* Eryng.; Ferr. mur.; Galium; Graph.; *Hedeoma; Hydrang.; Kali c.;* Kali iod.; Kreos.; *Lith. benz.; Lith. c.;* Lob. infl.; *Lyc.;* Merc. c.; Nat. m.; Nat. s.; *Nit.´ ac.;* Nit. mur. ac.; *Nux v.; Ocimum;* Pareira; Pariet.; Phos. ac.; Phos.; Physal.; Pichi; Piperaz.; Plumb. iod.; Puls.; *Sars.;* Selen.; Senna; *Sep.;* Skook. ch.; *Solid.;* Stigm.; *Thlaspi;* Tritic.; *Urt.;* Vesic. See Calculi.

Mucus, slime—Apoc.; Ars.; Aspar.; Bals. per.; *Baros.; Benz. ac.;* Berb. *v.;* Brachygl.; Calc. c.; *Can. s.; Canth.; Chimaph.;* Chin. s.; Cina; *Cub.; Dulc.;* Epig.; *Equis.;* Eup. purp.; *Hep.;* Hydrang.; *Kali bich.; Lyc.;* Menthol; Merc. c.; Nit. ac.; Nux v.; *Pareira;* Pichi; *Pop. tr.; Puls.; Sars.;* Senega; Sep.; *Solid.;* Stigm.; Sul.; *Tritic.; Uva.* See Cystitis.

Oxalates (oxaluria)—*Berb. v.;* Brachygl.; *Kali s.;* Lysidin; Nat. p.; Nit. ac.; *Nit. mur. ac.;* Ox. ac.; Senna.

Phosphates (phosphaturia)—*Alfal.;* Arn.; Avena; Bell.; Benz. ac.; Brachygl.; Calc. c.; *Calc. p.;* Can. s.; Chel.; Chin. s.; Graph.; Guaco; Guaiac.; Helon.; Hydrang.; Kali chlor.; Lecith.; Nit. ac.; *Phos. ac.; Picr. ac.;* Sang.; Senna; *Solid.;* Thlaspi; Uran. n.

Pus (pyuria)—*Ars.;* Aspar.; *Baros.; Benz. ac.;* Berb. v.; Bry.; Calc. c.;

Can. s.; Canth.; Chimaph.; Cop.; *Dulc.; Epig.;* Eucal.; *Hep.;* Hyos.;
Kali bich.; Lith. c.; *Lyc.; Merc. c.;* Nit. ac.; Nux v.; Ocimum; *Phos.;*
Pichi; *Pop. tr.;* Sars.; Sep.; Stigm.; Sul·; Tereb.; Thlaspi; Tritic.;
Uva.

Rose colored—Am. phos.

DIABETES—Sugar: *Acet. ac.; Adren.;* Am. acet.; *Arg. m.;* Arg. n.; Aristol.;
Arn.; *Ars. br.;* Ars. iod.; *Ars.;* Asclep. vinc.; *Aur.* ; Aur. mur.; Bell.;
Bor. ac.; Bov.; *Bry.;* Caps.; Carb. ac.; Ceanoth.; *Cham.;* Chel.;
Chimaph.; Chionanth.; Coca; Cod.; Colch.; *Crot.;* Cupr. ars.; *Cur.;*
Eup. purp.; Fel tauri; Ferr. iod.; Ferr. mur.; Fluor. ac.; Glon.; Gly-
cerin; Grind.; *Helleb.; Helon.;* Iod.; *Iris;* Kali acet.; Kali br.; *Kreos.;*
Lach.; *Lact. ac.;* Lecith.; Lycop.; Lyc.; Lyssin; Morph.; *Mosch.;*
Murex; Nat. m.; *Nat. s.;* Nit. ac.; Nux v.; *Op.; Pancreat.;* Phaseol.;
Phos. ac.; Phos.; Phlorid.; Picr. ac.; Plumb. iod.; Plumb.; Pod.; *Rhus
ar.;* Scilla; Sec.; *Sil.; Sizyg.;* Strych. ars.; Sul.; Tar. h.; Tarax.;
Tereb.; *Uran. n.;* Urea; Vanad.

Assimilative disorders—Uran. n.

Gastro-hepatic origin—*Ars. iod.;* Ars.; Bry.; Calc. c.; Cham.; Chel.;
Kreos.; *Lact. ac.;* Lept.; Lyc.; *Nux v.; Uran. n.*

Nervous origin—Ars.; Aur. mur.; Calc. c.; *Ign.; Phos. ac.;* Strych. ars.

Pancreatic origin—Iris; Pancreat.; Phos.

With debility—Acet. ac.; Op.

With gangrene, boils, carbuncles, diarrhœa—Ars.

With gouty symptoms—*Lact. ac.; Nat. s.*

With impotency—Coca; Mosch.

With melancholia, emaciation, thirst, restlessness—Helon.

With motor paralysis—Cur.

With rapid course—Cur.; Morph.

With ulceration—Sizyg.

MALE SEXUAL SYSTEM

BUBO—Acon.; Angust.; Apis; Aur. mur.; Bad.; *Bell.;* Calend.; *Carbo an.;* Carbo v.; Caust.; *Cinnab.;* Hep.; Jacar.; *Kali iod.;* Merc. *i. r.;* Merc. pr. rub.; *Merc. s.; Nit. ac.;* Phos. ac.; *Phyt.;* Sil.; Sul.; Syph.; Tar. c.

Bubo, chancroidal—Ars. iod.; Merc. c.; *Merc. i. r.; Merc. s.;* Sil.

Bubo, indurated—Alum.; Bad.; *Carbo an.;* Merc. s.

Bubo, phagedenic—*Ars.;* Graph.; Hydr.; *Kali iod.;* Lach.; *Merc. i. r.; Merc. s.; Nit. ac.;* Sil.; Sul.

CHANCROID—Coral.; *Jacar.;* Kali bich.; Merc. pr. rub.; *Merc. s.; Nit. ac.;* Thuya.

Chancroid, complications—*Ars.;* Hekla; *Hep.;* Lach.; *Sil.;* Sul.; Thuya.

COITUS—Aversion to: Arn.; Graph.; Lyc. See Desire.

Coitus, followed by backache—*Can. ind.;* Kali c.

Coitus, followed by irritability—Selen.

Coitus, followed by nausea, vomiting—Mosch.

Coitus, followed by pain in perineum—Alum.

Coitus, followed by pain in urethra—Canth.

Coitus, followed by prostration—Agar.; Calc. c.; *Cinch.;* Con.; Dig.; *Kali c.;* Kali p.; Nat. c.; Selen.; Thaspium. See Impotence.

Coitus, followed by pollution, increased desire—Nat. m.; Phos. ac.

Coitus, followed by toothache—Daphne.

Coitus, followed by urging to urinate—Staph.

Coitus, followed by vertigo—Bov.; Sep.

Coitus, followed by vomiting—Mosch.

Coitus, followed by weak vision—Kali c.

Coitus, painful—Arg. n.; Calc. c.; Sabal. See Impotence.

CONDYLOMATA—Aur. mur.; *Cinnab.;* Euphras.; Kali iod.; *Lyc.;* Merc.; Nat. s.; *Nit. ac.; Sab.;* Staph.; *Thuya.* See Syphilis.

CONTUSIONS—Of genitals: Arn.; Con.

DESIRE—Diminished, lost: *Agn.; Arg. n.;* Bar. c.; Berb. v.; *Calc. c.;* Caps.; *Con.;* Hep.; Ign.; Iod.; Kali br.; *Kali c.;* Lecith.; *Lyc.;* Nit. ac.; Nuph.; Onosm.; Oxytr.; Phos. ac.; *Sabal; Selen.;* Sil.; Sul.; X-ray. See Impotence.

Desire increased (erethism, satyriasis)—Alum.; Anac.; Bov.; Calad.; *Camph.; Can. ind.;* Can. s.; *Canth.; Dulc.;* Fluor. ac.; *Gins.;* Graph.; Hippom.; *Hyos.;* Ign.; *Kali br.;* Lach.; Lyc.; Lyssin; *Mosch.;* Nat. m.; *Nux v.;* Ol. an.; Onosm.; *Orig.; Phos.; Picr. ac.; Plat.;* Sab.; *Salix n.;* Stram.; *Tar. h.;* Thaspium; Thymol; Upas; Ver. a.; *Zinc. p.*

Desire increased in old men but impotent—Lyc.; Selen.

Desire perverted—Agn.; Nux v.; Plat.; Staph.

Desire suppressed, ill effect from—Con.

GENITALS—Burning, heat: Spong.; Sil. See Gonorrhœa.

Genitals, itching (pruritus)—Agar.; *Ambra;* Anac.; *Calad.;* Crot. t.; *Fagop.;* Rhus d.; *Rhus t.;* Sep.; Sul.; Tar. c. See Skin.

Genitals, relaxed, flabby, cold, weak—Absinth.; *Agn.; Calad.;* Caps.; *Cinch.; Con.; Diosc.; Gels.;* Ham.; *Lyc.;* Nuph.; *Phos. ac.;* Phos.; *Selen.;* Sep.; Staph.; Sul.; Uran. See Impotence.

GONORRHOEA—(specific urethritis) Remedies in general: *Acon.;* Agn.; Apis; *Arg. n.; Baros.;* Benz. ac.; *Camph.; Can. s.; Canth.; Caps.; Clem.; Cop.; Cub.;* Dig.; *Doryph.;* Echin.; Equis.; Erig.; Eucal.; Euphorb. pil.; Fabiana; Ferr.; *Gels.;* Hep.; *Hydr.;* Ichthy.; Jacar.; *Kali bich.;* Kali s.; Kreos.; Med.; *Merc. c.;* Merc. pr. rub.; *Merc. s.; Merc. v.;* Methyl. bl.; Naph.; Nat. s.; *Nit. ac.;* Nux v.; *Ol. sant.;* Pareira; *Petros.;* Pichi; Pin. c.; *Puls.;* Sabal; Sab. ; Salix n.; *Sep.;* Sil.; Stigm.; *Sul.;* Tereb.; *Thuya;* Tritic.; *Tussil.;* Zing.

Acute, inflammatory stage—*Acon.;* Arg. n.; Atrop.; *Can. s.; Canth.;* Caps.; *Gels.;* Petros.

Adenitis, lymphangitis—Acon.; Apis; *Bell.;* Hep.; *Merc.*

Chordee—Acon.; *Agave; Anac.;* Arg. n.; Bell.; Berb. v.; *Camph. monobr.; Can. ind.;* Can. s.; *Canth.;* Caps.; Clem.; Cop.; Gels.; Hyos.; Jacar.; *Kali br.; Lupul.;* Merc.; Œnanthe; Ol. sant.; Phos.; *Picr. ac.;* Pip. m.; Salix n.; Tereb.; Tussil.; Yohimb.; Zinc.; picr.

Chronic, subacute stage—Arg. n.; Can. s.; *Cop.; Cub.;* Erig.; *Hep.;* Hydr.; *Kali s.;* Merc. c.; Merc. i. r.; Merc.; Naph.; *Nat. s.; Ol. sant.;* Pin. c.; Psor.; *Puls.;* Rhod.; *Sabal;* Sep.; Sil.; Stigm.; *Sul.; Thuya.* See Gleet.

Cowperitis—Acon.; *Can. s.;* Gels.; *Hep.;* Merc. c.; Petros.; Pichi; *Sabal;* Sil. See Bladder.

DISCHARGE—Acrid, corroding: Cop.; Gels.; *Hydr.; Merc. c.;* Thuya.

Bloody—Arg. n.; *Canth.;* Cub.; *Merc. c.;* Millef.

Milky, glairy, mucus—Can. ind.; *Can. s.;* Cop.; Cupr. ars.; Graph.; *Hydr.; Kali bich.; Nat. m.; Petros.;* Puls.; Sep. See Gleet.

Muco-purulent, yellowish-green—Agn.; Alum.; *Arg. n.;* Baros.; *Can. s.;* Canth.; Caps.; Cob.; *Cop.; Cub.;* Dig.; *Hep.; Hydr.;* Jacar.; Kali iod.; *Kali s.; Merc. c.; Merc. s.;* Nat. m.; *Nat. s.;* Ol. sant.; *Puls.;* Sab.; Sep.; Sil.; Sul.; *Thuya;* Tussil.; Zing. See Gleet.

Watery—*Can. s.;* Fluor. ac.; Mez.; Millef.; *Nat. m.;* Sep.; Sul.; Thuya.

Folliculitis—Caps.; Hep.; Merc. s.; Sep.; Sil.

GLEET—Abies c.; *Agn.;* Arg. n.; Calad.; Calc. p.; *Can. s.; Canth.;* Caps.; Chimaph.; *Cinnab.;* Clem.; *Cub.;* Dorpyh.; Erig.; Graph.; *Hydr.;* Kali bich.; Kali iod.; *Kali s.;* Matico; Med.; Merc.; *Naph.; Nat. m.;* Nat. s.; *Nit. ac.;* Nux v.; *Ol. sant..;* Petros.; Pip. m.; Pop. tr.; *Puls.; Sabal;* Selen.; *Sep.;* Sil.; *Thuya;* Zinc. mur.

Ophthalmia—*Acon.;* Apis; Arg. n.; *Bell.;* Ipec.; Merc. c.

Orchitis, epididymitis—Aur. m.; Clem.; Gels.; Ham.; Puls.; Rhod.; *Spong.*

Prostatic involvement—Caps.; Cub.; Pareira; *Thuya.* See Prostatitis.

Rheumatism—*Acon.;* Arg. n.; Clem.; Cop.; *Daphne;* Gels.; Guaiac.; Iod.; *Irisin;* Kali iod.; *Med.; Merc.;* Nat. s.; *Phyt.; Puls.; Sars.;* Sul.; *Thuya.*

Stricture, organic—Acon.; *Arg. n.;* Calc. iod.; Canth.; Caps.; *Clem.;* Cop.; *Fluor. ac.;* Iod.; *Kali iod.;* Merc. pr. rub.; *Merc.;* Nux v.; Ol.

sant.; Pareira; Petros.; Puls.; Sep.; *Sil.;* Sul.; Sul. iod.; *Thiosin.;* *Thuya.*

Suppression ill effects—*Agn.;* Ant. t.; Benz. ac.; *Clem.;* Kali iod.; *Med.;* Nat. s.; *Puls.;* Sars.; *Thuya;* X-ray.

IMPOTENCE—*Agn.; Anac.;* Ant. c.; *Arg. n.;* Arn.; Ars.; Avena; Bar. c.; Berb. v.; *Calad.;* Calc. c.; Camph.; Carbon. s.; Chin. s.; *Cinch.; Cob.; Con.;* Damiana; Dig.; *Diosc.; Gels.;* Glycerin; Graph.; Hyper.; Ign.; Iod.; Kali br.; Kali iod.; Lecith.; *Lyc.;* Nat. m.; Nit .ac.; Nuph.; *Nux v.;* Onosm.; *Phos. ac.; Phos.; Picr. ac.;* Plumb. m.; *Sabal; Salix n.; Selen.;* Sep.; Sil.; Staph.; *Strych.;* Sul.; Thuya; Tribul.; *Yohimb.;* Zinc.; Zinc. p. See Spermatorrhœa.

MASTURBATION—Ill effects: Agn.; *Anac.;* Apis; Arg. m.; Bellis; *Calad.; Calc. c.; Calc. p.; Cinch.; Con.; Diosc.; Gels.;* Graph.; Grat.; *Kali br.; Lyc.;* Nat. m.; *Nux v.; Phos. ac.; Picr. ac.;* Plat.; *Salix n.;* Staph.; Still.; *Sul.;* Tab.; Thuya; Tribul.; Ustil.; Zinc. m.; Zinc. oxyd.

PENIS—Atrophy: Ant. c.; Arg. m.; Staph.

Glans: Epithelioma: Arg. n.; *Ars.;* Con.; Thuya.

Gangrene—Canth.; Lach.

Itching—*Acon.;* Ars.; Bell.; *Calad.; Canth.;* Caps.; Cinch.; Cinnab.; Coccus; *Con.;* Cop.; Coral.; *Crot. t.;* Graph.; Ham.; *Hep.;* Ign.; Kali bich.; Lyc.; *Merc.;* Nat. m.; Nux v.; *Puls.;* Selen.; Sep.; Staph.; *Sul.;* Thuya; *Viola tr.*

PAINS—Burning, sore: Anac.; *Ars.;* Bell.; *Can. s.; Canth.; Caps.;* Cinch.; *Cinnab.;* Con.; Cop.; Coral.; Crot. t.; *Gels.;* Ign.; Lyc.; *Merc. c.;* Mez.; *Nit. ac.;* Nuph.; Nux v.; Puls.; Rhus t.; Sep.; *Sul.; Thuya;* Viola tr.

Cutting, stitching, tearing—*Acon.;* Apis; *Arg. n.;* Calad.; *Can. s.; Canth.; Caps.;* Con.; *Hep.; Lyc.;* Naph.; Nat. m.; *Nit. ac.;* Papaya; *Pareira;* Petrol.; Phos. ac.; *Phyt.;* Prun. sp.; *Sars.;* Staph.; Sul.

Pressive, pinching—*Canth.;* Caps.; Graph.; Kali bich.; *Nit. ac.;* Puls.; *Rhod.*

Throbbing—Coccus; Ham.; Lith. c.; Nat. m.; *Nit. ac.*

Priapism—See Chordee.

Pustules—*Ars. hydr.;* Coccus; *Hep.; Kali bich.;* Merc.

Rash and spots—Antipyr.; *Bell.;* Bry.; Calad.; Can. s.; Caust.; *Cinnab.;* Gels.; Lach.; *Merc.;* Nat. m.; Petrol.; *Rhus t.;* Sep.; *Sul.;* Thuya.

Swollen, inflamed glans—*Acon.;* Antipyr.; *Apis; Arg. n.;* Arn.; Ars.; Calad.; *Can. s.; Canth.;* Cop.; Coral.; *Cub.;* Dig.; *Gels.;* Ham.; *Merc. c.;* Merc. s.; *Nit. ac.;* Phos. ac.; *Rhus t.;* Sars.; *Thuya.* See Gonorrhœa.

Ulcers, excoriations—*Ars.;* Can. s.; *Caust.;* Cop.; *Coral.;* Crot. t.; *Hep.; Merc. c.; Merc.;* Mez.; *Nit. ac.;* Osm.; Sep.; *Thuya.*

PREPUCE—Constriction (paraphimosis, phimosis): Acon.; *Apis;* Arn.; Bell.; Can. s.; *Canth.;* Caps.; Dig.; Euphras.; Ham.; *Merc. c.;* Merc. s.; *Nit. ac.;* Ol. sant.; Phos. ac.; *Rhus t.;* Sab.; Sul.; *Thuya.*

Herpes—Ars.; Carbo v.; Caust.; *Crot. t.;* Graph.; *Hep.;* Jugl. r.; *Merc.;* Mez.; *Nit. ac.;* Petrol.; Phos. ac.; *Rhus t.;* Sars.; *Thuya.*

Inflammation (balanitis, balano-postitis)—*Acon.;* Apis; Calad.; *Can. s.;*

Canth.; Cinnab.; Coccus; Con.; Crot. t.; Dig.; *Gels.; Jacar.;* Lyc.; Merc. c.; *Merc. s.; Nit. ac.;* Ol. sant.; *Rhus t.;* Sul.; *Thuya;* Viola tr.

Itching—Ars.; *Canth.; Caps.;* Cinnab.; *Con.;* Graph.; Ign.; Lyc.; *Merc. s.;* Nit. ac.; Nux v.; Puls.; *Rhus t.;* Sil.; *Sul.;* Thuya; Zing.

Pains—*Acon.;* Bell.; *Berb. v.;* Calad.; *Can. s.; Canth.;* Cinnab.; Coccus; Con.; *Cop.;* Coral.; Ign.; Merc. c.; *Merc.; Nit. ac.;* Nux v.; *Rhus t.;* Sep.; Sul.; *Thuya.*

Ulcers, exocriations—*Ars.;* Can. s.; *Caust.;* Cop.; *Coral.; Hep.;* Ign.; *Merc.; Nit. ac.;* Nux v.; Phos. ac.; Phyt.; Sep.; *Sil.; Thuya.*

Varices—Ham.; Lach.

Warts, condylomata—Apis; *Cinnab.;* Hep.; Kreos.; Lyc.; Nat. m.; *Nit. ac.;* Phos. ac.; *Sab.;* Sep.; Staph.; *Thuya.*

PROSTATE GLAND—Affections in general: Æsc.; Aloe; Baros.; Caust.; *Ferr. picr.;* Hep.; *Hydrang.; Iod.;* Kali iod.; *Melast.;* Merc. s.; Pareira; Phyt.; Pichi; Picr. ac.; Pop. tr.; *Sabal; Solid.;* Staph.; Sul. iod.; *Thuya;* Turnera.

Congestion—*Acon.; Aloe;* Arn.; Bell.; *Canth.;* Con.; Cop.; Cub.; Ferr. p.; Gels.; Kali br.; Kali iod.; Lith. c.; *Ol. sant.;* Puls.; *Sabal;* Thuya.

Hypertrophy—Alfal.; *Aloe;* Am. m.; *Arg. n.; Bar. c.;* Benz. ac.; Calc. fl.; Calc. iod.; *Chimaph.;* Chrom. s.; *Cim.;* Con.; Eup. purp.; *Ferr. picr.; Gels.;* Graph.; Hep.; *Hydrang.;* Ikshug.; Iod.; Kali bich.; Kali br.; Lyc.; Med.; Ol. sant.; Oxyden.; Pareira; Picr. ac.; Pip. m.; *Pop. t.;* Puls.; Rhus ar.; *Sabal;* Sars.; *Senec.; Solid.;* Staph.; *Sul.; Thiosin.; Thuya;* Thyr.; Tritic.

Inflammation (prostatitis): Acute: Acon.; Æsc.; Aloe; Apis; *Bell.;* Bry.; Canth.; *Chimaph.;* Colch.; *Cop.;* Cub.; Dig.; Ferr. p.; *Gels.; Hep.; Iod.;* Kali br.; Kali iod.; Merc. c.; *Merc. d.; Nit. ac.;* Nitrum; Ol. sant.; *Pichi;* Picr. ac.; *Puls.;* Sabad.; *Sabal;* Salix n.; Selen.; *Sil.;* Solid.; Staph.; *Thuya;* Tritic.; *Ver. v.;* Vesic.

Inflammation, chronic—Alum.; *Aur.;* Bar. c.; Brachygl.; Calad.; Carbon. s.; Caust.; Clem.; *Con.; Ferr. picr.;* Graph.; Hep.; Hydrocot.; Iod.; *Lyc.; Merc. c.; Merc.; Nit. ac.;* Nux v.; Phyt.; *Puls.;* Sabad.; *Sabal; Selen.; Sep.;* Sil.; Solid.; *Staph.;* Sul.; *Thuya; Tribul.* See Prostatitis.

Weakness (prostatorrhœa); discharge during stool, urination, straining: Acet. ac.; Æsc.; *Agn.; Alum.;* Anac.; *Arg. n.; Can. s.;* Caust.; *Chimaph.;* Con.; Cub.; Eryng.; Hep.; Junip.; Kali bich.; Lyc.; Nit. ac.; Nuph.; Nux v.; Petrol.; *Phos. ac.;* Phos.; Puls.; Sabal; *Selen.;* Sil.; *Sul.;* Tereb.; Thuya; Thymol; *Turnera;* Zinc. m.

PUBIC HAIR—Loss: Merc.; Nit. ac.; Selen.; Zinc.

SCROTUM—Cancer, epithelioma: Ars.; Fuligo; Thuya.

Cold, relaxed—*Agn.; Calad.;* Calc. c.; *Caps.;* Gels.; Lyc.; Merc.; *Phos. ac.;* Sep.; Staph.; Sul. See Impotence.

Eczema—Alumen; Ant. c.; Canth.; *Crot. t.; Graph.;* Hep.; Oleand.; Petrol.; Phos. ac.; *Rhus t.;* Sanic.; Sul.

HYDROCELE—Œdema: Abrot.; Ampel.; *Apis;* Ars.; *Aur.;* Bry.; Calad.; *Calc. c.;* Calc. fl.; Calc. p.; Canth.; Chel.; Cinch.; *Con.;* Dig.; Dulc.; *Fluor. ac.; Graph.;* Helleb.; *Iod.;* Kali iod.; Merc.; *Puls.; Rhod.;* Rhus t.; Samb.; Scilla; *Selen.; Sil.; Spong.;* Sul.

Induration—Calad.; Rhus t.

Inflammation—*Apis;* Ars.; Crot. t.; Euphorb.; *Ham.;* Rhus t.; Ver. **v.**

Itching—*Ambra;* Carbo v.; Caust.; *Crot. t.;* Euphorb.; *Graph.; Hep.;* Nit. ac.; Nux v.; Petrol.; Phos. ac.; Rhus t.; *Sars.;* Selen.; Sil.; Thuya; Urt. See Skin.

Hæmatocele, acute—Acon.; Arn.; Con.; Erig.; *Ham.;* Nux v.; *Puls.; Sul.*

Hæmatocele, chronic—Iod.; *Kali iod.;* Sul.

Nodules, hard, suppurating—Nit. ac. See Skin.

Numbness—*Ambra;* Am. c.; Sep. See Itching.

Pain—Am. c.; Berb. v.; *Clem.;* Iod.; Kali c.; *Merc.;* Nux v.; *Thuya.* See Inflammation.

Prurigo—*Ant. c.;* Aur.; *Graph.;* Mur. ac.; Nat. s.; *Nit. ac.;* Nux v.; *Rhus t.;* Staph.

Retraction—Plumb. m.

Spots, brown—Con.

Sweat—Bell.; *Calad.;* Calc. c.; Coral.; Cupr. ars.; *Diosc.;* Fagop.; Nat. m.; *Petrol.;* Sep.; *Sil.; Sul.;* Thuya; Uran. n.

Swelling—*Apis;* Ars.; *Bell.;* Brom.; *Canth.; Clem.;* Con.; Ign.; Nit. ac.; *Puls.;* Rhus d.; *Rhus t.;* Sep. See Inflammation.

Tubercles—Con.; *Iod.;* Sil.; Sul.; Teucr.

VARICOCELE—Acon.; Arn.; *Ferr. p.; Ham.;* Lach.; Nux v.; Plumb.; *Puls.;* Ruta; Sul.

SEMINAL VESICULITIS—Acute: Acon.; Æsc.; Aloe; *Bell.;* Canth.; Cub.; *Ferr. p.;* Hep.; Kali br.; *Merc.;* Phyt.; *Puls.;* Selen.; Sil.; Ver. v.

Chronic—*Agn.; Arg. n.;* Aur.; Bar. c.; Calad.; *Can. s.;* Cinch.; Clem.; Con.; *Cub.;* Ferr. picr.; Graph.; *Hep.; Iod.;* Kali br.; *Lyc.;* Merc.; Nux v.; *Ox. ac.;* Phos. ac.; Phyt.; *Puls.; Selen.;* Sep.; *Sil.;* Staph.; Sul.; Tribul.; Zinc. See Prostatitis.

SEXUAL EXCESSES—Ill effects: Agar.; *Agn.; Anac.;* Avena; Calad.; Calc. c.; *Cinch.;* Con.; Digitaline; *Gels.;* Graph.; Kali br.; Kali p.; Lyc.; Lyssin; Nat. m.; *Nux v.;* Phos. ac.; Phos.; Samb.; Selen.; Sil.; Staph.; Tribul. See Impotence, Spermatorrhœa.

SPERMATIC CORD—Pain in general: Anthem.; *Arg. n.;* Arundo; Aur.; *Bell.; Berb. v.;* Calc. c.; Cahinca; *Can. s.;* Caps.; *Clem.;* Cinch.; Con.; *Diosc.; Ham.;* Indium; Kali c.; Lith. c.; *Merc. i. r.;* Morph.; *Nit. ac.;* Nux v.; Ol. an.; Osm.; *Ox. ac.;* Oxytr.; *Phyt.;* Picr. ac.; *Puls.;* Sars.; *Senec.;* Sil.; *Spong.;* Staph.; Sul.; *Thlaspi; Thuya;* Tussil.; Ver. v.

Drawing—*Cahinca;* Calc. c.; *Clem.;* Con.; *Ham.;* Indium; Ol. an.; *Puls.;* Rhod.; Senec.; *Staph.;* Zinc. m.

Neuralgic—*Arg. n.;* Aur.; *Bell.; Berb. v.;* Clem.; Ham.; Menthol; Nit. ac.; Nux v.; *Ox. ac.;* Phyt.; *Spong.*

Swelling—Anthem.; *Can. s.;* Cinch.; *Ham.;* Kali c.; *Puls.; Spong.*

Tenderness—*Bell.; Clem.;* Ham.; Merc. i. r.; *Ox. ac.;* Phyt.; Rhod.; *Spong.;* Tussil.

SPERMATORRHOEA—(sexual debility, deficient physical power, nocturnal pollutions):—Absinth.; *Agn.; Anac.;* Arg. m.; *Arg. n.;* Arn.; Ars.;

Aur.; *Avena; Bar. c.; Calad.; Calc. c.; Calc. p.;* Camph. monobr.; Can. ind.; *Canth.;* Carbon. s.; Carbo v.; Chlorum; Cim.; *Cinch.; Cob.;* Coca; Cocc.; *Con.;* Cupr. m.; *Dig.; Digitaline; Diosc.;* Eryng.; *Ferr. br.;* Formica; *Gels.; Gins.; Graph.;* Hyper.; Ikshug.; Iod.; Iris; *Kali br.; Kali c.; Kali p.; Lyc.;* Lyssin; *Lupul.; Med.;* Mosch.; *Nat. m.;* Nit. ac.; *Nuph.; Nux v.;* Onosm.; Orchit; *Phos. ac.; Phos.; Picr. ac.;* Plumb. phos.; *Sabal; Salix n.;* Scutel.; *Selen.; Sep.; Sil.; Staph.; Strych.; Sul.;* Sul. ac.; Sumb.; Thuya; *Thymol;* Titan.; Turnera; Upas.; Ustil.; *Yohimb.; Zinc. picr.;* Viola tr.

With brain fag, mental torpidity—Phos. ac.

With debility, backache, weak legs—Aur.; Calc. c.; Calc. p.; *Cinch.; Cob.;* Con.; Cupr. m.; Dig.; *Diosc.;* Eryng.; Formica; Gels.; *Kali c.; Lyc.;* Med.; Nat. p.; *Nux v.; Phos. ac.; Picr. ac.;* Sars.; Selen.; *Staph.; Sul.;* Turnera; Zinc. m.

With dreams absent—Anac.; *Arg. n.;* Dig.; Gels.; Hep.; Nat. p.; *Picr. ac.* See Sleep.

With dreams amorous—Ambra; *Calad.;* Can. ind.; Cob.; Con.; Diosc.; Lyc.; *Nux v.; Phos.;* Sars.; Selen.; Senec.; Staph.; Thymol; Ustil.; Viola tr. See Sleep.

With emission and orgasm absent—Calad.; Calc. c.; Selen.

With emissions bloody—Ambra; Canth.; Led.; *Merc.;* Petrol.; Sars.

With emissions diurnal, straining at stool—*Alum.;* Canth.; Cim.; *Cinch.;* Digitaline; Gels.; Kali br.; *Nuph.; Phos. ac.;* Phos.; Picr. ac.; *Selen.;* Tribul. See Prostatorrhœa.

With emissions, premature—*Agn.;* Bar. c.; *Calad.; Calc. c.;* Carbo v.; *Cinch.; Cob.;* Con.; *Graph.; Lyc.;* Ol. an.; Onosm.; *Phos. ac.;* Phos.; *Selen.;* Sep.; Sul.; Titan.; Zinc. m.

With emissions profuse, frequent; after coitus—Phos. ac.

With emissions too slow—Calc. c.; Lyc.; Nat. m.; Zinc. m.

With erections deficient—Agar.; *Agn.;* Arg. m.; Arg. n.; Calad.; *Calc. c.;* Caust.; *Con.;* Graph.; Hep.; Kali c.; *Lyc.;* Mag. c.; Nit. ac.; Nuph.; *Phos. ac.;* Phos.; *Selen.;* Sul.; Zinc. m.

With erections painful—Can. ind.; *Canth.;* Ign.; Merc.; Mosch.; *Nit. ac.;* Nux v.; Picr. ac.; Puls.; Sabad.; Thuya.

With irritability, despondency—*Aur.;* Calc. c.; Calad.; Cim.; *Cinch.;* Con.; Diosc.; Kali br.; *Nux v.;* Phos. ac.; Phos.; *Selen.;* Staph.

With masturbatic tendency—Ustil.

With rheumatic pains—Gins.

With vision weak—Kali c.

With wasting of testes—*Iod.;* Sabal.

SYPHILIS—Remedies in general: *Æthiops;* Alnus; Anac.; Ant. c.; Arg. iod.; Ars.; Ars. br.; Ars. iod.; *Ars. m.;* Ars. s. fl.; Asaf.; *Aur. ars.;* Aur. iod.; *Aur.;* Aur. m. n.; Aur. mur.; Bad.; Bapt.; *Berb. aq.;* Calc. fl.; *Calop.;* Carbo an.; Carbo v.; Caust.; Chin. ars.; *Cinnab.;* Condur.; *Coryd.;* Echin.; *Fluor. ac.;* Francisca; Gels.; Graph.; Guaiac.; *Guaco;* Hekla; *Hep.;* Hippoz.; Hydrocot.; *Iod.; Jacar.; Kali bich.; Kali iod.;* Kali m.; *Kreos.; Lach.;* Lonic.; Lyc.; *Merc. aur.;* Merc. br.; *Merc. c.;* Merc. d.; *Merc. i. fl.; Merc. i. r.; Merc. nit.; Merc. pr. rub.; Merc. s.;*

Merc. tan.; *Merc. v.; Mez.; Nit. ac.;* Osm.; Phos. ac.; Phos.; *Phyt.;* Plat.; *Plat. mur.;* Psor.; Rhus gl.; Sars.; Staph.; *Still.;* Sul.; *Syph.; Thuya.*

Abuse of mercury—Angust.; *Aur.;* Calop.; Carbo an.; Fluor. ac.; *Hep.;* Kali iod.; *Nit. ac.;* Rhus gl.; Sul.

Adenopathy—*Bad.;* Carbo an.; Graph.; *Hep.;* Iod.; *Merc. i. fl.; Merc. i. r.;* Merc. s.; Phyt. See Glands (Generalities).

Alopecia—*Ars.;* Aur.; Carbo v.; Cinnab.; *Fluor. ac.;* Graph.; *Hep.;* Kali iod.; Lyc.; Merc. i. fl.; Merc. v.; *Nit. ac.; Phos.;* Sul. See Scalp.

Bone and cartilage lesions—Arg. m.; *Asaf.; Aur.;* Aur. mur.; Calc. fl.; Carbo v.; *Fluor. ac.;* Hep.; *Kali bich.; Kali iod.;* Lach.; *Merc.; Mez.; Nit. ac.;* Phos. ac.; *Phos.;* Phyt.; Sars.; *Sil.;* Staph ; Still.; Sul. See Bones (Generalities).

Cachexia, anæmia, emaciation—*Ars.; Aur.;* Calop.; Carbo an.; Carbo v.; Ferr. iod.; Ferr. lact.; *Iod.;* Merc.; Sars.

Chancre and primary lesions—Ananth.; Apis; Arg. n.; Ars.; Asaf.; *Cinnab.;* Coral.; Hep.; *Jacar.;* Kali bich.; *Kali iod.;* Lyc.; *Merc. c.; Merc. i. fl.; Merc. i. r.; Merc. s.; Merc. v.; Nit. ac.;* Phos. ac.; Phos.; Plat.; Piat. mur.; Sil.; Sul.

Chancre, gangrenous—Ars.; Lach.

Chancre, hard—Carbo an.; Kali iod.; Merc. i. fl.; *Merc. i. r.;* Merc. s.

Chancre, indurated, with lardaceous base; deep, round, penetrating; painful, bleeding; raw, everted edges—Merc. s.

Chancre, phagedenic—*Ars.; Cinnab.;* Hydr.; Lach.; *Merc. c.; Nit. ac.;* Sil.

Chancre, soft—Coral.; Merc. s.; Nit. ac.; Thuya.

Condylomata—Aur. mur.; *Cinnab.;* Euphras.; Kali iod.; Mercuries; Plat. mur.; Nat. s.; *Nit. ac.; Sab.;* Staph.; *Thuya.*

CONGENITAL, infantile—*Æthiops;* Ars. iod.; Ars. m.; *Aur.;* Calc. fl.; *Calc. iod.;* Coral.; Kali iod.; *Kreos.; Merc. d.; Merc. s.; Merc. v.; Nit. ac.;* Psor.; Syph.

Exotoses—*Calc. fl.;* Fluor. ac.; *Hekla;* Merc. phos.; Phos. See Bones.

Fever—*Bapt.; Chin. s.;* Cinch.; Gels.; *Merc.;* Phyt.

Gummata, nodes—Asaf.; *Aur.;* Berb. aq.; *Calc. fl.;* Carbo an.; Condur.; *Coryd.; Fluor. ac.;* Iod.; *Kali bich.; Kali iod.;* Merc.; Mez.; Nit. ac.; *Phyt.;* Sil.; Staph.; *Still.;* Sul.; Thuya.

Headache—*Kali iod.;* Merc.; Sars.; Still.; *Syph.* See Head.

Mucous patches—*Asaf.;* Aur.; Calc. fl.; Calop.; *Cinnab ; Condur.;* Fluor. ac.; *Hep.;* Iod.; *Kali bich.;* Kali iod.; Kali m.; *Merc. c.;* Merc. d.; *Merc. nit.; Merc. pr. rub.; Merc. s.; Nit. ac.;* Phyt.; Sang.; Staph.; Still.; *Thuya.*

Onychia, paronychia—*Ant. c.;* Ars.; Graph.; Kali iod.; *Mercuries.* See Whitlow (Skin).

Ozæna—*Aur.;* Kali bich.; Still. See Nose.

Nervous lesions—*Anac.;* Asaf.; *Aur.;* Iod.; *Kali iod.;* Lyc.; Merc. nit.; Merc. phos.; Mez.; *Phos.*

Nocturnal pains (osteocopic)—Asaf.; *Aur.;* Calc. fl.; Cinnab.; *Coryd.; Eup. perf.;* Fluor. ac.; Hep.; *Kali bich.; Kali iod.;* Lach.; Lyc.; *Merc.; Mez.;* Phos.; *Phyt.;* Sars.; Still.

Rheumatism—*Guaiac.;* Hekla; Hep.; *Kali bich.;* Kali iod.; *Merc.;* Nit. mur. ac.; *Phyt.;* Still. See Locomotor System.

Secondary stage—*Aur.;* Berb. aq.; Calop.; *Cinnab.;* Fluor. ac.; *Graph.;* Guaiac.; Iod.; *Kali bich.; Kali iod.;* Lyc.; Merc. br.; Merc. c.; *Merc. i. fl.; Merc. i. r.;* Merc. s.; *Merc. v.; Nit. ac.;* Osm.; Phos.; Phyt.; Rhus gl.; Sars.; *Still.;* Thuya.

Stomatitis, mercurial—Nit. ac.

SYPHILIDES—Bullæ:—Kali iod.; Syph.

Eczematous—*Ars.;* Graph.; Kreos.; Merc. s.; Petrol.; Phyt.; *Sars.* See Skin.

Papular—*Calop.;* Kali iod.; Lach.; Merc. c.; *Merc. i. r.;* Merc. s.

Pigmentary—Calc. s.; Nit. ac.

Psoriasis—Asaf.; *Graph.; Kali bich.;* Nit. ac.; Phos.

Pustular—*Ant. t.;* Asaf.; *Calop.;* Fluor. ac.; Hep.; Ign.; *Kali bich.;* Kali iod.; Lach.; *Merc. nit.;* Mez.; *Nit. ac.*

Roseolæ—Kali iod.; Merc. c.; Merc. i. r.; *Merc. s.;* Phos.; Phyt.

Rupia—Ars.; *Berb. aq.;* Kali iod.; *Merc.; Nit. ac.;* Phyt.; Syph.

Spots, copper-colored—*Carbo an.;* Carbo v.; *Coral.;* Kali iod.; Lyc.; Merc.; Nit. ac.; Sul.

Squamous—*Ars.;* Ars. iod.; *Ars. s. fl.;* Bor.; *Cinnab.;* Fluor. ac.; Kali iod.; Merc. c.; Merc. i. fl.; Merc. nit.; *Merc. pr. rub.;* Merc. s.; Merc. tan.; *Nit. ac.;* Phos.; Phyt.; Sars.; Sul.

Tubercular—*Ars.;* Aur.; *Carbo an.;* Fluor. ac.; Hydrocot.; *Kali iod.;* Merc. i. r.; Still.; Thuya.

Ulcerations—Ars.; *Asaf.;* Aur.; *Aur. mur.;* Carbo v.; *Cinnab.;* Cistus; *Condur.; Coral.; Fluor. ac.;* Graph.; Hep.; Iod.; *Kali bich.;* Kali iod.; Lach.; Lyc.; *Merc. c.;* Merc. cy.; Merc. d.; *Merc. pr. rub.;* Merc. v.; Mez.; *Nit. ac.; Phyt.;* Sil.; Staph.; Still.; Sul.; *Thuya.* See Mucous Patches.

Vesicular—*Cinnab.;* Merc. c.; *Merc. i. r.;* Thuya.

Tertiary stage—Ars. iod.; *Aur.;* Aur. mur.; Calcareas; Carbo v.; Cinnab.; *Fluor. ac.;* Graph.; Guaiac.; Hoang n.; Iod.; *Kali bich.; Kali iod.;* Lyc.; *Mercuries; Mez.; Nit. ac.;* Phos. ac.; *Phos.; Phyt.;* Psor.; Staph.; Sul.; Thuya.

Throat symptoms—Bor.; Calc. fl.; *Cinnab.;* Fluor. ac.; Kali bich.; Lyc.; *Merc. c.;* Merc. d.; Merc. i. fl.; Merc. i. r.; Merc.; *Nit. ac.; Phyt.;* Still.

Visceral symptoms—*Ars.;* Ars. iod.; Aur.; Ceanoth.; Hep.; *Kali bich.;* Kali iod.; Merc. aur.; *Merc. c.;* Merc. i. r.; *Merc. s.;* Merc. tan.; *Nux v.*

TESTICLES—Abscess:—Hep.; Merc.; Still.

Atrophy—Agn.; Ant. c.; *Arg. n.; Aur.;* Caps.; Carbon. s.; Cereus serf.; *Iod.;* Kali br.; Lyssin; *Rhod.; Sabal.*

Coldness—*Agn.;* Berb. v.; *Diosc.;* Merc.; Sil. See Impotence.

Cysts—*Apis;* Con.; *Graph.;* Sep.; Sul.

Hernia—Ars.; *Bar. c.;* Calc. c.; Carbo v.; Hep.; *Merc.;* Nit. ac.; *Sil.;* Thuya.

Hypertrophy—Bar. c.; *Berb. v.;* Cinnab.; Con.; *Ham.; Iod.;* Merc. i. r.; *Merc.;* Puls.; Stigm. See Inflammatory.

Induration, hard—Acon.; *Agn.;* Arg. n.; Arn.; *Aur.; Bar. c.;* Bell.;

Brom.; *Calc. fl.*; Carbo v.; *Clem.*; *Con.*; Cop.; *Iod.*; Kali c.; Merc.;
Ox. ac.; *Phyt.*; Plumb.; *Rhod.*; *Sil.*; *Spong.*; Sul. See Inflammation.

Inflammation of epididymis (epididymitis)—*Acon.*; Apis; Arg. n.; *Bell.*;
Can. s.; Cinch.; *Clem.*; *Gels.*; *Ham.*; *Merc.*; Phyt.; *Puls.*; *Rhod.*;
Sabal; *Spong.*; Sul.; Teucr. scor.; Thuya.

Inflammation of testes (orchitis)—Acute:—*Acon.*; Ant. t.; Arg. m.; Arg.
n.; *Bell.*; Brom.; Cham.; Chin. s.; Cinch.; *Clem.*; Cub.; Gels.; Ham.;
Kali s.; *Merc.*; Nit. ac.; Nux v.; Phyt.; Polyg.; *Puls.*; *Rhod.*; Spong.;
Teucr. scor.; Ver. v.

Inflammation, chronic—Agn.; *Aur.*; Bar. c.; *Calc. iod.*; Cinch.; *Clem.*;
Con.; Gels.; *Hep.*; Hyper.; Iod.; *Kali iod.*; Lyc.; Merc.; Nit. ac.;
Phyt.; *Puls.*; Rhod.; Rhus t.; *Spong.*; Sul.

Inflammation, metastatic—*Puls.*; Staph.

Inflammation, syphilitic—Aur.; *Kali iod.*; Merc. i. r.

PAINS—In general: *Acon.*; Agn.; *Apis*; Arg. m.; *Arg. n.*; *Aur.*; Bell.;
Berb. v.; *Brom.*; Cahinca; *Can. s.*; Caps.; Cereus bon.; Cham.; *Clem.*;
Con.; Eriod.; Gins.; *Ham.*; Hydr.; Ign.; Iod.; Kali c.; *Lycop.*; Lyc.;
Merc. i. r.; Merc.; Nit. ac.; Nux v.; *Ox. ac.*; *Oxytr.*; Papaya; Phos.
ac.; Picr. ac.; *Puls.*; *Rhod.*; Salix n.; Sep.; *Spong.*; Staph.; Sul.;
Thuya.

Aching, dragging, relaxed—Apis; *Aur.*; Can. s.; *Clem.*; *Con.*; Iod.; Nit.
ac.; Nux .v; Phos. ac.; *Puls.*; *Spong.*; Staph.; Sul.; *Thuya.*

Bruised, crushed, squeezed, contractive pain—*Acon.*; *Arg. m.*; *Arg. n.*;
Aur.; Cham.; Carbo v.; *Clem.*; *Con.*; Gins.; *Ham.*; Kali c.; Nit. ac.;
Ol. an.; Ox. ac.; *Puls.*; *Rhod.*; Sep.; *Spong.*; Staph.

Neuralgic (testalgia)—Arg. n.; *Aur.*; Bell.; Berb. v.; *Clem.*; *Col.*; Con.:
Euphras.; *Ham.*; Ign.; *Mag. p.*; Merc.; Nux v.; Ol. an.; *Ox. ac.*; Oxytr.;
Puls.; Spong.; Ver. v.; Zinc. m.

Sensitive, sore, tender—*Acon.*; Apis; *Bell.*; Berb. v.; Brom.; *Clem.*; Con.,
Cop.; *Ham.*; Indium; Merc. i. r.; *Phos. ac.*; *Puls.*; *Rhod.*; Sep.;
Spong.; Staph.

RETRACTION—Arg. n.; *Aur.*; Bell.; Brom.; Camph.; Cinch.; *Clem.*;
Col.; Euphras.; Nit. ac.; *Ol. an.*; Puls.; *Rhod.*; Zinc.

Swelling—*Acon.*; Agn.; *Apis*; Arg. m.; *Arg. n.*; Arn.; Ars.; *Aur.*; Aur.
m. n.; *Bell.*; *Brom.*; Calc. p.; Carbo v.; *Clem.*; *Con.*; Cop.; Dig.;
Graph.; *Ham.*; *Iod.*; *Kali c.*; Lyc.; *Merc. c.*; Merc.; Millef.; Ocimum;
Phos. ac.; *Puls.*; *Rhod.*; *Spong.*; Staph.; Tussil.; *Ver. v.*; Zinc. See
Inflammation.

TUBERCULOSIS—*Aur.*; Bac. test.; *Merc.*; Scrophul.; Spong.; *Teucr. scor.*

Tuberculosis, pseudo—*Aur.*; Calc. c.; Hep.; *Merc. i. r.*; *Sil.*; Spong.;
Sul.

Tumors (sarcocele)—*Aur.*; *Calc. c.*; Clem.; Merc. i. r.; Puls.; *Rhod.*;
Sil.; *Spong.*; Tub. See Hypertrophy.

Undescended testicle in boys—Thyr.

FEMALE SEXUAL SYSTEM

COITION—Fainting during: Murex; Orig.; *Plat.*

Coition, hæmorrhage after—Arg. n.; Kreos.; Nit. ac.; Sep.

Coition, painful—Apis; Arg. n.; Bell.; *Berb. v.;* Ferr.; Kreos.; Lyc.; Lyssin; Plat.; Sep.; *Staph.;* Thuya. See Vaginismus.

CONCEPTION, difficult (sterility)—*Agn.;* Alet.; Am. c.; Aur. m.; *Bar. m.; Bor.;* Calc. c.; Can. ind.; Caul.; *Con.;* Eup. purp.; Gossyp.; *Graph.;* Helon.; *Iod.;* Lecith.; *Med.;* Nat. c.; *Nat. m.;* Nat. p.; Phos.; *Plat.; Sabal.*

Conception easy—Merc.; Nat. m.

DESIRE, diminished or lost—*Agn.;* Am. c.; Berb. v.; Caust.; Ferr. mur.; Graph.; *Helon.; Ign.;* Nat. m.; *Onosm.;* Plumb.; *Sep.*

Desire, increased (nymphomania)—Ambra; *Aster.;* Arundo; *Bufo;* Calc. c.; *Calc. p.;* Camph.; *Canth.;* Cim.; Cinch.; Coca; Dulc.; *Ferrula; Grat.; Hyos.;* Kali br.; *Kali p.;* Kreos.; Lach.; Mosch.; *Murex;* Nux v.; *Orig.;* Phos.; Picr. ac.; *Plat.;* Raph.; *Robin.;* Sab.; Sil.; *Stram.;* Strych.; *Tar. h.; Ver. a.; Xerophyl.;* Zinc.

Desire increased, must keep busy to repress it—Lil. t.

Desire, suppressed, ill effects—*Con.;* Sabal.

GONORRHOEA—*Acon.;* Alumen; Apis; Arg. n.; *Can. s.; Canth.; Cop.; Cub.;* Jacar.; Kreos.; Med.; Merc. c.; *Merc.; Ol. sant.;* Petros.; Puls.; Sep.; Sul.; *Thuya.* See Leucorrhœa, Vaginitis, Vulvitis.

LEUCORRHOEA—Remedies in general: Agar.; *Agn.; Alet.;* Alnus; *Alum.; Ambra;* Am. c.; *Am. m.;* Arg. n.; Ars.; Asaf.; Aur. mur.; *Aur. m. n.;* Baros.; Bar. mur.; Bell.; *Bor.; Bov.;* Calc. c.; Calc. p.; *Canth.;* Carbo v.; *Caul.;* Caust.; Cham.; Cim.; *Cinch.; Cocc.; Con.; Cop.; Dictam.; Eucal.;* Eupion; Ferr. iod.; *Frax. am.;* Gels.; *Graph.;* Hedeoma; *Helon.;* Helonin; Hep.; *Hydr.;* Hydrocot.; Ign.; Iod.; Jacar.; Jonosia; *Kali bich.; Kali c.;* Kali m.; *Kali s.;* Kreos.; *Lil. t.; Lyc.;* Mag. c.; *Mag. m.;* Merc. pr. rub.; *Merc.;* Mez.; Murex; Naja; *Nat. m.; Nat. s.; Nit. ac.;* Nux v.; Orig.; *Ova t.;* Pall.; Picr. ac.; *Psor.;* Pulex; *Puls.; Sab.; Sec.;* Sil.; Spiranth.; *Stann.;* Sul.; Sul. ac.; Thlaspi; *Thuya;* Tilia; Trill.; Vib. op.; *Xanth.;* Zinc. m.

TYPE—Acrid, corroding, burning:—Æsc.: *Alum.;* Am. c.; Aral.; *Ars.;* Ars. iod.; Aur.; Aur. mur.; *Bor.; Bov.;* Calc. c.; Calc. iod.; Carb. ac.; Carbo an.; Carbo v.; Caul.; *Cham.; Con.;* Cop.; Eucal.; Ferr. br.; *Graph.;* Guaco; Helonin; Hep.; *Hydr.;* Ign.; *Iod.; Kreos.;* Lach.; *Lil. t.;* Lyc.; Med.; *Merc.; Nat. m.; Nit. ac.;* Phos.; Puls.; Sab.; *Sep.; Sil.; Sul.;* Sul. ac.; Thasp.

Albuminous, slimy, mucous—Agn.; *Alum.; Ambra; Am. m.;* Berb. v.; *Bor.;* Bov.; *Calc. c.; Calc. p.;* Ferr. iod.; Graph.; Hematox; Hydr.; Inula; Iod.; Kali m.; *Kali s.;* Kreos.; Mag. c.; Mez.; Plat.; *Puls.;* Sul. ac.; *Thuya;* Tilia.

Blackish—*Cinch.;* Thlaspi.

Bland—Bor.; Calc. p.; Eupion; *Frax. am.;* Kali m.; Puls.; Stann.

Bloody—Arg. n.; Ars.; Bufo; Calc. ars.; Carbo v.; *Cinch.;* Cocc.; Con.; *Kreos.; Merc. c.; Merc.;* Murex; Nit. ac.; Nux m.; *Sep.; Spiranth.;* Sul. ac.; *Thlaspi.*

Brown—Æsc.; Am. m.; Kreos.; *Lil. t.;* Nit. ac.; *Sec.; Sep.*

Flesh colored, like washing of meat, non-offensive—*Nit. ac.*

Greenish—*Bov.;* Carb. ac.; Carbo v.; *Kali s.;* Lach.; *Merc.; Murex;* Nat. s.; Nit. ac.; Phos.; Pulex; *Puls.;* Sec.; *Sep.;* Sul.; Thuya.

Gushing—Cocc.; *Eupion; Graph.; Sep.* See Profuse.

Intermittent—Con.; Sul.

Itching—*Ambra;* Anac.; Calc. c.; *Calc. iod.;* Carb. ac.; *Cinch.;* Hedeoma; Helonin; Hydr.; *Kreos.; Merc.; Sep.* See Pruritus.

Lumpy—Ant. c.; Hydr.; Psor.

Milky, white—Aur.; Bell.; *Bor.; Calc. c.; Calc. iod.;* Calc. p.; Canth.; Carbo v.; *Con.; Cop.;* Ferr. m.; *Graph.;* Hematox.; Iod.; *Kali m.;* Naja; *Ova t.;* Paraf.; *Puls.; Sep.; Sil.; Stann.;* Sul.

Offensive—Aral.; Ars.; Bufo; *Carb. ac.;* Cinch.; Eucal.; Guaco; *Helon.; Hep.; Kreos.; Merc.;* Med.; Nat. c.; Nit. ac.; Nux v.; *Psor.;* Pulex; Robin.; Sab.; Sang.; *Sanic.; Sec.; Sep.;* Thlaspi; Ustil.

Painful—Mag. m.; Sil.; Sul. See Concomitants.

Painless—Am. m.; Puls.

Profuse—*Alum.;* Ambra; Am. c.; *Arg. n.; Ars.;* Aur.; Bor.; *Calc. c.;* Calc. p.; Carb. ac.; *Caul.;* Caust.; Con.; Fluor. ac.; *Graph.;* Guaco; Helonin; *Hydr.;* Hydrocot.; Iod.; Kreos.; *Lach.;* Lil. t.; Mag. s.; *Merc.; Nat. m.; Ova t.;* Phos.; Pulex; *Puls.; Sep.;* Sil.; *Stann.; Syph.;* Thasp.; *Thuya;* Tilia; Trill.

Purulent, staining, yellow—Æsc.; *Agn.;* Alumen; Arg. n.; *Ars.;* Aur. mur.; *Bov.;* Calc. c.; *Can. s.;* Carbo an.; Ceanoth.; Cham.; *Cinch.;* Eupion; *Fagop.;* Helonin; *Hydr.;* Ign.; Iod.; *Kali bich.; Kali s.; Kreos.;* Lach.; Lil. t.; Lyc.; Merc. i. fl.; *Merc.;* Nat. s.; Pulex; *Puls.; Sep.; Stann.;* Sul.; Trill.; Ustil.

Thick—Æsc.; Aur.; *Bov.;* Canth.; Carbo v.; Con.; Helonin; *Hydr.; Iod.;* Kali m.; Kreos.; Mag. s.; Merc.; Murex; Nit. ac.; *Puls.;* Sab.; *Sep.;* Thuya.

Thin, watery—*Am. c.; Ars.;* Bell.; Bufo; Cham.; Frax. am.; *Graph.; Kali s.;* Kreos.; Lil. t.; *Merc. c.;* Merc.; Naja; Nat. m.; *Nit. ac.;* Plat.; Puls.; *Sep.; Syph.;* Sul.

Viscid, stringy, tough—*Æsc.; Alum.;* Asar.; Bov.; Dictam.; Ferr. br.; Graph.; *Hydr.;* Iris; *Kali bich.; Kali m.;* Nit. ac.; *Pall.;* Phyt.; Sab.; Trill.

OCCURRENCE—MODALITIES—After coitus: Nat. c.

After menses and between periods—Æsc.; *Alum.;* Bor.; *Bov.; Calc. c.;* Cocc.; Con.; *Eupion; Graph.;* Hydr.; *Iod.;* Kal.; *Kreos.; Nit. ac.;* Phos. ac.; *Puls.;* Sab.; *Sep.;* Thlaspi; *Xanth.*

After stool—Mag. m.

After urination—*Am. m.;* Con.; *Kreos.;* Mag. m.; Niccol.; Plat.; *Sep.;* Sil.

At climaxis—Psor.; Sang.

At night—Ambra; Caust.; *Merc.;* Nit. ac.

Before menses—*Alum.*; Bar. c.; Bor.; *Bov.; Calc. c.;* Calc. p.; Carbo v.; Con.; *Graph.*; Kreos.; Picr. ac.; *Puls.; Sep.*; Thlaspi.

Better from washing with cold water—Alum.

From motion, walking—*Bov.;* Carbo an.; Euphorb. pil.; Graph.; Helonin; *Mag. m.;* Tilia.

From rest—Fagop.

From sitting, relieved by walking—Cact.; *Cocc.;* Cycl.

From urine, contact of—Kreos.; *Merc.;* Sul.

In daytime—Alum.; Plat.

In infants, little girls—*Asperula; Calc. c.;* Can. s.; Carb. ac.; *Caul.; Cina; Cub.*; Hydr.; Merc. i. fl.; Merc.; *Millef.; Puls.; Sep.;* Syph.

In old, weak women—Ars.; *Helon.;* Nit. ac.; Sec.

In pregnant women—Cocc.; Kali c.; Sep.

Instead of menses—*Cocc.;* Graph.; *Iod.; Nux m.:* Phos.; Puls.; Senec.; *Sep.;* Xanth.

CONCOMITANTS—Abdominal pain, colic preceding and attending: Am. m.; Aral.; *Ars.;* Bell.; Calc. c.; *Con.;* Graph.; Ham.; Hematox.; Ign.; Lyc.; *Mag. m.;* Nat. c.; *Sep.;* Sil.; *Sul.:* Syph.

Backache and weak feeling, preceding and attending—*Æsc.; Eupion;* Graph.; *Helon.;* Kali bich.; Kreos.; Mag. s.; *Murex;* Nat. chlor.; *Nat. m.;* Ova t.; Psor.; *Stann.*

Cervical erosion, bleeding easily—Alum.; *Alnus;* Arg. n.; Dictam.; *Hydr.;* Hydrocot.; *Kali bich.*

Debility, weakness—*Alet.; Alum.;* Calc. c.; Carbo an.; Caul.; Caust.; Cinch.; *Cocc.;* Con.; Guaco; *Helon.;* Helonin; Hydr.; *Kreos.;* Onosm.; Phos.; Psor.; Puls.; Sep.; *Stann.*

Diarrhœa—Puls.

Feeling, as if warm water running—Bor.

Feeling of fulness, heat, relieved by cold water—Acon.

Hæmorrhage, obstinate, intermittent—Kreos.

Hepatic derangement, costiveness—Hydr.

History of abortion—Alet.; Caul.; *Sab.;* Sep.

Hysterical spasm in uterus and abdomen—Mag. m.

Mental symptoms—Murex.

Moth spots on forehead—Caul.; Sep.

Metorrhagia following—Mag. m.

Pruritus vulvæ—Agar.; Alum.; *Ambra; Anac.;* Calc. c.; *Fagop.; Helon.;* Hydr.; Kreos.; Merc.; *Sep.;* Sul.

Relaxation of genitals—Agn.; *Caul.;* Sec.; Sep.

Spasmodic contraction of vagina—Aur. m. n.

Urinary irritation—Berb. v.; *Erig.;* Kreos.; Sep.

MAMMAE—Abscess: Bry.; Crot. t.; Graph.; *Hep.; Phos.;* Phyt.; *Sil.;* Sul. See Mastitis.

Atrophy—Chimaph.; *Con.; Iod.;* Kali iod.; Nit. ac.; Onosm.; *Sabal.*

Cancer—*Arg. n.;* Ars. iod.; *Ars.; Aster.;* Bad.; Bapt.; Bar. iod.; Brom.; Bry.; Calc. iod.; *Carbo an.;* Carcinos.; Cic.; Clem.; *Condur.; Con.; Galium;* Graph.; Hep.; Hoang nan.; *Hydr.; Kali iod.;* Kreos.; Lach.;

Phos.; *Plumb. iod.;* Psor.; Sang.; *Scirrhin.;* Semperv. t.; Sil.; Sul.; Tar. c.; *Thuya.* See Tumors.

Cancer, bleeding—Hoang nan.; Kreos.; Lach.; *Phos.;* Sang.; Thuya.

Cancer, scirrhous—Ars.; Carbo an.; Condur.; *Con.;* Hydr.; Kreos.; Lapis alb.; Phyt.; *Scirrhin.; Sil.*

Induration, hardness—Alumen; Ananth.; *Aster.;* Bar. iod.; Bell.; *Bry.;* Bufo; *Calc. fl.; Carbo an.;* Carbo v.; Cham.; Cistus; Clem.; *Con.; Graph.; Iod.;* Kreos.; Lac c.; *Lapis alb.;* Merc.; Nit. ac.; *Phyt.; Plumb. iod.; Plumb. m.*

Inflammation (mastitis)—*Acon.;* Ant. t.; Apis; Arn.; Ars.; *Bell.; Bry.;* Calc. c.; *Cham.;* Cistus; *Con.; Crot. t.;* Ferr. p.; Galega; Graph.; *Hep.; Lac c.;* Lach.; *Merc.; Phell.; Phos.; Phyt.;* Plant.; *Puls.;* Sabad.; *Sil.;* Sul. See Pain, Swelling.

NIPPLES—Burning, itching: *Agar.;* Arundo; *Ars.;* Castor.; *Crot. t.;* Lyc.; Onosm.; Orig.; Petrol.; Puls.; Sil.; *Sul.*

Cracks, fissures, ulcerations—Ananth.; *Arn.;* Ars.; *Aur. sul.;* Calc. ox.; Calend.; Carbo v.; *Castor.;* Caust.; Cham.; *Condur.; Con.; Crot. t.; Eup. ar.;* Galium; Geran.; *Graph.;* Ham.; Hep.; Hippom.; Merc.; Nit. ac.; *Pæonia; Phell.;* Phos.; *Phyt.; Ratanh.: Sep.; Sil.;* Sul. See Soreness.

Inflamed, tender to touch—*Cham.;* Helon.; *Phyt.*

Retraction—Carbo an.; Hydr.; Lapis alb.; Nux m.; *Sars.;* Sil.

Soreness, tenderness—Apium gr.; *Arn.;* Bor.; Calend.; *Castor.; Cham.;* Cistus; *Con.; Crot. t.; Eup. ar.; Graph.;* Ham.; Helon.; *Hep.;* Hydr.; Lac c.; Med.; Ocimum; Orig.; Paraf.; *Phell.;* Phos.; *Phyt.; Ratanh.;* Sang.; Sil.; Sul.; Zinc.

PAIN IN BREASTS (mastodynia)—Acon.; Allium s.; Apis; Arg. n.; *Aster.;* Aur. sul.; *Bell.;* Brom.; *Bry.; Calc. c.;* Carbo an.; Cham.; *Chimaph.; Cim.; Con.;* Cotyled.; Croc.; *Crot. t.; Hep.;* Hydr.; Hyper.; Lac c.; Lach.; *Lact. ac.; Lapis alb.;* Lepid.; Med.; Merc. per.; *Merc.; Murex;* Nat. m.; Onosm.; Pall.; *Phell.; Phos.; Phyt.; Plumb. iod.;* Plumb. m.; Polyg.; Prun. sp.; Psor.; Puls.; *Sang.;* Sil.; Sumb.; Zinc.

Pain, inframammary—*Cim.;* Puls.; *Ran. b.;* Raph.; Sumb.; Ustil.; Zinc. m.

Pain relieved by supporting heavy mammæ—*Bry.; Lac c.;* Phyt.

Pain worse from jar, toward evening—Lac c.

SWELLING—Allium s.; Ananth.; *Asaf.; Aster.;* Aur. sul.; *Bell.;* Bellis; *Bry.;* Castor.; Dulc.; *Graph.;* Helon.; Lac c.; Merc. per.; *Merc.;* Onosm.; Phos.; *Phyt.;* Psor.; Puls.; Solan. ol.; Urt. See Mastitis.

Tenderness, soreness—Arg. n.; *Aster.; Bell.; Bry.;* Calc. c.; Carbo an.; *Cham.;* Clem.; *Con.;* Dulc.; *Helon.; Hep.;* Iod.; Kali m.; *Lac c.;* Lach.; *Med.;* Merc.; Onosm.; *Phyt.;* Plumb.; Radium; Sabal; Syph. See Pain.

TUMORS, nodosities—Ars. iod.; *Aster.; Bell.;* Berb. aq.; *Brom.;* Bry., Calend.; Calc. c.; *Calc. fl.; Calc. iod.;* Carbo an.; Cham.; *Chimaph.;* Clem.; Condur.; *Con.;* Ferr. iod.; Gnaph.; *Graph.;* Hekla; *Hydr.; Iod.;* Lach.; Lapis alb.; Lyc.; *Merc. i. fl.;* Murex; Nit. ac.; *Phos.;*

Phyt.; Plumb. iod.; Psor.; *Puls.;* Sab.; Sang.; *Scirrin.; Scrophul.; Sil.;* Thuya; *Thyr.;* Tub. See Cancer, Swelling, Inflammation.

Ulceration—Aster.; Calend.; Clem.; *Hep.; Merc.;* Pæonia; Phos.; *Phyt.; Sil.*

MASTURBATION—In children, due to pruritus vulvæ: *Calad.; Orig.;* Zinc. m.

MENOPAUSE—Climacteric period; change of life; Remedies in general: Acon.; Agar.; Alet.; *Amyl;* Aquil.; Arg. n.; Bell.; *Bellis;* Bor. ac.; *Cact.;* Calc. ars.; Calc. c.; Caps.; Carbo v.; *Caul.; Cim.;* Cocc.; Coff.; *Con.;* Cycl.; Ferr.; *Gels.; Glon.;* Graph.; Helon.; *Ign.; Jabor.;* Kah br.; *Kali c.; Kreos.; Lach.;* Mag. c.; *Mancin.; Murex; Nux m.; Nux v.; Oophor.;* Plumb.; *Puls.; Sang.;* Semperv. t.; *Sep.; Sul.;* Sul. ac.; Ther.; *Ustil.;* Val.; Vipera; Viscum; *Zinc. v.*

Anxiety—Acon.; *Amyl;* Sep.

Breasts enlarged, painful—Sang.

Burning in vertex—*Lach.;* Nux v.; Sang.; *Sul.*

Burning of palms and soles—Sang.; *Sul.*

Congestions—Acon.; *Amyl;* Calc. c.; *Glon.;* Lach.; Sang.; Sep.; *Sul.; Ustil.*

Cough, burning in chest, periodical neuralgia—Sang.

Earache—Sang.

Fainting spells—Cim.; Crotal.; Ferr.; *Glon.; Lach.;* Nux m.; Sep.; *Sul.;* Trill.

Falling of hair—Sep.

Fatigue, persistent tiredness, fagged womb—Bellis.

Fatigue without cause, muscular weakness, chilliness—Calc. c.

Flooding—Aloe; Amyl; Apoc.; *Arg. m.;* Arg. n.; Aur. mur.; Calc. c.; Caps.; *Cim.;* Cinch.; Ferr.; Hydrastinin; Kali br.; Lach.; Med.; Nit. ac.; *Plumb.;* Sab.; Sanguisorba.; *Sedum;* Sep.; Thlaspi; *Trill.; Ustil.;* Vinca. See Metrorrhagia.

Flushings—Acon.; *Amyl;* Bell.; Bor. ac.; Calc. c.; *Cim.;* Crotal.; Dig.; Ferr.; *Glon.; Ign.; Jabor.;* Kali br.; Kali c.; *Lach.; Mang. ac.;* Niccol. s.; Nux v.; Oophor.; Phos. ac.; Piloc.; *Sang.;* Sedum; *Sep.;* Stront.; *Sul.;* Sul. ac.; *Sumbul;* Tub.; *Ustil.;* Val.; Ver. v.; Vespa; Vinca; Zinc. v.

Globus hystericus—Amyl; *Lach.;* Val.; Zinc. v.

Headache—*Amyl;* Cact.; *Cim.; Cinch.;* Croc.; *Cyprip.;* Ferr.; *Glon.;* Ign.; Lach.; *Sang.; Sep.;* Stront. c.

Hysterical tendencies—*Ign.;* Val.; Zinc. v.

Inframammary pains—Cim.

Liver disorders—Card. m.

Mental depression or irritability—*Cim.;* Ign.; Kali br.; *Lach.;* Mancin.; Psor.; Val.; Zinc. v.

Nervous erethism—Absinth.; Arg. n.; Cim.; Coff.; Dig.; *Ign.;* Kali br.; *Lach.;* Oophor.; *Ther.;* Val.; *Zinc. v.*

Pains in uterus—Agar.; *Cim.;* Cocc.; Lach.; Puls.; Sep.

Palpitation—*Amyl; Calc. ars.;* Ferr.; Glon.; Kali br.; *Lach.;* Sep.; Trill.; Val.

Perspiration, profuse—Amyl; Bell.; Crotal.; Hep.; *Jabor.;* Lach.; Nux v.; *Sep.;* Tilia; Val.

Pruritus—Calad.

Salivation—Jabor.

Sexual excitement—Mancin.; *Murex.*

Sinking at stomach—Cim.; Crotal.; Dig.; Hydroc. ac.; *Ign.; Sep.;* Trill.

Ulcers, superficial, sores, on lower limbs—Polyg.

Vertigo, tinnitus—Glon.; Lach.; Trill.; Ustil.

Weakness—Dig.; Helon.; Lach.; *Sep.*

MENSTRUATION—TYPE: AMENORRHOEA: Remedies in general:
Acon.; Alet.; Alnus; *Apis;* Apoc.; Ars.; Avena; Bell.; Bry.; *Calc. c.;* Can. s.; *Caul.;* Caust.; *Cim.;* Con.; *Cycl.;* Dulc.; *Euphras.;* Ferr. ars.; *Ferr. m.; Ferr. red.;* Gels.; *Glon.; Graph.;* Hedeoma; *Helleb.; Helon.;* Jonosia; *Kali c.; Kali perm.;* Lil. t.; Mang. ac.; *Merc. per.; Nat. m.;* Nux v.; Op.; Ova t.; Parth.; Phos. ac.; Pinus lamb.; *Plat.;* Plumb.; *Polyg.; Puls.;* Sec.; *Senec.; Sep.;* Spong.; *Sul.;* Tanac.; Thyr.; Ustil.; *Xanth.*

Before the proper age—*Calc. c.;* Calc. p.; Carbo v.; Cinch.; Cocc.; *Sab.;* Sil.; Ver. a.

Delayed, first menses—Calc. c.; Calc. p.; Ferr.; *Graph.; Kali c.;* Kali per.; Polyg.; *Puls.; Senec.;* Sep.; Turnera.

Delayed, tardy flow—Acon.; Alet.; *Caust.; Cim.;* Con.; Cupr. m.; Dulc.; Euphras.; *Ferr. cit. strych.; Gels.;* Glon.; Gossyp.; *Graph.;* Helleb.; Iod.; Jonosia; *Kali c.;* Kali m.; *Kali p.;* Kali s.; Lac d.; *Mag. c.; Nat. m.;* Nux m.; Phos.; Pulex; *Puls.;* Radium; Sabad.; *Senec.; Sep.; Sul.;* Thasp.; Val.; *Vib. op.;* Zinc.

Intermittent—Coccus; Ferr. m.; *Kreos.; Lac c.;* Mag. s.; *Meli.;* Murex; Nux v.; Phos.; *Puls.; Sabad.; Sep.;* Sul.; Xanth.

Irregular—Ambra; Caul.; *Cim.; Cocc.; Cycl.; Graph.;* Iod.; Jonosia; Lil. t.; *Nux m.; Nux v.;* Phos.; Piscidia; *Puls.;* Radium; Sec.; Senec.; *Sep.;* Sul.

Protracted—Acon.; Calc. s.; Caust.; *Con.;* Crot.; *Cupr. m.;* Ferr.; Graph.; Iod.; Kreos.; *Lyc.;* Nat. m.; Nux m.; Nux v.; *Phos.;* Rhus t.

Scanty flow—Alet.; *Alum.;* Apis; Berb. v.; *Bor.;* Canth.; *Caul.;* Caust.; *Cim.; Cocc.;* Con.; Cycl.; Dulc.; *Euphras.;* Ferr. cit. ctrych.; *Gels.; Graph.;* Ign.; *Kali c.; Kali p.;* Kali s.; Lach.; Lamina; Lil. t.; *Mag. c.;* Mang. ac.; *Meli.;* Merc. per.; *Nat. m.;* Nux v.; *Ol. an.; Phos.;* Plat.; *Puls.;* Sang.; *Senec.; Sep.;* Sil.; *Sul.;* Val.; *Vib. op.;* Xanth. See Dysmenorrhœa.

Suppressed—*Acon.;* Apis; Bell.; *Bry.;* Calc. c.; Ceanoth.; Cham.; Chionanth.; *Cim.; Con.;* Croc.; Cupr.; *Cycl.; Dulc.;* Ferr.; Gels.; *Glon.;* Graph.; Helon.; Ign.; Kali c.; *Kali m.;* Lach.; Leonorus; Nat. m.; Nux m.; *Op.;* Pod.; *Puls.; Puls. nut.; Senec.;* Sep.; Sul.; *Tanac.;* Taxus; Tub.; *Ver. v.;* Zinc.

Suppressed, from anæmic conditions—Ars. iod.; Ars.; Caust.; Ferr. ars.; *Ferr. cit. strych.;* Ferr. red.; Graph.; *Kali c.;* Kali perm.; Kali p.; Mag. ac.; Nat. m.; Ova t.; *Puls.; Senec.*

Suppressed from anger with indignation—Cham.; Col.; Staph.

Suppressed, from cold water, exposure, chilling—*Acon.; Ant. c.;* Bell.; Calc. c.; Cham.; Cim.; *Con.; Dulc.;* Graph.; Lac c.; *Lac d.;* Phos.; *Puls.; Rhus t.;* Sul.; Ver. v.; Xanth.

Suppressed, from disappointed love—Helleb.

Suppressed, from fright, vexation—Act. sp.; *Acon.;* Cim.; Col.; Lyc.; Op.; Ver. a.

Suppressed, from transient, localized, uterine congestion, followed by chronic anæmic state—Sabal.

Suppressed, in emigrants—Bry.; Plat.

Suppressed, with asthma—Spong.

Suppressed, with cerebral congestion—*Acon.;* Apis; Bell.; Bry.; Calc. c. Cim.; *Gels.; Glon.;* Lach.; Psor.; Sep.; Sul.; *Ver. v.*

Suppressed, with congestion to chest—Acon.; Calc. c.; Sep.

Suppressed, with cramps to chest—Cupr. m.

Suppressed, with delirium, mania—Stram.

Suppressed, with dropsy—Apis; Apoc.; Kali c.

Suppressed, with fainting spells, drowsiness—Kali c.; *Nux m.;* Op.

Suppressed, with gastralgia or spasms—Cocc.

Suppressed, with jaundice—Chionanth.

Suppressed, with neuralgic pains about head, face—*Gels.*

Suppressed, with ophthalmia—Puls.

Suppressed, with ovaritis—*Acon.;* Cim.

Suppressed, with pelvic pressure, ovarian tenderness—Ant. c.; Bell.

Suppressed, with pelvic tenesmus—Pod.

Suppressed, with rheumatic pains—Bry.; Cim.; Rhus t.

Suppressed, with vicarious bleeding—*Bry.;* Crot.; Dig.; Erig.; Eupion; *Ferr.; Ham.;* Ipec.; Kali c.; Lach.; Millef.; Nat. s.; *Phos.; Puls.;* Sabad.; Sang.; *Senec.;* Sil.; Sul.; Trill.; Ustil.

DYSMENORRHOEA—Remedies in general: Acetan.; Acon.; Am. acet.; *Apioline;* Apis; Apium gr.; Aquil.; Atrop.; Avena; *Bell.; Bor.;* Bov.; Brom.; Bry.; *Cact.;* Calc. c.; Canth.; Castoreum; *Caul.; Cham.; Cim.; Cocc.; Coff.;* Collins.; *Col.;* Croc.; Cupr. m.; Dulc.; Epiph.; Ferr.; Ferr. p.; *Gels.;* Glon.; *Gnaph.;* Gossyp.; Graph.; *Guaiac.; Ham.;* Helon.; Hyos.; Ign.; *Kali perm.;* Lach.; Lil. t.; *Macrot.; Mag. c.;* Mag. m.; *Mag. p.;* Merc.; Millef.; Morph.; Nux m.; Nux v.; Op.; Plat.; *Puls.;* Rhus t.; Sab.; Sang.; Santon.; *Sec.; Senec.;* Sep.; Stram.; Thyr.; Tub.; Ustil.; *Ver. a.;* Ver. v.; *Vib. op.;* Vib. pr.; *Xanth.;* Zinc.

TYPE—Irregular, every two weeks, or so: Bor.; *Bov.; Calc. c.;* Calc. p.; Croc.; Ferr. p.; *Helon.;* Ign.; Mag. s.; Mez.; Murex; Nit. ac.; Nux v.; Phos. ac.; *Phos.;* Phyt.; Sab.; Sec.; Thlaspi; *Trill.;* Ust.

Irregular—Am. c.; *Bell.;* Bry.; *Calc. c.; Caul.;* Cim.; Cocc.; *Cycl.;* Guaiac.; Inula; Mag. s.; Murex; *Nat. m.; Nux v.;* Physost.; *Puls.;* Sec.; *Senec.; Sep.* See Amenorrhœa.

Membranous—*Ars.;* Bell.; *Bor.; Brom.;* Bry.; *Calc. acet.;* Calc. c.; Cham.; Collins.; Con.; Cycl.; Guaiac.; Heliotr.; Lac c.; *Mag. p.;* Merc.; Rhus t.; *Sul.;* Ustil.; *Vib. op.*

Nonobstructive, from ovarian irritation—*Apis;* Bell.; Ham.; Xanth.

Nonobstructive, from uterine irritation—*Cham.;* Coff.; Nit. ac.; Xanth.

Premature—Am. c.; *Calc. c.;* Caust.; Cocc.; Con.; Cycl.; Ign.; *Kali c.;* Lamina; Lil. t.; *Mag. p.;* Nat. m.; *Nux v.;* Ol. an.; Phos.; Sab.; Sep.; Sinap. n.; Sil.; *Sul.;* Xanth. See Irregular.

Rheumatic—Caul.; Caust.; *Cim.;* Cocc.; Guaiac.; Rham. c.

Spasmodic, neuralgic—Acon.; Agar.; *Bell.; Caul.;* Cham.; *Cim.;* Coff.; Collins.; *Gels.;* Glon.; Gnaph.; Mag. m.; *Mag. p.;* Nux v.; *Puls.;* Sab.; Santon.; *Sec.;* Senec.; Sep.; Ver. v.; *Vib. op.;* Xanth.

Spasmodic, with uterine congestion—Acon.; *Bell.;* Cim.; Collins.; Gels.; Puls.; *Sab.;* Sep.; Ver. v.

MENORRHAGIA—(profuse, premature flow): **Remedies in general:** Achill.; Agar.; *Alet.;* Aloe; Ambra; *Am. c.;* Apoc.; *Aran.; Arn.; Ars.; Bell.; Bor.;* Bov.; Bry.; *Cact.; Calc. c.;* Calc. p.; *Can. ind.; Canth.;* Carbo v.; Caul.; Ceanoth.; *Cham.;* Chin. s.; Cim.; *Cinch.; Cinnam.;* Collins.; Col.; *Croc.; Cycl.;* Dig.; *Erig.;* Ferr. m.; *Ferr. p.;* Ferr. red.; Ficcus; *Geran.;* Glycerin; *Ham.; Helon.;* Hydr.; Ign.; Jonosia; *Kali c.; Kali m.; Kreos.;* Lac c.; Lach.; Led.; Lil. t.; Mag. c.; Mez.; *Millef.;* Murex; *Nit. ac.; Nux v.;* Pall.; Paraf.; Phos. ac.; *Phos.;* Phyt.; *Plat.; Plumb.;* Ruta; *Sab.; Sec.;* Sedum; *Sep.;* Sil.; *Stann.;* Sul. ac.; Sul.; Thlaspi; *Trill.;* Ustil.; Vinca; *Xanth.*

After miscarriage, parturition—Apis; *Cim.;* .Cinch.; Helon.; Kali c.; *Nit. ac.; Sab.;* Sep.; Sul.; Thlaspi; *Ustil.;* Vib. op.

Every alternate period, profuse—Thlaspi.

Protracted, premature, profuse—*Aloe;* Asar.; *Bell.; Calc. c.;* Cal. iod.; Carbo an.; *Cinnam.;* Coff.; Ferr. ac.; Ferr. m.; Fluor. ac.; Glycerin; Grat.; Ign.; Kreos.; *Millef.;* Murex; *Nux v.;* Onosm.; *Plat.;* Raph.; Rhus t.; *Sab.;* Sanguisorba; *Sec.;* Sul.; *Thlaspi; Trill.;* Tub.; Xanth.

TYPE OF MENSTRUAL BLOOD—**Acrid, corroding:** Am. c.; Kali c.; Lach.; Mag. c.; Nat. s.; Nit. ac.; *Rhus t.;* Sab.; Sil.; *Sul.*

Bright-red—Acon.; *Bell.;* Brom.; Calc. p.; *Cinnam.; Erig.;* Glycerin; Ferr. p.; *Ipec.;* Lac c.; *Millef.;* Sab.; Sang.; *Trill.;* Ustil.

Changeable—Puls.

Coagulated—Am. m.; *Bell.;* Bov.; *Cham.;* Cim.; *Cinch.;* Cocc.; Coccus; Coff.; *Croc.; Cycl.;* Glycerin; Helon.; Jugl. r.; *Kali m.; Lil. t.;* Mag. m.; Med.; Murex; Nux v.; *Plat.;* Plumb.; *Puls.;* Sab.; Sang.; Sul.; *Thlaspi;* Trill.; Ustil.

Dark, blackish—Apis; *Asar.;* Bov.; Calc. p.; Canth.; Caul.; Cham.; Cim.; *Cinch.;* Cocc.; *Coccus;* Coff.; *Croc.; Cycl.;* Elaps; *Ham.;* Helon.; Ign.; *Kali m.; Kali n.;* Kreos.; Lach.; *Lil. t.;* Mag. c.; Mag. m.; Mag. p.; Med.; Nit. ac.; Nux v.; *Plat.;* Plumb.; *Puls.;* Sab.; Sec.; Sep.; *Thlaspi;* Trill.; *Ustil.; Xanth.*

Hot—Bell.

Membranous, shreddy, like meat washings—Brom.; *Cycl.;* Ferr. m.; Nat. c.; *Nit. ac.* See Coagulated.

Offensive—*Bell.;* Carbo v.; Cim.; Cop.; Helon.; *Kali c.;* Kali p.; *Lil. t.;* Mag. c.; *Med.;* Plat.; *Psor.;* Pyr.; *Sab.;* Sang.; *Sec.;* Sul.; Vib. op.

Pale—*Alum.;* Ars.; *Carbo v.;* Ferr. m.; Graph.; *Kali c.;* Nat. p.; *Puls.;* Sul. See Watery.

Partly fluid, partly clotted—*Ferr.;* Ham.; Plumb.; *Sab.; Sec.*

Pitch-like—Cact.; Cocc.; *Croc.;* Kali m.; *Mag. c.;* Med.; *Plat.*

Stringy, glairy, viscid, thick—Arg. n.; Coccus; *Croc.; Kali m.;* Kreos.; Lac c.; Mag. c.; Mag. p.; *Nit. ac.;* Nux m.; *Plat.;* Puls.; Sul.; *Trill.; Ust.; Xanth.*

Watery, thin—Æth.; Alumen; Eupion; Ferr. ac.; *Ferr. m.;* Gossyp.; Kali p.; Nat. p.; Phos.; *Sab.; Sec.*

COMPLAINTS, PRECEDING AND ATTENDING FLOW—Abdomen distended: Apoc.; Aran.; Cham.; *Cinch.; Cocc.;* Kali c.; Kreos.; Nux v. See Abdomen.

Abdomen sore—Ham.; Sep. See Abdomen.

Abdomen, weight—Aloe; Bell.; Glycerin; Kali s.; Puls.; *Sep.*

Anus, sore—Ars.; *Mur. ac.* See Anus.

Aphonia—*Gels.;* Graph.

Asthmatic seizures awaken her from sleep—Cupr.; *Iod.; Lach.;* Spong.

Axillæ, itching—Sang.

Backache, general bad feelings—Kali c.

Blindness—Cycl.; Puls.

Breasts, icy cold—Med.

Breasts, milk in them, in place of menses—Merc. v.

Breasts, tender, swollen—Bry.; Calc. c.; Canth.; *Con.;* Graph.; *Helon.;* Kali c.; *Lac c.;* Mag. c.; Merc.; *Murex; Phyt.; Puls.;* Sang.

Burning in hands and soles—Carbo v.

Catalepsy—Mosch.

Chilliness, coldness—Am. c.; Apis; Calc. c.; Cham.; Glycerin; Graph.; Nux v.; Plat.; *Puls.;* Sec.; Sep.; *Sil.; Ver. a.*

Cholera-like symptoms—*Am. c.;* Bov.; Ver. a.

Colds—Mag. c.; Sep.

Constipation—Am. c.; Collins.; *Graph.; Nat. m.;* Nux v.; Plat.; *Plumb.;* Sep.; *Sil.;* Sul.

Cough—*Graph.;* Lac c.; *Sul.*

Deafness, tinnitus—Kreos.

Diarrhœa—Am. c.; *Am. m.;* Ars.; *Bov.;* Cham.; Kreos.; Phcs.; *Puls.; Ver. a.*

Epistaxis—Acon.; *Bry.;* Dig.; Gels.; Nat. s.; Sep.; Sul.

Eruptions—Allium s.; *Bell.;* Bellis; Calc. c.; *Cim.;* Con.; *Dulc.;* Eug. j.; *Graph.; Kali ars.;* Kali c.; Mag. m.; Mang. ac.; *Med.;* Psor.; Sang.; *Sars.;* Sil.; Thuya; Ver. a.

Eyes, blindness or fiery spots—Cycl.; Sep.

Eyes, burning—Niccol.

Eyes, diplopia—Gels.

Eyes, ophthalmia—Puls.

Face flushed—*Bell.;* Calc. p.; Ferr. m.; *Ferr. p.;* Gels.; *Sang.*

Face pale, eyes sunken—Cycl.; Ipec.; Ver. a.

Feet and cheeks swollen—Apis; Graph.

Feet cold, damp—Calc. c.

Feet, pain in—Am. m.

Feet, swollen—Graph.; Lyc.; Puls.

Flushes of heat—Ferr.; Glon.; *Lach.; Sang.;* Sul.

Frenzy—Acon.

Genitals, sensitive—Am. c.; Cocc.; *Lach.;* Kali c.; *Plat.* See Vaginismus.

Headache, congestive symptoms—Aster.; *Bell.;* Bry.; Cim.; Cocc.; Croc.; *Cycl.;* Ferr. m.; Ferr. p.; *Gels.; Glon.;* Graph.; Kali p.; Kreos.; Lac c.; Lach.; Nat. c.; *Nat. m.; Nux v.;* Puls.; *Sang.; Sep.; Sul.; Ustil.;* Ver. v.; Xanth.

Heart, pain, palpitation, etc.—*Cact.;* Crot.; Eupion; Lach.; *Lith. c.;* Sep.; Spong.

Hoarseness, coryza, sweats—Graph.

Hunger—Spong.

Hysterical symptoms—Caul.. *Cim.;* Gels.; *Ign.; Mag. m.;* Nux v.; Plat.; Puls.; Senec.; Vib. op.

Inflammation of throat, chest, bladder—Senec.

Insomnia—Agar.; Senec.

Irritability—*Cham.;* Cocc.; Eupion; Kreos.; Lil. t.; Lyc.; Mag. m.; *Nux v.*

Joint pains—Caul.; Sab.

Labia burning—Calc. c.

Lachrymation, catarrhal state of eyes, nose—Euphras.

Leucorrhæa—Bar. c.; Bor.; *Calc. c.;* Carbo v.; Caust.; Graph.; Iod.; *Nat. m.;* Puls.

Leucorrhæa, acrid—Lach.; Sep.

Mania, chorea—Cim.

Mania, sexual—Can. ind.; *Dulc.;* Plat.; Stram.; Ver. a.

Morning sickness, nausea, vomiting—*Am. m.;* Bor.; *Cocc.; Cycl.;* Graph.; Ichth.; *Ipec.;* Kreos.; Meli.; Nat. m.; *Nux v.;* Puls.; *Sep.;* Thlaspi; Ver. a.

Mouth sore, swelling of gums, cheeks; bleeding ulcer—Phos.

Mouth, tongue, throat dry, especially during sleep—Nux m.; Tar. h.

Nervous disturbance, restlessness—*Acon.; Cham.;* Caul.; *Cim.;* Ign.; Kreos.; *Lach.;* Mag. m.; *Mag. p.;* Nit. ac.; Puls.; *Salix n.;* Senec.; Sep.; Trill.; Vib. op.; Xanth.

Nipples and breasts icy cold—Med.

Old symptoms aggravated—Nux v.

Pain, burning in left ovarian region, on motion—Croc.; *Thuya;* Ustil.

Pain, colicky, labor-like, spasmodic—*Alet.;* Aloe; *Am. c.;* Am. m.; Apis; *Bell.;* Bor.; *Bov.;* Brom.; Calc. c.;' *Caul.; Cham.; Cim.;* Cinch.; *Cocc.; Coff.; Col.;* Cupr. m.; *Cycl.;* Ferr. m.; Ferr. p.; *Gels.; Graph.;* Helon. *Hematox;* Ign.; Jonosia; *Kali c.;* Kreos.; Lil. t.; *Mag. c.; Mag. m.; Mag. p.;* Med.; Meli.; Nat. m.; Nit. ac.; Nux m.; *Nux v.;* Plat.; *Puls.; Sab.; Sec.;* Sep.; Stann.; Thlaspi; *Ver. a.;* Ver. v.; Vespa; *Vib. op.; Xanth.*

Pain, extending around pelvis, from sacrum to groin—Plat.; Puls.; Sep.; Vib. op.

Pain extending down hips, thighs, legs—*Am. m.;* Berb. v.; Bry.; Castor.; *Caul.;* Cham.; *Cim.;* Coff.; Col.; Con.; *Gels.;* Graph.; Lil. t.; Mag. c.; Mag. m.; Nit. ac.; Plat.; *Sep.;* Trill.; *Vib. op.;* Xanth.

Pain, extending through pelvis antero-posteriorly or laterally—Bell.

Pain, extending to back (sacrum, coccyx)—*Am. c.;* Am. m.; Asar.; Bell.; *Bor.;* Calc. c.; *Calc. p.;* Caust.; *Cham.;* Cic.; *Cim.;* Cupr. m.; Cycl.; *Gels.;* Graph.; *Helon.; Kali c.;* Kreos.; Mag. m.; Nit. ac.; *Nux v.*

Phos.; Plat.; Pod.; *Puls.;* Radium; Sab.; *Senec.; Sep.;* Spong.; Vib. op.; *Xanth.*

Pain, extending to chest—Caul.; Cham.; Cim.; *Cupr. m.*

Pain, extending to groins—Bor.; *Caul.;* Kali c.; Lil. t.; Plat.; Tanac.; *Ustil.*

Pain, extending to liver—Phos. ac.

Pain, extending to pubes—Alnus; Bov.; Col.; Cycl.; Radium; *Sab.;* Sep.; Vib. op.

Pain, extending to rectum—*Aloe;* Xerophyl.

Pain in feet—Am. m.

Pain in malar bones—Stann.

Pain in ovaries—*Apis;* Bell.; Bry.; Cact.; Canth.; *Cim.;* Col.; Ham.; Iod.; Jonosia; Kali n.; *Lach.; Lil. t.;* Picr. ac.; Salix n.; Tar. h.; *Thuya;* Vib. op.

Pruritus—Calc. c.; *Graph.;* Hep.; Inula; Kali c.; *Sil.;* Sul.

Rectal and vesical irritation—Sab.

Sadness—Am. c.; Aur.; Brom.; Caust.; *Cim.;* Cocc.; Ferr.; Helleb.; Helon.; *Ign.;* Lyc.; Nat. c.; *Nat. m.:* Nit. ac.; Phos.; Plat.; *Puls.; Sep.;* Stann.; Vespa.

Salivation—Pulex.

Sexual excitement—Plat.

Sore throat—Canth.; *Lac c.; Mag. c.*

Spasms—Artem.; *Bufo;* Calc. s.; Caul.; *Cim.;* Cupr. m.; Gels.; *Hyos.; Ign.;* Kali br.; Lach.; Mag. m.; Œnanthe; *Plat.;* Tar. h.

Stomach disturbances—Arg. n.; Ars.; *Bry.;* Kali c.; Lach.; *Lyc.;* Nux m.; *Nux v.; Puls.;* Sep.; Sul.

Stretching, yawning—Am. c.; Puls.

Syncope—Ars.; Cinch.; Ign.; *Mosch.;* Nux m.; *Nux v.;* Ver. a.

Tinnitus—*Ferr.;* Kreos.

Toothache—Am. c.; Calc. c.; Cham.; Mag. c.; *Puls.;* Sep.

Urinary symptoms—Calc. p.; *Canth.;* Coccus; *Gels.;* Hyos.; Mag. p.; Med.; Nux v.; Plat.; Pulex; Puls.; *Senec.;* Sep.; Ver. v.; Vib. op.

Vertigo—Calc. c.; Cycl.; Nux v.

Weakness—*Alum.; Am. c.;* Carbo an.; *Cinch.; Cocc.;* Ferr. m.; Glycerin; Graph.; *Helon.; Hematox.;* Ign.; Iod.; Niccol.; Puls.; *Ver. a.*

COMPLAINTS FOLLOWING MENSES—Diarrhœa: Graph.; Puls.

Erethism, neuralgic pains, inframammary pains, insomnia—Cim.

Eruption—Kreos.

Headache—Croc.; Lach.; Lil. t.; Puls.; Sep.

Headache, throbbing, with sore eyes—Nat. m.

Hemorrhoids—Cocc.

Hysterical symptoms—Ferr. m.

Leucorrhœa—Æsc.; Alum.; Graph.; *Kreos.;* Nit. ac. See Leucorrhœa.

Mammæ swollen, milky secretion—Cycl.

Old symptoms aggravated—Nux v.

Ovarian pain—Zinc. m.

Pains (intermenstrual)—*Bry.:* Ham.; Iod.; Kreos.; *Sep.*

Pruritus—Con.; Lyc.; *Tar. t*

Show occasional, every few days—Bor.; Bov.

Vomiting—Croc.

Weakness, profound—*Alum.*; Am. c.; Am. m.; *Ars.*; Calc. c.; *Carbo an.*; Carbo v.; Cim.; *Cinch.*; *Cocc.*; Ferr.; Glycerin; Graph.; Iod.; Ipec.; Kali c.; Mag. c.; Phos.; Thlaspi; *Trill.*; *Ver. a.*; Vinca.

MODALITIES—AGGRAVATION: At night: Am. c.; *Am. m.*; *Bor.*; *Bov.*; Coccus; *Mag. c.*; Mag. m.; Zinc.

During flow—*Cim.*; Ham.; Kreos.; *Puls.*; *Tub.*

From excitement—*Calc. c.*; *Sul.*; Tub.

From lying down, rest—*Am. c.*; Am. m.; *Bov.*; *Cycl.*; *Kreos.*; *Mag. c.*; *Zinc.*

From motion—Bov.; Bry.; Canth.; Caust.; Erig.; *Lil. t.*; Mag. p.; *Sab.*; *Sec.*; Thlaspi; *Trill.*

From sleep—Mag. c.

In morning, daytime—Bor.; Cact.; Carbo an.; *Caust.*; Cycl.; *Lil. t.*; *Puls.*; Sep.

AMELIORATION—From establishment of flow: Aster.; Cereum ox.; *Cycl.*; Eupion; *Lach.*; *Mag. p.*; *Senec.*; *Zinc.*

From cold drinks—Kreos.

From hot applications—Mag. p.

From lying down—Bov.; Cact.; Caust.; Lil. t.

From motion—Am. m.; *Cycl.*; Kreos.; *Mag. c.*; *Sab.*

NYMPHOMANIA—Ambra; Aster.; Bar. mur.; Calc. p.; Camph.; *Canth.*; Coca; Dulc.; *Ferrula gl.*; Fluor. ac.; *Grat.*; *Hyos.*; Kali br.; Lach.; *Lil. t.*; *Murex*; Orig.; Phos.; *Plat.*; Raph.; *Robin.*; *Salix n.*; Stram.; Strych.; *Tar. h.*; _Val.; *Ver. a.*

OVARIES—Abscess: Cinch.; *Hep.*; Lach.; *Merc.*; Phos. ac.; Pyr.; *Sil.*

Atrophy—*Iod.*; Oophor.; Orchit.

Complaints attending, or following, ovariotomy—Ars.; *Bell.*; Bry.; Cinch.; Coff.; *Col.*; Hyper.; Ipec.; Lyc.; Naja; Nux v.; *Oophor.*; Orchit.; *Staph.*

Congestion—*Acon.*; Æsc.; Aloe; Am. br.; *Apis*; Arg. n.; *Bell.*; *Bry.*; Canth.; *Cim.*; Col.; Con.; *Gels.*; *Ham.*; Iod.; *Lil. t.*; Merc.; Naja; *Nat. chlor.*; *Sep.*; Tar. h.; Ustil.; *Vib. op.* See Inflammation.

CYSTS, DROPSY—*Apis*; Apoc.; Arn.; Ars.; *Aur. iod.*; Aur. m. n.; Bell.; Bov.; Bry.; Cinch.; *Col.*; Con.; Ferr. iod.; Graph.; *Iod.*; Kali br.; Lach.; Lil. t.; *Lyc.*; Med.; *Oophor.*; Rhod.; Sab.; Tereb.; Zinc.

Induration—Aur.; Aur. m. n.; Carbo an.; *Con.*; Graph.; *Iod.*; Lach.; Pall.; Plat.; Ustil.

Inflammation (ovaritis)–Acute: Acon.; Am. br.; *Apis*; *Bell.*; Bry.; Cact.; *Canth.*; *Cim.*; *Col.*; Con.; Ferr. p.; Guaiac.; *Ham.*; Iod.; *Lach.*; Lil. t.; *Merc. c.*; Merc.; Phos. ac.; Plat.; *Puls.*; Sab.; Thuya; Viscum.

Acute, with peritoneal involvement—*Acon.*; Apis; Ars.; *Bell.*; Bry.; Canth.; Chin. s.; Cinch.; Col.; *Hep.*; *Merc. c.*; Sil.

Inflammation, chronic, with induration—*Con.*; Graph.; *Iod.*; Lach.; Pall.; Plat.; Sabal; Sep.; *Thuya.*

PAIN—Boring: *Col.;* Zinc. m.

Burning—*Apis; Ars.;* Bufo; *Canth.;* Con.; Eupion; *Fagop.;* Kali n.; Lil. t.; Plat.; Thuya; *Ustil.;* Zinc. v.

Crampy, constrictive—*Cact.;* Col.; Naja.

Cutting, darting, tearing—Absinth.; Acon.; *Bell.; Bry.;* Caps.; *Col.;* Con.; Croc.; *Lil. t.;* Naja; Puls.

Cutting, extending to thighs, legs—Bry.; *Cim.;* Croc.; Lil. t.; Phos.; Pod.; Wyeth.; *Xanth.;* Zinc. v.

Dull, constant—Aur. br.; Hydrocot.; Niccol.; Sep.

Dull, numb, aching—Pod.

Dull, wedge-like in uterus—Iod.

Neuralgic (ovaralgia)—Am. br.; *Apis;* Apium gr.; *Atrop.; Bell.;* Berb. v.; Bry.; *Cact.;* Canth.; *Caul.; Cim.; Col.; Con.;* Ferr.; Ferr. p.; *Gels.;* Gossyp.; Graph.; Ham.; Hyper.; Kali br.; *Lach.; Lil. t.; Mag. p.;* Meli; Merc. c.; Merc.; *Naja;* Phyt.; *Plat.;* Pod.; Puls.; *Sabal;* Salix n.; Sumb.; *Staph.;* Thea; *Ustil.; Vib. op.; Xanth.; Zinc. v.*

Neuralgic, intermittent—*Gossyp.;* Thaspium; Zizia.

Stinging—*Apis;* Canth.; Con.; Lil. t.; Merc.

Throbbing—Bell.; Brachygl.; Branca; *Cact.;* Hep.

Pain, in left ovary—Am. br.; Apis; Apium gr.; *Arg. m.;* Caps.; Carb. ac.; *Cim.; Col.;* Erig.; Eup. purp.; Frax. am.; Graph.; Iod.; *Lach.; Lil. t.;* Med.; Murex; *Naja;* Ov. g. pell.; Phos.; Picr. ac.; Thaspium; Thea; *Thuya;* Ustil.; *Vespa;* Wyeth.; *Xanth.;* Zinc.

Pain, in right ovary—Absinth.; *Apis;* Ars.; *Bell.;* Branca; *Bry.;* Col.; Eupion; Fagop.; Graph.; Iod.; Lach.; Lil. t.; *Lyc.; Pall.;* Phyt.; *Pod.;* Ustil.

Pain, with aggravation, from deep breathing—Bry.

Pain, with aggravation, from walking, riding, relieved by lying down—Carb. ac.; Pod.; Sep.; *Thuya;* Ustil.

Pain, with frequent urination—Vespa.

Pain, with numbness, shifting gases in ascending colon—Pod.

Pain, with relief, by drawing up leg—Apium gr.; Col.

Pain, with relief by flow—Lach.; Zinc. m.

Pain, with relief from pressure, tight bandage—Col.

Pain, with restlessness, can't keep still—Kali br.; Vib. op.; *Zinc.*

Pain, with sympathetic heart symptoms—Cim.; *Lil. t.;* Naja.

Swelling—*Am. br.; Apis; Bell.;* Brom.; Graph.; Ham.; *Lach.;* Pall.; *Tar. h.;* Ustil. See Congestion, Inflammation.

Tenderness, to touch, motion—Ant. c.; *Apis; Bell.; Bry.;* Canth.; Carbo an.; *Cim.; Ham.;* Hep.; Iod.; *Lach.;* Lil. t.; *Plat.;* Sabal; *Tar. h.;* Thea; Thuya; Ustil.; Zinc. v.

Traumatic conditions—Arn.; *Ham.;* Psor.

Tumors—*Apis;* Aur. m. n.; Bov.; *Col.;* Con.; Graph.; *Iod.; Kali br.;* Lach.; Oophor.; Pod.; *Sec.* See Cysts.

PELVIC—Abscess: Apis; Calc. c.; *Hep.;* Merc. c.; Pall.; *Sil.*

Pelvic cellulitis—Acon.; *Apis;* Ars.; Bell.; *Bry.;* Calc. c.; Canth.; *Cim.;* Hep.; Med.; *Merc. i. r.;* Merc. s.; Pyr.; *Rhus t.;* Sil.; Tereb.; Tilia; *Ver. v.*

Pelvic hæmatocele—Acon.; Apis; *Arn.;* Ars.; Bell.; Canth.; Cinch.; Col.; Dig.; *Ferr.; Ham.;* Ipec.; *Kali iod.;* Lach.; *Merc.;* Millef.; Nit. ac.; *Phos.;* Sab.; *Sec.; Sul.;* Tereb.; Thlaspi.

Pelvic peritonitis—*Acon.; Apis;* Arn.; Ars.; *Bell.; Bry.; Canth.;* Chin. s.; Cim.; Cinch.; *Col.;* Gels.; *Hep.;* Hyos.; *Lach.; Mere. c.;* Op.; Pall.; Rhus t.; Sab.; Sec.; *Sil.;* Tereb.; Ver. v. See Cellulitis, Metritis.

Pelvic peritonitis, with menorrhagia—Ars.; Ham.; Sab.; Thlaspi.

PREGNANCY AND LABOR—ABORTION: Remedies in general: Acon.; *Alet.;* Arn.; Bell.; Calc. fl.; *Caul.;* Cham.; *Cim.;* Cinnam.; Cinch.; Coff.; Croc.; Gossyp.; *Helon.;* Hyos.; Ipec.; *Kali c.;* Millef.; Nit. ac.; Nux v.; Op.; *Pinus lamb.;* Pyr.; Rhus t.; *Sab.; Sec.; Sep.;* Tanac.; Thlaspi; Trill.; *Vib. op.*

Abortion from debility—*Alet.;* Caul.; Chin. s.; Cinch.; *Helon.;* Sec.

From fatty degeneration of placenta—Phos.

From fright, emotions—*Acon.;* Cham.; Cim.; Op.

From mental depression, shock, watching, low fever—Bapt.

From ovarian disease—Apis.

From syphilitic taint—Aur.; Kali iod.; *Merc. c.*

From traumatism—Arn.; Cinnam.

With blood dark, fluid; formication—Sec.

With blood intermittent, pains spasmodic, excites suffocation, fainting; craves fresh air—Puls.

With blood light, fluid; painless—Millef.

With hæmorrhage persisting—Nit. ac.; Thlaspi.

With pains, frequent, labor-like; no discharge—Sec.

With pains, from small of back, around to abdomen, ending in crampy, squeezing, bearing down, tearing down thighs—Vib. op.

With pains, from small of back, to pubes, worse from motion; blood partly clotted—Sab.

With pains from small of back to thighs; weak back; pains worse from motion; also subsequent debility and sweat—Kali c.

With pains, flying across abdomen, doubling her up; chills; pricking in breasts; pains in loins—Cim.

With pains, irregular, feeble, tormenting; scanty flow, or long continued, passive oozing; backache, weakness, internal trembling—Caul.

With retained secundines—Cinch.; Pyr.

With septicæmia—Pyr.

With sequelæ—Kali c.; Sab.; Sul.

Tendency to abort—*Alet.;* Apis; Aur.; Bac.; Calc. c.; *Caul.; Cim.; Helon.;* Kali c.; Kali iod.; Merc. c.; Merc.; Plumb.; Puls.; *Sab.; Sec.; Sep.;* Sil.; Sul.; Syph.; *Vib. op.; Vib. pr.;* Zinc. m.

Tendency to abort at second or third month—*Cim.;* Kali c.; *Sab.; Sec.;* Vib. op.

Threatened—*Acon.;* Arn.; *Bapt.;* Bell.; *Caul.; Cham.;* Cim.; Cinch.; Coff.; Croc.; Eup. purp.; Ferr. m.; *Helon.;* Millef.; Plumb. m.; Puls.; *Sab.; Sec.;* Trill.; *Vib. op.;* Vib. pr.

COMPLAINTS DURING PREGNANCY—Abdomen, must lie on, during early months: Acet. ac.; Pod.

Acne—*Bell.;* Sab.; Sep. See Skin.

Albuminuria—*Apis;* Ars.; Aur. mur.; *Cupr. ars.;* Gels.; Glon.; *Helon.;* Indium; *Kali chlor.;* Kal.; *Merc. c.;* Phos.; Sab.; Thlaspi; Thyr.; Ver. v. See Kidneys (Urinary System).

Arms hot, sore, painful—Zing.

Backache—*Æsc.;* Kali c. See Locomotor System.

Bilious complications—Chel.

Bladder disturbances, tenesmus—*Bell.; Canth.; Caust.;* Equis.; Ferr.; Nux v.; Pop. tr.; *Puls.;* Staph.

Breasts, painful, inflammatory—*Bell.; Bry.*

Breasts, painful, neuralgic—*Con.;* Puls.

Congestion of brain—*Glon.* See Head.

Constipation—Alum.; *Collins.;* Lyc.; Nux v.; Op.; *Plat.;* Plumb.; *Sep.* See Abdomen.

Convulsions, spasms—Amyl; Cupr. m.; *Glon.;* Hyos.; Lyssin; *Œnanthe.* See Nervous System.

Cough—Acon.; *Apoc.; Bell.;* Bry.; *Cham.;* Caust.; *Con.;* Coral.; *Dros.;* Glon.; *Hyos.; Kali br.;* Ipec.; Nux v.; Vib. op.

Cramps, in calves—Cham.; *Cupr.;* Mag. p.; Nux v.; *Ver. a.*

Cravings, abnormal—*Alum.;* Calc. c.; Carbo v.; *Sep.* See Stomach.

Diarrhœa—Ferr. m.; Helleb.; Nux m.; Petrol.; Phos. ac.; *Puls.;* Sec.; *Sul.*

Discharge bloody—Erig.; Kali c.; Phos.; Rhus t. See Abortion.

Dyspepsia (heartburn, acidity)—Acet. ac.; Anac.; Calc. c.; Canth.; Caps.; Diosc.; *Nux v.; Puls.* See Stomach.

Dyspnœa—Apoc.; Lyc.; Nux v.; Puls.; *Viola od.* See Respiratory System.

False pregnancy—*Caul.;* Croc.; Nux v.; *Thuya.*

Gastralgia—Petrol.

Goitre—Hydr.

Hæmorrhoids—Collins.; Pod.; Sul. See Abdomen.

Herpes—Sep.

Hiccough—Cycl. See Stomach.

Insanity—Hyos. See Mind.

Mental symptoms—*Acon.;* Cham.; *Cim.;* Puls. See Mind.

Metrorrhagia—Cinch.; Cinnam.; Ipec.; Nit. ac.; Sec.; Trill. See Uterus.

Morning sickness (nausea, vomiting)—Acet. ac.; Acon.; Alet.; *Amyg. pers.;* Anac.; Ant. t.; *Apomorph.;* Arg. n.; *Ars.;* Bry.; Carb. ac.; *Cereum ox.; Cim.; Cocc.;* Colch.; *Cucurb.;* Cupr. ac.; Cycl.; Gnaph.; *Gossyp.;* Ingluv.; *Ipec.;* Iris; Kali m.; *Kreos.;* Lac d.; Lact. ac.; *Lob. infl.;* Mag. c.; Merc.; Nat. p.; Nux m.; *Nux v.;* Petrol.; Phos.; Piloc.; Psor.; *Puls.; Sep.;* Staph.; *Symphor.;* Tab.; Ther.; *Thyr.* See Stomach.

Mouth, sore—Hydr.; Sinap. a. See Mouth.

Nervous sensitiveness, extreme—Acon.; Asar.; Cim.; *Ther.*

Pain, false labor—*Caul.; Cham.; Cim.;* Gels.; *Puls.;* Sec.

Pain in abdomen, as if strained, left side—Am. m.

Pain, in lumbar region, dragging, distressful—Arn.; *Bell.; Kali c.;* Nux v.; Puls.; Rhus t.

Pain, rheumatic—Acon.; Alet.; *Cim.;* Op.; Rhus t.

Plethora—Acon.

Pruritus, vulvæ et vaginæ—Acon.; *Ambra;* Ant. c.; Bor.; *Calad.; Collins.;* Ichth.; *Sep.;* Tab. See Vulva.

Retinitis—Gels.

Salivation—Acet. ac.; Ars.; *Iod.; Jabor.;* Kreos.; **Lact. ac.;** *Merc. s.;* Nat. m.; *Piloc.;* Sul.

Sexual excitement—Plat. See Nymphomania.

Sleeplessness—*Acon.;* Cim.; *Coff.;* Nux v.; Puls.; Sul.

Toothache—Acon.; Bell.; *Calc. fl.; Cham.;* Coff.; *Kreos.; Mag. c.;* Nux v.; Ratanh.; Sep.; *Staph.;* Tab.

Toxæmic conditions—Kali chlor.

Uterine and abdominal soreness—Ham.; Puls.

Varicose veins—Arn.; Bellis; Calc. c.; Carbo v.; Ham.; Lyc.; Millef.; Sul.; Zinc. m.

Vertigo—Bell.; Cocc.; Nux v.

Weariness in limbs, cannot walk—Bellis.

PARTURITION—LABOR: CONVULSIONS (eclampsia): *Acon.;* Æth.; Amyl; Arn.; *Bell.;* Canth.; Cham.; *Chloral; Cic.;* Cim.; Coff.; *Cupr. ars.;* Cupr. m.; Gels.; Glon.; *Hydroc. ac.; Hyos.;* Ign.; Ipec.; Kali br.; Merc. c.; Merc. d.; *Œnanthe;* Op.; Piloc.; Plat.; Solan. n.; Spiræa; Stram.; *Ver. v.; Zinc. m.*

PAINS—Backache violent, wants it pressed—Caust.; *Kali c.*

Excessive—Bell.; Coff.

False labor pains—Bell.; Cham.; *Caul.; Cim.;* Gels.; Nux v.; *Puls.;* Sec.; Vib. op.

Hour glass contraction—Bell.; Sec.

Labor delayed—Kali p.; Pituitrin.

Labor premature—Sab.

Needle-like prickings in cervix—Caul.

Shifting, across abdomen, doubling her up; pricking in mammæ; shivers during first stage—Cim.

Shifting, all over, exhaustion; fretful; shivering—Caul.

Shifting, from back to rectum, with urging to stool, or urination—Nux v.

Shifting, from loins down legs—Aloe; *Bufo;* Carbo v.; Caul.; Cham.; *Nux v.*

Shifting upwards—*Cham.;* Gels.

Spasmodic, irregular, intermittent, ineffectual, fleeting—Arn.; Artem.; *Bell.;* Bor.; *Caul.;* Caust.; *Cham.;* Chloral.; *Cim.;* Cinnam.; *Cinch.;* Coff.; *Gels.;* Kali c.; Kali p.; Nat. m.; *Nux v.;* Op.; Pituitrin; *Puls.;* Sacchar. of.; *Sec.*

With dyspnœa from constriction of middle of chest arresting pains—Lob. infl.

With hypersensitiveness to pain—*Acon.;* Bell.; *Caul.;* Caust.; *Cham.; Cim.;* Cinch.; *Coff.; Gels.;* Hyos.; Ign.; *Nux v.;* Puls.

With relief from pressure in back—Caust.; *Kali c.*

With syncope—Cim.; Nux v.; Puls.; Sec.

PLACENTA—Retained: Arn.; Canth.; Caul.; Cim.; Cinch.; Ergotin; Gossyp.; *Hydr.; Ign.;* Puls.; Sab.; *Sec.;* Viscum.

RIGID OS—Acon.; *Bell.; Caul.;* Cham.; Cim.; *Gels.;* Lob. infl.; *Ver. v.*

PUERPERIUM—(Lying-in period): After-pains: *Acon.;* Amyl; *Arn.; Bell.;* Calc. c.; *Caul.;* Carbo v.; *Cham.; Cim.;* Cocc.; *Coff.;* Cupr. ars.; *Cupr. m.; Gels.;* Ign.; Kali c.; Lach.; Nux v.; *Puls.;* Pyr.; Rhus t.; *Sab.; Sec.;* Sep.; Vib. op.; *Vib. pr.; Xanth.*

After pains, across lower abdomen, into groins—Caul.; Cim.

After pains, extending into shins—Carbo v.; Cocc.

After pains severe, distressing, in calves and soles—Cupr. m.

Backache, debility, sweat—Kali c.

Complications prevented—*Arn.;* Calend.

Constipation—*Bry.; Collins.;* Nux v.; Ver. a.; Zinc. m.

Diarrhœa—*Cham.;* Hyos.; Puls.

Hemorrhage (flooding, post-partum)—*Acet. ac.;* Am. m.; Amyl; Arn.; Ars.; *Bell.;* Caul.; Cham.; *Cinch.; Cinnam.; Croc.;* Cycl.; Ferr.; Geran.; *Ham.;* Hyos.; Ign.; *Ipec.;* Kali c.; *Millef.;* Nit. ac.; Puls.; *Sab.; Sec.;* Trill.; Ustil.

With bright red fluid; painless flow—Millef.

With bright red, hot, profuse flow in gushes—Bell.

With bright red, hot, profuse flow; collapsic symptoms—Ipec.

With collicky, bearing-down pains, relieved by gush of blood—Cycl.

With dark, thick, paroxysmal flow; debility—Cinch.

With habitual tendency; profuse, dark, clotted—Trill.

With pain from back to pubes; dark, clotted, painless flow—Sab.

With passive, dark, fluid blood, worse from motion; thin females; relaxed uterus; formication—Sec.

With uterine inertia—Am. m.; Caul.; Puls.; Sec.

Hæmorrhoids—Acon.; *Aloe;* Bell.; Ign.; Puls.

LOCHIA—Acrid: Bapt.; Kreos.; *Nit. ac.;* Pyr.

Lochia bloody—Chrom. ac.; *Trill.*

Lochia bloody, dark—Caul.; Cham.; Kreos.; Nit. ac.; Pyr.; *Sec.*

Lochia bloody, in gushes, worse from motion—Erig.

Lochia hot, scanty—Bell.

Lochia intermittent—Con.; *Kreos.;* Pyr.; Rhus t.; Sul.

Lochia offensive—Bapt.; *Bell.;* Carb. ac.; *Carbo an.;* Carbo v.; Chrom. ac.; Crot. t.; Erig.; *Kreos.;* Nit. ac.; Pyr.; Rhus t.; *Sec.;* Sep.; Sul.

Lochia prolonged—Calc. c.; *Caul.;* Cinch.; Helon.; Millef.; *Rhus t.; Sab.; Sec.;* Trill.; *Ustil.*

Lochia scanty—Bell.; Cham.; Puls.

Lochia suppressed—*Acon.;* Aral.; Bell.; *Bry.;* Cham.; Echin.; Hyos.; Leonorus; Op.; *Puls.;* Pyr.; *Sec.; Sul.;* Zinc.

Nymphomania—Cinch.; *Plat.;* Ver. a.

Panaritium—Cepa.

Prolapsus recti—Ruta. See Abdomen.

Puerperal cellulitis—Hep.; *Rhus t.;* Ver. v.

Puerperal fever (milk fever)—Acon.; *Bry.; Calc. c.;* Cham.

Puerperal fever, septic (septicæmia)—*Acon.;* Ail.; Arn.; *Ars.; Bapt.; Bell.;* Bry.; Calc. c.; *Carb. ac.;* Canth.; Cham.; *Chin. s.;* Cim.; Crot.; *Echin.; Hydroc. ac.;* Hyos.; Kali c.; Kali p.; Lach.; Lyc.; *Merc. c.;* Merc. s.; Nux v.; *Puls.; Pyr.; Rhus t.;* Sec.; Sep.; Tereb.; *Ver. v.*

See Pyæmia (Generalities).

Puerperal mania—Bell.; *Can. ind.*; Cim.; *Hyos.*; Plat.; Senec.; *Stram.*; Ver. v.; Zinc. See Mind.

Puerperal melancholia—*Agn.*; Aur.; *Cim.*; Plat.; Puls. See Mind.

Puerperal metritis—Bell.; *Canth.*; Lach.; Nux v.; Tilia. See Uterus.

Puerperal peritonitis—Acon.; *Bell.*; Bry.; *Merc. c.*; Pyr.; Sul.; Tereb. See Abdomen.

Puerperal phlebitis after forceps delivery—Cepa.

Puerperal tympany—Tereb.

Sweating—Cham.; Samb.; Stram.

Urinary incontinence—Arn.; Bell.; Caust.; Hyos.; Trill.

Urinary retention, suppression—Acon.; *Arn.*; *Bell.*; Equis.; *Hyos.*; *Op.*; Staph.; Stram.

COMPLAINTS AFTER PUERPERIUM—Acne on chin: Sep.

Constipation—Lil. t.; *Lyc.*; Mez.; Ver. a. See Abdomen.

Hair falls out—Carbo v.; Nat. m.; *Sep.*

Hæmorrhoids—Ham. See Abdomen.

LACTATION—Discharge from vagina, bloody during nursing: Sil.

Excitement, sexual, during nursing—Calc. p.

Menses during—Calc. c.; Pall.

Milk, absent, or scanty, tardy (agalactea)—Acon.; *Agn.*; Asaf.; Bry.; *Calc. c.*; Caust.; Cham.; Chel.; Formica; Fragar.; *Lac c.*; Lac d.; *Phos. ac.*; Phos.; Phyt.; Piloc.; *Puls.*; *Ricinus*; Sec.; Sil.; Sticta; *Thyr.*; Urt.; X-ray.

Milk, bloody—Bufo.

Milk, bluish, transparent, sour, impoverished, or faulty, so child rejects it— Acet. ac.; Calc. c.; *Calc. p.*; Merc.; *Phos. ac.*; Sabal; *Sil.*; Sul.

Milk suppressed—*Acon.*; Agn.; Bell.; *Bry.*; Camph. monobr.; Cham.; Phyt.; *Puls.*; Sec.; Zinc. m.

Milk, too profuse (galactorrhœa)—Bell.; *Bor.*; *Calc. c.*; Cham.; Chimaph.; Con.; Erig.; Iod.; Lac c.; Lact. v.; *Medusa*; Parth.; Phos.; Phyt.; Pip. m.; Rheum; Ricinus; Sabal; *Salvia*; Sec.; *Solan. olec.*; Spiranth.; Ustil.

Milk, too profuse (to dry up during weaning)—Asaf.; Bry.; *Calc. c.*; Con.; Lac c.; *Puls.*; Urt.

Pain, drawing from nipple, all over body, during nursing—Phyt.; Puls.; Sil.

Pain, drawing from nipple through to back, during nursing; nipple very sore —Crot. t.

Pain, intolerable, between nursings—Phell.

Pain, in opposite breast—Bor.

Prolonged nursing, with anæmia, debility—*Acet. ac.*; Calc. p.; Carbo an.; *Cinch.*; Phos. ac.

Menorrhagia—*Calc. c.*; Phos.; *Sil.*

Milk leg (phlegmasia alba dolens)—Acon.; Apis; *Ars.*; Bell.; Bism.; Bry.; *Bufo*; Crot.; *Ham.*; Lach.; *Puls.*; *Rhus t.*; Sul.; Urt.

Nipples fissured from nursing—Graph.; Ratanh.; Sep.

Prolapsus uteri—Pod. See Uterus.

Sore mouth—Hydr.; Sinap. a.

Sub-involution—*Aur. m. n.*; Calc. c.; Caul.; Cim.; Croc.; *Epiph.*; Ferr iod.; *Frax. am.;* *Helon.;* Hydr.; *Kali b*; *Lil. t.;* Mer. c. sale; Nat. hypochl.; Pod.; *Sec.; Sep.;* Ustil.

Weakness—Chin. s.; Cinch.; Kali c.

Weaning, ill effects—Bry.; Cycl.; Fragar.; Puls.

PUBIC HAIR—Falls out: Nat. m.; Nit. ac.; Zinc. m.

TUBES, FALLOPIAN—Inflammation (salpingitis): Acon.; Apis; *Ars.;* Bry.; Canth.; Chin. s.; *Col.;* Eupion; Hep.; *Merc. c.;* Sabal. See Metritis, Peritonitis.

UTERUS—Atony, weakness, relaxation: Abies c.; *Alet.;* Aloe; Alston.; Alum; Bellis; *Caul.; Cinch.;* Ferr. iod.; *Helon.;* Lappa; *Lil. t.;* Puls.; Rhus ar.; *Sab.; Sec.; Sep.; Trill.;* Ustil. See Displacements.

CERVIX—Induration of, and os: Alumen; *Aur. m.; Aur. mur.;* Aur. m. n.; Carbo an.; Con.; Helon.; *Kali cy.; Iod.;* Kal.; Mag. m.; Nat. c.; *Plat.;* Sep.

Cervix, inflammation (endocervicitis)—Ant. t.; Arg. n.; *Ars.; Bell.;* Calend.; Hydr.; Lyc.; *Merc. c.;* Merc.; Nit. ac.; Sep. See Ulceration.

Cervix, redness—Hydrocot.; Mitchella.

Cervix, swelling, scirrhus-like—Ananth.

Cervix, swelling, with urinary symptoms—Canth.

Cervix, tenesmus—Bell.; Ferr. m.

Cervix, tumors, cancerous—Carbo an.; Iod.; Kreos.; Thuya.

Cervix, ulceration—Alnus; *Arg. m.;* Arg. n.; *Ars.; Aur. m. n.;* Bufo; *Carb. ac.;* Carbo an.; Fluor. ac.; *Hydr.;* Hydrocot.; Kali ars.; *Kreos.;* Lyc.; *Merc. c.;* Merc.; Murex; Phyt.; *Sep.;* Sul. ac.; Thuya; *Ustil.; Vespa.*

Cervix, ulceration, bleeding easily—Alnus; Arg. n.; Carbo an.; Kreos.

Cervix, ulceration, deep—Merc. c.

Cervix, ulceration, in aged—Sul. ac.

Cervix, ulceration, spongy—Arg. n.; Kreos.

Cervix, ulceration, superficial—*Hydr.;* Merc.

Cervix, ulceration, with fetid, acrid discharge—Ars.; Carb. ac.

Cervix, ulceration, with fetid, ichorous, bloody discharge—Carbo an.; Kreos.

CONGESTION—Acon.; *Aloe;* Aur.; *Bell.;* Bellis; *Caul.;* Cim.; *Collins.;* Croc.; *Frax. am.;* Gels.; Iod.; *Lil. t.;* Mag. p.; Mitchella; Murex; Puls.; Sabal; Sab.; *Sep.;* Stroph.; Sul.; Tar. h.; *Ver. v.* See Inflammation.

Congestion, chronic or passive—Æsc.; *Aur.;* Calc. c.; Cim.; *Collins.; Helon.;* Lach.; *Polymnia;* Sep.; Stann.; Sul.; *Ustil.*

Consciousness of a womb; very tender to jars—*Helon.;* Lyc.; Lyssin; *Med.;* Murex.

Disorders, with reflex heart symptoms—Cim.; Lil. t.

Disorders, with toothache, headache, salivation, neuralgia—Sep.

DISPLACEMENTS (flexions, versions)—*Abies c.;* Æsc.; *Bell.;* Carb. ac.; *Eupion;* Ferr. iod.; Ferr. m.; *Frax. am.;* Heliotr.; *Helon.;* Lappa; *Lil. t.;* Mel c. sale; Murex; Pall.; *Puls.;* Sabal; Sec.; Senec.; *Sep.; Stann.*

Displacements, prolapsus—Abies c.; Æsc.; Agar.; *Alet.;* Aloe; Arg. m.; Asperula; *Aur. m. n.; Bell.;* Benz. ac.; *Calc. c.;* Calc. p.; Calc. sil.; Caul.; *Collins.;* Con.; Ferr. br.; *Ferr. iod.;* Ferr. m.; *Frax. am.;* Graph.;

Helon.; Ign.; Kali bich.; Kreos.; Lach.; *Lil. t.;* Lyssin; *Mel c. sale; Murex;* Nat. chlor.; Nat. m.; Nux m.; *Nux v.;* Onosm.; Pall.; Plat.; *Pod.; Puls.; Rhus t.;* Sec.; Senec.; *Sep.; Stann.;* Staph.; Tilia; Trill.; Zinc. v.

HÆMORRHAGE (Metrorrhagia): Remedies in general—Acet. ac.; Achill.; Agar.; *Ambra;* Apis; Arg. n.; Arg. oxy.; *Arn.; Ars.;* Aur. mur. kali; *Bell.; Bov.;* Bry.; *Cact.; Calc. c.;* Canth.; *Caul.; Cham.;* Cim.; Cina; *Cinch.; Cinnam.;* Collins.; *Croc.;* Crot. casc.; Crot.; Dictam.; Elaps; *Erig.; Ferr. ac.;* Ferr. m.; *Ferr. p.;* Fuligo; *Ham.;* Helon.; Hydrast.; Iod.; *Ipec.;* Jonosia; Junip. v.; *Kali n.;* Kreos.; *Lach.;* Lil. t.; Mag. m.; Mangif. ind.; Millef.; Mitchella; Nat. chlor.; *Nit. ac.;* Nux v.; *Phos.;* Plat.; Plumb.; Puls.; *Pyr.; Rhus ar.;* Robin.; *Sab.; Sec.; Sep.;* Sul. ac.; Sul.; *Stram.;* Tereb.; *Thlaspi; Trill.;* Ustil.; *Vinca;* Viscum; Xanth.

From chlorosis; climacteric; cancer uteri—Med.; Phos.; Thlaspi; Ust.
From currettage—Nit. ac.
From fibroids—Calc. c.; Nit. ac.; *Phos.;* Sab.; Sec.; Sul. ac.; *Thlaspi; Trill.;* Vinca.
From mechanical injury, straining, undue exertion—*Ambra;* Arn.; *Cinnam.;* Ham.
From parturition, abortion—Caul.; Cham.; Cinch.; Croc.; Ipec.; Millef.; Nit. ac.; *Sab.; Sec.;* Thlaspi. See Pregnancy.
From retained placenta—Sab.; Sec.; Stram.
From uterine atony, malarial cases—Cinch.
Inter-menstrual—*Ambra;* Arg. n.; *Bov.; Calc. c.;* Cham.; Elaps; *Ham.; Ipec.;* Mag. s.; *Phos.;* Rhus t.; Robin.; *Sab.;* Vinca.
With backache, relieved by pressure, sitting—Kali c.
With blood, black—Caul.; *Croc.;* Elaps; Mag. c.; *Plat.*
With blood, bright red, profuse, gushing, from least motion—Acal.; *Bell.;* Bov.; Cham.; Erig.; *Ipec.;* Med.; *Millef.;* Mitchella; Phos.; *Sab.; Sec.; Trill.;* Ustil.; Viscum.
With blood, clotted or partly clotted—Acal.; *Bell.;* Cham.; *Cinch.;* Cocc.; *Croc.;* Cycl.; Erig.; *Ipec.;* Kali c.; Lach.; *Plat.; Plumb.;* Puls.; Rhus t.; *Sab.;* Thlaspi; Trill.; Ustil.; Viscum.
With blood clotted or fluid; paroxysmal or continual flow; nausea, vomiting; palpitation, pulse quick, feeble when moved; vital depression; fainting on raising head from pillow—Apoc.
With blood dark, fluid, offensive—Crot.
With blood, profuse, painless—Millef.; Nit. ac.
With blood, profuse, painless, dark, venous—*Ham.;* Mangif. ind.
With blood, profuse, passive, obstinate—Caul.; Cinnam.
With blood, profuse, passive, thin, fetid; in cachectic females—Sec.
With blood, profuse, very dark, thick, tarry; dragging, downward, pressing in pelvis and groins, followed by sacral pain; unnatural genital sensibility and irritability—Plat.
With blood thin; painless flow—Carbo an.; Cinch.; Sec.
With congestive headache—Bell.; Glon.
With fainting—Apis; *Cinch.;* Ferr. m.; *Trill.*

With faintness in stomach—Crct.; Trill.

With feeling, as if back and hips were falling to pieces, relieved by bandaging; fainting—Trill.

With feeling of enlarged head—Bad.

With flow in paroxysms, bright red; joint pains—Sab.

With flow in paroxysms, thin, light blood, firm coagula; severe labor-like pains—Cham.

With heavy abdomen, faintness, stinging pains—Apis.

With hysteria—Caul.; Cim.; Mag. m.

With labor-like pains—*Caul.; Cham.; Cim.;* Ham.; Sab.; Sec.; Thlaspi; Viscum.

With nausea—Apoc.; Caps.; *Ipec.*

With nervous erethism at menopause—Arg. n.; *Lach.*

With painful micturition; pallor; violent irritation of rectum, bladder; prolapsus—Erig.

With pain extending to navel; dyspnœa—Ipec.

With pain passing around pelvis, from sacrum to groin—Puls.; Sep.

With pain passing from sacrum to pubes—Sab.

With pain passing through pelvis, antero-posteriorly or laterally—Bell.

With septic fever—Pyr.

With sexual excitement—Ambra; Plat.; Sab.

With uterine congestion, inflammation—Sab.

With weak heart—Am. m.; Dig.

HYDROMETRA—Nat. hypochlor.; Sep.

Induration—Aur.; Aur. m. kali; *Aur. m. n.;* Carbo an.; *Con.;* Graph.; *Iod.;* Kal.; Kreos.; Mag. m.; Plat.; *Sep.*

INFLAMMATION (endometritis, metritis)—Acute: Acon.; Ant. iod.; *Apis;* Arn.; *Ars.;* Bell.; *Bry.;* Canth.; Cham.; *Cim.;* Cinch.; Con.; *Gels.;* Hep.; Hyos.; *Iod.;* Kali c.; Kali iod.; Lach.; Lil. t.; *Mel c. sale; Merc. c.;* Nux v.; Op.; Phos. ac.; Plat.; *Puls.;* Rhus t.; *Sab.;* Sec.; *Sep.; Sil.;* Stram.; Sul.; Tereb.; Tilia; *Ver. v.*

Inflammation, chronic—Alet.; Aloe; *Ars.; Aur. m.; Aur. m. n.;* Bor.; *Calc. c.; Carb. ac.;* Caul.; Chin. ars.; *Cim.; Con.;* Graph.; *Helon.; Hydr.;* Hydrocot.; Inula.; *Iod.; Kali bich.;* Kali c.; Kali s.; Kreos.; Lach.; *Mag. m.; Mel c. sale;* Merc.; *Murex;* Nat. m.; Nit. ac.; *Nux v.;* Phos. ac.; Phos.; Plumb.; *Puls.;* Rhus t.; *Sab.;* Sec.; *Sep.;* Sil.; Stram.; *Sul.*

Inflammation, chronic, follicular—*Hydr.;* Hydrocot.; Iod.; Merc.

Inflammation, chronic, with arterial congestion—Bell.; Lil. t.; *Sab.*

Inflammation, chronic, with venous congestion—Aloe; *Collins.;* Mag. m.; Murex; *Sep.*

Inflammation, hæmorrhagic cases—Ars.; Ham.; Led.; Phos.; *Sec.; Thlaspi.*

Inflammation, peri or para metritis—Acon.; *Bell.;* Canth.; Col.; Hep.; *Merc. c.;* Sil.

IRRITABLE uterus (hysteralgia)—Bell.; Caul.; *Cim.;* Ign.; *Lil. t.; Mag. m.;* Murex; Tar. h. See Pain.

MOLES, foreign bodies, promote expulsion—Canth.; Sab.

PAIN—Bruised, broken feeling, of pelvic bones:—*Æsc.;* Arn.; Bellis; Lappa; *Trill.*

Burning—Acon.; *Ars.; Bell.;* Bufo; Calc. ars.; *Canth.;* Carbo an.; Con.; Hep.; Kreos.; Lapis alb.; Murex; Pall.; *Sec.; Tereb.;* Xanth.

Colicky, cramps, labor-like, bearing down—*Agar.;* Apis; Arg. m.; Calad.; Calc. c.; Can. ind.; *Caul.;* Caust.; Cham.; *Cim.; Cocc.; Col.;* Con.; *Cupr.;* Diosc.; Ferr. iod.; Ferr.; *Gels.; Gossyp.;* Hedeoma; *Ign.;* Inula; *Ipec.; Lach.;* Mag. p.; Nat. m.; *Nux v.;* Onosm.; Op.; Plat.; *Puls.; Sab.; Sec.;* Sil.; Thlaspi; Tilia; *Vib. op.;* Xanth. See Labor.

Constricting, squeezing—*Bellis; Cact.;* Cham.; Cinch.; *Gels.; Mag. p.;* Nux v.; Polygon.; *Sep.;* Ustil.

Neuralgic, lancinating, spasmodic, tearing, shooting, cutting, stitching—Acon.; *Agar.;* Apis; *Aran.; Bell.;* Bry.; Bufo; Calc. c.; *Cim.;* Cinch.; *Col.; Con.;* Crot. casc.; Cupr. ars.; *Diosc.;* Ferr.; Graph.; Kali p.; Lach.; *Lil. t.;* Mag. m.; *Mag. p.;* Merc.; *Murex;* Op.; *Plat.;* Puls.; Sec.; Tar. h.; *Vib. op.;* Viscum. See Dysmenorrhœa.

Neuralgic, from back, circumferentially—Plat.; Sep.

Neuralige, from back to abdomen—Sep.; Viscum.

Neuralgic, from back to pubes—Bell.; Sab.

Neuralgic, from back to thighs, legs—Bufo; Carb. ac.; Cham.; *Cim.;* Puls.; *Sab.*

Neuralgic, from hip to hip—*Bell.;* Calc. c.; *Cim.;* Cinch.; *Col.;* Pall.

Neuralgic, from navel to uterus—Ipec.

Neuralgic, radiating to chest—Lach.; Murex; Vespa.

Neuralgic, right side, upward across body, thence to left mamma—Murex.

Pressing, as if viscera would protrude from vagina—*Agar.; Bell.;* Cim.; Cinnam.; Crot.; *Ferr. iod.;* Ferr. m.; *Frax. am.;* Gossyp.; Heliotr.; Kali ferrocy.; *Kreos.; Lac c.; Lil. t.;* Lyc.; Mosch.; *Murex; Nat. c.;* Nat. chlor.; Nat. m.; *Nux v.;* Onosm.; Ova g. pell.; Pall.; *Pod.; Puls.; Sanic.;* Sep.; *Stann.; Sul.; Tilia;* Trill.; Vib. op.; *Xanth.;* Xeroph.

Pressing, heaviness, fullness, dragging in pelvis—Agar.; Alet.; *Aloe;* Ant. c.; *Aur. m. n.; Bell.;* Calc. c.; Calend.; Carb. ac.; *Cim.;* Cinch.;ʹ *Cocc.; Collins.;* Con.; Ferr. br.; Frax. am.; Glycerin; Gnaph.; *Gossyp.; Helon.;* Kali bich.; Lappa; *Lil. t.;* Mag. c.; *Mag. m.;* Merc.; Murex; Nat. c.; Nat. chlor.; *Nux v.; Plat.;* Plumb.; *Pod.;* Polygon.; *Sep.;* Sul.; Trill.; Wyeth.; Zinc. v.

Pressing in back—Agar.; *Bell.;* Carb. ac.; Cham.; *Cim.; Gels.;* Gossyp.; Hedeoma; *Helon.;* Inula; *Kali c.;* Kreos.; Nat. m.; Onosm.; Trill.; Vespa; Vib. op.

Pulsating, throbbing—*Æsc.;* Bell.; *Cact.;* Hep.; Murex.

Splinter-like when walking or riding—Arg. n.

Ulcerative, between anus and perineum, when walking or sitting—Cycl.

HYSOMETRA—Bell.; Bry.; *Brom.;* Lac c.; *Lyc.;* Nux v.; Phos. ac.; Sang.

Soreness, tenderness of uterus—Abies c.; Acon.; *Apis;* Arg. m.; Arn.; *Bell.; Bellis; Bry.; Cim.;* Conv.; *Helon.;* Kreos.; *Lach.;* Lappa; *Lil. t.;* Lyssin; Mag. m.; *Mel c. sale;* Merc.; *Murex;* Plat.; Sanic.; *Sep.; Thlaspi; Tilia.*

TUMORS —Cancer, malignant disease: *Arg. m.; Ars. iod.; Ars.; Aur. m. n.;* Bell.; Bov.; Calc. ars.; Calc. s.; *Caltha; Carbo an.;* Carcinos; Cham.; Cinch.; *Con.; Graph.; Hydr.;* Iod.; Irid.; *Kali bich.;* Kali p.; Kali s.; *Kreos.;* Lach.; *Lapis alb.;* Mag. p.; Med.; Murex; Ova t.; *Phos.;* Phyt.; Rhus t.; *Sec.;* Sep.; *Sil.;* Staph.; Sul.; Tar. c.; Thlaspi; *Thuya;* Trill.; Zinc. m.

Cancer, hæmorrhage—Bell.; Crotal.; Kreos.; Lach.; Sab.; *Thlaspi;* Ustil.

Fibroids, polypi, myo-fibromata—*Aur. iod.; Aur. mur.;* Bell.; *Calc. c.; Calc. iod.;* Calc. p.; *Calend.;* Cinch.; *Con.;* Erod.; Ferr.; *Frax. am.;* Ham.; Hydr.; *Hydrocot.; Iod.;* Ipec.; *Kali iod.; Lach.;* Led.; Lyc.; Merc. c.; *Merc. i. r.; Nit. ac.; Phos.;* Plat.; Plumb.; Puls.; Sabal; *Sab.;* Sang.; Sec.; Sep.; Sil.; Solid.; Staph.; Sul.; *Thlaspi; Thuya; Thyr.;* Trill.

VAGINA—Aphthous patches, ulcers, erosions—Alumen; *Arg. n.;* Carbo v.; *Caul.; Graph.; Helon.; Hydr.;* Ign.; Kreos.; Lyc.; Lyssin; Merc.; Nat. m.; *Nit. ac.;* Rhus t.; Robin.; *Sep.;* Thuya.

Burning, heat—*Acon.;* Alum.; Antipyr.; Aur. mur.; *Bell.; Berb. v.;* Bov.; *Canth.;* Carbo an.; Carbo v.; Ferr. p.; *Hydrocot.;* Kali bich.; Kali c.; *Kreos.;* Lyc.; Lyssin; *Merc. c.;* Merc.; Nat. m.; *Nit. ac.;* Pop. c.; Pulex; *Sep.;* Spiranth.; *Sul.*

Burning, heat, after coitus—Lyc.; Lyssin.

Coldness—Bor. ac.

Cysts—Lyc.; Puls.; *Rhod.;* Sil.

Dryness—Acon.; Apis; *Bell.;* Ferr. p.; *Lyc.;* Lyssin; *Nat. m.;* Spiranth. See Inflammation.

Flatus, emission—*Brom.;* Lac c.; *Lyc.;* Nux m.; Sang.

Inflammation (vaginitis)—Acute:—*Acon.; Apis;* Arn.; Ars.; *Bell.;* Can. s.; *Canth.;* Cim.; Con.; *Crot. t.;* Gels.; *Helon.; Hydr.;* Kali c.; Kali m.; *Kreos.; Merc. c.;* Rhus t.; *Sep.;* Sul.; Thuya.

Inflammation, chronic—Ars.; Bor.; *Calc. c.;* Grind.; Hydr.; Iod.; *Kreos.;* Kali m.; *Merc.;* Nit. ac.; *Puls.; Sep.;* Sul. See Vulvitis.

Itching—Antipyr.; Arundo; Aur. mur.; *Calad.; Canth.; Con.; Helon.;* Hydrocot.; Hydr.; *Kreos.;* Merc.; Scrophul.; *Sep.;* Sil.; *Sul.* See Pruritus Vulvæ.

Pain, pressing—*Bell.;* Calc. c.; Chimaph.; Cinnab.; *Ferr. iod.;* Stann.

Pain, stinging, stitching, shooting, tearing—*Apis;* Cimex; Cim.; Col.; Kreos.; *Rhus t.;* Sab.; Sep.

Pain, throbbing—Bell.

Prolapsus vaginæ—Alum.; *Bell.;* Ferr.; Granat.; Kreos.; Lach.; *Lappa;* Nux m.; Nux v.; Ocimum; *Sep.; Stann.;* Staph.; Sul. ac.

Sensitiveness (vaginismus)—*Acon.;* Aur.; *Bell.; Berb. v.; Cact.; Caul.;* Caust.; Carbo v.; *Cim.; Cocc.; Coff.;* Con.; Ferr. iod.; Ferr. m.; Ferr. p.; *Gels.;* Ham.; *Ign.;* Kreos.; Lac c.; Lyssin; *Mag. p.; Murex;* Mur. ac.; Nit. ac.; Nux v.; Orig.; *Plat.; Plumb.;* Sil.; *Staph.;* Tar. h.; *Thuya.*

VULVA-LABIA—Abscess (vulvo-vaginal): *Apis; Bell.;* Bor.; *Hep.;* Kreos.; Iod.; Lach.; *Merc.;* Puls.; Rhus t.; Sep.; *Sil.;* Sul.

Burning—Acon.; Am. c.; Aur.; Bov.; *Canth.;* Carbo v.; *Graph.;* Helon.;

Kreos.; Lyc.; *Merc.;* Puls.; *Rhus t.;* Sep.; Sil.; *Sul.;* Thuya. See Pain.
Cancer—*Ars.;* Con.; Thuya.
Dryness—*Acon.; Bell.;* Calc. c.; Lyc.; Tar. h. See Vulvitis.
Eczema—Rhus t.
Erysipelas, with edema—*Apis.*
Hair falling out—Merc.; Nit. ac.
Hyperæsthesia, soreness—Acon.; *Bell.; Cim.;* Cocc.; *Coff.;* Ferr. iod.;
Gels.; Hep.; *Ign.;* Kali br.; *Kreos.;* Mag. p.; *Merc.; Murex; Nit. ac.;*
Nux v.; Petrol.; *Plat.; Sep.;* Sul.; *Thuya;* Tilia; Zinc. m.
Inflammation (vulvitis)—*Acon.;* Ambra; *Apis;* Ars.; *Bell.;* Brom.; *Calc.*
c.; Canth.; Carbo v.; Chimaph.; Coccus; Collins; *Cop.;* Eupion; Gos-
syp.; *Graph.;* Ham.; *Helon.; Hydr.; Kreos.;* Lyc.; Mag. p.; *Merc. c.;*
Merc.; Ocimum; Plat.; Puls.; Rhus divers.; *Rhus t.; Sep.;* Sil.; Sul.;
Thuya.
Vulvitis, follicular, herpetic—Ars.; Crot. t.; *Dulc.;* Merc.; Nat. m.; Robin.;
Sep.; Spiranth.; Thuya; *Xerophyl.*
Itching (pruritus)—Agar.; *Ambra;* Apis; *Ars.;* Arundo; Berb. v.; Bov.;
Calad.; Calc. c.; Canth.; Carb. ac.; *Carbo v.;* Caust.; *Coff.; Collins.;*
Con.; Conv.; Cop.; Crot. t.; Dulc.; *Fagop.;* Ferr. iod.; *Graph.;* Grind.;
Guaco; *Helon.;* Hydr ; Kali bich.; Kali br.; Kali c.; *Kreos.;* Lil. t.;
Lyc.; *Merc.;* Mez.; Nat. m.; Nit. ac.; *Orig.;* Petrol.; Picr. ac.; *Plat.;*
Radium; Rhus div.; *Rhus t.;* Rhus v.; Scrophul.; *Sep.;* Spiranth.;
Staph.; *Sul.;* Tar. c.; *Tar. h.;* Thuya; *Urt.;* Xerophyl.; Zinc. m.
Pain—Apis; Ars.; *Bell.; Berb. v.; Calc. c.; Can. s.;* Con.; Ferr.; Kali c.;
Kreos.; Lyc.; Meli.; *Merc. c.; Phos.;* Plat.; Sab.; *Sep.;* Sul. See
Vulvitis.
Papules, pustules—*Carb. ac.;* Graph.; *Sep.;* Sul.
Polypi—Bell.; Calc. c.; *Phos.;* Teucr.; *Thuya.*
Sensation, as if wet—Eup. purp.; Petrol.
Soreness, tenderness—*Acon.;* Ambra; *Bell.;* Caust.; Conv.; *Graph.;*
Helon.; Hep.; *Kreos.;* Ova g. pell.; *Plat.; Sep.;* Sul.; Tar. h.; Urt.
Soreness, with ulcers—Arg. n.; *Hep.;* Merc.; *Nit. ac.;* Thuya.
Sweat, offensive—*Calc. c.;* Fagop.; Lyc.; *Merc.;* Petrol.; *Sul.;* Thuya.
Ulcers—*Ars.; Aur. m. n.;* Graph.; Mur. ac.; *Nit. ac.;* Sep.; Syph.
Varices—Calc. c.; Carbo v.; Lyc.
Warts—Aur. mur.; Med.; *Thuya.*

CIRCULATORY SYSTEM

ARTERIES—AORTA—Inflamed, acute (aortitis): Acon.; Apis; Glon.; Tub.

Aorta, inflamed, chronically (aortitis chronica)—Adon. v.; *Adren.; Ant. ars.; Ars. iod.;* Aur. ars.; Aur.; *Cact.;* Chin. s.; Crat.; Cupr.; Glon.; Kali iod.; Lyc.; *Nat. iod.;* Spig.; Stroph.

Aortitis, ulcerative—Acon.; Ars.; Chin. s.

Aorta, pain—Adren.; Strych. See Angina Pectoris.

Arteritis—Ars.; Carbo v.; Echin.; *Kali iod.;* Lach.; *Nat. iod.;* Sec.

Atheroma of arteries (arterio-sclerosis)—Adren.; *Am. iod.;* Am. vanad.; Ant. ars.; Arn.; Ars.; *Ars. iod.; Aur. iod.;* Aur.; Aur. m. n.; *Bar. c.;* Bar. m.; Cact.; Calc. fl.; Chin. s.; Con.; Crat.; Ergotin; *Glon.;* Iodothyr.; *Kali iod.;* Kali sal.; Lach.; Lith. c.; *Nat. iod.;* Phos.; *Plumb. iod.;* Plumb. m.; *Polygon. av.;* Sec.; Stront. c.; *Stront. iod.;* Stroph.; Sumb.; *Vanad.* See Interstitial Nephritis.

Carotids, pulsate—*Acon.;* Amyl; *Bell.; Cact.;* Cinch.; Fagop.; *Glon.;* Lil. t.; Sab.; *Ver. v.* See Pulse.

Circulation, sluggish—Æth.; Calc. c.; *Calc. p.;* Carbo an.; *Carbo v.;* Cim.; Cinnam.; Ferr. p.; *Gels.;* Led.; Nat. m.; *Rhus t.;* Sil. See Heart.

Congestion of blood (local)—*Acon.;* Æsc.; Ambra; *Amyl;* Aur.; *Bell.; Cact.;* Calc. c.; Centaur.; Cupr. m.; Ferr. m.; *Ferr. p.;* Gadus mor.; *Glon.;* Kali iod.; Lil. t.; Lonic.; *Meli.;* Millef.; Phos.; *Sang.; Sep.;* Sil.; Spong.; Stellar.; *Sul.; Ver. v.*

Degeneration, fatty—Phos. See Heart.

Dilatation-Aneurism—Acon.; Ars. iod.; *Bar. c.; Bar. m.;* Cact.; Calc. fl.; Calc. p.; Glon.; Iod.; *Kali iod.;* Kal.; Lach.; Lith. c.; *Lyc.;* Lycop.; Morph.; *Nat. iod.;* Plumb.; Puls.; Spig.; Spong.; *Ver. v.*

Aneurism, capillary—*Calc. fl.;* Fluor. ac.; Tub.

Aneurism, pain—Cact. See Angina Pectoris.

RUPTURE of artery (apoplexy)—*Acon.;* Apis; Arn.; Aster.; Bar. c.; *Bell.;* Cact.; Camph.; Caust.; Chenop.; Cinch.; Croc.; Crotal.; Cupr. m.; Formica; *Glon.;* Hydroc. ac.; Hyos.; Junip. v.; Kali br.; Kali iod.; *Lach.; Laur.; Nux v.; Op.; Phos.;* Sep.; Stram.; Sul.; Ver. a.; *Ver. v.*

Rupture of artery; post-hemiplegia—Arn.; Ars.; *Bar. c.;* Bell.; Bothrops.; *Caust.; Cocc.;* Cupr. m.; Cur.; Lach.; Nux v.; Phos.; *Plumb.;* Rhus t.; Vipera; Zinc. m.

Rupture of artery: predisposition to, or threatened—*Acon.;* Arn.; Ars.; Bar. c.; *Bell.;* Calc. fl.; *Gels.; Glon.;* Guaco; Hyos.; *Lach.;* Laur.; *Nux v.; Op.; Phos.;* Stront. c.

HEART—Action tumultuous, violent, labored: Abies c.; Absinth.; *Acon.;* Æsc.; *Agar.;* Ammon.; *Amyl;* Ars.; *Aur.; Bell.;* Bry.; *Cact.;* Carb. ac.; Cim.; Colch.; Conv.; Ephedra; Gels.; *Glon.;* Helod.; Iberis; Kal.; *Lil. t.; Lycop.; Nat. m.;* Physost.; Prun. sp.; Pyr.; *Spig.;* Spong.; *Ver. v.* See Pulse.

AFFECTIONS in general—*Acon.; Adon. v.;* Am. c.; Am. m.; *Amyl;* Apoc.; Arn.; *Ars. iod.; Ars.;* Aur. m.; Aur. mur.; Bar. c.; Bell.; Benz. ac.;

Bry.; Cact.; Calc. ars.; Calc. fl.; Carbo v.; Cim.; Cinch.; Coca; Colch.;
Collins.; Conv.; Coronilla; *Crat.; Crot.; Digitaline; Dig.;* Ferr. m.;
Fer. p.; Gels.; *Glon.;* Grind.; *Hydroc. ac.; Iberis;* Ign.; Iod.; Kali c.;
Kali chlor.; *Kal.; Lach.;* Laur.; Lepid.; *Lil. t.;* Lith. c.; *Lycop.;* Merc.
c.; Mosch.; *Naja;* Nat. iod.; Nat. m.; Nux v.; *Ox. ac.; Phaseol.; Phos.;*
Piloc.; Scilla; *Spart.; Spig.; Spong.; Stroph.; Strych.;* Sumb.; Thyr.;
Val.; Ver. v.   See Separate Diseases of Heart.

Affections, rheumatic—Acon.; Aur.; Benz. ac.; *Bry.;* Cact.; Caust.;
Cim.; *Colch.;* Ign.; *Kal.;* Led.; Lith. c.; Lycop.; Naja; Phyt.; *Rhus
t.; Spig.;* Ver. v.

Affections, with hæmorrhoids—Cact.; *Collins.;* Dig.

CYANOSIS—Acetan.; Am. c.; *Ant. ars.; Ant. t.; Ars.;* Benz. nit.; Carbo
an.; *Carbo v.;* Crot.; Cupr.; *Dig.;* Hydroc. ac.; Lach.; *Laur.;* Lycop.;
Merc. cy.; Nat. nit.; Phos.; Piloc.; Psor.; *Rhus t.;* Samb.; Tab.; Zinc.
m.

DEBILITY, weakness—Acetan.; Acet. ac.; *Adon. v.;* Adren.; Am. c.; *Am.
m.;* Ant. ars.; *Ars.; Ars. iod.;* Aur.; *Cact.; Calc. ars.;* Camph.; Carb.
ac.; *Carbo v.;* Chin. ars.; Cinch.; *Conv.; Crat.; Dig.;* Diosc.; Eel
serum; Euphorbia; Ferr.; Grind.; Helod.; *Hydroc. ac.; Iberis;* Kali
c.; Kal.; Lach.; Lil. t.; Lycop.; Morph.; Mosch.; Nerium; Nit. ac.;
Nux m.; Phaseol.; Plumb.; Prun. sp.; Psor.; Pyr.; Sarcol. ac.; Scilla;
Spart.; Spig.; *Stroph.;* Tab.; Thyr.; *Ver. a.*

Debility, weakness, muscular, "heart failure"—Adon. v.; Adren.; Agaricin;
Alcohol; Amyl; Ant. t.; Atrop.; *Caffeine;* Camphorated oil; Cocaine;
Conv.; Crat.; *Digitaline; Dig.;* Ether; *Glon.;* Oxygen inhalation; Sac-
char. of.; Saline infusion; Serum ang.; Spart.; Stroph.; *Strych. s.;* Ver. a.

Debility, weakness, nervous—Adren.; Cact.; *Iberis;* Ign.; *Lil. t.;* Lith.
c.; *Mosch.; Naja;* Piloc.; Prun. v.; Spart.; *Spig.;* Tab.; *Val.*

Debility, weakness, with dropsy—*Acetan.; Adon. v.; Apoc.;* Ars. iod.; *Ars.;*
Asclep. syr.; Cact.; *Caffeine;* Collins.; *Conv.; Dig.;* Iberis; Lach.;
Lycop.; Oleand.; Scilla; Spart.; *Stroph.* See Generalities.

DEGENERATION, fatty—Adon. æst.; Adon. v.; Arn.; Ars. iod.; *Ars.;
Aur.; Bar. c.;* Cim.; Crat.; Cupr. ac.; Fucus; *Kali c.;* Kali feroc.; Kal.;
Phos. ac.; *Phos.;* Physost.; *Phyt.;* Sacchar. of.; Stroph.; Strych. ars.;
Strych. p.; *Vanad.*

DILATATION—Adon. v.; Am. c.; Ars. iod.; *Ars.; Bar. c.; Cact.;* Cim.;
Conv.; *Crat.; Dig.;* Gels.; Iberis; *Naja; Phaseol.;* Phos.; Physost.;
Prun. sp.; Spart. s.; *Spig.;* Stroph.; Tab.; Ver. v. See Debility, muscu-
lar.

DYSPNOEA (cardiac)—*Acon. fer.;* Acon.; Adon. v.; *Adren.;* Am. c.; Apis;
Arn.; Ars.; Ars. iod.; Aur. m.; *Cact.; Calc. ars.;* Carbo v.; *Chin. ars.;*
Cim.; Collins.; Conv.; *Dig.; Glon.; Iberis;* Kali n.; Kal.; Lach.; Laur.;
Lycop.; Magnol.; Naja; Ox. ac.; Op.; *Quebracho;* Spig.; Spong.; Stroph.;
Strych. ars.; Sumb.; Viscum. See Respiratory System.

Hydropericardium—Apis; Apoc.; Ant. ars.; Ars.; Iod.; Lach.

HYPERTROPHY—*Acon.; Arn.;* Ars.; Aur.; Bell.; *Brom.; Cact.;* Caffeine;
Caust.; Cereus; *Conv.; Crat.; Dig.;* Glon.; *Iberis;* Iod.; Kal.; Lil. t.;

Lycop.; *Naja;* Phos.; Phyt.; *Rhus t.;* Spig.; *Spong.;* Stroph.; Stryeh. ars.; *Ver. v.;* Viscum.

Hypertrophy uncomplicated, of athletes—Arn.; Brom.; Caust.; *Rhus t.*

Inflammation (ENDOCARDITIS)—Acute: *Acon.;* Ars.; Bell.; *Cact.; Colch.;* Conv.; Dig.; *Lach.;* Magnol.; *Naja;* Phos.; *Spig.;* Spong.; Tab.; Ver. v. See Pericarditis.

Endocarditis, malignant—Acon.; Ars.; *Chin. s.;* Crot.; Lach.; Vipera.

Endocarditis, rheumatic—Acon.; Adon. v.; Bell.; *Bry.; Colch.;* Kali c.; Kal.; Rhus t.; *Spig.*

MYOCARDITIS—Acon.; Adon. v.; *Ars. iod.;* Aur. mur.; Cact.; Chin. ars.; Crat.; *Dig.;* Galanth.; Iod.; Lach.; Phos.; Stroph.; *Vipera.* See Weakness, Degeneration.

PERICARDITIS, acute—*Acon.;* Adon. v.; Ant. ars.; *Apis; Ars.;* Asclep. t.; Bell.; *Bry.;* Cact.; Can. s.; *Canth.; Colch.;* Dig.; Iod.; Kali c.; *Kali iod.;* Kal.; Magnol.; Merc. c.; *Merc.;* Naja; Nat. m.; Phaseol.; Scilla; *Spig.; Spong.;* Sul.; Ver. a.; Ver. v.

Pericarditis, chronic—Apis; *Aur. iod.;* Calc. fl.; Kali c.; Scilla; Spig.; Sul.

Pericarditis, rheumatic—Acon.; Anac.; Bry.; *Colchicine;* Colch.; Crat.; Kal.; Rhus t.; *Spig.*

NEUROSES—*Acon.;* Adren.; Cact.; Cham.; Cinch.; *Coff.;* Ferr.; *Gels.; Iber.; Ign.;* Lach.; *Lil. t.;* Lycop.; *Mosch.; Nux v.;* Prun. v.; Scutel.; Sep.; *Spig.; Tab.;* Ver. a.; Zinc. m.

Neuroses, irritable from influenza—Iberis; Spart. s.

Neuroses, irritable from tea, coffee—Agaricine.

Neuroses, irritable from tobacco—*Agaricine;* Agn.; Ars.; Calad.; *Conv.;* Dig.; *Kal.;* Lycop.; Nux v.; *Phos.; Spig.;* Staph.; *Stroph.;* Tab.; Ver. a.

Neuroses, irritable from suppressed hæmorrhoids—Collins.

Neuroses, irritable from utero-ovarian disease—Cim.; Lil. t.

Neuroses, irritable tremulousness, from scarlet fever—Lach.

PAIN—Abies n.; *Acon.; Adon. v.; Amyl;* Apis; Arn.; *Ars.;* Aster.; *Bry.; Cact.;* Calc. fl.; Canth.; Cereus; Cereus serp.; *Cim.;* Coff.; *Colch.;* Conv.; Crat.; Daphne; *Dig.;* Diosc.; *Ferr. tart.; Hematox.; Hydroc. ac.;* Iberis; *Kal.;* Lach.; *Latrod.;* Lepid.; *Lil. t.; Lith. c.;* Lob. infl.; Lycop.; Magnol.; Med.; *Naja;* Onosm.; *Ox. ac.;* Ov. g. p.; *Pæonia;* Pip. nig.; Ptel.; *Spig.; Spong.; Stroph.;* Syph.; Tab.; *Ther.;* Thyr.; *Ver. v.;* Zinc. v.

Pain at apex—Lil. t.

Pain at base—Lob. infl.

Pain constricting, as if squeezed in vise—*Acon.;* Adon. v.; Amyl; Arn.; Ars.; *Cact.;* Cadm. s.; Calc. ars.; Coccus; Colch.; Iodof.; *Iod.;* Kali c.; Lach.; Laur.; *Lil. t.;* Lycop.; Mag. p.; Magnol.; Nux m.; Ptel.; Spong.; *Thyr.*

Neuralgic—ANGINA PECTORIS—*Acon.;* Adren.; *Amyl;* Arg. cy.; Arg. n.; *Arn.;* Ars. iod.; *Ars.;* Aur. mur.; Bism.; *Cact.;* Camph.; Cereus; Chin. ars.; *Cim.; Cocaine;* Conv.; *Crat.;* Crot.; *Cupr. ac.; Cupr. m.;* Dig.; Diosc.; *Glon.; Hematox.; Hydroc. ac.;* Kali c.; Kali iod.; Kal.; *Latrod.;* Lil. t.; Lith. c.; Lob. infl.; *Mag. p.;* Magnol.; Morph.; *Naja;*

Nat. iod.; Nat. nit.; *Nux v.;* Oleand.; *Ox. ac.;* Phos.; Phyt.; Pip. nig.; Prun. sp.; Samb.; Spart.; *Spig.; Spong.;* Staph.; Stront. c.; Stront. iod.; *Tab.;* Thyr.; Ver. v.; Zinc. v.

From abuse of coffee—Coff.

From abuse of stimulants—Nux v.; Spig.

From muscular origin—Cupr.; Hydroc. ac.

From organic heart disease—*Ars. iod.; Cact.;* Calc. fl.; Crat.; Kal.; Nat. iod.; Stront. iod.; Tab.

From rheumatism—Cim.; Lith. c.

From straining, overlifting—*Arn.;* Carbo an.; Caust.

From tobacco—Kal.; Lil. t.; Nux v.; Spig.; Staph.; Tab.

Pseudo-angina pectoris—Aconitine; Cact.; *Lil. t.; Mosch.;* Nux v.; Tar. h. See Pain.

Præcordial oppression, anxiety, heaviness—*Acon.; Adon. v.; Adren.;* Æsc.; Agar.; Am. c.; Amyl; Apis; *Ars.; Ars. iod.;* Aspar.; Aur.; Brom.; Bry.; *Cact.;* Calc. ars.; Calc. c.; *Camph.;* Carbo v.; Cereus; Cim.; *Colch.;* Collins.; Cotyled.; *Crat.;* Cupr.; *Dig.;* Diosc.; Ferr.; Glon.; Hematox.; *Hydroc. ac.; Iberis;* Ign.; *Iod.;* Ipec.; Kal.; *Lach.; Latrod.;* Laur.; *Lil. t.;* Lith. c.; *Lycop.;* Magnol.; Menyanth.; *Naja;* Nat. ars.; Primula v.; *Puls.;* Sapon.; *Spig.; Spong.;* Tab.; *Thea;* Thyr.; Vanad.; Ver. v.

Shooting, down left shoulder, arm to fingers—*Acon.;* Arn.; Asper.; Bism.; *Cact.;* Cim.; Crot.; *Kal.; Latrod.;* Lepid.; Naja; *Ox. ac.; Rhus t.; Spig.;* Tab.

Shooting, from apex to base—Med.

Shooting, from base to apex at night—Syph.

Shooting from back to clavicle, shoulder—Spig.

Shooting, lancinating, tearing—Ars.; Bell.; *Cact.;* Cereus; Cim.; Colch.; Daphne; Glon.; *Iberis; Kal.; Latrod.;* Lil. t.; Lith. c.; Magnol.; Menthol; *Ox. ac.;* Pæonia; Phyt.; *Spig.;* Syph.; Tab. See Neuralgia.

Stitching, cutting—Abies n.; *Acon.;* Anac.; Ars.; Asclep. t.; *Bry.; Cact.;* Can. ind.; Caust.; Cereus; Dig.; Iberis; *Kali c.;* Kali n.; Lith. c.; Naja; *Spig.*

PALPITATION—*Abies c.; Acon.; Adon. v.; Agar.;* Agaricine; Amyl; Apis; *Arg. n.; Ars.;* Asaf.; *Aur. m.;* Aur. mur.; Bar. c.; *Bell.; Cact.; Calc. ars.;* Calc. c.; Camph.; Canth.; Can. ind.; Carbo v.; Chin. ars.; *Cim.;* Cinch.; *Coca; Cocc.; Coff.;* Colch.; Con.; *Conv.;* Crat.; Cupr.; Digitaline; *Dig.;* Fagop.; Ferrum; Ferr. p.; *Gels.; Glon.;* Hydr.; *Hydroc. ac.; Iberis; Ign.; Iod.; Kali c.;* Kali ferr. cy.; *Kal.; Lach.;* Laur.; *Lil. t.;* Lob. infl.; *Lycop.; Mosch.;* Naja; *Nat. m.;* Nerium; Nux m.; *Nux v.;* Oleand.; Ol. j. as.; Ox. ac.; *Phaseol.;* Phos. ac.; *Phos.;* Plat.; *Puls.; Pyr.;* Sec.; Sep.; *Spig.; Spong.; Sul.; Sumb.; Tab.;* Thea; Thyr.; Val.; Ver. v.; Zinc.

CAUSE—**Anæmia, vital drains:** Ars.; *Cinch.;* Dig.; *Ferr. red.;* Kali c.; Kali ferrocy.; Nat. m.; *Phos. ac.;* Phos.; *Puls.;* Spig.; Ver. a.

Children, growing too fast—Phos. ac.

Dyspepsia—Abies c.; *Abies n.;* Arg. n.; Cact.; *Carbo v.; Cinch.;* Coca;

Coff.; Collins.; Diosc.; Hydroc. ac.; Lyc.; *Nux v.; Puls.;* Prun. v.; Sep.; Spig.; Tab.

Emotional causes—*Acon.;* Ambra; Am. val.; Anac.; Cact.; *Calc. ars.;* Cham.; *Coff.;* Gels.; Hydroc. ac.; *Ign.;* Iod.; Lach.; Lith. c.; *Mosch.;* Nux m.; Nux v.; Op.; Plat.; Sep.; Tar. h.

Eruption suppressed—Calc. c.

Exertion, even slightest—Bell.; Brom.; Cim.; Coca; Conv.; *Dig.; Iberis; Iod.;* Nat. m.; Sarcol. ac.; *Thyr.*

Grief—*Ign.;* Phos. ac.

Heart-strain—*Arn.;* Bor.; *Caust.;* Coca.

Nervous irritation—Atrop.; Cact.; *Coff.; Glon.;* Hydroc. ac.; Hyos.; Ign., Kali c.; Kali p.; Lil. t.; *Lycop.;* Mag. p.; *Mosch.; Naja;* Sep.; Spig.; *Sumb.*

Prolonged brain work, sexual excesses—Coca.

Tea drinking—Cinch.

Tobacco—Agar.; Ars.; Cact.; *Gels.;* Nux v.; Stroph.

Uterine disease—Conv.; Lil. t.

Worms—Spig.

CONCOMITANTS—**With anguish, restlessness:** *Acon.;* Æth.; Ars.; Calc. c.; Coff.; Ign.; Lach.; Nat. m.; Phaseol.; *Phos.; Puls.;* Sapon.; Spig.; *Spong.;* Ver. a.; Zinc. m.

With burning at heart—Kali c.

With choking in throat—Iberis; Lach.; Naja.

With dim vision—Puls.

With dyspnœa—Am. c.; *Cact.;* Dig.; *Glon.;* Glycerin; Lach.; Oleand.; Naja; Ox. ac.; *Phos.;* Spig.; *Spong.;* Ver. a.; Zinc. m.

With face red—Agar.; Aur.; Bell.; Glon.

With fainting—Acon.; *Cham.; Lach.;* Nat. m.; *Nux m.;* Petrol.; *Tab.*

With fetor oris—Spig.

With flatulence—*Arg. n.;* Cact.; Carbo v.; *Nux v.*

With headache—Æth.; Bell.; Lith. c.

With heart-labored, reverberates in head—Aur.; Bell.; *Glon.;* Spig.; Spong.

With heart weak—Coca; Dig.

With hot feeling, uncomfortable—Ant. t.; Calc. c.; Kali c.; Petrol.

With pain, præcordial—*Acon.;* Ars.; *Cact.;* Cham.; Caust.; *Coff.;* Hydroc. ac.; Laur.; Mag. m.; Naja; *Spig.;* Spong.

With piles or suppressed menses alternating—Collins.

With sleeplessness—Cim.; Coca; *Ign.;* Spig.

With stomach, heavy feeling in—Upas.

With stomach, sinking in—Cim.

With tinnitus, mental depression, anorexia, chest oppression—Coca.

With trembling—Asaf.; Lach.; Rhus t.; *Sul. ac.*

With urination copious—Coff.

With uterine soreness—Conv.

With vertigo—Adon. v.; Æth.; Cact.; Coronilla; *Iberis;* Spig.

With weakness, empty feeling in chest—Oleand.

AGGRAVATION—**After eating:** Calc. c.; Lil. t.; Lyc.; Nat. m.; *Nux v.,* Puls.

At approach of menses—*Cact.;* Crot.; Spong.

At night—*Ars.;* Cact.; Calc. c.; Iberis; Ign.; Lil. t.; Lyc.; Nat. m.; Phos.; Tab.

During sleep—Alston.; Am. c.; *Can. ind.;* Iberis; Phos. ac.; Spong.

From least motion—Acon.; Bell.; *Cact.; Calc. ars.;* Cim.; *Dig.;* Ferr.; Iberis; *Lil. t.;* Nat. m.; *Spig.*

From lying down—*Ars.;* Kali c.; Lach.; Lil. t.; Nat. m.; Nux v.; Sep.; Spig.; Thyr.

From lying on left side—Bar. c.; *Cact.;* Lac c.; *Lach.;* Lyc.; Nat. m.; *Phos.;* Puls.; *Tab.;* Thea.

From lying on right side—*Alumen;* Arg. n.

From mental exertion—Calc. ars.

From rising—Cact.

From sitting—Mag. m.; Phos.; Rhus t.

From sitting bent forward—Kal.

From stooping forward—Spig.

From thinking of it—Bar. c.; Gels.; *Ox. ac.*

In morning on waking—Kali c.; Nux v.

AMELIORATION—**Lying on right side:** Lac c.; Tab.

Motion—Ferr. m.; Gels.; *Mag. m.*

PULSE—**Full, round, bounding, strong, felt all over:** *Acon.;* Æsc.; Am. m.; *Amyl;* Antipyr.; Arn.; *Aur.;* Bar. c.; *Bell.;* Bry.; *Cact.;* Calc. c.; Canth.; Coff.; Cupr.; Fagop.; Ferr. m.; *Glon.; Iod.; Lil. t.;* Lycop.; Onosm.; *Op.; Physost.;* Piloc.; Poth.; Puls.; *Sab.;* Spig.; Spong.; *Ver. v.*

Intermittent—Acon.; *Apoc.;* Bapt.; *Cact.; Carbo v.;* Cinch.; Colch.; Conv.; *Crat.; Dig.;* Ferr. mur.; *Iberis;* Ign.; *Kali c.;* Kal.; Lil. t.; *Lycop.;* Merc. c.; Merc. cy.; *Nat. m.;* Nux m.; Phos. ac.; Pip. nig.; Rhus t.; Sec.; *Sep.; Spig.; Stroph.;* Tab.; Tereb.; Thea; Ver. a.; *Ver. v.;* Zinc. m.

Intermittent, every third to seventh beat—Dig.; *Mur. ac.*

Iregular—Acetan.; Acon.; Adon. v.; Adren.; *Agaricine;* Antipyr.; Apoc.; Arn.; *Ars.; Ars. iod.; Aur.;* Bell.; *Cact.;* Caffeine; Camph.; Cim.; *Cinch.; Conv.; Crat.; Dig.;* Eel serum; Ferr. m.; Gels.; *Glon.; Hydroc. ac.; Iberis;* Ign.; Kali c.; Kal.; *Lach.;* Laur.; *Lil. t.; Lycop.;* Mur. ac.; *Naja; Nat. m.;* Nux m.; *Phaseol.; Phos. ac.;* Pi.oc.; Puls.; Rhus t.; Sang.; Sec.; Serum an.;.; *Spart.; Spig.;* Stroph.; Strych. ars.; Strych. p.; Sumb.; *Tab.;* Thea; Ver. a.; *Ver. v.;* Zinc. m.

Rapid (tachycardia)—*Abies n.; Acon.;* Adon. v.; Adren.; *Agn.;* Am. val.; Ant. ars.; Ant. c.; *Ant. t.;* Antipyr.; Apoc.; Arn.; Ars. iod.; *Bell.;* Bry.; *Cact.;* Canth.; Carbo v.; Coff;. Colch.; Collins.; *Conv.; Crat.; Dig.;* Diph.; Eel serum; Ferr. p.; *Gels.;* Glon.; *Iberis;* Kal.; Kali chlor.; Lach.; Latrod.; Led.; *Lil. t.; Lycop.;* Merc. c.; *Morph.;* Mur. ac.; *Naja;* Nat. m.; Phaseol.; *Phos.;* Phyt.; Piloc.;ʲPyr.; Rhod.; Rhus t.; Sec.; Sep.; Spong.; Stroph.; Strych. p.; Tab.; Tereb.; Thea; *Thyr.;* Ver. a.; Ver. v. See Weak.

Rapid in morning—Ars.; Sul.

Rapid, out of all proportion to temperature—Lil. t.; *Pyr.*

Slow (brachycardia)—*Abies n.;* Adon. v.; Adren.; *Æsc.; Apoc.;* Cact.; *Camph.; Can. ind.;* Canth.; Caust.; Colch.; Cupr.; *Dig.;* Eserine; *Gels.;* Helod.; Helleb.; *Kal.;* Latrod.; *Lupul.;* Lycopers.; *Morph.;* Myr.; Naja; *Op.;* Pip. nig.; Rhus t.; Spig.; Tab.; Ver. a.; *Ver. v.* See Weak.

Slow, alternating with rapid—Cinch.; Dig.; *Gels.;* Iod.; Morph.

Soft, compressible—Acal.; *Ars.;* Bapt.; *Caffeine;* Conv.; Ferr. m.; *Ferr. p.; Gels.;* Kali c.; *Phos.;* Plumb.; Ver. a.; *Ver. v.* See Weak.

Weak, fluttering, almost imperceptible—Acetan.; *Acon.; Adon. v.;* Adren.; Æth.; *Agaricine;* Ail.; Am. m.; Ant. ars.; Ant. t.; Apis; Arn.; *Ars.; Ars. iod.; Aur.;* Aspar.; Bar. m.; *Cact.; Caffeine; Camph.;* Carb. ac.; Carbo v.; Cim.; Colch.; Collins.; *Conv.; Crat.;* Crot.; *Dig.;* Diph.; Eel serum; *Ferr. m.; Gels.; Hydroc. ac.;* Hysocin. hydrobr.; Iod.; *Kali c.;* Kali chlor.; *Kali n.;* Kal.; *Lach.;* Latrod.; *Laur.;* Lycop.; Merc. c.; *Merc. cy.;* Morph.; *Mur. ac.;* Naja; Op.; Ox. ac.; *Phaseol.; Phos. ac.; Phos.;* Physost.; Plumb.; Pyr.; Rhus t.; Sang.; *Sapon.;* Sec.; *Spart.; Spig.;* Sul.; *Tab.;* Tereb.; *Thyr.; Ver. a.; Ver. v.;* Viscum; Zinc. m.

SENSATIONS—**As if drops were falling from heart:** Can. s.

As if heart were burning—Kali c.; Op.; Tar. h.

As if heart were ceasing its beat—Antipyr.; Chin. ars.; Cim.; Crat.; *Dig.;* Lob. infl.; *Phaseol.;* Trifol.

As if heart were ceasing its beat, then started suddenly—*Aur.;* Conv.; Lil. t.; Sep.

As if heart were ceasing its beat when moving about, must keep still—Cocaine; *Dig.*

As if heart were ceasing its beat when resting, must move about—Gels.; Trifol.

As if heart were cold—Calc. c.; *Carbo an.;* Graph.; *Helod.;* Kali bich.; *Kali m.;* Kali n.; Lil. t.; *Nat. m.;* Petrol.

As if heart were fluttering—Absinth.; *Acon.;* Amyl; Apoc.; Asaf.; *Cact.; Cim.;* Conv.; Crot.; Ferr.; Glon.; *Iberis; Kal.;* Lach.; *Lil. t.;* Lith. c.; *Mosch.;* Naja; *Nat. m.;* Nux m.; *Phaseol.;* Phos. ac.; *Physost.;* Pyr.; *Spig.;* Sul. ac.; Thea. See Palpitation.

As if heart were purring—Pyr.; Spig.

As if heart were squeezed by iron hand—Arn.; *Cact.;* Iod.; *Lil. t.;* Sul.; Vanad.; Viscum.

As if heart were suspended by thread—Kali c.; Lach.

As if heart were too full, bursting—*Æsc.;* Amyl; Aur. m.; *Bell.;* Bufo; *Cact.;* Cenchris; Collins.; Conv.; *Glon.;* Glycerin; Iberis; Lact.; *Lil. t.;* Pyr.; *Spig.;* Stroph.; *Sul.;* Vanad.

As if heart were tired—Pyr.

As if heart were twisted—*Lach.;* Tar. h.

Soreness, tenderness of heart—Arn.; *Cact.;* Camph.; Gels.; Hematox.; Lith. c.; Lycop.; *Naja;* Sec.; *Spig.*

SYNCOPE—(fainting): Acetan.; Acet. ac.; *Acon.;* Alet.; Amyl; Apis; *Ars.;* Cact.; *Canth.;* Carbo v.; Cham.; Cim.; *Cinch.;* Collins.; Croc.; Cupr.; *Dig.;* Ferr.; Glon.; *Ign.;* Ipec.; Lach.; Lil. t.; *Linar.;* Mag. m.; Magnol.; *Mosch.; Nux m.;* Nux v.; Op.; Phaseol.; Phos. ac.; Phos.; Puls.;

Sep.; *Spig.;* Spong.; *Sul.; Sumb.;* Tab.; Thyr.; *Trill.; Ver. a.;* Zinc.
Syncope from odors, in morning, after eating—Nux v.
Syncope, lipothymia, hysterical—*Acon.;* Apium v.; Asaf.; Cham.; Cocc.;
Cupr.; *Ign.;* Lach.; *Mosch.;* Nux m.

VALVULAR DISEASE—Acon.; *Adon. v.;* Apoc.; *Ars.; Ars. iod.;* Aur. br.;
Aur. iod.; Aur. m.; *Cact.;* Calc. fl.; Camph.; *Conv.; Crat.; Dig.;* Ferr.;
Galanth.; *Glon.;* Iod.; Kal.; Lach.; Laur.; Lith. c.; *Lycop.; Naja;*
Ox. ac.; Phos.; Plumb.; Rhus t.; Sang.; Serum ang.; *Spig.; Spong.;*
Stigm.; *Stroph.;* Thyr.; Viscum.

VEINS—**Engorged, distended (plethora):** Adon. v.; *Æsc.; Aloe;* Arn.; Ars.;
Aur.; Bellis; Calc. c.; Calc. hypoph.; Camph.; *Carbo an.; Carbo v.;*
Chin. s.; *Collins.;* Conv.; *Dig.;* Fluor. ac.; *Ham.;* Lept.; Lyc.; *Nux*
v.; Op.; Plumb.; *Pod.; Puls.; Sep.;* Spong.; Stellar.; *Sul.;* Verb.
Veins engorged (pelvic)—*Aloe;* Collins.; *Sep.;* Sul.
Veins engorged (portal)—*Æsc.; Aloe; Collins.;* Lept.; Lyc.; *Nux v.;*
Sul.
Veins inflamed (phlebitis)—Acon.; Agar.; *Apis;* Arn.; *Ars.;* Bell.; Crot.;
Ham.; Kali c.; *Lach.;* Lyc.; Merc.; Phos.; *Puls.;* Stront. c.; Vipera.
Veins inflamed, chronic—Arn.; Merc.; *Puls.;* Ruta.
Veins varicosed—Acet. ac.; *Æsc.;* Alumen; Apis; Ars.; Bellis; Calc. c.;
Calc. fl.; Calc. iod.; Carbo v.; *Card. m.;* Caust.; Collins.; Ferr. p.; *Fluor.*
ac.; Graph.; *Ham.;* Kali ars.; Lach.; *Lyc.;* Magnif.; Mur. ac.; Nat.
m.; Pæonia; Plumb.; Polyg.; *Puls.;* Ran. s.; Ruta; Scirrhin; Sep.;
Staph.; Stront. c.; Sul.; Sul. ac.; *Vipera; Zinc. m.*

LOCOMOTOR SYSTEM

AXILLAE—Abscess: *Hep.;* Irid.; Jugl. r.

Acne—Carbo v.

Eczema—Elaps; Nat. m.

Herpes—Carbo an.

Pain, in muscles, right side—Prim. v.

Pain, with, or without swelling—Jugl. c.

Sweat, profuse, offensive—Bov.; *Calc. c.;* Hep.; *Kali c.;* Lyc.; *Nit. ac.;* Osm.; Petrol.; Sep.; Sil.; *Strych. p.;* Sul.; *Tellur.;* Thuya.

BACK—Bent, arch-like, opisthotonos: Angust.; *Cic.;* Nat. s.; *Nicot.;* Op.; Phyt.; *Strych.* See Convulsions (Nervous System.)

Burning between scapulæ—Glon.; *Lyc.;* Phos.; Sul.

Burning—*Alum.;* Ars.; Aur. mur.; Berb. v.; Calc. fl.; Carbo an.; Helod.; *Helon.;* Kali p.; Lyc.; Med.; Nit. ac.; *Phos.;* Picr. ac.; Sep.; Tereb.; Ustil.; Xerophyl.

Burning in small spots—Agar.; *Phos.;* Ran. b.; Sul.

Coldness between scapulæ—*Abies c.;* Am. m.; Helod.; *Lachnanth.;* Sep.

Coldness—*Abies c.;* Acon.; Ars.; Benz. ac.; *Gels.;* Gins.; Quass.; Raph.; Sep.; *Strych.;* Ver. a.

Curvature (scoliosis)—Bar. c.; *Calc. c.;* Phos. ac.; Phos.; *Sil.;* Sul.

Eruption—Sep.

Lameness, stiffness—Abrot.; Acon.; Æsc.; Agar.; Am. m.; Bell.; *Berb. v.;* Bry.; Calc. c.; Camph. monobr.; *Caust.;* Cim.; *Cupr. ars.;* Diosc.; Dulc.; Gettysburg Water; Gins.; *Helon.;* Hyper.; Kali c.; Kali p.; Kal.; Lachnanth.; Led.; Lyc.; Nicot.; Physost.; *Phyt.;* Rhus t.; Ruta; Sarcol. ac.; *Sep.;* Spong.; Staph.; *Strych.;* Sul. ac.; *Sul.;* Zing.

Numbness—*Acon.;* Berb. v.; Calc. p.; *Ox. ac.;* Oxytr.; Sec.; Sil.

PAIN in general—Abrot.; *Acon.;* Æsc.; *Agar.;* Arn. c.; Angust.; *Ant. t.;* Apis; Arg. m.; Arg. n.; *Arn.;* Bar. c.; Bell.; *Berb. v.;* Bry.; Calc. c.; Calc. p.; Can. ind.; Carb. ac.; Caul.; *Caust.;* Cham.; Chin. s.; Cic.; *Cim.;* Cinch.; *Cob.;* Cocc.; Colch.; Col.; Dulc.; *Eup. perf.;* Graph.; *Guaco;* Ham.; *Helon.;* Homar.; Kali bich.; *Kali c.;* Kali m.; Lach.; Lil. t.; Lyc.; Mag. m.; Mag. s.; Med.; *Merc.;* Mez.; Mormord.; Nat. c.; *Nat. m.;* Nit. ac.; *Nux v.;* Ox. ac.; Paraf.; Petrol.; Phos. ac.; *Picr. ac.;* Puls.; *Radium;* Ran. ac.; Rhod.; *Rhus t.;* Ruta; Sab.; Sang.; Sarrac.; Scolop.; Sec.; Selen.; *Sep.;* Sil.; Staph.; *Stellar.;* Strych.; *Sul.;* Tar. h.; *Tellur.;* Ther.; Triost.; *Upas; Variol.;* Wyeth.; Xerophyl.; *Zinc. m.*

Aching, as if it would break and give out—*Æsc.;* Æth.; Am. m.; *Bell.;* Can. ind.; Cham.; *Chel.;* Dulc.; *Eup. perf.;* Eupion; Graph.; *Ham.;* Kali bich.; *Kal.;* Kreos.; *Nat. m.;* Ol. an.; Ova t.; *Phos.;* Plat.; *Puls.;* Rhus t.; Sarcol. ac.; Sanic.; Senega; Sil.; *Trill.*

Aching, dull, constant (backache)—Abies n.; *Æsc.;* Agar.; Aloe; Am. m.; *Ant. t.;* Apoc.; Arg. m.; Arg. n.; *Arn.;* Bapt.; Bellis; *Berb. v.;* But. ac.; *Calc. c.;* Calc. fl.; Canth.; *Cim.;* Cob.; Coccinel.; *Cocc.;* Colch.; Con.; Conv.; Cupr. ars.; *Dulc.;* Euonym.; Eupion; Ferr. p.; Gels.;

Glycerin; *Helon.;* Hyper.; Inula; Ipomœa; *Kali c.;* Kali iod.; *Kal.;* Kreos.; Lach.; Lith. benz.; Lycoper.; *Lyc.;* Morph.; *Nat. m.; Nux v.;* Ol. an.; *Ol. j. as.; Ox. ac.;* Pall.; Petrol.; Phos. ac.; *Phyt.;* Picr. ac.; Piscidia; *Pulex; Puls.; Radium; Rhus t.;* Ruta; *Sabal;* Sab.; Senec.; *Sep.;* Solan. lyc.; Solid.; *Staph.; Still.; Sul.;* Symphyt.; *Tereb.;* Upas; *Vib. op.;* Viscum; Zinc. m.

Between scapulæ—*Acon.;* Apomorph.; Asclep. t.; Bar. c.; *Calc. c.;* Can. ind.; Con.; Guaco; Guaiac.; Jugl. c.; Kali c.; Med.; *Pod.;* Radium; *Rhus t.;* Sep.; Sul.; Zinc. m.

Bruised—*Acon.;* Æsc.; Agar.; Ant. t.; *Arn.;* Bar. c.; *Berb. v.;* Bry.; Cina; *Dulc.;* Gins.; Graph.; *Ham.;* Mag. s.; *Merc.;* Nat. m.; *Nux v.;* Phos. ac.; Phyt.; *Rhus t.; Ruta;* Sil.; Sul.; Tellur.

Crampy—*Bell.;* Cim.; Cinch.; *Col.;* Graph.; Iris; Mag. p.; Ova t.; Sep.

Digging, cutting—Sep.

Drawing—Anac.; Carbo v.; *Caust.; Kali c.;* Lyc.; Nux v.; Rhus t.; *Sab.;* Sul.

Falling apart sensation, involving small of back, Sacro-iliac synchondroses; relieved by bandaging tightly—Trill.

Heaviness, dragging, weight—Æsc.; *Aloe; Am. m.;* Anac.; Ant. c.; Benz. ac.; *Berb. v.;* Bov.; Colch.; *Eup. purp.; Helon.;* Hydr.; Kali c.; *Kreos.; Lil. t.;* Nat. s.; Picr. ac.; *Sep.* See Female Sexual System.

Lancinating, drawing, tearing—Alum.; Asclep. t.; *Berb. v.;* Colch.; Col.; Kali m.; Lyc.; Mimosa; Nux v.; *Scolop.;* Sep.; Sil.; Stellar.; *Strych.*

Lancinating, extends down thighs, legs—*Æsc.;* Aur. mur.; Bapt.; *Berb. v.;* Carb. ac.; Cocc.; *Col.;* Cur.; Ham.; *Helon.;* Kali c.; Kali m.; Lac c.; *Ox. ac.;* Phyt.; *Scolop.; Stellar.;* Tellur.; Xerophyl.

Lancinating, extends to pelvis—*Arg. n.;* Aur. mur.; Berb. v.; Cham.; *Cim.;* Eupion; Ham.; Sil.; *Variol.;* Viscum.

Lancinating, extends to pubes—*Sab.;* Vib. op.; Xanth.

Lancinating, extends upwards—Aspar.; Gels.

Paralytic—Cocc.; Kali p.; Nat. m.; Sil.

Pressing, plug-like—*Æsc.; Agar.; Anac.;* Aur. mur.; Benz. ac.; *Berb. v.;* Colch.; Hyper.; Nat. m.; *Nux v.;* Sep.; Tellur.

Sensitiveness extreme of sacrum—Lob. infl.

Stitching, piercing, pricking—Agar.; Aloe; Alum.; Apis; *Berb. v.;* Bry.; Guaiac.; Hyper.; *Kali c.; Merc.;* Nat. s.; Sul.; Tellur.; Ther.

MODALITIES—AGGRAVATION: After emission: Cob.

After masturbation—Nux v.; Phos. ac.; Staph.

At night—Aloe; Calc. c.; Lyc.; *Merc.;* Mez.; Nat. m.; *Staph.;* Viscum.

From cold exposure—Acon.; Bry.; *Rhod.;* Sul.

From damp exposure—Dulc.; Phyt.; *Rhus t.*

From eating—Kali c.

From exertion—Agar.; *Berb. v.;* Cocc.; Hyper.; Kali c.; Kali p.; Ox. ac.; Sul. See Motion.

From jar, touch—*Acon.;* Berb. v.; *Bry.;* Kali bich.; *Lob. infl.;* Mez.; Sil.; *Tellur.*

From lying down—Bell.; *Berb. v.;* Niccol. s.; Nux v.; Rhus t.

From motion, beginning—Lac c.; *Rhus t.*

From motion, walking—*Æsc.;* Aloe; *Ant. t.;* Bell.; *Bry.; Caust.;* Chel.; Cinch.; *Colch.;* Kali bich.; *Kali* ʋ. · Mez.; *Nux v.;* Ox. ac.; Paraf.; Petrol.; Phyt.; Ran. ac.; Sep.; *Sul.*

From resting, sitting—*Agar.;* Alum.; Ant. t.; Bell.; *Berb. v.;* Can. ind.; Cob.; Ferr. mur.; Kali p.; Kreos.; *Lac c.;* Merc.; Nux v.; Puls.; *Rhus t.;* Sep.; Sul.; *Zinc. m.*

From standing—*Æsc.;* Bell.; Nux v.; Sarcol. ac.; Sep.

From stooping—*Æsc.;* Berb. v.; Diosc.; Guaco; Tellur.

From warmth—*Kali s.;* Puls.; Sul.

In morning—Agar.; *Berb. v.;* Bry.; Conv.; Kali c.; Nat. m.; Nux v.; Petrol.; Phyt.; Ruta; Selen.; *Staph.*

When rising from seat—Æsc.; Arg. n.; *Berb. v.; Caust.;* Kali p.; *Lach.;* Sil.; Sul.; Tellur.

AMELIORATION—After rising: Kali c.; Ruta; Staph.

From bending backward—Rhus t.

From bending forward—Lob. infl.

From emission—Zinc. m.

From lying on abdomen—Acet. ac.

From lying on back—*Æsc.; Cob.;* Gnaph.; Nat. m.; Rhus t.; Ruta.

From lying on something hard, or firm support—Eupion; *Nat. m.; Rhus t.;* Sep.

From lying, sitting—Sep.

From motion, walking—Arg. n.; Bell.; Caust.; Cob.; Ferr. mur.; *Helon.;* Kali m.; Kreos.; Merc.; *Puls.;* Radium; *Rhus t.;* Sep.; Staph.; *Sul.; Zinc. m.*

From rest—*Æsc.;* Colch.; Nux v.; Sil.

From sitting—Bell.

From standing—Arg. n.; Caust.; Sul.

From urination—*Lyc.;* Med.

WEAKNESS—Of back: Abrot.; *Æsc. gl.; Æsc.;* Alum.; Ant. t.; Arn.; Berb. v.; But. ac.; Calc. c.; *Calc. p.; Cinch.; Cocc.;* Glycerin; Graph.; Guaco; *Helon.;* Ign.; Irid.; Jacar.; *Kali c.;* Merc.; Nat. m.; Nux v.; Ox. ac.; Petrol.; Phos. ac.; Phos.; *Picr. ac.;* Pod.; Sarrac.; *Sep.; Sil.;* Staph.; *Zinc. m.*

BODY—Bruised, sore feeling, all over: Abrot.; Ampel.; Apis; *Arn.; Bapt.; Bellis;* Caust.; Cic.; Cim.; *Cinch.; Eup. perf.; Gels.;* Ham.; Hep.; Iberis; Lil. t.; *Mang. ac.;* Med.; Morph.; Nux m.; *Phyt.;* Psor.; *Pyr.; Radium; Rhus t.; Ruta;* Sarcol. ac.; Solan. lyc.; Staph.; Tellur.; *Thuya;* Wyeth.

Burning, in various parts—Acon.; *Agar.;* Apis; *Ars.; Canth.;* Caps.; *Carbo an.;* Phos. ac.; *Phos.;* Sul.

Coldness—Acon.; *Æth.;* Ant. t.; Ars.; Atham.; *Bar. m.; Bor. ac.;* Cadm. s.; *Camph.;* Camph. monobr.; *Chloral;* Cupr.;] *Helod.; Jatropha;* Lachnanth.; Luffa; *Sec.;* Tab.; *Ver. a.;* Zinc .m.

Constriction, as if caged—Cact.; Med.

Numbness—*Acon.;* Ars.; Cic.; Con.; *Ox. ac.; Phos.;* Plumb. m.; *Sec.*

Swelling—*Apis;* Doryph.; Frag. See Dropsy (Generalities).

Trembling—*Agar.;* Cod.; *Con.; Gels.;* Hyos.; Iberis; Lonic.; *Myg.;* Phos.; Sarcol. ac.

COCCYX—Burning on touch: Carbo an.

Itching—Bov.; Graph.

Neuralgia, worse rising from sitting posture—Lach.

Numbness—Plat.

Pain (coccygodynia)—Ant. t.; Arn.; *Bell.; Bry.; Calc. caust.;* Castorea; *Caust.; Cic.; Cim.;* Cistus; Con.; *Ferr. p.;* Fluor. ac.; *Graph.; Hyper.;* Kali bich.; Kali c.; Kali iod.; *Kreos.;* Lac c.; *Lach.;* Lobel. infl.; Mag. c.; *Mag. p.; Merc.; Paris;* Petrol.; Phos.; *Rhus t.;* Sil.; *Tar. h.;* Tetradym.; Xanth.; Zinc. m.

Bruised—Am. m.; *Arn.;* Caust.; Ruta; Sul.

Bruised from injury—Hyper.

Dragging, drawing—*Ant. t.; Caust.;* Graph.; Kreos.

Tearing, lancinating—*Bell.;* Canth.; *Cic.;* Kali bich.; *Mag. p.;* Merc.

Ulcer—Pæonia.

EXTREMITIES—Coldness: Acon.; Agar.; *Agar. ph.; Bell.; Calc. c.;* Calc. hypoph.; *Calc. p.; Camph.; Coccinel.;* Crat.; Dulc.; *Ferr. m.;* Hedeoma; *Helod.; Hydroc. ac.;* Ign.; Kal.; Lol. tem.; Lonic.; Meli.; Merc.; *Mur. ac.;* Nat. m.; Nux m.; Oleand.; Op.; *Phyt.;* Quass.; Sang.; *Sec.;* Sulphon.; Trill.; *Ver. a.;* Zinc. m.

Itching—*Arundo;* Kali c.; Lyc.; Pall.; *Phos.;* Prun. v.; Val.

Lameness, stiffness—*Agar.;* Agaricine; Aloe; *Calc. p.;* Carbo v.; *Cocc.; Eucal.;* Gins.; Ipec.; Kali p.; *Lith. c.; Rhus t.;* Triost.; Xerophyl.; Zinc. m.

Numbness, tingling, fall asleep—Absinth.; *Acon.;* Alum.; Aran.; *Arg. n.;* Avena; Bar. c.; Calc. c.; *Calc. p.;* Camph.; *Carbo v.; Caust.;* Cham.; Cic.; Cinch.; *Cocc.; Gels.;* Helod.; *Kali c.;* Kal.; *Lonic.; Morph.;* Nat. m.; *Onosm.;* Op.; *Ox. ac.; Phos.; Picr. ac.; Plat.;* Plumb. m.; *Sec.; Sil.;* Solan. n.; Sul.; *Thall.;* Ver. a.; *Zinc. m.*

PAIN—Aching: Æsc.; Apis; *Arn.;* Ars.; Azadir.; *Bry.;* Calc. c.; Carbo v.; Caust.; Cepa; *Cim.;* Cinch.; *Con.;* Cur.; Cycl.; Echin.; Eucal.; *Gels.;* Hedeoma; *Kal.; Merc.;* Myr.; *Pyr.;* Quass.; *Radium;* Ran. sc.; *Rhod.; Rhus t.;* Sec.; Sil.; Staph.; *Stellar.;* Strych. p.; Thyr.

Bone-pains—Aran.; Aur.; Calc. p.; *Eup. perf.; Gels.; Kali bich.;* Kali iod.; Mag. mur.; Mang. ac.; *Merc.; Mez.; Phos. ac.; Ran. sc.;* Rhus ven.; Ruta; *Sang.;* Sars.; *Still.;* Stront. c.; Triost.

Cramp-like, constricting—Abrot.; Alumen; Ant. t.; Antipyr.; *Asaf.;* Calc. c.; Canth.; Carbon. s.; *Cocc.; Col.;* Croc.; *Cupr. m.;* Gins.; Mag. p.; Menyanth.; *Plat.;* Sec.; Sil.; *Strych.;* Ver. a.

Drawing—Camph.; Caust.; Graph.; Hep.; Kali c.; Lyc.; Nat. m.; Rhus t.

Erratic, fly about—*Caul.;* Iris; Kali bich.; *Kali s.;* Kal.; *Lac c.;* Magnol.; *Mang. ac.;* Phyt.; *Puls.;* Rhod.; Sal. ac.; *Stellar.*

Growing pains—Apium gr.; Calc. p.; *Guaiac.;* Hippom.; Phos. ac. See Bones (Generalities).

Hysterical contractures—Bell.; *Cocc.; Cupr.;* Hyos.; *Ign.;* Lyc.; Merc.; Nux v.; Stram.; Zinc. m.

Neuralgic, lancinating, tearing, shooting—Absinth.; *Acon.;* Alum.; *Bell.;*

Branca; *Carbon. s.;* Caul.; *Cham.;* Daphne; Elat.; Eucal.; Gels.; Guaiac.; Kali c.; Kal.; Lyc.; *Mag. p.;* Magnol.; *Mimosa;* Nit. ac.; *Ox. ac.;* Phos.; Phyt.; *Rhod.;* Rhus t.; Sars.; Sil.; Strych.

Rheumatico-gouty—*Acon.;* Anag.; Ant. t.; Apis; *Arn.;* Aspar.; Bell.; Branca; *Bry.;* Calc. c.; *Calc. p.;* Caul.; Caust.; Cham.; *Colch.;* Dulc.; Eucal.; Guaiac.; Iod.; Kali c.; *Kal.;* Lac c.; Lyc.; *Merc.;* Prun. v.; *Radium; Rhod.; Rhus t.;* Sang.; *Stellar.;* Sticta.

Shock-like, paralytic—Cina; Colch.; *Phyt.; Thall.;* Veratrin; Ver. v.; Xanth.

Sprained, dislocated feeling—*Arn.;* Bellis; Calc. c.; Carbo v.; *Cinch.;* Rhus t.; *Ruta.* See Joints.

Paralysis—*Acon.;* Alum.; *Bar. ac.; Caust.; Cocc.; Con.;* Cur.; Dub.; *Dulc.;* Hedeoma; Kal.; *Lol. tem.;* Nux v.; Oleand.; *Op.; Phos.;* Picr. ac.; Rhus t.; Sec.; Sil. See Nervous System.

Sprains, chronic—Graph.; Petrol.; *Stront. c.* See Generalities.

Stretching continually—Alum.; Amyl; Angust.; *Ars.;* Cinch.; Quass.; Sep.

Trembling, twitching, jerking—Acon.; *Agar.;* Alum.; Apis; *Arg. n.;* Ars.; Bell.; Calc. p.; Carbo v.; Caust.; *Cim.;* Cinch.; *Cina; Cocc.; Con.;* Cupr. ars.; *Cupr. m.; Gels.;* Helod.; *Hyper.; Hyos.; Ign.;* Kali c.; *Lach.; Lol. tem.;* Lonic.; Lyc.; Mag. p.; *Merc.; Morph.; Myg.; Op.;* Phos. ac.; *Phos.;* Physost.; Rhus t.; *Sec.;* Sep.; Sil.; Stram.; *Strych.;* Sulphon.; Sul.; *Tar. h.;* Thall.; *Val.;* Viola od.; Xerophyl.; *Zinc. m.;* Zinc. s. See Weakness.

Weakness, debility—Æth.; Agar.; *Alum.; Am. caust.;* Am. m.; Anac.; Apis; Arg. n.; *Ars.;* Asar.; Bellis; Bism.; *Calc. c.; Caust.; Cinch.; Cocc.; Con.;* Cupr. m.; Cur.; Cyprip.; Dig.; Eucal.; *Gels.;* Gins.; Helon.; Hippom.; *Kali bich.;* Kal.; Lecith.; Lyc.; Mag. p.; Med.; Merc.; *Mur. ac.;* Myr.; Nat. c.; Nat. m.; Niccol. s.; Nux v.; *Onosm.;* Ox. ac.; *Phos. ac.; Phos.; Picr. ac.; Plat.;* Prim. v.; Puls.; *Sarcol. ac.;* Scutel.; Selen.; Sep.; Sil.; *Stann.;* Strych. p.; Sulphon.; *Thall.;* Thuya; Ver. a.; *Zinc. m.* See Neurasthenia (Nervous System).

UPPER EXTREMITIES—ARM: See Extremities in general.

Coldness—Apis; Carbo v.; Raph.; Ver. a.

Eruptions—Arundo; Caust.; Phos. ac.; Sul.

Gangrenous ulceration—Ran. flam.

Heaviness—*Acon.; Alum.;* Can. ind.; Cim.; *Cur.;* Ham.; Hep.; *Latrod.;* Lyc.; Nat. m.; Ver. a.

Intolerant of band around—Ov. g. p.

Itching—Fagop.

Jerking, involuntary motion—*Agar.;* Ant. c.; *Cic.; Cina;* Cocc.; *Ipec.;* Lact. v.; Lyc.; Op.; Tar. h.; *Thlasp.*

Jerking, or involuntary motion, of one arm, and leg—Apoc.; *Bry.; Helleb.; Myg.;* Zinc. m.

Lameness, stiffness—Acon.; Am. c.; Bapt.; Can. ind.; *Caust.;* Paris; *Rhus ven.;* Thasp.; Ver. a.

Nodules—Hippoz.

Numbness, fall asleep—Acon.; Ambra; Aran.; Aster.; Bar. c.; *Cact.;* Cham.; Cim.; *Cocc.;* Dig.; *Graph.;* Iberis; Ign.; Kali c.; *Latrod.;*

Lil. t.; Lyc.; *Mag. m.;* Magnol.; *Nux v.;* Paris; Phos.; *Rhus t.;* Sep.; Sil.; Xanth.

Numbness, left arm—Acon.; Dig.; Kal.; Puls.; *Rhus t.;* Sumb.

Numbness, right arm—Phyt.

PAINS—Æsc.; *Alum.;* *Anag.;* Calc. c.; *Caust.;* Cepa; Cic.; Cinnab.; *Eup. perf.;* Ferr. picr.; Gels.; Guaco; *Guaiac.;* Indium; Mag. m.; Nat. m.; Phos.; *Phyt.;* *Rhus t.;* *Sang.;* Solan. lyc.; *Stellar.;* Sticta; *Sul.;* Wyeth.; *Zinc. m.*

Pain in left arm—Acon.; Agar.; Aster.; *Cact.;* *Cim.;* Colch.; Crot.; Iberis; Kal.; *Latrod.;* Magnol.; Mag. s.; *Rhus t.;* *Spig.;* Tab.; Xanth.

Pain in right arm—*Ferr. mur.;* Ferr. picr.; Pip. m.; Rhus v.; *Sang.;* Solan. lyc.; Viola od.; Wyeth.

Aching—Bapt.; Berb. v.; *Caust.;* Gels.; Jal.; Lith. c.; Nat. ars.; Ol. j. as.; Sarrac.

Aching, weakness, when singing, using voice—Stann.

Bruised, cramp-like—Acon.; Arg. n.; *Cocc.;* Cupr. m.; Oleand.; *Phos. ac.;* Sec.; Sul. ac.; Ver. v.; *Zinc. s.*

Drawing—Calc. c.; *Caust.;* Lyc.; *Mag. m.;* Mur. ac.; Oleand.; Sep.; Sil.; Zinc. m.

Neuralgic (brachyalgia)—*Acon. rad.;* Alum.; Bry.; *Hyper.;* Kali c.; *Kal.;* Lyc.; Merc.; *Nux v.;* Pip. m.; *Puls.;* *Rhus t.;* Scutel.; Sul.; Teucr.; Ver. a.; Viscum.

Paralysis—Cocc.; Ferr.; Gels.; Nux v.; Rhus t.

Sensibility, diminished—Carbon. s.; Phos.

Tearing, stitching—Calc. c.; Ferr.; Hep.; Phos.; Sep.; Sil.

Trembling—Cod.; Cocc.; *Gels.;* Kali br.; *Phos.;* Sil. See Weakness.

Weakness—*Alumen;* Anac.; *Cur.;* Dig.; Iod.; Kali c.; Lach.; Lyc.; Mag. p.; Med.; *Nat. m.;* Sarcol. ac.; Sep.; *Sil.;* _Stann.;_ Sul.

FOREARM—See Extremities.

Coldness—Arn.; Brom.; Med.

Pain—Anac.; Cinnab.; *Eup. perf.;* Ferr. mur.; Ferr. picr.; Gels.; Guaco; *Hyper.;* Kali c.; *Kal.;* Phyt.; *Rhus t.;* Sep.; Stann.

Paralysis—Arg. n.; Nux v.; Plumb.; Sil. See Nervous System.

Soreness of flexor carpi ulnaris—Brachygl.

Unsteadiness of muscles of forearm, hands—Caust.

HAND—**Automatic motion of hand and head**—Apoc.; Bry.; Helleb.; Zinc. m.

Blueness, distended veins: Am. c.; Amyl; *Ant. t.;* *Carbo an.;* Dig.; Elaps; Laur.; *Nit. ac.;* Oleand.; Samb.; Stront. c.; *Ver. a.* See Cyanosis (Circulatory System).

Burning, heat—*Acon.;* Agar.; Carbo v.; Cocc.; *Lach.;* Lyc.; *Med.;* Ol. j. as.; *Phos.;* Sang.; Sil.

Chapping—Alum.; *Calc. c.;* Castor.; Cistus; *Graph.;* Lyc.; Mag. c.; Nat. ars.; *Nat. c.;* *Petrol.;* Sars.; Sulphurous ac.

Coldness—Abies c.; Acon.; *Ant. t.;* Apis; Ars.; Cact.; Calc. c.; *Camph.;* *Carbon. ox.;* Cic.; *Cinch.;* Con.; *Cupr.;* *Dig.;* Iod.; *Menyanth.;* Nat. m.; Nit. ac.; Scilla; *Tab.;* Thuya; Trifol.; *Ver. a.*

Coldness of one, warmth of the other—Cinch.; Dig.; Ipec.; Puls.

Cramps—Bell.; Calc. c.; *Sec.;* Sil.

Cramps (writers'); piano or violin players, typists—Ambra; *Arg. m.; Arg. n.;* Brachygl.; *Caust.; Cim.;* Cupr.; Cycl.; *Gels.;* Graph.; Hep.; *Mag. p.;* Ruta; *Stann.;* Sul. ac.; Sul. See Nervous System.

Dryness—Lyc.; Zinc. m.

Enlarged feeling—*Aran.;* Caust.; *Cocc.;* Gins.; Kali n.

Eruption—Bor.; Cistus; Pedic.; *Pix l.* See Skin.

Fidgety— *Kali br.; Myg.;* Tar. h.; Zinc. m.

Hypothenar eminences bright red—Acon.

Itching—Agar.; Tellur.

Nodotities, gouty, on dorsum—*Am. phos.;* Eucal.; Med. See Fingers.

Numbness, go asleep—*Acon.;* Arg. n.; Ars.; Bor.; Can. ind.; *Caust.; Cocc.;* Cod.; *Colch.;* Graph.; *Hyper.;* Iberis; Laburn.; Lach.; Lil. t.; Lyc.; Mag. p.; Nat. c.; Nux v.; *Phos.;* Physost.; Pyr.; Raph.; Sec.; Tela ar.

Pains—Bruised: *Ruta;* Ver. a.

Lancinating—*Cepa;* Lappa; Selen.; Sul.

Rheumatic—Ambra; Berb. v.; *Caul.; Caust.;* Chel.; Guaiac.; Led.; *Puls.; Rhus t.; Ruta;* Sang.; Solan. lyc.

Paralysis—Ferr.; Laburn.; Merc.; Plumb. ac.; Ruta; Sil.

PALMS—Blisters: Bufo.

Burning—*Azadir.;* Bolet.; Ferr. m.; Ferr. p.; Gadus; *Lach.;* Lachnanth.; Limul.; Nat. m.; *Ol. j. as.;* Petrol.; *Phos.;* Prim. v.; Puls. nut.; *Sang.;* Sep.; *Sul.*

Chapping, fissuring—Calc. fl.; *Ran. b.*

Cramps—*Cupr. m.;* Scrophul.; Zing.

Desquamation—Elaps.

Eruption, dry, bran-like, itching—Anag.; *Ars.;* X-ray.

Injury with intolerable pain—Hyper.

Itching—Ant. s. a.; *Fagop.; Granat.;* Limulus; Ran. b.; Tub.

Pains—Azadir.; Trifol.

Stiffness of hands while writing—Kali m.

Sweating—*Calc. c.;* Cocc.; Con.; Dulc.; Fagop.; *Fluor. ac.;* Nat. m.; Picr. ac.; Sep.; *Sil.; Strych. p.; Sul.;* Wyeth.

Swelling—Æsc.; Agar.; *Apis;* Arg. n.; Ars.; Arundo; Bry.; *Cact.;* Calc. c.; Crot.; Elaps; Ferr. p.; Nat. chlor.; *Rhus div.* See Dropsy (Generalities).

Twitching, trembling, weakness—Act. sp.; Anac.; Ant. c.; Ant. t.; *Arg. n.;* Arn.; Avena; Calc. c.; *Cic.; Cina;* Cocc.; *Con.; Cur.; Gels.;* Hippom.; Lach.; Lact. v.; Lol. tem.; *Mag. p.;* Merc.; *Phos.;* Sars.; *Sarcol. ac.;* Sil.; *Stann.; Stram.;* Sul.; Tab.; *Zinc. m.*

Warts—*Anac.;* Ant. c.; Calc. c.; *Dulc.;* Ferr. mag.; *Ferr. picr.;* Nat. c.; Nat. m.; *Ruta.*

Yellow color—Chel.; Sep. See Skin.

FINGERS—Blueness, coldness: Chel.; Crat.; Cupr. m.; Ver. a. See Hands
Blue, numb, shrivelled, spread apart, or bent backward—Sec.

Burning—*Azadir.;* Gin.; Oleand.; Sars.; *Sul.*

Chapped tips, cracks, fissures—Alum.; *Graph.;* Nat. m.; *Petrol.; Ran. b.; Sanic.;* Sars.

Cramp-like, contracted, clenching—*Æth.*; Ambra; Anag.; *Arg. n.*; Bism.; *Brachygl.*; Can. s.; Caust.; *Cic.*; *Cina*; Cocc.; Colchicine; *Cupr. ac.*; *Cupr. m.*; Cycl.; Diosc.; *Helleb.*; Kali bich.; Laur.; Lyc.; Paris; Ruta; *Sec.*; Solan. t.; Stann.; *Sul. ac.*

Crooked—Kali c.; Lyc.

Crushed, mashed tips—Hyper.

Eruptions—Alnus; Anac.; *Bov.*; *Graph.*; Limul.; *Lob. er.*; Nat. c.; Nit. ac.; *Petrol.*: Prim. far.; *Rhus t.*; Sars.; Selen.; Veronal. See Skin.

Exostoses—Calc. fl.; *Hekla.*

Fidgety, must move constantly—Kali br.

Hypertrophy—Aur. mur.

Impression deep, from scissors—Bov.

Itching between—Phos. ac. See Skin.

Jerking, when holding pen—*Caust.*; Cina; Cycl.; Kali c.; *Stann.*; Sul. ac.

Joints, inflamed, painful—*Benz. ac.*; Berb. v.; *Bry.*; Fluor. ac.; Lyc.; Med.; *Nat. p.*; Pip. m.; Prim. sylv.; Puls.; *Rhus t.*; Staph.; *Stellar.* See Rheumatism.

Joints, nodosities on—*Am. phos.*; *Benz. ac.*; Benzoin; Calc. c.; Calc. fl.; *Caul.*; *Colch.*; Graph.; Led.; Lith. c.; *Lyc.*; *Med.*; Staph.; Stellar. See Joints.

Joints, pain in—Bry.; Graph.; Led.; Lyc.; Sil.; Sul.

Joints, stiff—Carbo v.; *Caul.*; Lyc.; Prim. sylv.; Puls. See Joints.

Numbness, tingling of fingers—Acon.; Æsc.; Ambra; Apis; Ars.; Aster.; Bar. c.; Calc. c.; *Cocaine*; Con.; *Dig.*; Lathyrus; Lyc.; Mag. p.; Mag. s.; Nat. m.; Nit. ac.; *Ox. ac.*; *Paris*; Phos.; Propyl.; Sarcol. ac.; *Sec.*; Sil.; *Thall.*; Upas; Verbasc.; Zinc. m.

Pains, at root of nails—Berb. v.; Bism.; *Cepa*; Myrist. seb.

Pains in general—Abrot.; Azadir.; Lil. t.; Sec.

Pains in tips—Am. m.; Bor.; Chel.; *Hyper.*; Kali c.; *Sec.*; Sil.; Teucr.

Pains, rheumatic—*Act. sp.*; *Ant. c.*; Berb. v.; *Caul.*; Colch.; Fagop.; Granat.; Graph.; Guaco; Hyper.; Lappa; *Led.*; Lith. c.; Lyc.; Med.; Pæonia; Puls.; Ran. sc.; *Rhus t.* See Rheumatism.

Pains, tearing—*Act. sp.*; Am. m.; *Caul.*; Caust.; Ced.; Led.; Lyc.; *Puls.*; Rhus t.

Pains, throbbing—Amyl; Bor.

Panaritium—Alum.; Am. c.; Diosc.; Myrist. seb.; Sil.

Sensibility, diminished—*Carbon. s.*; Pop. c.; Sec.

Sensitive to cold—*Cistus*; Hep.

Skin, dry, shrivelled—Æth. See Skin.

Skin peels off—Elaps. See Skin.

Soreness between—Nat. ars. See Skin.

Stiffness, rigidity—Am. c.; Carbon. s.; *Caul.*; Cocc.; Lyc.; Oleand.; Puls.; Sil. See Joints.

Swelling—*Am. c.*; Bry.; Carbon. s.; Cinnam.; Hep.; Kali m.; *Lith. c.*; Mang.; Oleand.; *Puls.*; *Thuya.*

Thick, horny tips—*Ant. c.*; Pop. c.

Trembling—Bry.; Iod.; Kali br.; Lolium; Merc.; Oleand.; Rhus t.; Zinc. m.

Ulcers—Alum.; Arundo; Ars.; Bor.; Sep.

Weariness—Bov.; Calc. c.; *Cur.;* *Gels.;* Hippom.; Phos.; Sil. See Hand.

LOWER EXTREMITIES—BUTTOCKS (glutei): Cold feeling: Daphne.
   Cold feeling, fall asleep—Calc. p.
   Cramp—Graph.
   Emaciation—Lathyr.
   Pain to hips, small of back—Staph.
   Pricking—Guaiac.
   Swelling—Phos. ac.

LOINS—LUMBAGO: *Acon.;* Act. sp.; *Æsc.;* Agar.; *Aloe; Ant. t.; Arn.;*
   Bell.; *Berb. v.;* Bry.; *Calc. fl.; Calc. p.;* Carb. ac.; Carbon. s.; *Caul.;*
   Cham.; Chel.; *Cim.;* Cina; Colch.; Col.; Diosc.; *Dulc.; Eup. perf.;*
   Ferr. m.; *Gins.; Gnaph.:* Guaiac.; Hydr.; *Hymosa;* Ipomoea; Kali bich.;
   Kali c.; Kali iod.; Kali ox.; Lathyr.; Led.; Lith. benz.; Lyc.; *Macrot.;*
   Merc. s.; Nat. m.; *Nux v.;* Pampin.; Picr. ac.; Phyt.; Puls.; Radium;
   Rham. c.; Rhod.; *Rhus t.;* Ruta; *Sabal;* Senec.; Sep.; Spiranth.; *Sul.;*
   Tereb.; Vib. op.
   Alternates, with headache, piles—Aloe.
   With aggravation in open air—Agar.
   With aggravation on beginning to move—Anac.; Con.; Glycerin; *Rhus t.*
   With aggravation, on beginning to move, relieved by continued motion—
      Calc. fl.; *Rhus t.*
   With aggravation on exertion; during day; while sitting—Agar.
   With aggravation on lying down—Bell.; Murex.
   With chronic tendency—Æsc.; Berb. v.; *Calc. fl.; Rhus t.;* Sil.
   With masturbatic origin; sexual weakness—Nux v.
   With numbness, in lower part of back, weight in pelvis—Gnaph.
   With relief from lying down—Euonym.; Sep.
   With relief, from slow walking—Ferr. m.
   With retching, cold, clammy sweat, from least motion—Lathyr.
   With sciatica—*Rhus t.*

THIGS-LEGS—Blue, painful, swollen, if hanging down: Lathyr.
   Burning—*Ars.;* Arundo; Bar. c.; Kali c.; Led.; Lyc.; Mez.; Still.
   Coldness—Acon.; Alum.; Astrag.; Berb. v.; Bism.; *Calc. c.;* Calc. p.;
      Carbo an.; Carbo v.; Colch.; Crot.; Lact. ac.; Lact. v.; *Laur.;* Lyc.;
      Merc.; Mez.; *Nat. m.;* Nit. ac.; Ox. ac.; Sep.; Sil.; *Tab.; Ver. a.;*
      Zinc. m.
   Contractions of hamstrings, tendons—*Am. m.; Caust.;* Cimex; Col.;
      Graph.; Guaiac.; Lach.; Med.; Nat. m.; Ruta; Sul.
   Curved limbs, cannot be straightened, and vice versa—Cic.
   Emaciation—*Abrot.;* Acet. ac.; Kali iod.; *Lathyr.;* Pin. sylv.
   Enlargement of femur, in rachitic infants—Calc. fl.
   Eruptions—Calc. c.; Chrysar.; Gins.; *Graph.;* Mag. c.; *Petrol.;* Sul. See
      Skin.
   Erysipelas—Sul. See Skin.
   Excoriation, itching over tibia—Bism.
   Heaviness—*Alum.;* Bry.; Calc. c.; Can. ind.; Cim.; *Con.;* Gins.; *Guaco;*
      Helleb.; Med.; Nux v.; Pall.; *Picr. ac.;* Sep.; Sulphon.; *Sul.;* Verbasc.;
      Vib. op.

Itching—Bellis; Bov.; *Fagop.*; Nit. ac.; *Rumex*; Stellar.

Motion involuntary—Bry.; Helleb.; Lyc.; *Myg.*; Tar. h. See Trembling.

Numbness, formication, "going asleep"—*Agar.*; *Alum.*; Aran.; Calc. c.; *Calc. p.*; *Caust.*; Carbon. s.; *Cocc.*; Col.; Crot.; *Gnaph.*; Graph.; Kali c.; Kali iod.; Lact. v.; Mez.; *Nux v.*; Onosm.; *Phos.*; *Rhus t.*; Sarcol. ac.; *Sec.*; Sep.; *Sul.*; Tar. h.; Tela ar.; *Triost.*; Zinc. m.

PAINS—**In general**: Agar.; Can. ind.; *Caps.*; *Carbon. s.*; Carbo an.; Chel.; Cic.; Diad.; *Diosc.*; Euphorb.; Ferr. m.; *Gels.*; *Gnaph.*; Helod.; Illic.; Indigo; Iod.; Irid.; *Kali c.*; *Kal.*; Lach.; Mag. m.; Mang. ac.; Mang. ox.; Menisp.; Murex; Nat. s.; Nit. ac.; Phos. ac.; *Phos.*; Picr. ac.; *Plumb. m.*; Puls.; *Rhus t.*; Sab.; Sil.; Tongo; Trifol.; Vib. op.; *Vipera.*

Aching, bruised—Arg. n.; *Arn.*; *Bapt.*; Calc. c.; Cim.; Cocc.; *Colch.*; Diosc.; *Eup. perf.*; *Gels.*; Guaiac.; Laur.; Lil. t.; Mag. c.; Med.; *Phos. ac.*; *Pyr.*; Sab.; Sarcol. ac.; Sep.; Solan. lyc.; Staph.; Ulnus; *Variol.*

Cramps, contractions—Abrot.; Æsc. gl.; Agar.; Ambra; Am. br.; *Am. m.*; Anac.; *Arn.*; Bapt.; Bar. c.; *Calc. c.*; *Camph.*; Carb. ac.; Carbo an.; Carbo v.; *Caust.*; Cholas ter.; *Cimex*; Cim.; Cinch.; *Cocc.*; Colch.; *Col.*; Con.; *Cupr. ars.*; *Cupr. m.*; Eupion; Ferr. m.; *Gels.*; Hyper.; Hyos.; Irid.; Jatropha; Lathyrus; Lol. tem.; *Lyc.*; *Mag. p.*; Med.; Nit. ac.; *Nux v.*; Ox. ac.; Pin. sylv.; Plumb. m.; Puls.; *Rhus t.*; Sarcol. ac.; *Sec.*: Sep.; *Sil.*; Solan. t.; *Sul.*; Ustil.; *Ver. a.*; Vipera; Zinc. s.

Cramps (tailor's)—Anac.; Anag.; Mag. p.

Pains in tibia—Ars.; Bad.; Carbo an.; *Dulc.*; Ferr. m.; *Kali bich.*; *Lach.*; Mang. ox.; *Mez.*; Phos.; Sep.

Rending, tearing, lancinating—*Am. m.*; Ars.; Bapt.; Bar. ac.; *Bell.*; Bellis; Cob.; Col.; *Diosc.*; *Hyper.*; Kali bich.; Kali c.; *Kal.*; Lyc.; Nit. ac.; *Plumb. m.*; Puls.; *Rhus t.*; Sep.; *Sul.*; Teucr.; Viscum.

Rheumatic—Berb. v.; *Bry.*; Chel.; Colch.; Daphne; *Dulc.*; Led.; *Phyt.*; Merc.; *Rhus t.*; Sang.; Stellar.; Val. See Rheumatism.

Paralysis—*Agar.*; Alum.; Bry.; *Can. ind.*; Chel.; Cocc.; *Crot.*; Dulc.; Gels.; *Guaco*; Kali iod.; Kali tart.; *Lathyr.*; Nux v.; Oleand.; *Plumb. m.*; *Rhus t.*; Sec.; Sulphon.; Tab.; *Thall.*; Ver. a.; Zinc. m. See Nervous System.

Restless, fidgety—Ars.; Carbo v.; *Caust.*; Cim.; Cinch.; Con.; Crot.; Graph.; Kali br.; Lil. t.; Lyc.; *Med.*; *Menyanth.*; Merc. c.; Myg.; Nit. ac.; *Phos.*; *Rhus t.*; Ruta; Scutel.; *Sep.*; Sulphon.; Tar. h.; *Tarax.*; Thasp.; *Zinc. m.*; Zinc. v.

Rigidity, stiffness, lameness—Alum.; Angust.; *Arg. n.*; Bapt.; Bar. m.; Calc. c.; *Cic.*; Colch.; *Con.*; Diosc.; *Eup. perf.*; Guaiac.; *Lathyr.*; Physost.; Plat.; *Rhus t.*; Sarcol. ac.; Sep.; *Strych.*; Xerophyl.

Sensibility, diminished—Ox. ac.; Phos. See Nervous System.

Sensibility, increased—Lach.; Lathyr. See Nervous System.

Spots on, red—Calc. c.; Sul.

Stretching—Am. c.; *Amyl*; Helleb.; Helod. See Fever.

Sweat, cold, clammy, at P. M.—Calc. c.; Merc.

Sweat extending below knees in A. M.—Sul.

Sweat on thighs, exhausting at P. M.—Carbo an.

Swelling—*Acet. ac.*; *Apis*; *Ars.*; Aur.; *Cact.*; Chel.; Colch.; *Dig.*; Eup.

perf.; *Ferr. m.*; Fluor. ac.; Graph.; Kali c.; Lathyr.; *Lyc.*; Merc.; Phos.; *Rhus t.*; Samb.; Sep.; Stront. c.; *Stroph.*; Sul.; Thyr.; Viscum. See Dropsy (Generalities).

Trembling—Æsc. gl.; Arg. m.; *Cob.*; *Cocc.*; Cod.; Colch.; *Con.*; Cur.; Doryph.; *Gels.*; Lol. tem.; *Mimosa*; Nit. ac.; Phos. ac.; Phos.; Tab.; Zinc. m.

Trickling, as from drops of water—Acon.

Ulcers—*Ars.*; Calc. c.; Carbo v.; Cistus; Echin.; Lyc.; Phos. ac.; Rhus t.; Sacchar. of.: *Sil.*; Trifol. See Generalities.

Weakness, easily fatigued—Æsc.; *Alumen; Alum.*; Am. c.; Arg. m.; Arg. n.; Bar. m.; Berb. v.; *Calc. p.*; *Can. ind.*; Cim.; Cob.; *Cocc.*; Colch.; *Con.*; Cupr. m.; Cur.; Dig.; Ferr. m.; *Formica; Gels.*; Ham.; Kali c.; Kal.; Lach.; Med.; *Nat. m.*; *Nux v.*; *Oleand.*; Onosm.; Pœonia; Phell.; *Phos. ac.*; *Phos.*; *Picr. ac.*; Rhus t.; Ruta; Sarrac.; *Sarcol. ac.*; Sil.; *Stann.*; Sul.; Vib. op.

FEET—Affections of ball, and dorsum of toes: Can. s.

Bunions—Agar.; *Benz. ac.*; Hyper.; *Kali iod.*; Rhod.; *Sil.*; Ver. v. See Skin.

Burning—Agar.; Am. c.; *Apis*; Azadir.; Branca; Bor.; Graph.; Helod.; Kali c.; *Lach.*; Led.; *Med.*; Nat. m.; Phos. ac.; *Phos.*; Puls.; Sec.; Sep.; Sil.; *Sul.*

Chilblains—*Abrot.*; Agar.; Petrol.; Sul.; Tamus; Zinc. m. See Skin.

Coldness—*Acon.*; Alum.; *Ars.*; *Calc. c.*; Camph.; Carbo an.; *Carbo v.*; Caust.; Chel.; Cistus; Con.; Dig.; *Dulc.*; Elaps; Helod.; Kali c.; *Lach.*; *Lyc.*; *Menyanth.*; *Mur. ac.*; Oleand.; Petrol.; *Picr. ac.*; *Plat.*; Puls.; Samb.; Scilla; *Sec.*; Sep.; *Sil.*; Sul. ac.; Sul.; Trifol.; *Ver. a.*

Coldness, clammy—Bar. c.; *Calc. c.*; Laur.; *Sep.*; Strych. p.

Coldness during day, burning soles at night—Sul.

Coldness of one, warmth of other—Chel.; *Cinch.*; Dig.; Ipec.; *Lyc.*

Enlarged feeling—Apis.

Eruptions—Bism.; Elaps; Graph.; *Petrol.* See Skin.

Fidgety—*Cina*; Kali p.; *Med.*; Sul.; Tar. h.; *Zinc. m.*; *Zinc. v.*

Itching, worse from scratching, warmth of bed—Led.; Puls.; Rhus t.

Spasmodic motion of left foot—Cina.

Tender feet with shop girls—Scilla.

HEELS—Blisters: Scilla.

Burning—Cycl.; Graph. See Feet.

Numbness—*Alum.*; Ign.

Os Calcis, pain—Aran.

Purring sensation, extending to right toes—Astrag.

PAINS—In general—*Agar.*; Am. c.; Am. m.; Brom.; *Calc. caust.*; Caul.; Caust.; Colch.; Cycl.; Ferr. m.; *Graph.*; Kali iod.; Led.; *Mang. ac.*; Nat. ars.; Nit. ac.; *Phos. ac.*; Phyt.; Ran. b.; *Rhus t.*; Sab.; Sep.; *Sil.*; Tetradyn.; Thuya; Upas; *Val.*; Zinc. m.

Aching, bruised—Agar.; Arn.; Lauy.; Led.; *Phyt.*; *Rhus t.*

Soreness—Agar.; Ant. c.; Caust.; Cepa; *Cycl.*; Jal.; Kali bich.; Med.; Phos. ac.; Phyt.; Val.

Soreness, as if stepping on pebbles—Hep.; Lyc.

Tendo-Achilles, pain—Aristol.; *Benz. ac.;* Calc. caust.; Caust.; *Cim.;* Ign.; Med.; *Mur. ac.;* Nat. ars.; Ruta; Tetradyn.; Thuya; Upas; *Val.*

Ulcerative—Am. m.; Berb. v.; *Phos. ac.;* Puls.; *Ran. b.*

Ulcers on heels—Ars.; Arundo; Cepa; Lamium.

Itching of feet—*Agar.;* Am. m.; Ant. s. a.; *Bov.;* Caust.; Magnol.; Nat. s.; Sul.; *Tellur.*

Itching, worse on scratching, warmth of bed—Led.; *Puls.;* Rhus t.

Joints, gouty, enlarged—Eucal.; Puls. nut.; Tar. c.; *Zinc. m.* See Joints.

Numbness, formication, go asleep—Æth.; Am. m.; Ars.; Calc. c.; *Carbo v.;* Cob.; *Cocc.;* Cod.; Colch.; *Con.;* Fagop.; Gels.; *Hyper.;* Lact. v.; Mag. s.; Mez.; Nux v.; Onosm.; *Physost.;* Phos.; Pyr.; *Sec.;* Sil.; Ulnus; Upas; Viola od.; *Zinc. m.*

PAINS—Aching, bruised: *Am. m.;* Arn.; Azadir.; Brom.; Dros.; Euonym.; Prun. sp.; *Ver. a.*

Cramps—Bism.; Cholas ter.; Cinch.; *Colch.; Cupr. m.;* Frax. am.; Jatropha; Lyc.; Nat. c.; *Sec.;* Sep.; Verbasc.; Zinc. m.

Lancinating—Abrot.; *Act. sp.;* Apis; Ced.; Led.; Lyc.; Nat. c.; Sep.

Rheumatic—*Act. sp.;* Apis; Berb. v.; *Caul.; Caust.; Colch.;* Graph.; *Led.; Lith. c.;* Mang. ac.; Myr.; Phyt.; *Puls.;* Ran. b.; *Rhus t.;* Ruta.

Sensibility, diminished—Carbon. s.

SOLES—Blistered: Bufo; Calc. c.; Cepa.

Burning—Anac.; Apoc. andr.; Arundo; Calc. c.; *Calc. s.;* Canth.; *Cham.;* Cupr.; Ferr. m.; Graph.; Ign.; Kreos.; *Lach.;* Lachnanth.; Limul.; Lyc.; Mang.; *Med.;* Niccol. s.; Petrol.; Phos. ac.; Puls.; *Sang.;* Sanic.; *Sul.*

Callosities—Anac. oc.; *Ant. c.;* Lyc.; Ran. b.; Sil. See Skin.

Injury, with intolerable pain—Hyper.

Itching—*Agar.;* Ananth.; Anthem.; *Calc. s.; Hydrocot.;* Indium; Nat. s.; Sil.

Numbness—*Cocc.;* Limul.; Raph.; Sep.

PAINS—In general: *Apoc. andr.;* Bor.; Can. ind.; Ferr.; *Guaco;* Kali iod.; *Led.;* Limul.; Mur. ac.; Nat. c.; Petrol.; Phos. ac.; *Puls.;* Verbasc.

Aching—Limul.; Puls.

Cramps—Agar.; Am. c.; Apoc. andr.; Carbo v.; *Colch.; Cupr.;* Med.; *Nux v.;* Stront.; Sul.; Verbasc.; Zinc.

Cramps, worse at P. M.—Cupr.; *Eug. j.;* Zing.

Pains, when walking—*Aloe;* Caust.; Graph.; Lyc.; Mur. ac.; *Petrol.;* Phos. ac.

Ulcerative, unable to walk—Canth.; Ign.; Phos.

Rawness, soreness, tenderness—Æsc.; Alum.; *Ant. c.;* Arn.; Bar. c.; *Calc. c.; Graph.;* Kali c.; *Led.;* Lyc.; *Med.;* Nat. c.; Nit. ac.; *Petrol.;* Phos. ac.; *Ruta; Sanic.;* Sil.

Swelling—Agar.; Alum.; Arundo; Calc. c.; Led.; Lyc.; Petrol. See Feet.

Ulcer—Ars.

Weakness—Hippom. See Feet.

SWEATING OF FEET—Alum.; Am. c.; *Am. m.;* Ananth.; Apoc. andr.; Arundo; Bar. ac.; *Bar. c.; Calc. c.; Carbo v.;* Cob.; *Graph.;* Iod.; Lact.

ac.; *Lyc.;* Mag. m.; *Nil. ac.;* Ol. an.; *Petrol.;* Phos. ac.; *Psor.;* Rhus t.; Sal. ac.; *Sanic.; Sep.; Sil.; Sul.; Tellur.;* Thuya; Zinc. m.

Sweating, fetid—Alum.; Am. m.; *Bar. c.; But. ac.;* Calc. c.; Graph.; Kali c.; Nit. ac.; Petrol.; *Psor.; Sanic.; Sil.;* Zinc. m.

Sweating, suppressed—*Cupr.;* Sep.; Sil.; *Sul.;* Zinc. m.

Sweating, suppressed, then throat affections—*Bar. c.;* Graph.; Psor.; Sanic.; Sil.

Sweating, with soreness of toes—Bar. c.; Iod.; Lyc.; Nit. ac.; *Petrol.;* Sanic.; *Sil.;* Zinc. m.

Swelling—*Acet. ac.;* Æsc.; Am. c.; *Apis; Ars.;* Arundo; Bry.; *Cact.;* Caust.; Cinch.; Colch.; *Dig.;* Ferr.; *Graph.; Ham.;* Helod.; Led.; Lyc.; *Merc. c.;* Merc.; Nat. m.; Nat. s.; Phos. ac.; Plumb. m.; *Prun. sp.;* Puls.; Sacchar. of.; Samb.; Sep.; Sil.; *Stroph.;* Ver. a. See Dropsy (Generalities).

Tenderness, soreness—*Ant. c.;* Arn.; Bar. c.; Cepa; Led.; Petrol.; Phos. ac.; *Sil.;* Zinc. See Pain.

Trembling—*Gels.; Phos.;* Sars.; Sep.; Stram.

Ulcer—Bar. c.

Varices—*Ferr. act.;* Ham. See Generalities.

Weakness—Acon.; *Æsc.;* Ant. c.; Ars.; Bov.; Can. s.; *Gels.;* Hippom.; Ign.; Lyc.; Mag. c.; Ran. rep.

TOES—Bunion on big toe—Agar.; *Benz. ac.;* Bor.; Hyper.; Iod.; Kali iod.; *Rhod.;* Sang.; Sars.; *Sil.;* Ver. v. See Skin.

Burning—Alum.; Sars.

Callosities—Acet. ac.; *Ant. c.;* Calc. c.; Cur.; *Ferr. picr.;* Graph.; Hyper.; Lyc.; Nit. ac.; *Ran. b.;* Ran. sc.; Semperv. t.; Sep.; *Sil.;* Sul. ac. See Skin.

Chilblains—*Nit. ac.;* Sal. ac. See Skin.

Coldness—Sul.

Cracks of skin—Eug. j.; *Graph.; Petrol.;* Sabad.; Sars.

Crooked—Graph.

Crushed, with intolerable pain—Hyper.

Festering—Graph.

Itching—*Agar.;* Kali c.; Maland.

Joints inflamed—Am. c.; *Benz. ac.;* Bor.; Bothrops; Carbo v.; *Colch.;* Daphne; *Led.; Rhod.;* Teucr. See Joints.

Nails, deformed, thick—Ant. c.; Graph.; Sil.

Nails, inflamed—Sabad.

Nails, ingrowing—*Caust.;* Graph.; Hep.; Mag. p.; *Mag. pol. aust.; Nit. ac.; Sil.;* Staph.; Teucr.; Thuya.

Nails, pain around—Ant. c.; *Fluor. ac.;* Hep.; Nit. ac.; Teucr.

Numbness—Con.; Nat. m.; Phos.; Sil.; Sul.; *Thall.*

PAINS—Big toe: Am. c.; Ars.; Bar. c.; Calc. c.; Elat.; Eup. perf.; Kali c.; Led.; Plumb. m.; Prim. c.; Sep.; Sil.

Cramps—*Cupr. ac.;* Cupr. m.; Dig.; *Diosc.;* Hyos.; Lyc.; Rhus t.; Sec.; Sep.; Sul.

Rheumatic—*Act. sp.;* Apoc. andr.; *Benz. ac.;* Bor.; Bothrops; *Caul.;*

Caust.; *Colch.*; Daphne; *Gnaph.*; Hyper.; Kali c.; *Led.*; *Lith. c.*; Nit. ac.; Pæonia; Phos. ac.; *Puls.*; Sab.; *Sil.* See Gout.

Rheumatic, in big toe—Am. benz.; Arn.; *Benz. ac.*; Bor.; Bothrops; *Colch.*; Conv.; Gnaph.; Kali c.; *Led.*; Rhod.; Sil.

Rheumatic, in tips of toes—Am. m.; *Hyper.*; Kali c.; *Sil.*; Syph.

Tearing—*Act. sp.*; Am. m.; Benz. ac.; Brom.; *Caul.*; *Colch.*; Pall.; Sil.; Syph.

Soreness—Bar. c.; Brom.; Nat. ars.; Phos. ac. See Feet.

Stiffness—*Caul.*; Graph.; Led.; Sec. See Joints.

Ulcer of big toe—Sil.

Ulcer, pemphigus—*Ars.*; Graph.; Petrol.; Sep.

Wheals, eroding—Sul.

GAIT—Agility: Coff.

Ataxic—*Arg. n.*; Bell.; Helod.; Ign.; Nux v.; *Sec.*; *Sulphon.* See Locomotor Ataxia (Nervous System).

Sluggish, slow—Gels.; Phos. ac.; Phos.

Spastic; knees knock against each other when walking—Lathyr.

Staggering, unsteady, difficult walking—Acon.; *Agar.*; Agrost.; Angust.; *Arg. n.*; Asar.; Aster.; Astrag.; *Bell.*; Calc. p.; *Carbon. s.*; *Caust.*; *Cocc.*; Colch.; *Con.*; Dub.; *Gels.*; Helod.; Ign.; Lact. ac.; *Lathyr.*; Lil. t.; Lcl.; Mang. ac.; Merc.; Morph.; Mur. ac.; *Myg.*; Nat. c.; Nux m.; *Nux v.*; Onosm.; *Oxytr.*; Pæonia; Phos. ac.; *Phos.*; Rhus t.; *Sec.*; Sep.; Stram.; Sulphon.; Tab.; Trion.; *Zinc. m.*

Staggering, unsteady, when unobserved—Arg. n.

Staggering, unsteady, when walking in dark, or with eyes closed—*Alum.*; *Arg. n.*; Carbon. s.; Dub.; *Gels.*; Iodof.; *Stram.*

Staggering, unsteady, with muscular inco-ordination—Alum.; Arag.; Arg. n.; Aster.; Astrag.; *Bar. m.*; Bell.; Cocc.; *Gels.*; Kali br.; Med.; Onosm.; Phos. ac.; *Physost.*; Picr. ac.; Plumb.; Sec.; Sil.; Trion.; *Zinc. m.*

Walking backward—Oxytr.

Walking backward, on metacarpo-phalangeal joint—Mang. ac.

Walking, child slow to learn—Bar. c.; Calc. c.; Calc. p.; Caust.; Nat. m.; Sil.

When walking, drags feet—*Myg.*; Nux v.; Tab.

When walking, foot shoots out, or turns—Acon.

When walking, heels do not touch ground—Lathyr.

When walking, joints feel painfully tense, as from ham-strings shortened—Am. m.; Caust.; Cimex.

When walking, legs feel heavy as lead—Med.

When walking, legs feel as if made of wood, or glass—Thuya.

When walking, legs involuntarily thrown forward—Merc.

When walking, lifts feet higher than usual, and brings them down hard—Helod.

When walking, limps involuntarily—Bell.

When walking, must stoop—Arn.; *Lathyr.*; Mang. ac.; Phos.; Sul.

When walking on uneven ground, very difficult—Lil. t.

When walking or standing, suddenly falling to ground—Mag. c.

When walking, seems to be walking on air—Dub.; Lac c.

When walking, stumbles easily, makes missteps—Agar.; Phos. ac.

When walking, tendency to fall forward; falls when walking backward—Mang. ac.

When walking, trembles all over—Lact. ac.

JOINTS—Burning:—Apis; Ars.; *Caust.*; Colch.; Mang. ac.; Merc.; *Rhus t.;* Sul.

Bursæ—Benz. ac.; Kali m.; *Ruta;* Sil.

Contraction, painful, of tendons, hamstrings—Abrot.; *Am. m.; Caust.; Cimex;* Col.; Formica; *Guaiac.;* Kali iod.; *Nat. m.; Tellur.*

Cracking, on motion—Acon.; Angust.; *Benz. ac.;* Calc. fl.; Camph.; *Caust.;* Cocc.; Gins.; *Graph.;* Kali bich.; Kali m.; Led.; Nat. m.; *Nat. p.; Nit. ac.;* Petrol.; Thuya; Zinc. m.

Dropsy (hydarthrosis)—*Apis;* Bov.; Canth.; Chin. s.; Cinch.; Iod.

Hysterical joints—*Arg. n.;* Cham.; Cotyled.; Hyper.; *Ign.;* Zinc. m.

Inflammation (ARTHRITIS)—Acute: Abrot.; *Acon.;* Arbut.; Benz. ac.; Berb. v.; *Bry.;* Caust.; Cim.; Cinch.; *Colch.;* Gnaph.; *Guaiac.;* Iod.; Kali bich.; Kali iod.; Kal.; *Led.;* Lil. t.; Lith. c.; Mang. ac.; *Merc.;* Nat. sil.; Nit. ac.; Phyt.; *Puls.;* Radium; Rhod.; *Rhus t.;* Sab.; Sal. ac.; Solid.; *Stellar.;* Sul. tereb.; Viola tr. See Rheumatism.

Inflammation, chronic (arthritis deformans)—Am. phos.; Ant. c.; Arbut.; Arn.; *Ars.;* Benz. ac.; Calc. c.; Calc. ren.; Caul.; *Caust.;* Cim.; Cinch.; Colch.: Colchicine; Ferr. iod.; Ferr. picr.; *Guaiac.; Iod.; Kali br.; Kali iod.;* Lact. ac.; Led.; Lyc.; Merc. c.; Nat. br.; Nat. p.; Nat. s.; *Piperaz.; Puls.;* Radium; Sab.; Sal. ac.; Sep.; Sul.; *Sul. tereb.;* Thyr.

Inflammation—GOUT—Abrot ; *Acon.; Am. benz.;* Apis; *Arn.; Ars.;* Aur. mur.; Aur. m. n.; Bell.; *Benz. ac.;* Berb. v.; *Bry.; Cajup.;* Calc. c.; Carls.; Cham.; *Chin. s.; Cinch.; Colch.; Colchicine;* Cupr.; Daphne; Dulc.; Ferr. picr.; Formica; *Guaiac.;* Irid.; Jabor.; Kali bich.; Kali iod.; Kal.; *Led.; Lith. c.; Lyc.;* Mang. ac.; Med.; *Merc. s.;* Nat. lact.; Nat. m.; Nat. sal.; Nux v ; Ox. ac.; Pancreat.; Phyt.; *Puls.;* Querc.; Rhod.; Rhus t.; *Sab.;* Sil.; Spig.; Stellar.; *Sul.;* Taxus; *Uric ac.;* Urt.

Debility after attack—Bellis; Cyprip.

Gout of chest—Colch.

Gout of eyes—Nux v.

Gout of hands, feet, little swelling, subacute—Led.

Gout of heart—Aur. mur.; Cact.; Conv.; Cupr. m.; Kal.

Gout of nerves (neuralgia)—*Colch.;* Col.; Sul.

Gout of stomach—Hydroc. ac.; Nux m.; Nux v.; Puls.

Gout of throat—Colch.; Merc. s.

Metastases to heart—Colch.; Kal.

Metastases to stomach—Ant. c.; Nux v.

Nervous restlessness—Ign.

Retrocedent or suppressed—*Cajup.;* Nat. m.; Ox. ac.; Rhus t.

Sub-acute—Guaiac.; *Led.;* Puls.

Uterine disorders—Sab.

Inflammation-SYNOVITIS—Acute: Acon.; *Apis;* Arn.; *Bell.;* Berb. v.; *Bry.;* Canth.; Fluor. ac.; Hep.; *Iod.;* Led.; *Puls.; Rhus t.;* Ruta; *Sab.; Sil.;* Slag; Sticta.

Inflammation, chronic—*Am. phos.; Benz. ac.; Berb. v.;* Calc. c.; Calc. fl.; Calc. p.; Caust.; Hep.; *Iod.; Kali iod.; Merc. s.;* Phyt.; Puls.; *Rhus t.; Ruta;* Sil.; Staph.; *Stellar.;* Sul.; Tub.

Itching in bends of joints—Phos. ac.

Lameness—Abrot.; Cepa; *Rhus t.;* Ruta; Sul. See Stiffness.

NODOSITIES, tophi—Agn.; Am. benz.; *Am. phos.;* Ant. c.; Aur.; *Benz. ac.;* Berb. v.; Calc. c.; *Calc. ren.;* Caul.; Caust.; Cim.; *Colch.;* Elat.; Eucal.; Eup. perf.; Formica; Graph.; Guaiac.; *Hekla;* Iod.; Kali ars.; *Kali iod.: Kali sil.:* Led.; *Lith. c.; Lyc.;* Med.; Nat. lact.; Nat. ureat.; Piperaz.; Rhod.; Ruta; *Sab.; Staph.;* Sul.; Urea; Uric ac.

PAINS—In general: Am. c.; Am. m.; *Arg. m.;* Bar. c.; *Bry.; Calc. p.;* Ced.; Diosc.; Dros.; Euonym.; *Iod.;* Kreos.; Lappa; Mang.; Sil.; Sul.; Zinc. m.

Bruised—*Arn.;* Bry.; Hyper.; Kal.; Mez.; *Rhus t.;* Ruta.

Cutting—Acon.; Bry.; *Caul.;* Cim.; Kal.

Digging at P. M.—Kali iod.; Mang. ac.; *Merc. s.*

Drawing, tensive—*Aloe;* Am. c.; Am. m.; Apoc. andr.; Caust.; Cimex; Cinch.; *Colch.; Gins.;* Mez.; *Puls.; Rhus t.; Sul.*

Neuralgic—Arg. m.; *Ced.;* Col.; Plumb.; Zinc. m.

Rheumatic—Abrot.; *Acon.;* Asclep. t.; Benz. ac.; Berb. v.; *Bry.; Caul.;* Caust.; Cim.; Cinch.; *Colch.;* Dig.; Diosc.; Ferr.; Formica; *Guaiac.;* Iod.; Kali bich.; *Kal.;* Lact. ac.; Led.; *Merc. s.;* Pinus sylv.; *Puls.; Radium;* Rham. c.; Rhod.; *Rhus t.; Ruta; Sab.;* Salol; Staph.; Stront. See Rheumatism.

Soreness, tenderness—*Acon.;* Am. m.; Apis; *Arn.;* Bell.; Bellis; *Bry.; Colch.;* Guaiac.; *Ham.;* Hep.; Kal.; Led.; Lith. c.; Meli.; *Phyt.;* Puls.; *Rhus t.;* Sab.; Sticta; Ver. a.; *Verbasc.*

Stitching, tearing, shifting, erratic—Apis; Benz. ac.; *Bry.;* Caust.; *Cim.;* Cinch.; *Colch.;* Guaiac.; Kali iod.; *Kal.;* Led.; Lith. c.; Magnol.; *Merc. s.;* Phos. ac.; *Puls.; Rhus t.;* Sul.; Ver. v.

Stiffness—Abrot.; Angust.; Apis; Apoc. andr.; Arn.; Asclep. t.; Bar. m.; *Bry.;* Caul.; *Caust.; Colch.;* Col.; Diosc.; Formica; *Gins.; Guaiac.;* Iod.; *Kali iod.;* Lyc.; Magnol.; Med.; *Merc. s.;* Mez.; Nux v.; Ol. j. as.; Petrol.; *Phyt.;* Pinus sylv.; *Rhus t.;* Sep.; *Stellar.;* Strych.; *Sul.;* Thiosin.; Triost.; Verbasc.

Swelling—Abrot.; *Acon.; Act. sp.;* Anag.; *Apis;* Ars.; *Bell.;* Benz. ac.; *Bry.;* Caust.; Cinch.; *Colch.;* Dig.; *Guaiac.;* Iod.; *Kali m.;* Kal.; Led.; *Lith. c.;* Mang. ac.; Med.; *Merc. s.; Phyt.; Puls.;* Rham. c.; Rhod.; *Rhus t.;* Sab.; *Stellar.;* Sticta.

Swelling, dark red—Bry.; Kal.; *Rhus t.*

Swelling, pale, white—*Apis;* Aur.; Bry.; *Calc. c.;* Calc. p.; Cistus; *Colch.;* Con.; Dig.; Iod.; Led.; *Merc. c.; Merc. s.;* Phos. ac.; Phos.; *Puls.;* Rhod.; *Sil.;* Sul.; Symphyt.; Tub. See Knee.

Swelling, shining—*Acon.; Apis; Bell.; Bry.;* Dig.; Mang. ac.; Sab.

Ulceration of cartilages—Merc. c.

Weakness—Acon.; Bar. m.; Bov.; *Carbo an.; Caust.;* Cinch.; Euphorb.; Hippom.; *Led.; Phos.;* Psor.; Mez.; *Rhus t.;* Zing.

Weakness, sprained easily—Carbo an.; Hep.; Led.

ANKLES—Itching: Puls.; Rhus t.; Selen.

Itching, worse from scratching, warmth of bed—Led.

Pain in general—Abrot.; Alum.; Am. c.; But. ac.; Caust.; Euonym.; Lappa; Lathyr.; Nat. m.; Sil.; Tetradyn.; Verbasc.; *Viscum.*

Bruised, dislocated feeling—Bry.; Led.; Prun. sp.; *Ruta;* Sil.; Sul.

Rheumatic—Abrot.; *Act. sp.; Caul.;* Caust.; Colch.; Guaco; Guaiac.; *Led.;* Mang. ac.; Mang. mur.; Med.; *Prophyl.; Puls.;* Radium; *Rhod.; Ruta;* Sil.; Stellar.; Sul.; Urt.

Sprains—Carbo an.; *Led.;* Nat. ars.; *Nat. c.; Ruta;* Stront. c.

Sprains, chronic—Bov.; *Stront. c.*

Stiffness—Kali c.; Med.; Sep.; Sul.; Zinc. m.

Swelling—Apis; *Arg. n.;* Ferr.; Ham.; *Led.;* Lyc.; Med.; Mimosa; Plumb.; Stann.; Stront. c. See Dropsy.

Ulcer, itching—Sul.

Weakness, "foot turns under"—Calc. c.; *Calc. p.; Carbo an.; Caust.; Cham.;* Ham.; *Led.;* Mang. ac.; Mang. mur.; Med.; *Nat. ars.; Nat. c.;* Nat. m.; Phos.; *Pinus sylv.; Ruta;* Sil.; Sul.

ELBOWS—Numbness: Puls.

Pains—Ant. c.; *Arg. m.;* Ars.; *Caust.;* Cinnab.; Colch.; *Ferr. mur.;* Guaco; Kali c.; *Kal.; Lyc.; Menisp.;* Ol. j. as.; Phos.; Solan. lyc.; Sul.; *Viscum;* Zinc. ox.

HIPS—Morbus Coxarius: Diseases of: Acon.; *Arg. m.;* Ars.; Ars. iod.; Calc. c.; Calc. hyphos.; Calc. iod.; *Calc. p.; Caust.;* Cinch.; *Cistus; Col.;* Ferr. m.; Ferr. p.; Fluor. ac.; Hep.; Hippoz.; Hyper.; Iod.; *Kali c.; Kali iod.;* Merc. i. r.; Merc.; *Phos. ac.;* Phos.; Rhus t.; *Sil.;* Staph.; Still.; *Sul.;* Tub. See Coxalgia.

Luxation—Col.

Pain (coxalgia)—*Æsc.;* Allium s.; Arg. m.; *Ars.;* Berb. v.; *Bry.;* Calc. c.; *Calc. p.;* Carbo an.; Caust.; Cham.; Chel.; Cistus; Colch.; *Col.;* Con.; Dros.; Elat.; Ferr. m.; Formica; *Gels.;* Glycerin; Guaco; *Hyper.;* Kali c.; *Kali iod.;* Led.; Lil. t.; Limul.; Lyc.; Mag. mur.; Mez.; Murex; Nat. m.; Nat. s.; Nux m.; *Puls.;* Radium; Solan. n.; *Stram.;* Thuya; Tongo; Tromb.

Pain, as if broken; as if pelvis was falling apart—Æsc.; *Trill.*

Pain, as if sprained—*Æsc.;* Am. m.; *Calc. p.;* Caust.; *Col.;* Laur.; Nat. m.; *Puls.;* Rhus t.; Sarrac.

Pain, in left hip—Am. m.; Col.; Irid.; Ov. g. p.; Sang.; Solan. n.; *Stram.*

Pain, in right hip—Agar.; Ant. t.; *Chel.;* Graph.; Kali c.; Led.; *Lil. t.;* Limul.; Nux m.; Pall.; Stram.

KNEES—Coldness: Agn.; Apis; Calc. c.; *Carbo v.;* Nat. c. See Extremities·

Cracking, on motion—*Benz. ac.;* Caust.; *Cocc.;* Croc.; Diosc.; Nat. ars.; Nux v.

Dislocation of patella, on going upstairs—Can. s.

Dropsy—Caust.; Ced.; Iod.

Herpes—Carbo v.; Graph.; Petrol.

Hygroma patella—Arn.; Calc. p.; *Iod.*

Inflammation (synovitis, bursitis: housemaid's knee): **Acute:** *Acon.; Apis;* Arn.; Bell.; *Bry.;* Canth.; Cistus; Helleb.; *Hep.;* Iod.; **Kali** c.; *Kali iod.;* Phos.; *Puls.;* *Rhus t.;* Ruta; *Sil.;* *Slag; Sticta;* Sul. See Swelling.

Inflammation, chronic—Ant. t.; *Benz. ac.;* Berb. v.; *Calc. fl.;* Calc. p.; Hep.; *Iod.; Kali iod.; Merc. s.;* Phyt.; Rhus t.; Ruta; *Sil.;* Tub.

Numbness—Carbo v.; Meli.

Numbness, extends to scrotum, relieved by sitting—Bar. c.

PAINS—**In general:** Angust.; *Apis;* Bell.; Benz. ac.; *Berb. v.;* Calc. c.; Can. ind.; Diosc.; *Elaps;* Kali iod.; Keros.; Lappa; Mag. m.; *Meli.;* Mez.; Mur. ac.; Phos.; Sul.; Xerophyl.

Aching—Anac.; Con.; Led.; *Meli.;* Ol. j. as.

Boring, relieved by walking—Indigo.

Bruised—Ars.; *Berb. v.;* Bry.; Sarrac.

Digging, in left knee—Aur.; Caust.; Col.; Rhus t.; Spig.; Tarax.

Drawing—Calc. c.; Mag. m.; Mur. ac.; Phos.; Sul.

Rheumatic—Arg. m.; *Benz. ac.;* Berb. v.; *Bry.; Cinch.;* Cop.; Daphne; Elaps; Diosc.; *Dulc.;* Guaiac.; Jacar.; *Kali c.; Kali iod.; Lact. ac.; Led.; Mang. ac.:* Meli.; *Merc.;* Nat. p.; *Puls.;* Puls. nut.; Radium; Sab.; Sticta; Viscum.

Tearing—Calc. c.; *Caust.;* Col.; Granat.; Lyc.; *Merc.;* Petrol.; Sticta; Tarax.; Tongo; Ver. v.

Tensive, crampy—Anac.; Caps.; Lathyr.; Pæonia; *Puls.;* Sil.; *Verbasc.*

POPLITEAL SPACE, Itching—Lyc.; Sep.

Popliteal space, pain—Caust.; Lyc.; Physost.; Radium.

Popliteal space, prurigo—Ars.

REFLEXES—**Diminished, lost:** *Cur.;* Oxytr.; Plumb. m.; *Sec.;* Sulphon.

Reflexes increased—Anhal.; Can. ind.; Lathyr.; Mang. ac. See Nervous System.

Stiffness of knees—*Berb. v.; Bry.;* Lyc.; Mimosa; Petrol.; Sep.; Sul.

Swelling—*Apis;* Arn.; Bell.; Benz. ac.; Berb. v.; *Bry.; Calc. c.; Cinch.;* Cocc.; *Kali iod.;* Lyc.; Mag. c.; *Rhod.;* Sal. ac.; Sil.

Swelling, white—Acon.; *Apis;* Arn.; *Calc. c.;* Calc. p.; *Cistus; Kali iod.;* Led.; Phos. ac.; Phos.; *Puls.;* Rhus t.; Sil.; Slag; *Sticta;* Sul.; Tub.

Tenderness—Apis; Berb. v.; *Bry.;* Cinch.; *Rhus t.* See Joints.

Ulceration of cartilage—Merc. d.

Weakness—Acon.; Anac.; Aur.; *Cob.; Cocc.;* Diosc.; Hippom.; Lact. ac.; Nat. m.; Nit. ac.; Sul.

SHOULDERS-SCAPULÆ—**Deltoid, pain, rheumatism:** Ferr. p.; Glycerin; Lycopers.; Med.; Nux m.; Ox. ac.; Rhus t.; *Sang.:* Sticta; *Syph.;* Urt.; Viola od.; Zinc. ox.; Zing.

PAINS—**In general:** Alum.; *Am. phos.;* Anag.; Arn.; Azadir.; Bar. c.; Can. ind.; *Chel.;* Cocc.; Con.; Fagop.; Jugl. r.; Kreos.; Lyc.; Menisp.; Myr.; Nat. ars.; Nat. c.; Nit. ac.; *Ran. b.;* Sep.; Ver. a.; Viscum.

Pain, between scapulæ—Æsc.; Ars.; Bry.; Camph.; *Chenop.:* Euonym.; Granat.; Guaiac.; Mag. s.

Pain burning, in small spots—Agar.; *Phos.;* Ran. b.; *Sul.*

Pain, drawing—Ars.; Berb. v.; Cham.; Col.; Sul.

Pain, in left—*Acon.;* Æsc.; *Agar.;* Ant. t.; *Aspar.;* Cham.; Chenop. gl.;

Col.; Eup. purp.; Ferr. m.; Led.; Lob. syph.; Nux m.; *Onosm.;* Rhodium; Stram.; Sul.

Pain, in left, lower angle—*Chenop. gl.;* Cupr. ars.; Ran. b.

Pain, in right—Abies c.; Am. m.; Bry.; *Chel.;* Chenop. gl.; *Col.;* Ferr. p.; Ferr. mur.; *Guaeo;* Ichthy.; Ipomœa; Jugl. c.; *Kali c.;* Kal.; Mag. c.; Pall.; Phyt.; Puls. nut.; Ran. b.; *Sang.;* Solan. lyc.; *Sticta;* Stront. ; *Urt.*

Pain, in right, lower angle—*Chel.;* Chenop. anth.; Kali c.; *Merc.;* Pod.

Pains, rheumatic—Acon.; Am. caust.; *Berb. v.;* Bry.; Colch.; Ferr. mur.; *Ferr. p.;* Guaiac.; Ham.; *Kali c.;* Kal.; Lact. ac.; *Led.;* Lith. c.; *Lith. lact.;* Med.; Ol. an.; Pall.; *Phyt.;* Prim.; Radium; *Ran. b.;* Rhod.; *Rhus t.; Sang.;* Stellar.; *Sticta;* Stront.; Sul.; Syph.; Urt.; Viola od.

Pains, worse singing, using voice—Stann.

Stitches, tearing—Am. m.; *Bry.;* Hyper.; Kali c.; Lyc.; Mag. c.; Nit. ac.

Stiffness—Cocc.; *Dulc.;* Granat.; Indium; *Phyt.;* Prim. v.; *Sang.;* Senec. jac.

WRISTS—Ganglion, on back: *Benz. ac.;* Calc. fl.; Phos.; Rhus t.; *Ruta; Sil.;* Thuya.

Gouty deposits—Calc. c.; Ruta.

PAINS—In general: Abrot.; *Act. sp.;* Am. c.; Bism.; Carbo an.; *Caul.;* Chel.; *Hippom.; Kali c.;* Nat. p.; Pæonia; *Prophyl.;* Rhod.; *Ruta;* Sep.; Sil.; Sul.; Urt.; *Viola od.*

Cramps, spasms, painful (writer's cramp)—*Arg. m.;* Arn.; Bell.; Bellis; *Caust.; Con.; Cupr.;* Cycl.; Ferr. iod.; *Gels.; Mag. p.;* Nux v.; Picr. ac.; Ran. b.; *Ruta;* Sec.; Sil.; *Stann.;* Staph.; *Strych.;* Sul. ac.; Viola od.; Zinc. m.

Rheumatic—Abrot.; *Act. sp.;* Benz. ac.; Calc. c.; *Caul.; Caust.;* Colch.; Hippom.; Lact. ac.; Lyc.; Prophyl.; *Rhod.;* Rhus t.; Rhus v.; *Ruta;* Sab.; Sep.; Solan. lyc.; Stellar.; Ulnus; Variol.; *Viola od.;* Wyeth.

Sprained, dislocated feeling—Bry.; Cistus; *Eup. perf.; Hippom.;* Ox. ac.; *Rhus t.; Ruta;* Ulnus.

Paralysis—*Con.; Cur.;* Hippom.; *Plumb. ac.; Plumb. m.;* Picr. ac.; Ruta; Stann. See Nervous System.

NECK—Burning: Guaco.

Cracking of cervical vertebræ, on motion—Aloe; *Cocc.; Nat. c.;* Niccol.; Ol. an.; Thuya.

Emaciation—Nat. m. See Generalities.

Eruption—Anac.; Clem.; Lyc.; Nat. m.; Petrol.; *Sep.*

Fullness, must loosen collar—*Amyl;* Fel tauri; *Glon.; Lach.;* Pyr.; Sep.

Itching—Ant. c.

Muscles, cervical, contraction, rigidity—*Cic.;* Cim.; Nicot.; *Strych.*

Muscles, cervical, shooting—Sul. ac.

Muscles, cervical, twitching—Agar.

Muscles, sterno-cleido-mastoid—*Gels.;* Rhod.; Tarax.; Trifol. See Torticollis.

NAPE OF NECK: PAINS—In general: Acon.; Æsc.; Am. c.; *Bell.;* Chin. ars.; *Cim.;* Col.; Fel tauri; Ferr. picr.; *Gels.;* Graph.; Hyper.; Jugl.

c.; Lach.; Lyc.; Myr.; *Nat. cholein;* Nat. s.; Paris; Ver. a.; Vib. op.; X-ray; Zinc. v.

Aching—Adon. v.; Æsc.; Angust.; Bapt.; Caust.; *Con.; Gels.; Guaiac.:* Paris; Radium; Ver. v.; Ver. v.; Zinc. m.

Dislocated, bruised feeling—Bell.; Caust.; Fagop.; *Lachnanth.*

Rheumatic—Acon.; *Bry.;* Calc. p.; Caust.; *Cim.;* Colch.; *Dulc.; Guaiac.;* Iod.; Kali iod.; *Lachnanth.:* Petrol.; Puls.; Radium; Rhod.; *Rhus t.;* Sang.; Stellar.; *Sticta.*

Tearing, shooting, stitching—*Acon.;* Asar.; Bad.; Bar. c.; Bell.; *Berb. v.; Bry.;* Chin. ars.; Colch.; Ferr. picr.; *Mag. p.;* Nux v.; *Strych.;* Xanth.

Tension—Con.; Sep.; Sul.; Tub.

Tensive numbness—Plat.

Stiffness—*Acon.;* Ant. t.; Bell.; *Bry.;* Calc. c.; Calc. caust.; Calc. p.; *Caust.;* Cham.; Chel.; *Cim.;* Cocc.; Colch.; *Dulc.;* Ferr. p.; Gels.; Guaiac.; Hyper.; Jugl. c.; Kali c.; Lac c.; *Lachnanth.;* Lyc.; Mag. c.; Med.; Menthol; *Merc. i. r.;* Nicot.; Nit. ac.; Nux v.; Pampin.; Petrol.; Phos.; Phyt.; *Puls.;* Radium; Rhodium; Rhod.; Rhus v.; Sep.; Stellar.; *Sticta;* Sul.; Trifol.; Vinca m.; X-ray.

Swelling—Calc. c.; Iod.; Lyc.; Phos.; Sil.

Tenderness—Amyl; *Bry.;* Cim.; Kali perm.; *Lach.;* Tarax.

Tumor, fatty—Bar. c.

Veins, swollen—Op.

Weakness, unable to hold head up—*Abrot.;* Æth.; Colch.; Fagop.; Kali c.; Sil. See Head.

Wry neck (torticollis)—*Acon.;* Agar.; Atrop.; *Bell.;* Bry.; *Cim.; Colch.;* Guaiac.; Hyos.; Ign.; *Lachnanth.;* Lyc.; Mag. p.; Myg.; Nux v.; Strych.; Thuya.

RHEUMATISM: TYPE—Articular, acute, **RHEUMATIC FEVER:** *Acon.;* Agar.; Am. benz.; Am. caust.; Ant. t.; *Apis; Arn.;* Ars.; *Bell.;* Benz. ac.; Berb. v.; *Bry.; Cact.; Calc. c.;* Calc. p.; Camph.; *Cascara; Cham.; Chin. s.; Cim.;* Cinch.; Clem.; *Colch.; Colchicine;* Col.; *Dulc.; Eup. perf.; Ferr. p.;* Formica; Franciscea; Gaulth.; Gels.; Gins.; *Guaiac.;* Ham.; Hymosa; *Kali bich.;* Kali c.; Kali iod.; Kali m.; Kal.; *Led.;* Lyc.; Macrot.; Merc. s.; *Merc. v.;* Methyl. sal.; Nat. lact.; Nat. sal.; Nux v.; Nyctanth.; Ox. ac.; Petrol.; Phyt.; *Prophyl.; Puls.;* Ran. b.; *Rham. c.;* Rhod.; *Rhus t.;* Ruta; Sal. ac.; Sang.; Spig.; *Stellar.;* Sticta; Still.; Strych.; *Sul.;* Syph.; Thuya; Tilia; Ver. a.; *Ver. v.; Viola od.*

Ascending pains—Arn.; *Led.*

Descending pains—Cact.; *Kal.*

Erratic, wandering pains—Apoc. andr.; *Caul.;* Cim.; Colch.; Kali bich.; Kal.; Kali s.; *Lac c.;* Mang.; Phyt.; *Puls.;* Puls. nut.; Rhod.; *Stellar.;* Sul.

Fibrous tissues (sheaths, tendons)—Arn.; Formic acid; Gettysburg Water; Phyt.; Rhod.; *Rhus t.*

Joints, large—*Acon.;* Arbut.; Arg. m.; Asclep. s.; *Bry.;* Dros.; *Merc.;* Mimosa; Rhus t.; Sticta; Ver. v.

Joints, small—*Act. sp.;* Benz. ac.; Bry.; *Caul.; Colch.;* Kali bich.; Lact. ac.; *Led.;* Lith. c.; Lith. lact.; *Puls.;* Rhod.; Ruta; *Sab.;* Viola od.

Mono-articular—Acon.; Apis; *Bry.;* Caust.; Cinch.; Cop.; *Merc.* See Joints.

Poly-articular—Arn.; *Bry.;* Guaiac.; *Puls.* See Erratic Pains.

CONCOMITANTS—**Alternates with diarrhœa, dysentery:** *Abrot.; Dulc.;* Gnaph.; *Kali bich.*

Alternates, with indigestion—Kali bich.

Alternates, with urticaria—Urt.

Auricular fibrillation following—Dig.

Debility—*Ars.;* Calc. p.; Chin. s.; *Cinch.; Colch.;* Ferr. carb.; Sul.

Fever, adynamic—Bry.; *Rhus t.*

Fever, remittent—Chin. s.

Metastases, to brain—Bell.; Op.

Metastases, to heart—Adon. v.; Avena; Cact.; *Kal.;* Lith. c.; Prophyl.; *Spig.*

Mild cases, in nervous persons—Viola od.

Nervousness, intense pains—Cham.; Coff.; Rhus t.

Numbness—Acon.; Cham.; Led.; *Rhus t.*

Restlessness—*Acon.;* Caust.; Cim.; Puls.; *Rhus t.*

Secretions checked—Abrot.

Sensitiveness to cold—Led.; *Merc.*

Sleeplessness—Bell.; Calc. c.; Coff.; Ign.

Skin diseases, acute, after—Dulc.

Sweating—*Calc. c.;* Hep.; Lact. ac.; *Merc.;* Rham. c.; Sal. ac.; Tilia.

Urticarial eruption—Urt.

AGGRAVATIONS—**At night:**—*Acon.;* Arn.; Cham.; *Cim.; Colch.;* Eucal.; *Kali iod.;* Kali m.; *Kal.;* Lact. ac.; Led.; *Merc.;* Phyt.; *Puls.;* Rhod.; Rhus t.; Sars.; Sil.; *Sul.*

Before storm—Puls.; *Rhod.;* Rhus t.

Colchicum, abuse—Led.

Crosswise, side to side—Lac c.

Every other day—Cinch.

From cold, dry weather—*Acon.;* Bry.; Caust.; Nux m.; *Rhod.*

From damp, wet weather—Arn.; Ars.; *Calc. p.;* Cim.; *Colch.; Dulc.;* Kali iod.; *Merc.;* Nat. s.; Nux m.; *Phyt.;* Ran. b.; *Rhod.; Rhus t.;* Sars.; Ver. a.

From melting snow—Calc. p.

From motion—Act. sp.; Apis; *Arn.; Bry.; Calc. c.;* Cim.; Clem.; *Cinch.,* Colch.; Formica; Gettysburg Water; Guaiac.; Iod.; *Kali m.;* Kal.; Lac c.; Led.; *Merc.;* Nux v.; Phyt.; Ran. b.; Sal. ac.; *Stellar.*

From rest—Euphorb.; Puls.; Rhod.; *Rhus t.*

From sweating—Hep.; *Merc.;* Tilia.

From touch—Act. sp.; Acon.; Apis; *Arn.;* Bry.; *Cinch.; Colch.;* Iod.; Lac c.; Ran. b.; Rhus t.; Sal. ac.

From warmth—Cham.; Kali m.; *Led.; Merc.; Puls.*

AMELIORATIONS—**From motion, walking:**—Cham.; Cinch.; Dulc.; Ferr. m.; Lyc.; *Puls.;* Rhod.; *Rhus t.;* Ver. a.

From pressure—Bry.; Formica.

From rest—Bry.; Gettysburg Water.

From warmth—*Ars.;* Bry.; Caust.; Kali bich.; Nux m.; Rhus t.; *Sil.*

From water, cold to feet—*Led.;* Sec.

In damp weather—Caust.

In open air—Kali m.; Puls.

ARTICULAR, CHRONIC—*Am. phos.;* Ant. c.; Anthrok.; Benz. ac.; Berb. v.; *Bry.;* Calc. c.; *Calc. caust.;* Carbon. s.; Caul.; *Caust.;* Cim.; Colch.; *Dulc.;* Euonym.; Ferr.; Guaiac.; Hep.; Iod.; Kali bich.; Kali c.; *Kali iod.;* Led.; *Lith. c.;* Lyc.; Med.; Merc.; Mez.; *Ol. j. as.;* Petrol.; Phyt.; *Puls.;* Rhod.; *Rhus t.;* Ruta; Sil.; *Stellar.;* Still.; *Sul.;* Sul. tereb.; Taxus. See Joints.

ARTHRITIS DEFORMANS—Arbut.; *Arn.; Ars.;* Benz. ac ; Calc. c.; Caps.; Caul.; *Caust.; Cim.; Colch.;* Colchicine; *Dulc.;* Ferr. iod.; Ferr. picr.; *Guaiac.; Iod.;* Kali c.; *Kali iod.;* Lact. ac.; Led.; Lyc.; Mang. ac.; Methyl. bl.; *Merc. c.;* Nat. p.; Pip. menth.; *Puls.;* Rhod.; *Sab.;* Sal. ac.; Sep.; *Sul.;* Sul. tereb.; Thymus Ext.; Thyr. See Joints.

Chronic, secondary to uterine disorder—Caul.; *Cim.; Puls.;* Sab.

Gonorrhœal—Acon.; *Arg. m.;* Arn.; Bry.; Caust.; Cim.; Clem.; Cop.; *Daphne;* Guaiac.; Iod.; *Irisin;* Jacar.; Kali bich.; Kali iod.; Kal.; *Med.;* Merc.; Nat. s.; Phyt.; *Puls.;* Rhus t.; *Sars.;* Sul.; *Thuya.*

Intercostal—Arn.; *Cim.;* Phyt.; *Ran. b.;* Rhus t.

Muscular (myalgia)—*Acon.;* Ant. t.; Apis; Arn.; *Bry.;* Calc. c.; *Cascara;* Caust.; Chin. s.; *Cim.;* Cinch.; Colch.; Dulc.; *Ferr.;* Gels.; Glycerin; Gnaph.; Ham.; Hyper.; Jacar.; Lyc.; *Macrot.;* Merc.; Phos.; **Phyt.;** *Ran. b.;* Rhod.; Rhus t.; Sang.; Sil.; Sul.; Syph.; Ver. v.

Paralytic—*Caust.;* Lathyr.; Phos. See Chronic.

Periosteal—Bell.; Cham.; Colch.; Cycl.; Guaiac.; *Kali bich.;* Kali iod.; Merc.; *Mez.;* Phos.; Phyt.; Sars.; Sil.

Subacute—Dulc.; *Led.;* Merc.; *Puls.;* Rhus t.

Syphilitic—See Periosteal.

RESPIRATORY SYSTEM

BRONCHIAL TUBES—ASTHMA: Remedies in general: *Acon.;* Alumen; Ambros.; Amyl; Ant. ars.; *Ant. t.;* Apis; *Aral.; Ars.;* Ars. iod.; Atrop.; *Bac.;* Bell.; *Blatta orient.;* Brom.; Bry.; Cinch.; Coff.; *Carbo v.;* Chin. ars.; Chlorum; Cic.; *Coca;* Cocaine; *Crot. t.; Cupr. ac.;* Cupr. ars.; *Dros.;* Dulc.; Egg Vaccine; Glon.; *Grind.;* Hep.; *Hydroc. ac.;* Illic.; Iod.; *Ipec.; Kali bich.; Kali c.;* Kali chlor.; *Kali iod.; Kali n.;* Kali p.; Lach.; Led.; *Lob. infl.;* Lyc.; Magnolia; Meph.; Morph.; Naja; *Naph.; Nat. s.; Nux v.; Passifl.; Pothos;* Psor.; *Ptel.;* Puls.; Quebr.; Sabad.; *Samb.;* Sang.; Scilla; Scrophul.; Silph.; *Stercul.;* Stram.; Strych.; *Sul.;* Syph.; Tab.; Tela ar.; *Thuya;* Tub.; Ver. a.; Ver. v.; *Viscum;* Zinc. m.; *Zing.*

TYPE—OCCURRENCE—Alternates with eruptions: Calad.; Caust.; Rhus t.; *Sul.*

Alternates, with itching rash—Calad.

Alternates, with spasmodic vomiting—Cupr. m.; Ipec.

Anger, from—Cham.; Nux v.

Cardiac—*Cact.;* Digitaline; Grind. sq.; Stroph. See Heart.

Epiglottis, spasm or weakness—Med.

Eruptions, suppressed, from—Ars.; Hep.; Psor.; *Sul.*

Foot sweat, suppressed, from—Ol. an.

Hay asthma—Aral.; *Ars.;* Ars. iod.; Chin. ars.; *Ipec.; Lob. infl.;* Naph.; Nat. s.; Nux v.; *Sabad.;* Sang.; Sticta; Sul. iod. See Rhinitis (Nose).

Hebdomadal—Cinch.; Ign.

Humid—Acon.; *Ant. iod.;* Ars.; *Bac.;* Bry.; *Can. ind.;* Cochlear.; Cupr.; *Dulc.;* Eucal.; Euphorb. pil.; Grind.; Hyper.; Iod.; *Kali bich.; Nat. s.;* Pulmo v.; Sabal; *Senega;* Stann.; *Sul.;* Thuya.

Humid, in children—*Nat. s.;* Samb.; Thuya.

Millar's—Arum drac.; *Arundo;* Coral.; Cupr.; Guarea; Hep.; Ipec.; Lach.; Lob. infl.; Mosch.; Poth.; *Samb.* See Laryngismus stridulus.

Miner's—Card. m.; Nat. ars.

Nervous—Acon.; Ambra; Amyl; *Asaf.;* Chin. s.; Cina; Coff.; *Cupr.;* Grind.; *Hydroc. ac.; Ipec.;* Kali p.; Lob. infl.; *Mosch.;* Nux m.; *Nux v.;* Sumb.; Tela ar.; Thymus; *Val.;* Ver. a.

Periodical—*Ars.;* Chin. ars.; *Cinch.;* Ipec.

Preceded by coryza—Aral.; Naja; Nux v.

Preceded by formication—Cistus; Lob. infl.

Preceded by rose cold—Sang.

Recent, uncomplicated cases—Hydroc. ac.

Sailors on shore—Brom.

Senile cases—Bar. m.

Tetter recedes with attack—Sul.

CONCOMITANTS—With bronchial catarrh:—Acon.; *Ant. t.;* Ars.; Blatta am.; *Bry.;* Cupr. ac.; *Eriod.;* Eucal.; *Grind.; Ipec.;* Kali iod.; Lob. infl.; Nat. s.; Oniscus; Sabal; Sul. See Humid.

With burning in throat and chest—Aral.

With constriction of throat—Cham.; Dros.; *Hydroc. ac.;* Lob. infl.; *Moseh.*
With cramp, muscular spasm of various parts—Cupr. m.
With cyanosis—Ars.; Cupr.; Samb.
With despondency, thinks he will die—*Ars.;* Psor.
With diarrhœa following—Nat. s.
With dysuria, nocturnal—Solid.
With every fresh cold—Nat. s.
With gastric derangement—Arg. n.; *Bry.;* Carbo v.; Ipec.; Kali m.; *Lob. infl.;* Lyc.; *Nux v.;* Puls.; Sang.; Ver. v.; Zing.
With gout, rheumatism—Led.; Sul.; *Viscum.*
With hæmorrhoids—Juncus; Nux v.
With hydrothorax—Colch.
With insomnia—Chloral; Telea ar.
With nausea, cardiac weakness, vertigo, vomiting, weak stomach, cold knees —Lob. infl.
With palpitation—Ars.; Cact.; Eucal.; Puls.
With thirst, nausea, stitches, burning in chest—Kali n.
With urine supersaturated with solids—Nat. nit.

MODALITIES—AGGRAVATION: After sleep: Aral.; Grind.; *Lach.;* Samb.
At night, lying down—*Aral.;* Ars.; Cistus; Con.; Ferr. ac.; *Grind.;* Lach.; Merc. pr. rub.; Naja; Puls.; *Samb.;* Sul.
From cold, damp weather—Ars.; *Dulc.;* *Nat. s.* See Humid.
From cold, dry weather—Acon.; Caust.; Hep.
From falling asleep—Am. c.; *Grind.;* Lac c.; *Lach.;* *Merc. pr. rub.;* Op.
From food -Kali p.; *Nux v.;* Puls.
From inhaling dust—*Ipec.;* Kali c.; Pothos.
From odors—Sang.
From sitting up—Ferr. ac.; Laur.; Psor.
From talking—Dros.; Meph.
In early A. M.—Am. c.; Ant. t.; *Ars.;* Grind.; Kali bich.; *Kali c.;* Nat. s.; Nux v.; Zing.
In spring—Aral.
In summer—Syph.

AMELIORATION—At sea: Brom.
From bending forward, rocking—Kali c.
From eructation—*Carbo v.;* Nux v.
From expectoration—Aral.; *Eriod.;* Grind.; Hyper.; *Ipec.;* Kali bich.; Zinc. m.
From lying down, keeping arms spread apart—Psor.
From lying on face, protruding tongue—Med.
From motion—Ferr. m.; Lob. infl.
From sitting up—Ars.; Kali c.; Merc. pr. rub.; Nux v.; *Puls.*
From sitting up, with head bent backward—Hep.
From stool—Pothos.
From vomiting—Cupr. m.
In damp weather—Caust.; Hep.
In open air—Naph.

BRONCHIECTASIS: BRONCHORRHOEA—Dilatation, with profuse, fetid, purulent sputum: Acet. ac.; Allium s.; Alumen; Ant. t.; *Bac.; Bals. per.;* Benz. ac.; *Calc. c.;* Eucal.; Ferr. iod.; Grind.; *Hep.;* Ichth.; *Kali bich.; Kali c.;* Kreos.; Lyc.; Myos.; Myrt. ch.; *Puls.;* Sang.; *Sil.; Stann.;* Sul.; Tub. See Chronic Bronchitis.

BRONCHITIS—**Inflammation, acute:**—*Acon.;* Am. c.; Am. iod.; Am. phos.; Ant. ars.; Ant. iod.; *Ant. t.;* Ars. iod.; Ars.; Asclep. t.; Aviare; *Bell.;* Blatta or.; *Brom.; Bry.; Caust.;* Cham.; Cinch.; Colch.; Cop.; *Dulc.;* Eup. perf.; Euphras.; *Ferr. p.;* Gels.; Grind.; *Hep.;* Hyos.; *Ipec.; Kali bich.;* Lob. infl.; Mang. ac.; *Merc. s.;* Naph.; Nat. ars.; Nit. ac.; *Phos.; Piloc.; Puls.;* Rhus t.; *Rumex; Sang.; Sang. n.; Scilla;* Solid.; Spong.; *Sticta; Sul.;* Sul. ac.; Thuya; Tub.; Ver. a.; Ver. v.; Zinc. m.

Capillary—Am. c.; Am. iod.; Ant. ars.; *Ant. t.;* Ars.; Bac.; *Bell.;* Bry.; Calc. c.; Camph.; *Carbo v.;* Chel.; Cupr. ac.; *Ferr. p.; Ipec.;* Kali c.; Kali iod.; *Kaolin;* Nit. ac.; Phos. ac.; Phos.; *Senega; Solanine;* Sul.; *Tereb.;* Ver. a.

Chronic (winter catarrhs)—Alumen; Alum.; *Ammon.; Am. c.;* Am. caust.; Am. iod.; Am. m.; Ant. ars.; Ant. iod.; *Ant. s. a.; Ant. t.; Ars. iod.; Ars.;* Bac.; *Bals. per.;* Bar. c.; *Bar. m.; Calc. c.;* Calc. iod.; Calc. sil.; Canth.; Carbo an.; *Carbo v.;* Ceanoth.; Chel.; *Cinch.;* Coccus; Con.; *Cop.;* Cub.; Dig.; Dros.; *Dulc.;* Eriod.; Eucal.; Grind.; *Hep.;* Hydr.; Hyos.; Ichth.; Iod.; *Ipec.; Kali bich.;* Kali c.; Kali hypophos.; *Kali iod.;* Kali s.; Kreos.; Lach.; *Lyc.; Merc. s.;* Myos.; Myrt. ch.; Nat. m.; Nat. s.; *Nit. ac.;* Nux v.; Phos.; Pix l.; *Puls.;* Rumex; Sabal; Sang.; *Scilla;* Sec.; *Senega;* Sep.; *Sil.;* Silph.; Spong.; *Stann.;* Strych.; *Sul.;* Taxus; Tereb.; Tub.; Ver. a.

Fibrinous—*Calc. acet.;* Bry.; Brom.; *Kali bich.;* Phos.

Toxemic—Am. c.; Ant. t.; Bry.; Colch.; Diphtherotox.; *Merc. c.*

Irritation of tubes—Acet. ac.; *Acon.;* Alumen; Ambros.; Brom.; *Bry.;* Chlorum; Ferr. p.; *Hep.; Phos.;* Piloc.; *Rumex;* Sang. n.; Spong. See Bronchitis.

Sensitiveness, to cold air—Allium s.; *Aral.;* Bac.; Calc. sil.; *Cham.;* Cinch.; *Coral.; Dulc.; Hep.;* Iod.; Kali c.; Mang. ac.; *Merc. s.;* Naja; *Psor.; Sil.; Tub.*

CHEST—**Affections, after brain fag**—Phos. ac.

Affections, after operations, for fistulæ—Berb. v.; Calc. p.; Sil.

Affections, after operations, for hydrothorax, empyema—Abrot.

Affections, after suppressed skin eruptions—Hep.

Affections, in circumscribed spots, persistent after inflammation—Senega.

Affections, in stone cutters with adynamia—Sil.

Burning—Acet. ac.; *Acon.;* Am. c.; Am. m.; Ant. t.; Apis; Aral.; *Ars.;* Bell.; *Brom.;* Bry.; *Calc. c.; Carbo v.;* Cic.; Euphorb.; Kreos.; Lyc.; Mag. m.; Mang. ac.; *Merc.;* Merc. sul.; Mez.; Myrtis; Ol. j. as.; Op.; *Phos.;* Primula; Ran. sc.; *Sang.;* Sang. n.; *Spong.; Sul.;* Wyeth.; Zinc. m.

Coldness—Abies c.; *Am. m.; Brom.;* Carbo an.; Cistus; *Coral.; Elaps;* Helod.; *Kali c.;* Lith. c.

Eruptions on—Arundo; Jugl. c.; Kali br.; Lyc.; Petrol.

Inability to lie down (orthopnœa)—Acon. fer.; *Ars.; Conv.;* Dig.; Grind.; Lach.; Mag. p.; Puls.; Viscum.   See Respiration.

Inability, to lie on left side—*Phos.;* Puls.

Inability, to lie on right side—Merc.

Injury followed by phthisis—Millef.; Ruta.

Itching, extending to nares—Coccus; Con.; Iod.; *Ipec.;* Puls.

Lightness, emptiness, eviscerated feeling—Cocc.; Nat. s.; *Phos.; Stann.*

PAINS—In general: Abrot.; Acal.; *Acon.; Apis;* Arg. n.; *Arn.;* Ars.; *Bell.;* Bor.; Brom.; Bry.; *Cact.;* Calc. c.; Caul.; *Caust.;* Chel.; *Cim.;* Collins.; Commocl.; Crot. t.; Dig.; Elaps; Eriod.; Gadus; *Hydroc. ac.;* Jugl. c.; *Kali c.;* Kali n.; *Kreos.;* Med.; Morph.; Myrtis; *Ox. ac.; Phos.;* Pothos.; Psor.; Puls.; *Ran. b.; Rumex; Sang.;* Solan. lyc.; Sticta; Strych. p.; Succin.; Sul.

Bruised, ulcerative—Ampel.; *Arn.;* Calc. c.; Eup. perf.; Kreos.; Lyc.; Phaseol.; *Psor.; Puls.; Ran. b.;* Ran. sc.; Sang.

Constriction, must frequently breathe deeply to expand lungs: Adon. v.; Asaf.; *Bry.; Dig.;* Ign.; Iod.; Lach.; Meli.; Millef.; *Mosch.;* Nat. s.; *Phos.;* Scilla; Xanth.

Constriction, spasmodic, tightness, fullness, oppression—Abies n.; *Acon.;* Adren.; Ambros.; Am. c.; *Ant. t.;* Apis; *Apoc.; Apium gr.; Aral.;* Arg. n.; *Ars.;* Asaf.; *Bac.;* Bell.; Brom.; *Bry.; Cact.;* Calc. ars.; *Calc. c.; Caps.;* Carbo v.; Cham.; *Chlorum;* Cic.; Coca; Cocc.; Coff.; *Cupr. ac.;* Cupr. m.; *Dig.;* Diosc.; Dulc.; *Ferr. m.;* Ferr. p.; Glon.; Glycerin; *Grind.;* Hematox.; Hep.; *Hydroc. ac.; Ipec.; Justicia;* Kali bich.; *Kali c.; Kali n.; Kreos.;* Lach.; Lact. v.; Laur.; *Lob. infl.;* Lyc.; Magnol.; Med.; Morph.; *Mosch.;* Naja; Naph.; *Nat. ars.; Nat. s.; Nit. sp. d.; Nux v.;* Ornothog.; Ox. ac.; *Phos.; Puls.;* Ran. b.; Ruta; *Samb.;* Sang.; Senega; Sep.; Sil.; Silph.; Solan. n.; Spig.; Spong.; Stram.; Strych.; Sul. ac.; *Sul.;* Ver. v.

Cutting—*Bry.;* Kali c.; Kali n.; Sul.; Zinc. m.

Pressing, heaviness, weight—*Abies n.;* Abrot.; Acon.; Am. c.; *Anac.;* Arg. n.; Arn.; *Ars.;* Aur.; Bry.; *Cact.; Calc. c.;* Cham.; Chel.; Ferr. iod.; Hematox.; Ipec.; Kali n.; *Kreos.; Lil. t.; Lob. infl.;* Lyc.; Phos. ac.; *Phos.;* Prun. pad.; Ptel.; *Puls.;* Ran. b.; Ruta; Samb.; Sang. n.; Senega; Sil.; *Spong.; Sul.;* Ver. v.

Stitching, tearing, darting, shooting—*Acon.;* Agar.; Allium s.; Am. c.; Ant. t.; Apium gr.; Ars.; *Asclep. t.;* Bell.; Berb. v.; *Bor.;* Brom.; *Bry.;* Calc. c.; Canth.; Caps.; *Carbo an.;* Carbo v.; *Caust.; Chel.;* Cim.; *Cinch.;* Coccus; Colch.; Crot. t.; *Elaps;* Formica; *Guaiac.;* Hematox.; Inula; *Kali c.;* Kali iod.; Kal.; *Lob. card.;* Lyc.; Menthol; Merc. c.; Merc.; Myrtis; *Nat. s.;* Nit. ac.; Nux v.; *Ol. an.;* Ol. j. as.; Pæonia; Phell.; *Phos.; Ran. b.;* Rhod.; Rhus t.; Rhus r.; Rumex; Sang.; *Scilla;* Sep.; *Sil.;* Spig.; Stann.; *Sticta; Sul.; Ther.;* Thuya; Trill.; Zing.

LOCATION—Cartilages, costal: Perichondritis: Arg. m.; Bell.; Cham.; *Cim.;* Guaiac.; Oleand.; Plumb.; *Ruta.*

Infra-mammary—*Cim.;* Puls.; Ran. b.; Ustil.   See Female Sexual System.

Intercostal (pleurodynia)—*Acon.;* Am. c.; Aristol.; *Arn.;* Ars.; *Asclep. t.;* Azadir.; Bor.; *Bry.;* Caust.; Chel.; *Cim.; Colch.;* Echin.; Gaulth.;

Guaiac.; *Kali c.; Nux v.;* Ox. ac.; *Phos.; Puls.; Ran. b.;* Rham. c.; Rhod.; Rhus r.; *Rhus t.;* Rumex; Senega; Sinap. n.; Sul. ac.

Lung, left: Apex and middle portion—Acon.; Am. c.; *Anis.;* Ant. s. a.; Crot. t.; Illic.; *Lob. card.; Myrtis;* Pæonia; Phos.; *Pix l.;* Puls.; *Ran. b.;* Rumex; Sil.; Spig.; Stann.; Sticta; *Sul.; Ther.;* Tub.; Ustil.

Lower portion—Agar.; Ampel.; Asclep. t.; Calc. p.; Cim.; *Lob. syph.;* Lyc.; Myos.; *Nat. s.; Ox. ac.; Rumex;* Scilla; Sil.

Lung, right: Apex and middle portion—Abies c.; *Ars.;* Bor.; *Calc. c.;* Commocl.; Crot. t.; *Elaps;* Eriod.; *Illic.;* Iodof.; *Phell.;* Sang.; Upas.

Lower portion—Am. m.; Berb. v.; Bry.; Cact.; Card. m.; *Chel.;* Diosc.; Kali c.; Lyc.; *Merc.*

Substernal—Apium gr.; Ars.; *Asclep. t.;* Aster.; Aur.; Azadir.; *Bry.;* Card. m.; *Caust.;* Chel.; Con.; *Diosc.;* Jugl. r.; Kali n.; Kal.; *Kreos.;* Lact. v.; Morph.; Nit. ac.; Nit. sp. d.; Osm.; Phell.; Phos. ac.; Phos.; Psor.; Puls.; *Ran. b.;* Ran. sc.; *Rumex;* Ruta; Samb.; *Sang.;* Sang. n.; Sep.; Sil.; Spig.; Sul.; Trill.

MODALITIES—AGGRAVATIONS: From ascending: Ars.; Sep.

From bending forward—Sul.

From breathing, coughing—Am. m.; Arn.; *Bry.;* Colch.; Menthol; Nat. m.; Phos.; *Ran. b.;* Senega; Sep.; Sil.; Sul.

From cold drinks—Thuya.

From cold weather—Petrol.; Phos.

From damp weather—Ran. b.; Rhus t.; Spig.

From lying down, at night—Calc. c.; Sep.

From lying on affected side—Nux v.; Phos.; Stann.

From lying on left side—Phos.

From lying on right side—Kali c.; *Merc.*

From motion—Arn.; Ars.; *Bry.;* Calc. c.; Card. m.; Jugl. r.; Kali c.; Mag. c.; Phos.; *Ran. b.;* Senega; Sep.; Spig.; Sul.

From pressure—Arn.; Ars.; *Bry.;* Colch.; Nux v.; *Phos.; Ran. b.*

From spinal irritation—Agar.; Ran. b.

From talking—Alum.; Hep.; *Stann.*

From working—Am. m.; Lyc.; Sep.

AMELIORATIONS—From bending forward: Asclep. t.; Hyos.

From eructation—Bar. c.

From lying down—Psor.

From lying on affected side—Bry.; Puls.

From motion—Ign.; Puls.

From rapid walking—Lob. infl.

From rest—Bry.

In open air—Anac.; *Puls.*

Snesitiveness, tenderness, rawness of chest—Ant. t.; Aral.; *Arn.;* Ars.; *Asclep. t.;* Bry.; Calc. c.; Calc. p.; Calc. sil.; *Carbo v.;* Caust.; Cim.; Cur.; *Eup. perf.;* Ferr. p.; Ham.; *Iod.;* Kali c.; *Kaolin; Merc.;* Naph.; *Nat. s.; Nit. ac.; Ol. j. as.; Phos.;* Pop. c.; Puls.; *Ran. b.; Ran. sc.; Rumex; Sang.; Sen·ga;* Sep.; Spong.; Stann.; Sul.

Spots on, brown—Sep.

Spots on, yellow—Phos.

Weakness, from least exertion, even talking, laughing, singing—Alumen; Am. c.; *Arg. m.; Calc. c.;* Canth.; *Carbo v.;* Cocc.; *Dig.;* Iod.; Kali c.; Lob. infl.; *Phos. ac.;* Phos.; Psor.; Ran. sc.; Rhus t.; Ruta; Spong.; *Stann.; Sul.*

COUGH—Remedies in general: Acal.; *Acet. ac.;* Acon.; *Allium s.; Alum.; Ambra;* Am. br.; *Am. c.;* Am. caust.; Am. m.; Ant. ars.; Ant. s. a.; *Ant. t.;* Aral.; Arn.; Ars.; *Ars. iod.;* Asclep. t.; Bals. per.; *Bell.; Bism.; Brom.; Bry.; Calc. c.;* Canth.; *Caps.;* Carb. ac.; *Carbo v.;* Caust.; *Cepa;* Cham.; Chel.; *Cim.⸗ Cina; Coccus; Cod.;* Con.; *Coral.; Crot.;* Cupr. ac.; Cupr. m.; *Dros.;* Dulc.; *Eup. perf.;* Euphras.; *Ferr. p.; Hep.;* Hydroc. ac.; *Hyos.;* Hyosc. hydrobr.; Ign.; *Iod.; Ipec.; Kali bich.; Kali c.;* Kali chlor.; *Lach.; Lact. v.; Laur.; Lob. infl.; Lyc.; Mag. p.;* Mang. ac.; *Mentha;* Meph.; Merc. s.; *Merc. v.;* Myrtis; *Naja;* Nat. m.; *Nit. ac.; Nux v.;* Op.; *Osm.;* Phell.; *Phos.;* Pop. c.; *Puls.;* Rhus t.; *Rumex; Samb.; Sang.;* Santon.; *Scilla; Senega; Sil.; Spong.; Stann. iod.;* Stann.; *Sticta; Sul.;* Trifol.; Tub.; *Verbasc.; Viola od.;* Wyeth.

CAUSE, OCCURRENCE, AGGRAVATION—Abdomen, irritation from: Sep.

After anger in children—Anac.; Ant. t.

After anger, vexation, cleaning teeth—Staph.

After diarrhœa—Abrot.

After falling asleep, especially, in children, constant tickling cough without waking—*Acon.;* Agar.; *Aral.; Cham.;* Cycl.; Lach.; Nit. ac.; Sul.; Tub.; Verbasc. See Evening.

After sleep—Brom.; Lach.; Spong.

Afternoon, in—Am. m.; Lyc.; Thuya.

Air, hot—Kali s.

Arsenical wall paper—Calc. c.

Ascending—Am. c.

Bathing—Nux m.

Catarrh—Am. m.; Caust.; *Ipec.;* Kreos.; *Scilla;* Sticta.

Catarrh, post-nasal, in children and adults—Hydr.; Pop. c.; Spig.

Chest, feeling as if lump in—Abies n.

Cold air—*Acon.;* Alum.; Am. c.; Ars.; Bar. c.; Brom.; Calc. sil.; *Carbo v.; Cepa; Hep.;* Lach.; *Mentha;* Nit. ac.; *Phos.;* Rhus t.; *Rumex;* Scilla; Senega; *Spong.;* Trifol.

Cold air, to warm—Ant. c.; *Bry.;* Ipec.; *Nat. c.;* Scilla; Ver. a.

Condiments, vinegar, wine—Alum.

Dampness—Ant. t.; Calc. c.; *Dulc.; Nat. s.;* Nux m.

Daytime only—*Euphras.; Ferr.;* Nat. m.; Stann.; Staph.; Viola od.

Drinking—Ars.; *Bry.; Carbo v.;* Dros.; Hyos.; Lyc.; Phos.; Staph.

Drinking, cold—*Carbo v.; Hep.;* Merc.; Rhus t.; Scilla; Sil.; *Spong.;* Ver. a.

Eating—Anac.; Ant. ars.; Ant. t.; *Bry.; Calc. c.; Carbo v.; Cinch.;* Hyos.; Kali bich.; *Lach.; Mez.;* Myos.; *Nux v.;* Phos.; Staph.; Taxus; Zinc. m.

Eczema or itch suppressed—Psor.

Entering, warm room—Acon.; *Ant. c.;* Anthem.; *Bry.; Caust.;* Cham.; Merc.; *Nat. c.; Puls.;* Ran. b.; Ver. a.

Evening, night—Acal.; *Acon.; Am. br.*; Am. c.; Ant. t.; Arn.; *Ars.; Bell.; Bry.; Calc. c.;* Caps.; *Carbo v.; Caust.; Cim.; Cod.; Colch.; Con.; Dros.; Eup. perf.; Hep.;* Hydroc. ac.; *Hyos.*; Kali br.; Ign.; Laur.; Lyc.; Mentha; Meph.; *Merc.; Nit. ac.*; Op.; Passifl.; *Phos.; Prun. v.; Psor.;* Puls.; *Rhus t.; Rumex;* Samb.; Sang.; *Sanic.*; Santon.; Sep.; Sil.; *Spong.; Stann.; Sticta; Sul.*; Tub.; *Verbasc.*

Before midnight—Aral.; *Bell.*; Carbo v.; Mag. m.; *Phos.*; Samb.; *Spong.*; Stann.

After midnight, early A. M.—*Acon.*; Am. br.; Am. c.; *Ars.*; Cupr. m.; *Dros.; Hep.; Kali c.; Nux v.*; Phell.; Rhus t.

Constriction in larynx, trachea—Ign.

Excitement—Ambra; Coral.; Ign.; Spong.; Tar. h. See Nervous.

Expiration—*Acon.; Caust.; Nux v.*

Exposure even of hand from under cover—Bar. c.; Hep.; Rhus t.

Heart disease—Arn.; Hydroc. ac.; Lach.; Laur.; Lycop.; *Naja; Spong.*

Influenza—Cepa; *Eriod.*; Hyos.; *Kali bich.*; Kali s.; *Kreos.*; *Pix l.; Sang.*; Senega; Stann.; Strych.

Injuries—Arn.; Millef.

Inspiration—*Acet. ac.*; Acon.; *Bell.; Brom.*; Bry.; Cina; Iod.; *Ipec.*; Kali bich.; Lach.; Mentha; Nat. m.; *Phos.; Rumex*; Scilla.; *Spong.; Sticta.*

Intermittent, suppressed—Eup. perf.

Liver affections—Am. m.

Lying down—Ant. ars.; *Aral.*; Ars.; *Bell.*; Bry.; *Caust.*; Cochlear.; *Con.*; Croc.; Crot. t.; *Dros.*; Dulc.; *Hyos.*; Ign.; Inula; Lith. c.; Meph.; Nit. ac.; Nux v.; Petrol.; *Phos.; Prun. v.*; Psor.; *Puls.; Rumex;* Sabad.; *Sang.; Sil.*; Sticta; Tub.; Verbasc.

Lying on back—Am. m.; Ars.; Iod.; *Nux v.*; Phos.

Lying on left side—Dros.; *Phos.*; Ptel.; Rumex; Stann.

Lying on right side—Am. m.; Benz. ac.; *Merc.*

Lying with head low—Am. m.; *Spong.*

Measles—Dros.; Dulc.; Eup. perf.; Euphras.; Ipec.; Kali bich.; *Puls.*; Sang.; Scilla; *Sticta.* See Skin.

Menses, or piles, suppressed—Millef.

Mental exertion—Nux v.

Morning—Acal.; Allium s.; *Alum.*; Ambra; Calc. c.; Cina; *Coccus; Hep.; Iod.*; Kali bich.; Kali iod.; Kali n.; Lyc.; Nat. m.; *Nit. ac.; Puls.*; Rhus t.; Selen.; Sep.; Sticta; Sil.; Tab.

Morning, early—*Am. br.; Am. c.; Ars.*; Caust.; Cupr. m.; Hep.; *Kali c.; Nux v.*; Phell.; Puls.; Sul.

Morning, on waking—Alum.; Ambra; *Bry.; Coccus*; Kali bich.; Psor.; Rhus t.

Motion—Ars.; Bell.; *Bry.; Cina*; Hep.; Iod.; *Ipec.*; Nux v.; Puls.; Senega; Spong.; Ver. a.

Odors strong; presence of strangers—Phos.

Old people—Ant. iod.; Ant. t.; Bar. c.; Bar. m.; *Carbo v.; Hyos.*; Kreos.; Myrtis; Rhus t.; *Senega;* Sil.; Sticta.

Operations for fistulæ, after—Berb. v.; Calc. p.; Sil.

Periodic, recurring in spring, autumn—Cina.

Pertussis after; from least cold—Caust.; Sang.

Physical exhaustion—Scilla; *Sticta.*

Pregnancy—*Apoc.;* Bry.; Caust.; *Con.; Kali br.;* Nux m.; Vib. op.

Reading, laughing, singing, talking—Alum.; *Ambra;* Anac.; *Arg. m.; Arg. n.;* Arum; Carbo v.; *Caust.;* Cim.; Collins.; *Con.; Dros.; Hep.; Hyos.;* Iridium; Lach.; *Mang. ac.;* Mentha; Nux v.; *Phos.; Rumex;* Sil.; Spong.; *Stann.;* Sul.

Reflex—Ambra; Apis; Phos.

Sciatica in summer alternating—Staph.

Standing still during a walk—Astac.; Ign.

Stomach, irritation, from—Bism.; *Bry.;* Calad.; Cereum ox.; Kali m.; *Lob. infl.;* Nat. m.; Nit. ac.; Nux v.; Phos.; *Sang.;* Sep.; Sul.; Ver. a.

Swallowing, from—Spong.

Sweets—Med.; *Spong.;* Zinc. m.

Tickling, as from dust, feather—Am. c.; Ars.; *Bell.; Calc. c.;* Caps.; Caust.; *Carbo v.;* Cina; Dros.; Euphorb. dath.; *Ign.;* Lac c.; Lach.; *Lact. v.;* Nat. m.; Nux v.; Paris; *Phos.; Rumex;* Sep.

Tickling, in chest (substernal, suprasternal fossa)—*Ambra;* Am. br.; *Ant. c.;* Apis; Arn.; Ars.; Brom.; *Bry.; Calc. c.;* Caps.; *Carbo v.; Caust.;* Cham.; Coccus; *Con.;* Ferr. ac.; *Ign.; Iod.;* Ipec.; Kali bich.; Kreos.; *Lach.; Mentha;* Myrtis; *Nux v.; Osm.;* Paris; Phos. ac.; *Phos.;* Puls.; Radium; Rhus t.; *Rumex;* Sang.; Sep.; · *Sil.;* Spong.; *Stann.;* Sul.; Ver. a.

Tickling, in larynx—Alum.; *Arg. m.; Bell.;* Brom.; *Calc. c.;* Caps.; *Carbo v.;* Caust.; *Cepa;* Cochlear.; *Coccus; Con.;* Crot.; *Dros.;* Dulc.; Eryng.; Hep.; *Ign.;* Iod.; Ipec.; Kreos.; *Lach.;* Menthol; Nit. ac.; Phos.; Puls.; *Rumex;* Sang.; *Sil.;* Spong.; *Sul.*

Tickling, in throat—Alum.; Ambra; Am. br.; Am. c.; *Aral.; Arg. n.;* Bell.; *Calc. c.; Caps.;* Cham.; Cim.; Cina; *Con.; Dros.; Hep.;* Hepat.; *Hyos.; Ign.; Iod.;* Kali c.; Lact. v.; *Lob. infl.;* Meli.; Menthol; Nux v.; *Phos.;* Rumex; Stann. iod.; Sul.; Wyeth.

Tobacco smoke—Mentha; Merc.; Spong.; *Staph.*

Tonsils, enlarged—Bar. c.; Lach.

Touch, pressure—Lach.; *Rumex.*

Undressing, or uncovering body—Bar. c.; *Hep.;* Kali bich.; *Rhus t.; Rumex.*

Uvula, relaxed—Bar. c.; *Hyos.;* Kali c.; Merc. i. r.

Warmth—*Ant. c.; Bry.;* Caust.; Dros.; Dulc.; Ipec.; *Merc.;* Nat. c.; Nux m.; Puls.; Scilla.

Weeping—Arn.

Winter—Aloe; *Ant. s. a.;* Bry.; Cham.; Ipec.; Kreos.; Lippia; *Psor* See Chronic Bronchitis.

Worms—Cina; Tereb.

Young, phthisical persons with constant, distressing night cough—Dros.

TYPE—**Barking:** *Acon.;* Ambra; *Bell.;* Coral.; *Dros.;* Hep.; Iod.; *Kali bich.;* Phos.; Samb.; Sinap. n.; *Spong.;* Ver. a. See Dry; Hoarse; Spasmodic.

Chronic (phthisical)—*Allium s.; Ant. t.;* Ars. iod.; Bar. c.; Bry.; Calc. iod.; Calc. p.; Cham.; *Cod.;* Crot.; *Dros.;* Dulc.; Eup. perf.; Hyos. hydrobr.; Kreos.; Laur.; Lob. infl.; Lyc.; Mang.; Merc.; Naja; *Nit. ac.;* Phell.; *Phos.;* Psor.; Puls.; Rumex; *Sang.;* Scilla; Sil.; *Spong.;* Sticta; Sul. See Tuberculosis.

Croupy—*Acon.;* Brom.; Gels.; *Hep.;* Iod.; *Kali bich.;* Nit. ac.; Phos.: *Spong.;* Staph. See Croup.

Dry, hard, racking, hacking, short, tight, tickling—*Acal.; Acon.;* Alumen; *Alum.; Am. br.;* Am. c.; Ant. s. a.; *Ars.;* Ars. iod.; *Arum;* Asclep. t.; Aviare; *Bell.; Brom.; Bry.; Calc. c.;* Calc. iod.; Canth.; *Caps.;* Carb. ac.; Carbo v.; *Caust.; Cepa; Cham.;* Cim.; *Cina;* Cochlear.; *Cod.;* Coff.;] *Con.; Coral.;* Dig.; Dros.; Euphras.; Ferr. p.; Glycerin; *Hep.; Hydroc. ac.; Hyos.;* Hyosc. hydrobr.; *Ign.; Iod.;* Justicia; *Kali bich.; Kali br.; Kali c.;* Kali m.; Kreos.; *Lach.; Laur.; Lob. infl.;* Lyc.; Lycop.; Lycopers.; Mang.; Med.; *Mentha;* Menthol; Merc.; *Morph.; Naja;* Nat. m.; *Nit. ac.; Nux v.;* Ol. j. as.; *Onosm.;* Op.; *Osm.;* Petrol.; *Phos.; Puls.; Rhus t.;* Rumex; Salvia; Samb.; Sang.; *Sang. n.;* Scilla; *Senega; Sep.; Sil.; Spong.;* Stann.; *Sticta;* Sul.; Sul. ac.; Tela ar.; Tub.; Vanad.; Ver. a.; *Verbasc.;* Wyeth.

Explosive, noisy—*Caps.;* Dros.; *Osm.;* Solan. lyc.; Strych. See Spasmodic.

Fatiguing, exhausting, irritating—*Acon.;* Am. c.; Ant. iod.; *Ars.; Arum;* Aviare; Bals. per.; *Bell.;* Bry.; Calc. c.; *Caust.;* Cham.; Chel.; *Cod.;* Collins.; Con.; *Coral.; Dros.;* Eucal.; Hep.; *Hyos.;* Hydroc. ac.; *Ign.;* Iod.; *Ipec.;* Kali br.; Kreos.; Lact. v.; Laur.; *Lob. infl.;* Lyc.; *Mentha;* Menthol; Merc.; Myrtis; *Naja;* Nit. ac.; Op.; Phell.; *Phos.;* Psor.; Rumex as.; Rumex; Sang.; *Scilla; Senega; Sep.; Sil.;* Silph. cyr.; *Sticta;* Strych.; Tela ar. See Spasmodic.

Hoarse, hollow, deep, metallic—*Acon.; Ambra;* Am. phos.; Ant. t.; Apoc.; Ars. iod.; *Arum;* Bell.; Brom.; Bry.; *Carbo v.; Caust.; Cina; Dros.;* Dulc.; Euphorb.; Euphras.; *Hep.;* Ign.; Iod.; Irid.; *Kali bich.;* Lippia; Lyc.; Mang.; Med.; Meph.; Myrtis; Nit. ac.; *Phos.;* Samb.; *Spong.;* Stann.; Ver. a.; *Verbasc.* See Spasmodic.

Laryngeal, nervous—Acon.; *Ambra;* Asar.; *Bell.; Brom.;* Caps.; Carbo v.; *Caust.;* Cina; *Coral.; Cupr.; Dros.;* Gels.; *Hep.;* Hydroc. ac.; *Hyos.; Ign.;* Ipec.; Kali br.; Kali m.; Lach.; Med.; Merc.; *Nit. ac.;* Nux v.; *Phos.;* Puls.; *Rumex; Santon.; Spong.;* Sul.; Tar. h.; Terebene; Ver. a.; Viola od.

Loose, rattling, gagging, choking, strangling—Am. br.; Am. m.; Ant. s.; *Ant. t.;* Ars.; Asclep. t.; Bals. per.; *Brom.; Calc. ac.; Calc. c.; Chel.;* Cina; Coccus; Cupr. m.; Dros.; *Dulc.;* Eup. perf.; *Hep.; Ipec.;* Kali bich.; Kali c.; Kali m.; Kali s.; Lyc.; *Merc.; Nat. s.;* Nit. ac.; Phos.; *Puls.;* Rhus t.; Samb.; Sang.; Scilla; *Senec.;* Senega; Sep.; Sil.; *Stann.·* Sticta; *Sul.;* Tereb.; Ver. a.

Spasmodic, paroxysmal, nervous, violent, suffocative—*Acon.;* Agar.; *Ambra; Am. br.;* Ant. ars.; Ant. t.; Aral.; *Arn.; Ars.;* Asar.; *Bell.; Brom.; Bry.;* Caps.; Carb. ac.; *Carbo v.; Caust.;* Cham.; *Chel.; Cina;* Coccus; Con.; *Coral.;* Crot. t.; *Cupr. ac.; Cupr. m.; Dros.;* Dulc.; Gels.; Glycerin; *Hep.; Hydroc. ac.; Hyos.; Ign.;* Iod.; *Ipec.; Justicia; Kali br.; Kali c.; Kreos.; Lach.; Lact. v.;* Laur.; Led.; *Lyc.; Mag. p.: Meph.;*

Merc.; Naph.; *Nat. m.; Nit. ac.;* Nux m.; *Nux v.;* Op.; *Osm.:* Pertussin; *Phos.;* Radium; *Rumex; Samb.;* Sang.; Santon.; *Scilla;* Sep.; *Sil.; Spong.; Stann.;* Sticta; *Sul.;* Trifol.; Ver. a.; *Viola od.*

Successive, in two paroxysms—Merc.; Puls.

Successive, in three paroxysms—Cupr. m.; Stann.

Wheezing, asthmatic—Ambros.; Ant. t.; *Ars.;* Benz. ac.; Croc.; Hep.; Iod.; *Ipec.;* Kali bich.; *Lob. infl.;* Meph.; Nit. ac.; Rhodium; Samb.; *Sang.;* Senega; *Spong.* See Spasmodic.

WHOOPING (pertussis)—*Acon.;* Alumen; Ambra; *Ambros.;* Am. br.; Am. m.; Am. picr.; Ant. c.; *Ant. t.; Arn.;* Bad.; *Bell.;* Bry.; Brom.; Caps.; Carb. ac.; Carbo v.; Caust.; *Castanea;* Cereum ox.; *Chel.; Cina;* Cinch.; Cocaine; *Coccus♦* Con.; *Coral.;* Coquel.; *Cupr. ac.; Cupr. m.; Dros.; Dulc.;* Eucal.; Euphorb. dath.; Euphras.; *Formal.;* Grind.; Hep.; *Hydroc. ac.; Hyos.; Ipec.; Justicia; Kali bich.;* Kali br.; *Kali c.; Kali m.;* Kali p.; Kali s.; Led.; *Lob. infl.;* Lob. m.; *Mag. p.; Meph.;* Merc.; *Naph.;* Nit. ac.; Ol. j. as.; Op.; Passifl.; Pertussin; Phos.; Pod.; *Puls.;* Samb.; Sang. n.; *Sep.;* Sil.; Solan. c.; Sticta; Sul.; Thymus; Tongo; *Trifol.; Ver. a.;* Viola od. See Spasmodic.

Whooping at night, "minute gun" during day—Coral.

Whooping, convulsions—*Bell.;* Cina; *Cupr. ac.;* Cupr. m.; Hydroc. ac.; Hyos.; Kali br.; Mag. p.; Narcissus; Solan. c.

Whooping, early stage (spasmodic)—*Acon.; Bell.;* Carb. ac.; Carbo v.; *Castanea;* Chel.; *Cina;* Coccus; Coral.; Cupr.; *Dros.;* Hyos.; Ipec.; Mag. p.; Meph.; Naph.; Narcissus; Samb.; Stann.; Thymus.

Whooping, hæmorrhage—*Arn.; Cereum ox.;* Coral.; Cupr.; *Dros.;* Ind.; *Ipec.;* Merc.

Whooping, later stages (catarrhal)—*Ant. t.;* Cinch.; Hep.; *Ipec.;* Puls.

Whooping, vomiting—Ant. t.; Bell.; Carbo v.; *Cereum ox.; Coccus; Cupr. m.; Dros.; Ipec.;* Lob. infl.; Ver. a.

Whooping—Concomitants: Body stiff, rigid, cyanosis: Am. c.; *Ant. t.;* Carbo v.; Cina; Coral.; *Cupr. ac.; Cupr. m.;* Iod.; *Ipec.;* Mag. p.; Meph.; Op.; Samb.; *Ver. a.*

Coryza—Alum.; Lyc.; Nat. c.

Crowing inspiration absent—Ambra.

Crying—*Arn.;* Bry.; *Caps.;* Samb.

Diarrhœa—Ant. t.; *Cupr. ars.;* Euphorb. dath.; Ipec.; *Rumex;* Ver. a.

Dyspnœa—Ambra; Am. c.; *Ant. t.;* Bell.; Brom.; *Carbo v.;* Cina; Coral.; *Cupr. m.; Dros.;* Euphorb.; Hep.; Hippoz.; Iod.; *Ipec.;* Kali bich.; *Lob. infl.;* Meph.; Naph.; Op.; *Samb.;* Senec.; *Ver. a.; Viola* od See Respiration.

Epistaxis, bleedings—*Arn.;* Bell.; Cereum ox.; Coral.; *Cupr.; Dros.; Ind.; Iod.;* Ipec.; Merc.

Paroxysms follow each other rapidly and violently—Dros.

Paroxysms wakes child at 6-7 A. M., vomiting of ropy mucus—Coccus.

Paroxysms with flow of tears—Nat. m.

Spasm of glottis—Cupr.; Meph.; Mosch.

Sublingual ulcer—Nit. ac.

Vomiting of solid food after regaining consciousness—Cupr. m.

With every cold, severe cough returns—Sang.

EXPECTORATION: TYPE—Acid: Carbo an.; Nit. ac.; Puls.

Albuminous, clear, white—*Arg. m.;* Ars.; Bry.; Coccus; Eucal.; Kali m.; Scilla; *Selen.;* Sul.

Bitter—Bry.; Calc. c.; Cham.; Dros.; Kali n.; Nit. ac.; *Puls.*

Bloody, blood streaked—*Acon.;* Arg. n.; *Arn.; Ars.; Bell.; Bry.; Calc. c.;* Can. s.; Canth.; *Cetrar.;* Coral.; Crot.; *Dig.;* Dros.; Dulc.; *Elaps;* Ferr. p.; *Hep.;* Hyos.; Iod.; Ipec.; Kali c.; *Kali n.; Laur.; Led.;* Lyc.; Merc. c.; Merc.; *Millef.;* Nit. ac.; Nitrum; Nux v.; Op.; *Phos.;* Puls.; *Rhus t.;* Selen.; Sil.; Sul.; *Trill.*

Casts—*Calc. ac.;* Kali bich.

Daytime—Ambra; Bry.; Calc. c.; Hyos.; Stann.

Easy, raising—*Arg. m.;* Carbo v.; Dulc.; Eriod.; Kali s.; *Nat. s.;* Puls.; Scilla; *Stann.;* Tub.

Fetid, offensive—Ars.; Bor.; *Calc. c.;* Caps.; Carbo v.; Cop.; Euphras.; Kali c.; *Kali hypophos.;* Lyc.; Nit. ac.; *Phell.;* Phos. ac.; *Pix l.;* Psor.; *Sang.;* Sep.; *Sil.; Stann.;* Sul.

Globular, lumpy—*Agar.;* Arg. m.; Am. m.; Ant. t.; *Bad.;* Calc. c.; Calc. fl.; *Chel.; Kali c.;* Mang.; Nat. selen.; Rhus t.; *Sil.*

Gray, greenish, mucus—Am. phos.; Ant. s. a.; Ars.; *Benz. ac.;* Calc. c.; Calc. iod.; Calc. p.; Calend.; Can. s.; *Carbo v.; Cop.;* Dros.; Dulc.; Ferr. ac.; *Kali iod.;* Kali m.; Kali s.; Kaolin; *Lyc.;* Nat. c.; *Nat. s.; Paris;* Phos.; Psor.; *Puls.;* Senega; Sep.; Silph.; Spong.; *Stann.;* Sul.; Thuya.

Herby taste—Bor.

Liver-colored—Graph.; Lyc.; Puls.; Sep.; Stann.

Profuse—Allium s.; *Ammon.; Am. m.;* Ant. ars.; *Ant. iod.;* Ant. t.; Arg. m.; *Ars. iod.;* Asclep. t.; *Bals. per.;* Calc. c.; Calc. sil.; Canth.; *Carbo v.;* Ceanoth.; Chel.; Cinch.; *Coccus;* Cop.; Dros.; *Dulc.;* Eucal.; Grind.; *Hep.;* Hepat.; Hydr.; Ipec.; *Kali bich.;* Kali c.; Kali iod.; *Kreos.; Laur.; Lyc.;* Merc.; Myos.; Myrt. ch.; Nat. ars.; Nat. s.; Phell.; Phos. ac.; Piloc.; *Puls.;* Ruta; Sang.; *Scilla; Senega; Sep.; Sil.;* Silph.; *Stann.; Sul.;* Tereb.; Trill.; Zing.

Purulent, muco-purulent—Ammon.; Ant. iod.; Ars. iod.; Asclep. t.; *Bac.; Bals. per.; Calc. c.;* Calc. p.; Calc. sil.; Calc. s.; *Carbo v.;* Cinch.; Cop.; Dros.; Eucal.; Eryng.; Hep.; Hepat.; *Hydr.;* Iod.; *Kali bich.;* Kali c.; Kali iod.; *Kali p.;* Kali s.; *Kreos.;* Laur.; *Lyc.;* Merc.; Myos.; Myrtis; Myrt. ch.; Nat. c.; Nit. ac.; Phos. ac.; *Phos.;* Pix l.; Psor.; Ruta; Sang. n.; Sang.; Scilla; Sep.; *Sil.;* Solan. n.; *Stann.; Sul.;* Tereb.; Tereb. scor.; Trill.

Rust-colored—*Bry.;* Ferr. p.; *Phos.;* Rhus t.; *Sang.*

Salty—Ambra; Ars.; Calc. c.; *Kali iod.; Lyc.; Mag. c.;* Nat. c.; Nat. m.; Phos. ac.; Phos.; Psor.; Puls.; Scilla; *Sep.;* Sil.; Stann.

Scanty—Alum.; Am. m.; *Ant. t.; Ars.;* Asclep. t.; Brom.; Bry.; *Caust.;* Cim.; Kali c.; Kali hypophos.; Ign.; Lach.; Morph.; Nit. ac.; *Nux v.;* Op.; *Phos.;* Rumex; Sang.; Scilla; Spong.; Zinc. m. See Viscid.

Serous, frothy, watery—*Acon.;* Am. c.; *Ant. ars.;* Ars.; Bry.; Carbo v.; Croc.; Ferr. p.; Grind.; *Kali iod.;* Lach.; Merc.; Nat. m.; Œnanthe; Phos.; Piloc.; Silph.; Tanac.

Slips back, or must be swallowed—Arn.; *Caust.;* Con.; Iod.; *Kali e.;* Lach.; Nux m.; Spong.

Soapy—Caust.

Sour—Calc. c.; Iris; Lach.; Nit. ac.; Nux v.; Phos. ac.; Phos.; Stann.; Zinc.

Sweetish—Hepat.; Phos.; Sang. n.; *Stann.;* Sul.

Viscid, tenacious, difficult of raising—Allium s.; *Alum.;* Ammon.; *Am. c.; Am. m.;* Ant. iod.; Ant. s. a.; *Ant. t.;* Aral.; *Ars.;* Asclep. t.; Bals. per.; Bar. c.; Bar. m.; Bell.; Bov.; *Bry.;* Calc. c.; Can. s.; *Canth.; Carbo v.; Caust.;* Chel.; Cinch.; *Coccus;* Cupr. m.; Dulc.; Eucal.; Grind.; *Hydr.; Ipec.; Kali bich.;* Kali c.; *Kali hypophos.;* Kali m.; *Lach.;* Laur.; Lyc.; Mang. ac.; Merc.; Morph.; Myrtis; Naph.; Nat. s.; Nux v.; Osm.; *Paris;* Phos.; Psor.; Quill.; Rumex; *Sang.;* Sang. n.; Scilla; *Senega; Sep.; Sil.;* Silph.; Sul.; Stann.

EMPTY FEELING IN CHEST—Phos. ac.; *Stann.*

Eructations—Ambra; Caps.

Faintness—Sep.

Gaping, alternates with cough—Ant. t.

Grasps genitals—Zinc. m.

Grasps throat—Acon.; *Cepa; Iod.;* Lob. infl.

Gurgling, from throat to stomach—Cina.

Herpes facialis—Arn. See Skin.

Hiccough—Tab.

Hoarseness—Ambra; Am. c.; *Brom.;* Calc. c.; Calend.; Carbo v.; *Caust.; Dros.; Eup. perf.; Hep.;* Iod.; Lach.; Meph.; *Merc.;* Phos.; Sil.; *Spong.;* Sul.

Hyperesthesia of mucosæ—*Bell.;* Con.; *Hyos.;* Lach.; Phos.; *Rumex;* Sticta.

Lachrymation—Caps.; *Cepa;* Cina; *Euphras.;* Nat. m.; *Scilla.*

Left breast, feels cold—Nat. c.

PAIN—Chest: Abies n.; Ars.; *Bell.;* Brom.; *Bry.;* Caps.; Carbo v.; *Caust.;* Chel.; Cinch.; Cina; Commocl.; *Dros.;* Dulc.; Elaps; *Eup. perf.;* Euphorb.; Ign.; *Iod.;* Justicia; Kali bich.; *Kali c.;* Kali iod.; Kali n.; *Kreos.; Lact. v.;* Lyc.; Meph.; *Merc.;* Myrtis; Nat. c.; *Nat. s.; Niccol.;* Nux v.; Phell.; *Phos.;* Phyt.; *Rumex;* Senega; Sil.; Spong.; *Sticta; Sul.;* Thasp.

Distant parts—Agar.; Am. c.; Bell.; *Bry.; Caps.; Caust.;* Chel.; Lach.; Nat. m.; Senega.

Head—Æth.; Anac.; Asclep. t.; Bell.; *Bry.;* Carbo v.; Eup. perf.; Ferr. m.; Formica; Lyc.; *Nat. m.; Nux v.;* Sep.; Sul.

Head, he places hands to it—*Bry.;* Caps.; Nat. m.; Nat. s.

Larynx—*Acon.;* Ant. t.; Arg. m.; Arum; Asclep. t.; *Bell.;* Caust.; *Cepa;* Hep.; Inula; *Iod.;* Nit. ac.; *Phos.;* Rumex; *Spong.*

Stomach, abdomen—Asclep. t.; *Bry.;* Calc. c.; *Nux v.;* Puls.; Sep.; Sil.; Sul.; Thuya.

Throat—*Bell.; Lach.;* Merc. i. r.; Sil.

POLYURIA—Scilla.

Prostration—Am. c.; *Ant. t.; Ars.;* Coral.; *Cupr. m.;* Cur.; Hep.; Iod.; *Ipec.;* Meph.; Nit. ac.; Phos. ac.; Rumex; *Ver. a.*

Rawness, soreness of chest—Amyg. am.; Ant. s. a.; Ars.; *Bry.;* Calc. c.; Carbo v.; *Caust.;* Coral.; Dig.; *Eup. perf.;* Ferr. p.; Gels.; Graph.; Mag. m.; Meph.; *Merc.; Phos.;* Rhus t.; *Rumex;* Selen.; Senega; *Stann.*

Rubs face, with fists—Scilla.

Sleepiness, between attacks—Euphorb. dath.

Sneezing, at end—Agar.; Bell.; Cina; Dros.; *Justicia; Scilla;* Senega.

Spasms—*Bell.;* Cina; *Cupr. ac.; Cupr. m.;* Hydroc. ac.; Œnanthe; *Solan. c.*

Spasm of chest—Samb.

Tingling, in chest—Acon.

Urine, involuntary, spurting—Alum.; Caps.; *Caust.;* Colch.; *Ferr.; Ferr. mur.;* Ferr. p.; Nat. m.; *Puls.;* Rumex; *Scilla;* Ver. a.; Verbasc.; *Yerba;* Zinc. m.

Vomiting; retching, gagging—Alumen; Anac.; *Ant. t.; Bry.;* Carbo v.; Coccus; *Cupr. ac.;* Cupr. ars.; Cupr. m.; Cur.; *Dros.;* Euphorb. dath.; Euphras.; *Ferr. m.; Hep.; Ipec.; Kali c.;* Kreos.; Meph.; Myos.; Nit. ac.; *Nux v.;* Phos.; Puls.; Sep.; *Sil.;* Ver. a.

AMELIORATIONS—**From drinking, cold things:** *Caust.; Cupr. m.;* Phos.; Tab.

From drinking, warm things—Spong.

From eating—Anac.; Bism.; Ferr.; *Spong.*

From eructations—Ambra; Angust.; Sang.

From expectoration—Zinc. m.

From lying down—Calc. p.; Ferr. m.; *Mang. ac.;* Sinap.

From lying on right side—Ant. t.

From lying on stomach—Med.

From placing hands, on chest—*Bry.;* Caps.; Cina; Dros.; *Eup. perf.;* Lact. v.; *Nat. s.*

From resolute suppression of cough—Ign.

From resting, on hands and feet—Eup. perf.

From resting, with hands on thighs—Niccol.

From sitting up—*Bry.;* Crot. t.; *Dros.;* Hep.; *Hyos.;* Nat. s.; Phell.; *Puls.;* Sang.

From warming air by covering head with bedclothes—Hep.; Rhus t.; *Rumex.*

From warmth—Bad.

LARYNX—**Anesthesia:** Kali br.

Burning—Am. caust.; Am. m.; Arg. m.; Ars.; Canth.; Mang.; *Merc.;* Mez.; *Paris;* Phos.; *Rumex; Sang.;* Spong.; Zing. See Pain.

Cancer—Nit. ac.; Thuya.

Coldness—*Brom.;* Rhus t.; Sul.

Constricted feeling—Acon.; *Bell.;* Brom.; Calad.; *Chlorum; Cupr.;* Dros.; Guaco; Hydroc. ac.; *Iod.;* Mang. ac.; Med.; *Mosch.;* Naja; Ox. ac.; Phos.; *Spong.;* Still.; Ver. a. See Spasms.

Dryness—Ars.; *Bell.;* Carbo v.; Caust.; Dros.; Dub.; Hep.; Iod.; Kali bich.; Kali iod.; Lemna; *Mang. ac.;* Mez.; *Phos.;* Pop. c.; *Sang.;* Senega; *Spong.* See Inflammation.

Edema of glottis—*Apis; Ars.;* Bell.; Chin. ars.; Chorum; *Kali iod.;* Lach.; Merc.; Piloc.; *Sang.;* Stram.; *Vipera.*

Epiglottis, affections—Cepa; Chlorum; Hepat.; Wyeth.

INFLAMMATION—LARYNGITIS—Acute, catarrhal: Acon.; Æsc.; Ant. t.; Apis; Arg. m.; Ars. iod.; *Arum; Bell.;* Brom.; Bry.; Canth.; Carbo v.; *Caust.; Cepa;* Cub.; Dros.; *Dulc.;* Eup. perf.; *Ferr. p.;* Guaiac.; *Hep.;* Iod.; Ipec.; *Kali bich.;* Kali iod.; *Merc.;* Menthol; Osm.; *Phos.; Rhus t.; Rumex; Samb.;* Sang.; *Spong.;* Sticta; Sul.

Inflammation, atrophic—Am. m.; *Kali bich.;* Kali iod.; Lach.; Mang. ac.; Phos.; Sang.

Inflammation, chronic, catarrhal—Am. br.; Am. iod.; Ant. s. a.; Ant. t.; *Arg. m.; Arg. n.;* Bar. c.; Bar. m.; Calc. c.; Calc. iod.; *Carbo v.; Caust.;* Coccus; Cotyled.; *Dros.; Hep.;* Iod.; Irid.; *Kali bich.;* Kali c.; *Kali iod.; Lach.; Mang. ac.;* Merc. c.; *Merc.;* Nat. m.; Nat. selen.; Nit. ac.; *Nux v.; Paris; Phos.; Puls.;* Rhus t.; Sang. n.; *Selen.; Senega; Stann.;* Still.; *Sul.;* Thuya.

Inflammation, follicular—Arg. n.; Hep.; *Iod.;* Kali iod.; Selen.; *Sul.*

Inflammation, membranous exudate—MEMBRANOUS CROUP—*Acet. ac.;* Acon.; Ammon.; *Am. caust.;* Ant. t.; Ars.; Ars. iod.; Bell.; *Brom.;* Calc. iod.; Con.; Dros.; Ferr. p.; Hep.; *Iod.; Kali bich.;* Kali chlor.; *Kali m.;* Kali n.; *Kaolin;* Lach.; Merc. cy.; *Merc.;* Phos.; Samb.; *Sang.; Spong.* See Diphtheria (Throat).

Inflammation—SPASMODIC CROUP—Acon.; Ant. t.; Ars.; Bell.; Benzoin; *Brom.;* Bry.; *Calc. fl.; Calc. iod.; Chlorum;* Cupr.; Euphorb.; Ferr. p.; *Hep.;* Ign.; *Iod.;* Ipec.; *Kali bich.;* Kali br.; *Kali n.;* Kaolin; Lach.; Meph.; Merc. i. fl.; Mosch.; Naja; Petrol.; *Phos.;* Poth.; Samb.; Sang.; *Spong.; Ver. v.*

Inflammation, syphilitic, associated with, secondary symptoms—Merc. c.; Merc. s.; Nit. ac.

Inflammation, syphilitic, associated with, tertiary symptoms—*Aur.;* Cinnab.; Iod.; *Kali bich.; Kali iod.;* Lach.; *Merc. c.;* Merc. i. fl.; Merc. i. r.; Mez.; *Nit. ac.;* Sang.; Thuya. See Syphilis (Male Sexual System).

Inflammation, syphilitic, hereditary—*Aur.;* Fluor. ac.; *Hep.;* Kreos.; Merc. i. fl.; *Merc. i. r.;* Merc.; *Nit. ac.; Phyt.;* Sul.; Thuya.

Inflammation, tuberculous—*Arg. n.;* Ars.; *Ars. iod.;* Atrop.; Bapt.; Brom.; *Calc. c.;* Calc. p.; Canth.; Carbo v.; *Caust.;* Chrom. oxy.; Cistus; *Dros.;* Ferr. p.; Hep.; *Iod.;* Ipec.; Jabor.; Kali c.; Kali m.; Kreos.; Lyc.; *Mang. ac.;* Merc. nit.; Naja; *Nat. selen.;* Nit. ac.; *Phos.; Selen.;* Spong.; *Stann.;* Sul.

Irritation—*Arg. m.;* Bar. c.; Caust.; Chlorum; *Hep.;* Kali bich.; Kali iod.; Kali perm.; *Lach.;* Mang. ac.; Nux v.; *Phos.* See Rawness.

Motion, up and down, violent—*Sul. ac.*

Mucus—Ant. t.; *Arg. m.;* Arg. n.; *Brom.; Bry.;* Canth.; Dros.; *Hep.; Kali bich.;* Kali c.; Lach.; *Mang. ac.;* Ox. ac.; Paris; Phos.; Rumex; *Samb.;* Sang.; Selen.; Senega; Stann. See Inflammation.

Pains—Acon.; Alum.; Arg. n.; Arum; *Bell.;* Bry.; *Cepa; Hep.; Iod.;* Justicia; Kreos.; Lach.; *Mang. ac.;* Med.; Merc. c.; Nit. ac.; *Osm.; Phos.;* Sang.; *Spong.* See Inflammation.

Polypus—Berb. v.; Psor.; Sang.; *Sang. n.; Teucr.;* Thuya.

Rawness, roughness, soreness, sensitiveness—Acon.; Alum.; Am. caust.; *Arg. m.;* Arn.; *Arum; Bar. c.; Bell.;* Benzoin; Brom.; Bry.; *Caust.; Cham.;* Cistus; Dros.; Eup. perf.; *Hep.;* Iod.; Kali bich.; *Kali iod.;* Kali perm.; Kaolin; *Lach.;* Lyc.; *Mag. p.; Mang. ac.;* Med.; *Merc.;* Nux v.; Osm.; Phos. ac.; *Phos.;* Puls.; Rhus t.; *Rumex;* Sang.; *Spong.; Sul.;* Zinc. m.

Spasm (laryngismus stridulus)—*Acon.;* Agar.; Am. caust.; Ars. iod.; Arum; *Bell.;* Brom.; *Calc. c.;* Calc. iod.; Calc. p.; Chel.; *Chlorum;* Chloral; Cic.; Cinch.; *Coral.; Cupr. ac.; Cupr. m.; Formal.; Gels.;* Granat.; Ign.; *Iod.; Ipec.;* Kali br.; *Lach.;* Meph.; *Mosch.;* Phos.; *Samb.;* Spong.; Stram.; *Strych.;* Vespa; Zinc. m.

Suffocative catarrh—Ambra; Ars.; Calc. c.; Coff.; Sang.; Spong.

Tickling—Alum.; *Ambra;* Ant. s. a.; *Bell.;* Calc. c.; Caps.; Carbo v.; Cepa; *Coccus;* Cop.; Dros.; Dulc.; *Iod.;* Kali bich.; *Phos.* See Cough.

Tumors, benign—Caust.; Kali bich.; Sang.; Thuya.

Tumors, malignant—*Ars.;* Ars. iod.; Bell.; Carbo an.; Clem.; *Con.;* Hydr.; Iod.; Kreos.; Lach.; Morph.; *Phyt.;* Sang.; Thuya.

Vocal cords, ulceration—Aur. iod.; Iod.; Lyc.; Merc. nit.

Vocal cords, weak—*Carbo v.; Caust.;* Coca; Dros.; Graph.; Penthor.; Phos. See Voice.

VOICE—**Deep, bass:** Brom.; Camph.; Carbo v.; *Caust.;* Dros.; Phos.; Pop. c.; Sang. n.; Stann.; Sul.; *Verbasc.*

High, piping—*Bell.*

Hoarse, aphonia—*Acon.;* Alumen; Alum.; Am. c.; *Am. caust.; Am. m.;* Ant. c.; Antipyr.; Arg. iod.; *Arg. m.; Arg. n.;* Arn.; Ars. iod.; *Arum;* Asclep. t.; Bar. c.; *Bell.;* Benzoin; *Brom.; Bry.; Calc. c.;* Calc. caust.; Camph.; *Carbo v.; Caust.;* Cham.; Chlorum; Cina; *Coca;* Cochlear.; Coccus; Cub.; *Dros.;* Dub.; *Dulc.; Eup. perf.;* Ferr. p.; Gels.; Graph.; *Hep.;* Hyos.; Ign.; Iod.; *Ipec.;* Justicia; *Kali bich.; Kali c.;* Kali chrom.; Kreos.; Mag. p.; *Mang. ac.; Merc.; Nit. ac.;* Nux m.; *Nux v.;* Op.; Osm.; *Ox. ac.;* Paris; Penthor.; Petrol.; *Phos.;* Plat.; *Pop. c.;* Puls.; *Rhus t.; Rumex; Samb.;* Sang.; Sang. n.; *Selen.;* Senega; Sep.; Sil.; *Spong.;* Stann.; Sticta; *Still.; Sul.;* Thuya; Ver. v.; *Verbasc.;* Viola od.

Hoarseness, capricious—Hep.; Puls.

Hoarseness, chronic—Ampelop.; *Arg. n.;* Bar. c.; Calc. c.; *Carbo v.; Caust.;* Graph.; *Mang. ac.;* Phos.; *Sul.*

Hoarseness, croupy—Acon.; Ail.; Brom.; Caust.; *Cepa; Hep.;* Kali s.; *Spong.*

Hoarseness, from cold weather—Carbo v.; Caust.; Rumex; Sul.

Hoarseness, from overheating—Ant. c.; Ant. t.; Brom.

Hoarseness, from overusing voice, especially public speakers, professional singers—Alum.; *Arg. m.; Arg. n.;* Arn.; *Arum;* Carbo v.; *Caust.;* Coca; Ferr. p.; Ferr. picr.; *Hep.;* Iod.: Mang. ac.; Med.; Merc. cy.;

Merc. s.; Nat. selen.; Phos.; *Rhus t.; Selen.;* Spong.; Still.; Sul.; Tab.; Terebene.

Hoarseness, hysterical—Cocc.; *Gels.; Ign.;* Nux m.; Plat.

Hoarseness, painless—Bell.; *Calc. c.;* Carbo v.; Paris.

Hoarseness, paretic—Am. caust.; Bell.; *Caust.; Gels.;* Lach.; *Ox. ac.;* Phos.; Rumex; Sil.

Hoarseness, relieved temporarily by coughing or expectoration—Stann.

Hoarseness, worse, at end of cold—Ipec.

Hoarseness, worse, in A. M.—*Arum;* Benz. ac.; Calc. c.; *Caust.;* Eup. perf.; Hep.; *Mang.;* Nit. ac.; *Nux v.;* Sul.

Hoarseness, worse, in P. M.—*Carbo v.;* Kali bich.; Phos.; *Rumex.*

Hoarseness, worse, in damp weather—Carbo v.

Hoarseness, worse talking, singing, swallowing—Spong.

Hoarseness, worse, walking against wind—Acon.; Arum; *Euphras.;* Hep.; *Nux m.*

Hoarseness, worse when crying—Acon.; *Bell.;* Phos.; Spong.

Menstrual—Gels.

Nervous aphonia with cardiac disorder—Coca; Hydroc. ac.; Nux m.; Ox. ac.

Timbre, varies continually—Ant. c.; Arg. m.; *Arum;* Bell.; Carbo v.; Caust.; Dros.; Lach.; Rumex.

Voice producer, instantaneous—Arum; Caust.; *Coca;* Ferr. p.; *Pop. c.*

Voice, low, monotonous; economical speech—Mang. ac.; Mang. oxy.

Whispering, weak voice—Arg. m.; Camph.; Canth.; Carbo v.; *Caust.;* Dub.; *Phos.; Pop. c.;* Primula; Puls.; Ver. a.

LUNGS—Abscess: Acon.; *Ars. iod.;* Bell.; Caps.; Chin. ars.; *Cinch.;* Hep.; Iod.; Kali c.; Merc.; *Sil.*

Congestion—*Acon.;* Adren.; Ars. iod.; *Bell.;* Bothrops; *Cact.;* Conv.; *Ferr. p.;* Iod.; Kali n.; Lyc.; Nux v.; Op.; Phos.; Stroph.; Sulphon.; Upas; *Ver. v.* See Inflammation.

Congestion, passive—Carbo v.; *Dig.;* Ferr. m.; Hydroc. ac.; Nux v.; Phos.; *Sul.*

Dilation of cells (emphysema)—*Am. c.; Ant. ars.;* Ant. t.; *Ars.; Aur. mur.;* Bell.; Bry.; Calc. c.; *Calc. p.;* Carbo v.; Chin ars.; Cinch.; Dig.; *Dros.;* Eucal.; Glon.; Grind.; Hep.; Ipec.; Kali c.; *Lob. infl.; Lyc.;* Myrtis; Naph.; Nux v.; Phell.; *Phos.;* Puls.; Sep.; Spong.; *Strych.;* Sul. See Asthma.

Distended feeling—Tereb.

Edema—*Am. c.;* Am. iod.; Ant. t.; *Apis; Ars.;* Cochlear.; *Kali c.;* Kali iod.; Lach.; *Phos.;* Piloc.; Pulmo v.; *Sang.;* Senec.; Stroph.; Tub.

Gangrene—Arn.; *Ars.; Caps.;* Carbo an.; *Carbo v.; Crot.;* Eucal.; Dulc.; Hep.; Kreos.; *Lach.;* Lyc.; *Sec.;* Sil.

HAEMORRHAGE (hæmoptysis)—*Acal.;* Acet. ac.; *Achillea; Acon.; Allium s.; Arn.; Cact.;* Carbo v.; Chin. ars.; *Cinch.;* Cinnam.; Dig.; Erecht.; Ergot.; *Erig.;* Ferr. ac.; Ferr. m.; *Ferr. p.;* Gelat.; *Geran.; Ham.;* Helix t.; *Hydrast. mur.; Ipec.;* Kali c.; Kreos.; *Lamina; Led.;* Mangif.

ind.; Meli.; *Millef.;* Nat. nit.; *Phos.;* Rhus t.; Sang.; Stroph.; *Sul. ac.;* Tereb.; *Trill.;* Ver. *v.*

Hæmorrhage, bright, red, blood—Acal.; *Acon.;* Aran.; Cact.; Ferr. ac.; *Ferr. p.;* Geran.; Led.; *Millef.;* Nit. ac.; Rhus t.; Trill.

Hæmorrhage, dark, clotted blood—Arn.; Crot.; *Elaps;* Ferr. mur.; *Ham.;* Sul. ac.

Hæmorrhage, during menopause—Lach.

Hæmorrhage, bæmorrhoidal—Mez.; Nux v.

Hæmorrhage, in drunkards—Hyos.; *Led.;* Nux v.; *Op.*

Hæmorrhage, in periodical attacks—Kreos.

Hæmorrhage, in puerperal fevers—Ham.

Hæmorrhage, traumatic—Millef.

Hæmorrhage, tubercular—Acal.; Ferr. p.; Millef.; Nux v.; Trill.

Hæmorrhage, vicarious—Bry.; Ham.; Phos.

Hæmorrhage, with cough—*Acon.;* Acal.; *Ferr. ac.;* Ferr. p.; *Ipec.; Led.;* Phos. See Cough.

Hæmorrhage, without cough, or effort—*Acon.;* Ham.; Millef.; Sul. ac.

Hæmorrhage, with valvular disease—Cact.; Lycop.

Hot feeling—Acon. See Congestion.

Inflammation—BRONCHO-PNEUMONIA—*Acon.;* Am. iod.; Ant. ars.; *Ant. t.;* Ars.; *Ars. iod.;* Bell.; Bry.; *Chel.;* Ferr. p.; Glycerin; Iod.; *Ipec.;* Kali c.; *Koch's lymph;* Phos.; Puls.; *Scilla;* Solania; *Tub.*

Inflammation—CROUPOUS PNEUMONIA—*Acon.;* Agar.; Am. iod.; Ant. ars.; Ant. iod.; Ant. s. a.; *Ant. t.;* Apomorph.; Arn.; Ars.; *Bell.;* Brom.; *Bry.;* Caffeine; Camph.; Carb. ac.; Carbo v.; *Chel.;* Cinch.; Dig.; *Ferr. p.;* Gels.; Hep.; *Iod.;* Ipec.; Kali bich.; *Kali c.;* Kali iod.; Lach.; *Lyc.; Merc.;* Millef.; Nat. s.; Nit. ac.; Op.; Ox. ac.; *Phos.;* Puromococcin; Pneumotoxin; Pyr.; Ran. b.; Rhus t.; *Sang.;* Scilla; Senega; Strych.; *Sul.;* Tub.; Ver. a.; *Ver. v.*

Stages of pneumonia—Congestive: Acon.; Æsc.; Bell.; Bry.; Ferr. *p.; Iod.;* Sang.; Ver. *v.*

Consolidation—Ant. t.; *Bry.; Iod.;* Kali iod.; Kali m.; *Phos.;* Sang.; Sul;

Resolution—*Ant. t.;* Ant. s. a.; Ars.; Ars. iod.; Carbo v.; *Hep.;* Iod.. *Kali iod.;* Kali s.; *Lyc.;* Nat. s.; *Phos.; Sang.;* Sil.; Stann. iod.; *Sul.*

Type—Bilious—Ant. t.; *Chel.;* Lept.; Merc.; Phos.; Pod.

Latent—Chel.; Phos.; *Sul.*

Neglected, lingering, cases—Am. c.; Ant. iod.; Ant. s. a.; *Ant. t.;* Ars. iod.; Bry.; *Carbo v.;* Cinch.; Hep.; Kali iod.; Lach.; *Lyc.;* Phos.; Plumb.; Sul.

Secondary—Ant. ars.; *Ant. t.; Ferr. p.;* Phos.

Senile—Ant. ars.; *Ant. t.;* Dig.; Ferr. p.

Sycotic—Nat. s.

Typhoid—*Hyos.;* Lach.; Laur.; Merc. cy.; Op.; *Phos.; Rhus t.;* Sang.; Sul.

PARALYSIS of lungs—Am. c.; *Ant. ars.; Ant. t.;* Arn.; Bac.; Carbo v.; Cur.; Diphtherotox.; Dulc.; *Grind.;* Hydroc. ac.; Ipec.; Lach.; *Laur.; Lob. purp.;* Lyc.; Merc. cy.; Morph.; Mosch.; Phos.; *Solania.*

Tired feeling—Ail.; Arum.

TUBERCULOSIS (phthisis pulmonalis)—Acal.; Acon.; Agaricin; *Allium s.;* Ant. ars.; *Ant. iod.; Ars.; Ars. iod.;* Aur. ars.; Atrop.; Aviare; *Bac.;* Bals. per.; *Bapt.;* Bell.; Blatta or.; *Bry.;* Calc. ars.; *Calc. c.;* Calc. chlor.; Calc. hypophos.; *Calc. iod.; Calc. p.;* Calop.; Can. s.; *Cetrar.; Chin. ars.;* Cim.; Coccus; Cod.; *Crot.;* Cupr. ars.; *Dros.;* Dulc.; Eriod.; Ferr. ac.; *Ferr. ars.;* Ferr. iod.; Ferr. m.; *Ferr. p.;* Form. ac.; Formica; *Gall. ac.; Guaiacol;* Guaiac.; Ham.; Hep.; Helix; Hippoz.; Hydr.; Hyosc. hydrobr.; Hysterion; Ichth.; *Iod.;* Iodof.; Ipec.; Kalag.; Kali bich.; *Kali c.;* Kali n.; *Kreos.;* Lach.; *Lachnanth.;* Lact. ac.; Laur.; Lecith.; *Lyc.;* Mang. ac.; Med.; Millef.; *Myos.;* Myrtis; Naph.; *Nat. cacodyl.; Nat. selen.;* Nat. s.; *Nit. ac.;* Nux v.; Ox. ac.; *Phell.;* Phos. ac.; *Phos.;* Piloc.; Pineal gland ext.; *Polygon. av.;* Puls.; Rumex; Ruta; Salvia; *Sang.;* Sep.; *Sil.;* Silph. cyr.; *Spong.; Stann.;* Stann. iod.; Sticta; Succin.; *Sul.;* Teucr. scor.; Thea; Ther.; *Tub.;* Urea; Vanad.; Yerba.

Acute (phthisis florida)—Ant. t.; *Ars.;* Calc. c.; Calc. iod.; Ferr. ac.; Ferr. m.; Ferr. mur.; *Iod.; Phos.;* Piloc. mur.; *Sang.;* Ther.; Tub.

Cough—Allium s.; Ars.; *Ars. iod.;* Aviare; Bapt.; *Bell.;* Calc. c.; Caust.; Cinch.; *Cod.;* Con.; *Coral.;* Crot.; *Dros.;* Ferr. ac.; *Hep.; Hyos.;* Ipec.; *Kali c.;* Lach.; Laur.; Lob. infl.; Myos.; *Nit. ac.; Phos.;* Rumex; Sang.; *Sil.;* Silph. cyr.; Spong.; *Stann.;* Sticta.

Debility—Acal.; Ars.; *Ars. iod.;* Aviare; *Chin. ars.;* Phos.; Sil. See Nervous System.

Diarrhœa—Acet. ac.; Arg. n.; Arn.; *Ars.;* Ars. iod.; Calc. c.; *Cinch.; Coto;* Iod.; Iodof.; *Phos. ac.; Phos.;* Sil. See Abdomen.

Digestive disorders—Ars.; Aviare; Calc. c.; Carbo v.; *Cupr. ars.;* Ferr. ac.; Ferr. ars.; Gall. ac.; *Hydr.;* Kreos.; *Nux v.;* Strych. See Stomach.

Dyspnœa—Carbo v.; Ipec.; Phos.

Emaciation—Allium s.; Ars.; *Ars. iod.;* Calc. p.; Eriod.; *Iod.;* Myos.; Phos.; Sil.; Silph. cyr.; *Tub.* See Generalities.

Fever—Acon.; Allium s.; Ars.; Ars. iod.; *Bapt.;* Calc. iod.; *Chin. ars.;* Chin. s.; Cinch.; *Ferr. p.;* Iod.; Lyc.; Nit. ac.; Phos.; Sang.; Sil.; Stann.

Fibroid—Bry.; Calc. c.; Sang.; *Sil.*

Hemoptysis—*Acal.; Achillea; Acon.;* Calc. ars.; *Ferr. ac.;* Ferr. m.; *Ferr. p.; Ham.; Ipec.;* Millef.; Nit. ac.; *Phos.;* Piloc. mur.; *Trill.* See Hemoptysis.

Incipient—Acal.; Agar.; *Ars. iod.; Calc. c.;* Calc. iod.; Calc. p.; *Dros.; Ferr. p.;* Iod.; Kali c.; Kali iod.; Lachnanth.; Mang. ac.; Med.; Myrtis; Ol. j. as.; *Phos.;* Polygon.; Puls.; Sang.; Sec.; Succin.; Sul.; Trill.; *Tub.;* Vanad.

Insomnia—Allium s.; *Coff.;* Dig.; Sil. See Nervous System.

Liver disturbance—Chel.

Mechanical injury, after—Millef.; Ruta.

Night sweats—*Acet. ac.; Agaricin; Ars.;* Ars. iod.; Atrop.; *Cinch.;* Eriod.; Gall. ac.; Hep.; *Jabor.;* Kali iod.; Lyc.; Myos.; *Phos. ac.; Phos.;* Piloc.; Piloc. mur.; Salvia; Samb.; Sec.; *Sil.;* Silph. cyr.; Stann.; Yerba. See Fever.

Pains in chest—Acon.; *Bry.*; Calc. c.; Cim.; Guaiac.; *Kali c.*; Myrtis; Phos.; Pix liq. See Chest.

Sore mouth—Lach.

PLEURÆ—EMPYEMA: Arn.; *Ars.*; Calc. c.; *Calc. s.*; Cinch.; Echin.; Ferr. m.; *Hep.*; Ipec.; Kali c.; *Merc.*; Nat. s.; Phos.; *Sil.*

Hydrothorax—*Adon. v.*; Ant. t.; *Apis*; Apoc.; *Ars.*; Ars. iod.; Canth.; Carbo v.; Cinch.; Colch.; *Dig.*; Fluor. ac.; Helleb.; *Iod.*; *Kali c.*; Kali iod.; *Lact. v.*; Lyc.; *Merc. sul.*; Phaseol.; Phos.; Piloc.; *Ran. b.*; Scilla; *Senega; Sul.*

PLEURISY—Abrot.; *Acon.*; Ant. ars.; Ant. t.; *Apis*; Arn.; *Ars.*; *Asclep. t.*; Bell.; Bor.; *Bry.*; *Canth.*; Carbo an.; Cinch.; *Dig.*; Eriod.; Ferr. mur.; *Ferr. p.*; Formica; *Guaiac.*; Hep.; *Iod.*; *Kali c.*; Kali iod.; Led.; Lob. card.; *Merc.*; Nat. s.; Op.; Phos.; Ran. b.; Rhus t.; Sabad.; *Scilla; Senega*; Sep.; Sil.; Spig.; *Sul.*; Tub.

Adhesions—Abrot.; Carbo an.; Hep.; Ran. b.; Sul.

Chronic—Ars. iod.; *Hep.*; *Iod.*; Kali iod.; Scilla; *Sul.*

Diaphragmatic—Acon.; *Bry.*; Cact.; Cupr.; Mosch.; *Ran. b.*

Rheumatic—Acon.; Arn.; *Bry.*; Ran. b.; Rhod.; Rhus t.

Tuberculosis—Ars. iod.; Bry.; Hep.; *Iod.*; Iodof.; Kali c.

With Bright's disease—Ars.; *Merc. c.* See Urinary System.

RESPIRATION—Arrested (apnœa): Ars.; Bov.; Camph.; Hydroc. ac.; *Latrod.*; Lyssin; Upas.

Arrested, on falling asleep—*Am. c.*; Dig.; *Grind.*; *Lach.*; Lac c.; Merc. pr. rub.; Op.; *Samb.*

Cheyne-Stokes—*Acon. fer.*; Antipyr.; Atrop.; Bell.; Carbo v.; Cocaine; *Grind.*; Kali cy.; *Morph.*; Op.; Parth.; *Spart. s.*

DYSPNŒA (difficult, embarrassed, oppressed, anxious): *Acet. ac.*; *Acon. fer.*; *Acon.*; Adren.; *Am. c.*; Amyl; *Ant. ars.*; Ant. iod.; *Ant. t.*; *Apis*; Apoc.; *Aral.*; *Ars.*; Ars. iod.; *Aur.*; *Bac.*; Bell.; *Blatta or.*; *Brom.*; *Bry.*; *Cact.*; Cajup.; *Calc. ars.*; *Calc. c.*; Canth.; Caps.; *Carbo v.*; Caust.; *Cepa*; Cham.; Chel.; *Chlorum*; Cinch.; *Coca*; Collins.; *Conv.*; *Crat.*; *Cupr. ac.*; Cupr. m.; *Cur.*; Dig.; Diosc.; Dros.; *Ferr. m.*; Ferr. p.; Fluor. ac.; *Formal.*; Glon.; *Grind.*; Hep.; Hydroc. ac.; Ign.; *Iod.*; *Ipec.*; Justicia; Kali bich.; *Kali c.*; Kali n.; Lach.; Laur.; *Lob. infl.*; Lyc.; Merc. c.; *Merc. sul.*; Mosch.; Naph.; Nat. ars.; *Nat. s.*; *Nux v.*; Op.; *Phos.*; Phyt.; Pothos; *Puls.*; Pulmo v.; *Quebracho*; Ran. b.; Ruta; *Samb.*; Sang.; *Scilla*; Senec.; *Senega*; Serum ang.; *Sil.*; *Spig.*; Spong.; Stann.; *Stroph.*; Strych.; *Sul.*; Tab.; Ver. a.; Ver. v.; *Viela od.*; *Zinc. m.* See Asthma.

Dyspnœa, aggravated at P. M.—Act. spic.; *Ars.*; Aur.; Cahinca; Calc. c.; Carbo v.; *Dig.*; Phos.; Puls.; *Samb.*; Sep.; *Sul.*; Trifol.

Dyspnœa, aggravated during damp, cloudy weather—Nat. s.

Dyspnœa, aggravated from ascending stairs—Am. c.; Ars.; Bor.; Calc. c.; Chin. ars.; Iod.; Ipec.; Lob. infl.; Nat. m.; Sep.

Dyspnœa, aggravated from exposure to cold air—Act. spic.; Lob. infl.

Dyspnœa, aggravated from foreign bodies—Ant. t.; Sil.

Dyspnœa, aggravated from least thing coming near mouth or nose—Lach.

Dyspnœa, aggravated from lying down—Abies n.; Act. spic.; Aral.; *Ars.*;

Cahinca; Dig.; Grind.; Lach.; Merc. sul.; Puls.; Sep.; Strych. ars.; Sul.

Dyspnœa, aggravated from lying on left side—Naja; Spig.; Tab.; Viscum.

Dyspnœa, aggravated from lying on right side—Viscum.

Dyspnœa, aggravated from lying with head low—Cinch.; Nitrum; Spong.

Dyspnœa, aggravated from myocardial disease—Sarcol. ac.

Dyspnœa, aggravated from nervous causes—Ambra; Arg. n.; Ars.; Asaf.; *Cajup.; Mosch.;* Nux m.; Puls.; *Val.;* Viola od.

Dyspnœa, aggravated from rest—Sil.

Dyspnœa, aggravated from sinking sensation in abdomen—Acet. ac.

Dyspnœa, aggravated from sitting up—Carbo v.; Laur.; Psor.; Sep.

Dyspnœa, aggravated from sleep—Dig.; *Lach.;* Samb.; Sep.; Spong.

Dyspnœa, aggravted from sleep; sitting indoors; relieved by rapid motion—Sep.

Dyspnœa, aggravated from stooping—Calc. c.; Sil.

Dyspnœa, aggravated from walking—*Acon.;* Am. c.; Carbo v.; Con.; *Ipec.;* Kali c.; Nat. m.; Sep.; Sil.

Dyspnœa, aggravated from working—Am. m.; Calc. c.; Lyc.; Nat. m.; Nit. ac.; Sep.; Sil.; Sumb.

Dyspnœa, aggravated in aged, alcoholics, athletics—Coca.

Dyspnœa, aggravated in children—Lyc.; Samb.

Dyspnœa, aggravated in lower chest—Lob. syph.; Nux v.

Dyspnœa, aggravated in morning—Ant. t.; Con.; Kali bich.; Kali c.; Nat. s.

Dyspnœa, aggravated in warm room—Am. c.; Puls.; Sep.

Dyspnœa, relieved from bending forward—Ars.; Kali c.

Dyspnœa, relieved from bending shoulders backwards—Calc. c.

Dyspnœa, relieved from eructating—Ambra; Ant. t.

Dyspnœa, relieved from expectoration—*Ant. t.;* Ars.; Kali bich.; Zinc. m.

Dyspnœa, relieved from fanning rapidly—Carbo v.

Dyspnœa, relieved from fanning slowly and at a distance—Lach.

Dyspnœa, relieved from lying down—Kali bich.; *Psor.*

Dyspnœa, relieved from lying on right side—Ant. t.

Dyspnœa, relieved from lying on right side, head high—Cact.; Spig.; Spong.

Dyspnœa, relieved from motion—Lob. infl.; Sep.

Dyspnœa, relieved from sitting up—Acon. fer.; Ant. t.; *Ars.;* Dig.; Laur.; Merc. sul.; Nat. s.; *Samb.;* Sul.; Tereb.　　6

Dyspnœa, relieved from standing up—Can. s.

Dyspnœa, relieved from stretching arms apart—Psor.

Dyspnœa, relieved in open air—Calc. c.; Lach.; *Sul.*

Gasping—Brom.; Hydroc. ac.; *Ipec.;* Phos.; Samb.

Hoarse, hissing—Acet. ac.

Inspiration difficult—Brom.; Cact.; Chel.; Iod.; Nicot.; *Ox. ac.* See Dyspnœa.

Inspiration free, expiration impeded—*Chlorum;* Med.; Meph.; *Samb.*

Irregular—Ail.; *Ant. t.;* Bell.; Crat.; *Dig.;* Helleb.; Hippoz.; *Hydroc. ac.;* Op.; Trill.

Rapid, short, superficial—*Acon. fer.;* Acon.; Am. c.; *Ant. t.;* Apis; *Apoc.;* Aral.; *Ars.;* Bell.; *Bry.;* Calc. c.; Carbo v.; Cupr. ac.; Cupr.; Cur.; *Ferr. p.;* Hippoz.; Kali bich.; Lach.; Lob. purp.; Lyc.; Mag. p.; Merc.

cy.; Merc. sul.; Nat. s.; *Nux v.;* Ox. ac.; Phos. ac.; *Phos.;* Prun. sp.; Senega; Sil.; *Spong.;* Stann.; Sul. ac.

Rattling—Allium s.; *Ammon.;* Am. c.; Am. caust.; Am. m.; *Ant. ars.; Ant. t.;* Bals. per.; Bar. c.; Bar. m.; *Brom.;* Calc. ac.; Calc. c.; Can. s.; Carbo v.; Cham.; *Chel.;* Chlorum; *Cinch.;* Cupr. m.; Dulc.; Ferr. p.; Grind.; *Hep.; Ipec.;* Kali bich.; Kali c.; Kali m.; Kali n.; *Kali s.;* Lyc.; Meph.; *Nat. s.;* Œnanthe; *Op.;* Phos.; Pix l.; *Puls.;* Scilla; *Senega;* Sil.; *Stann.; Sul.;* Ver. a.

Sawing—Brom.; Iod.; Samb.; *Spong.*

Sighing—Ail.; Apoc.; Cact.; *Calc. p.;* Carb. ac.; Cereus bon.; *Dig.;* Gels.; Granat.; Helleb.; *Ign.; Lach.;* Led.; Naph.; Nat. p.; *Op.;* Phaseol.; Piloc.; Samb.; Sec.; Sulphon.

Slow, deep—Am. c.; Aur.; Benz. din.; Cact.; Can. ind.; Cinch.; Dig.; Gadus; Gels.; *Helleb.; Hydroc. ac.;* Laur.; Lob. purp.; *Op.;* Phaseol.; Piloc.; *Ver. v.*

Stertorous—Acon.; Am. c.; Arn.; Bell.; Bry.; Can. ind.; *Cinch.;* Euphorb. dath.; Helleb.; Hippoz.; *Hydroc. ac.;* Lob. purp.; Naja; Nat. sal.; *Œnanthe; Op.;* Phaseol.; Phos.; Piloc.; Sec.; *Sulphon.;* Tanac.; Trion.; Ver. v.; Viscum.

Suffocative—*Acon. fer.; Ant. t.; Apis; Ars.;* Bell.; Brom.; Cact.; *Calc. c.;* Camph.; *Chlorum; Cinch.;* Coral.; Cupr. m.; *Dig.;* Graph.; *Grind.; Guaiac.;* Hep.; Hydroc. ac.; Iod.; *Ipec.;* Kali bich.; Kali iod.; *Lach.; Latrod.;* Led.; Lil. t.; Lob. infl.; Lyc.; Meli.; Meph.; Merc. cy.; *Merc. pr. rub.;* Morph.; *Mosch.;* Naja; Puls.; *Samb.; Spong.; Sul.;* Tub.; Trifol.; Ver. a.; Viscum.

Wheezing—Alum.; Am. c.; Ant. iod.; *Ant. t.;* Aral.; *Ars.;* Can. s.; Carbo v.; Card. m.; Eriod.; *Grind.; Hep.;* Iod.; Iodof.; *Ipec.;* Justicia; Kali bich.; *Kali c.;* Lob. infl.; Lycop.; Nux v.; Prun. sp.; Samb.; Senega; *Spong.* See Asthma.

Whistling—Ars.; Ipec.; Samb.

TRACHEA—Burning: *Ars.;* Kali bich.; Sang. See Irritation.

Catarrh—Alum.; *Ant. t.;* Arg. n.; Ars.; *Bry.;* Calc. c.; Can. s.; Carbo v.; *Caust.;* Coccus; Conv.; Cotyled.; Ferr. iod.; Hep.; Iberis; Illic.; *Kali bich.;* Mang.; *Merc.;* Naph.; Nat. m.; Nux v.; Paris; *Rumex;* Sil.; *Stann.;* Sticta; Sul.; Tab.

Constricted feeling—Brom.; Cistus; Guaco; *Mosch.; Nux v.;* Xerophyl.

Dryness—Ars.; Bell.; Carbo v.; *Rumex;* Sang.; Spong. See Irritation.

Irritation, rawness, hypersensitiveness—Acet. ac.; Æsc.; Ambros.; Apis; Arg. m.; *Arg. n.;* Ars.; *Bell.;* Brom.; *Bry.;* Can. s.; Carbo an.; Carbo v.; *Caust.;* Ferr. p.; *Hyos.;* Kali bich.; Kaolin; *Lach.;* Mentha; *Osm.;* Phos.; *Rumex; Sang.;* Stann.; Still.; Sul.; Syph.; Xerophyl.

Tickling—Ambros.; Brom.; Calc. c.; Caps.; *Carbo v.;* Cop.; Ipec.; *Lach.;* Nux v.; *Phos.; Rumex.* See Cough.

SKIN

ACNE ROSACEA—Agar.; Ars.; *Ars. br.;* Ars. iod.; Bell.; *Carbo an.;* Caust.; Chrysar.; Eug. j.; *Hydrocot.;* Kali br.; Kali iod.; Kreos.; Nux v.; Oophor.; Petrol.; Psor.; Radium; Rhus r.; Rhus t.; Sep.; Sul.; *Sul. iod.;* Sulphurous ac.

ACNE SIMPLEX—*Ant. c.;* Ant. s. a.; *Ant. t.;* Ars.; *Ars. br.;* Ars. iod.; Ars. sul. rub.; Asimina; *Aster.; Bell.;* Bellis; *Berb. aq.; Bov.; Calc. picr.;* Calc. sil.; *Calc. s.;* Carb. ac.; *Carbo an.; Carbo v.;* Cic.; Cim.; Cob.; Echin.; *Eug. j.;* Granat.; Graph.; *Hep.; Hydrocot.; Jugl. c.; Jugl. r.; Kali br.;* Kali bich.; *Kali iod.;* Kali m.; Lappa; *Led.; Lyc.;* Nabul. s.; Nat. br.; Nat. m.; Nit. ac.; *Nux v.;* Oleand.; Phos. ac.; Psor.; Puls.; Radium; Selen.; Sep.; Sil.; Staph.; *Sul.; Sul. iod.;* Sumb.; Thuya.

From abuse of KI—Aur.

From abuse of mercury—Kali iod.; Mez.; Nit. ac.

From cheese—Nux v.

From cosmetics—Bov.

From syphilis—Aur.; *Kali iod.;* Merc. s.; Nit. ac. See Male Sexual System.

In anaemic girls at puberty, with vertex headache, flatulent dyspepsia, better by eating—Calc. p.

In drunkards—Ant. c.; Bar. c.; *Led.; Nux v.;* Rhus t.

In fleshy young people, with coarse habits; bluish red, pustules on face, chest, shoulders—Kali br.

In scrofulous—Bar. c.; Brom.; *Calc. c.;* Calc. p.; Con.; *Iod.;* Merc. s.; Mez.; Sil.; *Sul.*

In tubercular children—Tub.

With cachexia—Ars.; Carbo v.; Nat. m.; Sil.

With gastric derangements—*Ant. c.; Carbo v.;* Cim.; Lyc.; *Nux v.;* Puls.; Robin.

With glandular swellings—Brom.; Calc. s.; Merc. s.

With indurated papules—Agar.; Arn.; Ars. iod.; Berb. v.; Bov.; Brom.; *Carbo an.;* Cob.; Con.; *Eug. j.;* Iod.; *Kali br.; Kali iod.;* Nat. br.; Nit. ac.; Robin.; *Sul.;* Thuya.

With menstrual irregularities—Aur. m. n.; Bell.; Bellis; *Berb. aq.;* Berb. v.; Calc. c.; *Cim.;* Con.; Eug. j.; *Graph.;* Kali br.; Kali c.; Kreos.; Nat. m.; Psor.; *Puls.; Sang.;* Sars.; Thuya; Ver. a.

With pregnancy—Bell.; Sab.; Sars.; Sep.

With rheumatism—Led.; Rhus t.

With sexual excesses—*Aur.;* Calc. c.; Kali br.; *Phos. ac.;* Rhus t.; Sep.; Thuya.

With scars unsightly—Carbo an.; Kali br.

With symmetrical distribution—Arn.

ACTINOMYCOSIS—Hekla; Hippoz.; Kali iod.; Nit. ac.

ALOPECIA—Alum.; Anthrok.; *Ars.;* Calc. s.; *Fluor. ac.;* Mancin.; *Nat. m.; Phos. ac.; Phos.;* Piloc.; *Pix l.;* Selen.; *Sep.;* Tub.; Vinca. See Scalp (Head).

ANIDROSIS (deficient sweat, dry skin)—Acet. ac.; Acon.; *Æth.; Alum.;* Apoc.; Arg. n.; Ars.; *Bell.; Berb. aq.;* Crot. t.; *Graph.;* Iod.; *Kali ars.; Kali c.;* Kali iod.; Lach.; Mag. c.; *Malandr.;* Nat. c.; *Nux m.;* Op.; *Petrol.;* Phos.; Plumb. m.; *Psor.;* Sanic.; Sars.; Sec.; *Sul.;* Thyr.

ARTHRAX—Carbuncle; Malignant pustule: Acon.; *Anthrac.; Apis;* Arct. l.; Arn.; *Ars.;* Bell.; Bothrops; Bry.; Bufo; Calc. chlor.; *Carb. ac.;* Carbo v.; *Cinch.;* Crot.; Cupr. ars.; *Echin.;* Euphorb.; Hep.; Hippoz.; *Lach.; Led.;* Mur. ac.; Nit. ac.; Phyt.; *Pyr.;* Rhus t.; *Scolop.;* Sec.; *Sil.;* Sul.; Sul. ac.; *Tar. c.*

ATROPHY—of skin:—Ars.; Cocc.; Graph.; Sabad.; Sul.

BLISTERS, small—Apis; *Canth.;* Nat. m.; *Rhus t.;* Sec.

BLOOD BOILS—*Anthrac.;* Arn.; Ars.; Crot.; *Lach.;* Phos. ac.; Pyr.; Sec.

BLUENESS—Lividity: Agar.; *Ail.; Ant. t.;* Arn.; *Ars.;* Cadm. s.; Camph.; *Carbo an.; Carbo v.;* Cinch.; Crat.; Crot.; *Cupr.; Dig.;* Helleb.; Ipec.; Kali iod.; *Lach.; Laur.; Morph.;* Mur. ac.; *Sec.;* Sul. ac.; *Tar. c.; Ver. a.;* Vipera. See Face.

BROMIDROSIS (offensive sweat)—Art. v.; *Bapt.;* Bry.; Carbo an.; Cinch.; Con.; Graph.; *Hep.; Lyc.; Merc. s.; Nit. ac.;* Osm.; *Petrol.;* Phos.; *Psor.;* Pulex; Sep.; *Sil.;* Stann.; *Staph.;* Sul.; *Tellur.;* Thuya; Variol.
Bromidrosis, sour odor of body—*Calc. c.;* Cham.; Colost.; Graph.; *Hep.;* Kreos.; Lac d.; *Mag. c.; Rheum; Sul. ac.;* Sul.

BURNING—Acet. ac.; *Acon.; Agar.;* Anac.; *Apis; Ars.;* Bapt.; *Bell.;* Bry.; *Canth.;* Caps.; Caust.; Dulc.; Euphorb.; *Formica;* Grind.; Kali c.; Kreos.; Medusa; *Nux v.;* Phos.; Radium; *Ran. b.; Rhus t.;* Sang.; *Sec.; Sul.;* Vespa. See Pruritus.

CALLOSITIES (corns)—*Ant. c.;* Elaeis; *Ferr. picr.; Graph.;* Hydr.; Lyc.; *Nit. ac.;* Petrol.; *Ran. b.;* Rhus t.; Sal. ac.; Sars.; Sep.; Sil.; *Thuya.* See Feet (Locomotor System).

CHILBLAINS. *Abrot.; Agar.;* Apis; Ars.; Bor.; Calc. c.; Calend.; *Canth.;* Carbo an.; Crot. t.; Cycl.; Ferr. p.; Fragar.; Ham.; *Hep.;* Lach.; Led.; Merc.; *Mur. ac.; Nit. ac.; Petrol.;* Plant.; *Puls.; Rhus t.;* Sil.; Sul. ac.; *Sul.; Tamus; Tereb.;* Thyr.; Ver. v.; Zinc. m.

CHLOASMA—Liver spots, moth patches: *Arg. n.;* Aur.; Cadm. s.; Card. m.; *Caul.;* Cob.; Cur.; Guar.; Laur.; *Lyc.; Nat. hyposul.;* Paul.; Petrol.; Plumb. m.; *Sep.;* Sul.; Thuya. See Spots, copper-colored.

CICATRICES—Affections:—*Caust.; Fluor. ac.;* Graph.; Iod.; Nit. ac.; Phyt.; Sil.; Sul. ac.; *Thiosin.*

COLDNESS—Abies c.; *Acet. ac.;* Acon.; Agar.; *Ail.;* Ant. chlor.; Ant. c.; *Ant. t.; Ars.;* Bothrops; Calc. c.; *Camph.; Carbo v.;* Chel.; Chin. ars.; *Cinch.;* Crat.; *Crot.;* Dig.; Ipec.; *Jatropha;* Lach.; *Latrod.; Laur.;* Med.; Pyr.; Rhus t.; *Sec.; Tab.; Ver. a.* (See Collapse Nervous System.) Coldness (Fever).

COMEDO—*Abrot.; Bar. c.;* Bell.; Calc. sil.; Cic.; *Dig.; Eug. j.;* Mez.; *Nit. ac.;* Sab.; *Selen.;* Sep.; *Sul.; Sumb.*

DECUBITUS (bed sores)—Arg. n.; *Arn.;* Bapt.; Carb. ac.; Carbo v.; Cinch.;

Echin.; Fluor. ac.; Hippoz.; *Lach.; Mur. ac.;* Nux m.; Pæonia; Petrol.; Pyr.; Sil.; *Sul. ac.;* Vipera. See Ulcer.

DERMAL (trophic lesions)—Thallium.

DERMATALGIA (pain, sensitiveness, soreness)—Agar.; Apis; Ars.; *Bad.;* Bell.; Bellis; Bov.; Chin. s.; *Cinch.;* Con.; Crot. t.; *Dolich.;* Euphorb.; Fagop.; *Hep.; Kali c.; Lach.;* Lyc.; Nux m.; *Oleand.;* Osm.; Pæonia; *Petrol.;* Phos.; *Psor.;* Ran. s.; Rhus d.; *Rhus t.;* Rumex; Semperv. t.; Sep.; *Sil.; Sul.;* Tar. c.; *Ther.; Vinca;* Xerophyl.

DRYNESS—*Acon.; Alum.; Ars.; Bell.;* Calc. c.; *Graph.;* Hydrocot.; Iod.; Lyc.; Nat. c.; Nit. ac.; *Nux m.;* Piloc.; *Plumb.; Psor.;* Sabad.; Sars.; Sec.

ECCHYMOSES—Æth.; *Arn.;* Ars.; Bellis; Bothrops; Carbo v.; Chloral; *Crot.; Ham.;* Kreos.; *Led.; Phos.;* Rhus t.; Sec.; *Sul. ac.;* Supraren. ex.; Tereb.

ECHTHYMA—Ant. c.; *Ant. t.; Ars.;* Bell.; *Cic.;* Cistus; *Crot. t.;* Hydr.; Jugl. c.; *Jugl. r.;* Kali bich.; Kreos.; *Lach.; Merc. s.;* Nit. ac.; Petrol.; Rhus t.; *Sec.; Sil.;* Sul.; Thuya.

ECZEMA—*Æthiops;* Alnus; Alum.; *Anac.;* Anthrok.; *Ant. c.;* Arbut.; *Ars.;* Ars. iod.; Berb. aq.; *Berb. v.;* Bor.; *Bov.;* Calc. c.; *Canth.;* Caps.; *Carb. ac.;* Carbo v.; *Castor eq.;* Caust.; Chrysar.; *Cic.; Clem.;* Commocl.; Con.; *Crot. t.;* Dulc.; Euphorb.; Fluor. ac.; Frax. am.; Fuligo; *Graph.; Hep.;* Hippoz.; Hydrocot.; Jugl. c.; *Kali ars.;* Kali m.; Kreos.; Lyc.; *Mang. ac.; Merc. c.;* Merc. d.; Merc. pr. rub.; *Merc. s.; Mez.;* Mur. ac.; Nat. ars.; Nat. m.; Nux v.; *Oleand.;* Persicaria; *Petrol.;* Piloc.; *Plumb.;* Pod.; Prim. v.; *Psor.; Rhus t.; Rhus v.;* Sars.; *Sep.;* Skook. ch.; *Sul.; Sul. iod.;* Thuya; Tub.; Ustil.; *Vinca; Viola tr.;* Xerophyl.; X-ray.

Acute form—Acon.; Anac.; Bell.; Canth.; *Chin. s.; Crot. t.;* Mez.; *Rhus t.;* Sep.

Eczema, behind ears—Ars.; Arundo; Bov.; *Chrysarob.; Graph.; Hep.;* Jugl. r.; Kali m.; Lyc.; *Mez.; Oleand.; Petrol.;* Psor.; Rhus t.; Sanic.; *Scrophul.;* Sep.; Staph.; Tub. See Ears.

Eczema, of face—Anac.; Ant. c.; Bac.; Calc. c.; *Carb. ac.;* Cic.; Col.; Cornus c.; *Crot. t.;* Hyper.; Kali ars.; Led.; Merc. pr. rub.; Psor.; Rhus t.; Sep.; Staph.; *Sul.; Sul. iod.; Vinca.* See Face.

Eczema, of flexures of joints—*Æth.;* Am. c.; Caust.; *Graph.;* Hep.; Kali ars.; Lyc.; Mang. ac.; *Nat. m.;* Psor.; *Sep.;* Sul.

Eczema, of hands—Anag.; Bar. c.; *Berb. v.; Bov.;* Calc. c.; *Graph.; Hep.;* Hyper.; Jugl. c.; Kreos.; Malandr.; *Petrol.; Pix l.;* Plumb.; Rhus v.; Sanic.; Selen.; Sep.; Still. See Hands (Locomotor System).

Eczema, of neurasthenic persons—*Anac.;* Ars.; Phos.; *Strych. ars.;* Strych. p.; Viola tr.; Zinc. p.

Eczema, of pudendum—Am. c.; Ant. c.; Ars.; Canth.; *Crot. t.;* Hep.; Plumb. m.; Rhus t.; Sanic.; Sep. See Female Sexual System.

Eczema, of rheumatico-gouty persons—Alum.; Arbut.; Lact. ac.; *Rhus t.;* Uric. ac.; Urea.

Eczema, of scalp—Astac.; Berb. aq.; *Calc. c.;* Cic.; Clem.; Fluor. ac.;

Hep.; Kali m.; Lyc.; Mez.; Nat. m.; *Oleand.;* Petrol.; Psor.; Sep.; *Selen.;* Staph.; Sul.; Tub.; *Vinca;* Viola od. See Head.

Eczema, of strumous persons—*Æthiops;* Ars. iod.; Calc. c.; *Calc. iod.;* Calc. p.; Caust.; Cistus; Crot. t.; *Hep.;* Merc. c.; Merc. s.; Rumex; Sep.; Sil.; Tub.

Eczema, of whole body—Crot. t.; Rhus t.

Eczema, madidans—Cic.; Con.; Dulc.; Graph.; Hep.; Kali m.; Merc. c.; Merc. pr. rub.; Mez.; Sep.; Staph.; Tub.; Viola tr.

Eczema, with pigmentation in circumscribed areas following—Berb. v.

Eczema, with urinary, gastric, hepatic disorders—Lyc.

Eczema, worse after vaccination—Mez.

Eczema, worse at menstrual period, menopause—Mang. ac.

Eczema, worse at seashore, ocean voyage, excess of salt—Nat. m.

ELEPHANTIASIS—Anac. or.; *Ars.;* Calop.; Card. m.; *Elaeis;* Graph.; Ham.; *Hydrocot.;* Iod.; Lyc.; *Myrist. s.;* Sil.

EPHELIS (sunburn)—Bufo; Canth.; Kali c.; Robin.; Ver. a.

EPITHELIOMA—Acet. ac.; Alumen; *Ars.;* Ars. iod.; Cic.; *Condur.;* Con.; Euphorb.; Fuligo; *Hoang. n.;* Hydr,; Jequir.; Kali ars.; Kali s.; Lapis alb.; Lob. erin.; Lyc.; Nat. cacodyl.; Radium; Scrophul.; *Sep.;* Sil.; *Thuya.* See Face.

ERUPTIONS—Copper-colored: Ars.; Calc. iod.; *Carbo an.;* Kreos.; Nit. ac.

Eruptions, dry, scaly—Alumen; *Anag.;* Ant. c.; *Ars.;* Ars. iod.; *Berb. aq.;* Bov.; Cadm. s.; Canth.; Corydal.; Euphorb. d.; Graph.; *Hydrocot.; Iod.; Kali ars.;* Kali m.; Kali s.; Lith. c.; Lyc.; *Malandr.;* Merc. s.; Nat. m.; Nit. ac.; Petrol.; Phos.; Phyt.; Pip. m.; Pix l.; *Psor.; Sars.;* Selen.; Sep.; *Sul.;* Tub.; Xerophyl.

Eruptions, humid, moist—*Æthiops;* Ant. c.; Ant. t.; Bar. c.; Bov.; Caust.; Chrysarob.; *Clem.; Crot. t.;* Dulc.; *Graph.; Hep.;* Lyc.; Mancin.; Merc. s.; *Mez.;* Nat. m.; *Oleand.;* Petrol.; *Psor.; Rhus t.;* Sep.; Staph.; Stront.; Variol.; Viola tr.

Eruptions, pustular—Alnus; *Ant. c.;* Ant. t.; Bell.; *Berb. v.;* Bufo; Chel.; Cic.; *Crot. t.;* Echin.; Euphorb.; *Hep.;* Hippoz.; Iris; Jugl. r.; *Kali bich.;* Kali iod.; Kreos.; Lach.; Merc. c.; *Merc. s.;* Nit. ac.; Phyt.; *Psor.;* Ran. b.; Rhus v.; Sep.; *Sil.;* Sul.; Sul. iod.; Taxus; Variol.

Eruptions, scabby—Ant. c.; Ars.; Calc. c.; Chrysarob.; *Cic.;* Dulc.; Graph.; *Hep.; Lyc.;* Merc.; *Mez.;* Mur. ac.; Nat. m.; Petrol.; Staph.; *Sul.;* Viola tr.; Vinca.

Eruptions, better in winter—Kali bich.; Sars.

Eruptions, worse in spring—Nat. s.; Psor.; Sang.; *Sars.*

Eruptions, worse in winter—Aloe; *Alum.:* Ars.; *Petrol.; Psor.;* Sabad.

ERYSIPELAS—*Acon.;* Anac. oc.; Ananth.; *Apis; Arn.;* Ars.; Atrop.; Aur.; *Bell.;* Camph.; *Canth.;* Carb. ac.; Carbo v.; *Cinch.;* Commocl.; Cop.; Crot.; *Crot. t.; Echin.;* Euphorb.; *Graph.;* Hep.; Jugl. r.; *Lach.;* Led.; Nat. m.; Nat. s.; Prim. ob.; Ran. c.; *Rhus t.; Rhus v.;* Samb.; Sul.; Taxus; Ver. v.; *Xerophyl.*

Afebrile—*Graph.;* Hep.; Lyc.

Biliary, catarrhal duodenal symptoms—Hydr.

Constitutional tendency—Calend.; *Graph.;* Lach.; Psor.; Sul.

Edema, persisting—*Apis;* Ars.; Aur.; Graph.; Hep.; Lyc.; Sul.

Facial—Apis; Arn.; *Bell.;* Bor.; Canth.; Carbo an.; *Euphorb.; Graph.;* Hep.; *Rhus t.;* Solan. n.; Sul.

Leg, below knee—Sul.

Mammæ—Carbo v.; Sul.

Neonatorum—Bell.; Camph.

Phlegmonous—Acon.; Anthrac.; Arn.; *Ars.;* Bell.; Bothrops; Crot.; Ferr. p.; Graph.; *Hep.;* Hippoz.; *Lach.;* Merc.; *Rhus t.;* Sil.; *Tar. c.;* Ver. v.

Recurrent and chronic—Ferr. p.; *Graph.;* Nat. m.; *Rhus t.; Sul.*

Repercussion—Cupr. ac.

Senile—*Am. c.;* Carbo an.

Swelling marked, burning, itching, stinging—Rhus t.

Traumatic—Calend.; Psor.

Traumatic: umbilical, of new born—Apis.

Vesicular—Anac. oc.; Arn.; *Canth.;* Carb. ac.; Caust.; Crot. t.; *Euphorb.;* Mez.; *Rkus t.; Rhus v.;* Tereb.; Urt.; Verb.; Ver. v.

Wandering—Apis; *Ars.;* Cinch.; *Graph.;* Hep.; Hydr.; Puls.; Sul.

ERYTHEMA—**Intertrigo (chafing):** *Æth.;* Agn.; Ars.; Bell.; Bor.; Calc. c.; *Caust.; Cham.;* Fagop.; *Graph.;* Jugl. r.; Kali br.; *Lyc.;* Merc. s.; Mez.; Oleand.; Ox. ac.; *Petrol.;* Psor.; Sul. ac.; *Sul.;* Tub.

Erythema multiforme—Antipyr.; Bor. ac.; Cop.; Vespa.

Erythema nodosum—Acon.; Ant. c.; *Apis; Arn.;* Ars.; Chin. ars.; *Chin. s.;* Cinch.; Ferr.; Led.; Nat. c.; Ptel.; *Rhus t.; Rhus v.*

Erythema simplex—*Acon.; Antipyr.;* Apis; *Arn.;* Ars. iod.; *Bell.;* Bufo; *Canth.;* Chloral.; Echin.; *Euphorb. d.;* Gaulth.; Grind.; Kali c.; Lact. ac.; *Merc.; Mez.;* Narcissus; Nux v.; Plumb. chrom.; *Rhus t.;* Robin.; Tereb.; Urt.; Ustil.; Ver. v.; Xerophyl.

Fibroma—Calc. ars.; *Con.; Iod.;* Kali br.; Lyc.; Sec.; Thuya.

FISSURES—**Rhagades, chaps:** *Alum.;* Anthrok.; Ars. s. fl.; Bad.; Bar. c.; Cact. fl.; *Cistus; Condur.;* Eug. j.; *Graph.; Hep.;* Kali ars.; Led.; *Lyc.; Malandr.;* Mang. ac.; Merc. i. r.; Merc. pr. rub.; *Nat. m.;* Nit. ac.; Oleand.; *Petrol.;* Pix l.; Ran. b.; Ratanh.; Rhus t.; Sars.; *Sil.;* Sul.; Xerophyl.; X-ray.

FLABBINESS—**Non-tonicity:** *Abrot.;* Aster.; Bar. c.; Ars.; Calc. c.; Chel.; *Hep.;* Ipec.; *Merc. v.;* Morph.; Op.; Nat. m.; Sanic.; Sars.; Salvia; Thyr.; Ver. a.

FOREIGN BODIES—**To promote expulsion of fish bones, splinters, needles:** Anag.; Hep.; Sil.

FORMICATION—**Tingling, numbness:** *Acon.;* Ambra; Apium gr.; Arundo; Calend.; *Cocaine;* Cod.; Medusa; *Mez.; Morph.;* Oleand.; Phos. ac.; Plat.; Rumex; Sec.; *Selen.;* Sil.; Staph.; *Sul. ac.;* Val.; Zinc. m.

FUNGUS HEMATODES—*Ars.;* Lach.; Lyc.; Mancin.; *Phos.; Thuya.*

FURUNCLE (boil)—Abrot.; Æth.; Ananth.; Anthrac.; Ant. c.; *Arn.;* Ars.: *Bell.; Bellis;* Calc. hypophos.; *Calc. picr.;* Calc. s.; Carbo v.; Echin.; *Ferr. iod.;* Gels.; *Hep.;* Hippoz.; *Ichth.;* Lach.; Lyc.; *Med.; Merc. s.;*

Ol. myr.; Operc.; *Phos. ac.; Phyt.;* Picr. ac.; Rhus r.; Sec.; *Sil.; Sul.;* Sul. iod.; Sul. ac.; *Tar. c.;* Tub.; Zinc. ox.

Furuncle, recurrent tendency—*Arn.;* Ars.; Berb. v.; Calc. c.; *Calc. mur.;* Calc. p.; *Calc. picr.;* Echin.; Hep.; *Sul.;* Tub.

GANGRENE—Ail.; Anthrac.; Ant. c.; Apis; *Ars.;* Bothrops; Brass.; Brom.; Calend.; Canth.; Carb. ac.; Carbo an.; *Carbo v.;* Chlorum; Chrom. oxy.; Cinch.; Crot.; Cupr. ars.; *Echin.; Euphorb.;* Ferr. p.; Kali chlor.; Kali p.; Kreos.; *Lach.; Polygon. pers.;* Ran. ac.; Sal. ac.; *Sec.; Sul. ac.;* Tar. c.

Gangrene, senile—Am. c.; Ars.; Cepa; Sec.; Sul. ac.

Gangrene, traumatic—Arn.; Lach.; Sul. ac.

HERPES (tetter)—Acon.; Æthiops; Alnus; Anac.; Ananth.; Anthrok.; Apis; Arn.; *Ars.;* Bar. c.; Bor.; Bry.; Bufo; Calc. c.; *Canth.; Carb. ac.;* Caust.; Chrysarob.; Cistus; Clem.; Commocl.; *Crot. t.; Dulc.;* Eucal.; *Graph.; Kali bich.;* Lith. c.; *Merc. s.;* Mez.; Nat. c.; *Nat. m.; Nit. ac.;* Petrol.; Phos. ac.; Psor.; Ran. b.; Ran. sc.; *Rhus t.; Sars.;* Sep.; Sil.; Sul.; Tellur.; Variol.; Xerophyl.

Herpes, between fingers—Nit. ac.

Herpes, chronic—Alnus.

Herpes, Circinatus, tonsurans—Ars. s. fl.; Bar. c.; Calc. ac.; Calc. c.; Chrysar.; Equis. arv.; Hep.; Nat. c.; Nat. m.; *Sep.; Tellur.;* Tub. See Trichophytosis.

Herpes, Circinatus, in isolated spots—Sep.

Herpes, Circinatus, in intersecting rings—Tellur.

Herpes, dry—Bov.; Fluor. ac.; Mang.; Sep.; Sil.

Herpes, of chest, nape of neck—Nat. m.; Petrol.

Herpes, of chin—Ars.; Caust.; Graph.; Mez.; Sil.

Herpes, of face—Apis; *Ars.;* Calc. fl.; Caps.; Caust.; Clem.; Con.; Lach.; Limulus; *Nat. m.;* Ran. b.; *Rhus t.;* Sep.; Sul. See Face.

Herpes, of flexures of knees—Graph.; *Hep.; Nat. m.; Sep.;* Xerophyl.

Herpes, of genitals—Aur. mur.; Calc. c.; *Caust.;* Crot. t.; Dulc.; *Hep.;* Jugl. r.; *Merc. s.; Nit. ac.;* Petrol.; Phos. ac.; *Sars.;* Tereb. See Male Sexual System.

Herpes, of hands—Cistus; Dulc.; *Limul.;* Lith. c.; Nit. ac.

Herpes, of knees—Carbo v.; Petrol.

Herpes, of thigh—Graph.; Petrol.

Herpes, neuralgia after—Kal.; *Mez.;* Ran. b.; Still.; Variol.

Herpes, with glandular swelling—Dulc.

Herpes, with pimples or pustules surrounding; spread by coalescing—Hep.

HERPES ZOSTER—Zona; shingles—Apis; Arg. n.; *Ars.;* Aster.; *Canth.;* Carbon. ox.; *Caust.;* Ced.; *Cistus;* Commocl.; Crot. t.; *Dolich.;* Dulc.; Graph.; Grind.; Hyper.; Iris; Kali ars.; Kali m.; Kal.; Merc. s.; *Mez.;* Morph.; Pip. m.; *Prun. sp.; Ran. b.;* Ran. sc.; *Rhus t.;* Sal. ac.; Semperv. t.; Staph.; Strych. ars.; Sul.; Thuya; Variol.; Zinc. p.; Zinc. v.

Chronic—Ars.; Semperv. t.

Neuralgia, persisting—Ars.; Dolich.; *Kal.; Mez.;* Ran. b.; Still.; Zinc. m.

HYDROA—Kali iod.; Kreos.; Mag. c.; *Nat. m.;* Rhus v. See Herpes.

HYPERIDROSIS (excessive sweating)—*Acet. ac.*; Æth.; *Agaricin*; Am. c.; Ant. t.; Ars. iod.; *Bapt.*; Bell.; Bolet.; *Calc. c.*; Cham.; *Cinch.*; Eser.; Ferr.; Graph.; *Jabor.*; Lact. ac.; *Merc. s.*; Nat. c.; Nit. ac.; Nux v.; Op.; *Phos. ac.*; Phos.; Piloc.; *Samb.*; Sanic.; Selen.; *Sep.*; *Sil.*; Sul. ac.; Sul.; Thuya; Ver. a. See Fever.

ICHTHYOSIS (fish skin disease)—*Ars.*; *Ars. iod.*; Aur.; Clem.; Graph.; *Hydrocot.*; Iod.; Kali iod.; Merc. s.; Nat. c.; Œnanthe; Phos.; Platanus; Plumb. m.; *Syph.*; Sul.; Thuya; *Thyr.*

IMPETIGO—Alnus; *Ant. c.*; Ant. s. a.; *Ant. t.*; *Ars.*; Arum.; Calc. mur.; *Cic.*; Clem.; *Dulc.*; Euphorb.; Graph.; Hep.; Iris; Jugl. c.; *Kali bich.*; Kali n.; Lyc.; *Mez.*; *Rhus t.*; Rhus v.; Sep.; Sil.; Sul.; Thuya; *Viola tr.*

KELOID—*Fluor. ac.*; *Graph.*; Nit. ac.; Sab.; Sil.

LENTIGO (freckles)—Am. c.; Bad.; Calc. c.; Graph.; *Kali c.*; *Lyc.*; Mur. ac.; Nat. c.; *Nit. ac.*; Petrol.; Phos.; *Sep.*; *Sul.*; Tab.

LEPRA, leprosy—Anac.; *Ars.*; *Bad.*; Calopt.; Carb. ac.; *Chaulmugra*; Commocl.; Cupr. ac.; Cur.; *Dipterocarpus*; Elaeis; Graph.; Guano; *Gynocardia*; *Hoang n.*; Hura; *Hydrocot.*; Jatropha goss.; Lach.; Merc. s.; Œnanthe; Phos.; *Pip. m.*; Sec.; Sep.; *Sil.*; Thyr.

LEUCODERMA—*Ars. s. fl.*; Nat. m.; Nit. ac.; Sumb.; Zinc. p. See Face, pale.

LICHEN PLANUS—Agar.; Anac.; *Ant. c.*; Apis; *Ars.*; *Ars. iod.*; Chin. ars.; Iod.; *Jugl. c.*; *Kali bich.*; Kali iod.; Led.; Merc.; Sars.; Staph.; *Sul. iod.*

LICHEN SIMPLEX—Alum.; Am. m.; *Ananth.*; *Ant. c.*; Apis; *Ars.*; *Bell.*; Bov.; Bry.; *Calad.*; Castan.; Dulc.; *Jugl. c.*; Kali ars.; *Kreos.*; *Led.*; *Lyc.*; Merc. s.; Nabul. s.; Nat. c.; *Plant.*; *Phyt.*; *Rumex*; Sep.; *Sul.*; Sul. iod.; Tilia. See Acne.

LUPUS ERYTHEMATOSUM—Apis; Cistus; Guarana; *Hydrocot.*; *Iod.*; *Kali bich.*; *Phos.*; Sep.; *Thyr.*

LUPUS VULGARIS—Apis; *Ars.*; *Ars. iod.*; *Aur. ars.*; Aur. iod.; *Aur. mur.*; Calc. c.; Calc. iod.; Calc. s.; *Cistus*; Condur.; Ferr. picr.; Form. ac.; Formica; Graph.; Guarana; *Hep.*; *Hydr.*; *Hydrocot.*; Irid.; Jequir.; *Kali bich.*; *Kali iod.*; Lyc.; Nit. ac.; Phyt.; Staph.; *Sul.*; Thiosin.; Thuya; *Tub.*; Urea; X-ray.

MILIARIA (prickly heat)—*Acon.*; Am. m.; Ars.; *Bry.*; Cact.; Centaurea; Hura; *Jabor.*; Led.; Raph.; Syzigium; Urt.

MILIUM—*Calc. iod.*; Staph.; Tab. See Acne.

MOLLUSCUM—*Brom.*; Bry.; *Calc. ars.*; Calc. c.; Kali iod.; Lyc.; Merc. s.; Nat. m.; *Sil.*; Sul.; Teucr.

MORBUS SUDATORIUS—Acon.; Ars.; Carbo v.; Jabor.; Merc.

MORPHÆA—Ars.; *Phos.*; Sil. See Scleroderma.

NÆVUS—Acet. ac.; Calc. c.; *Carbo v.*; Condur.; *Fluor. ac.*; Lyc.; Phos.; Radium; *Thuya.*

NAILS—Affections in general: Alum.; *Ant. c.;* Castor eq.; *Graph.;* Hyper.; Nit. ac.; *Sil.;* Upas; X-ray.

Affections of pulp, nails recede, leave raw surface—Sec.

Atrophy—Sil.

Biting of—Am. br.; Arum.

Blueness—Dig.; Ox. ac. See Cyanosis (Circulatory System).

Deformed—brittle, thickened (onchogryposis)—Alum.; Ananth.; *Ant. c.; Ars.;* Caust.; Diosc.; Fluor. ac.; *Graph.;* Merc.; Nat. m ; Sabad.; Sec.; Senec.; Sep.; *Sil.;* Thuya; X-ray.

Eruptions—Around nails: Graph.; Psor.; Stann. mur.

Falling off—Brass.; But. ac.; Helleb. fort.; Helleb.

Hangnails—*Nat. m.;* Sul.; Upas.

Hypertrophy (onychauxis)—Graph.

Inflammation—Around root (paronychia): Alum.; Bufo; Calc. s.; *Diosc.;* Graph.; Hep.; *Nat. s.* See Felon.

Inflammation of pulp (onychia)—Arn.; Calend.; *Fluor. ac.; Graph.;* Phos.; Psor.; Sars.; Sil.; Upas.

Inflammation, under toe nail—Sabad.

Ingrowing toe nail—Caust.; Magnet. aust.; Nit. ac.; *Sil.;* Staph.; Teucr.; Tetradyn.

Injury to matrix—Hyper.

Irritable feeling under finger nails, relieved by biting them—Am. brom.

Itching—About roof of: Upas.

Pains—Burning under: Sars.

Pains, gnawing, beneath finger nails—Alum.; Sars.; Sep.

Pains, neuralgic, beneath finger nails—Berb. v.

Pains, neuralgic—Alum.; *Cepa;* Colch.

Pains, smarting at roots—Sul.

Pains, splinter-like, beneath toe nails—Fluor. ac.

Pains, ulcerative, beneath toe nails—Ant. c.; Graph.; Teucr.

Skin around, dry, cracked—Graph.; Nat. m.; Petrol.

Skin around, pigmented—Naph.

Softening—Plumb.; Thuya.

Spots, white on—Alum.; Nit. ac.

Trophic changes—Radium.

Ulceration—Alum.; Graph.; Merc.; *Phos.;* Psor.; Sang.; Sars.; Sil.; Teucr.; Tetradyn.

Yellow color—Con.

ŒDEMA, SWELLING—Acal.; *Acet. ac ;* Acon.; *Agar.; Anac.; Apis; Ars.;* Bell.; Bellis; Bothrops; Bry.; *Dig.;* Elat.; Euphorb.; Ferr. m.; *Helleb.;* Hippoz.; Lach.; Lyc.; Nat. c.; Nat. sal.; Oleand.; Prim. ob.; *Prun. sp.; Rhus t.;* Samb.; *Thyr.*

ŒDEMA, ANGIONEUROTIC—Agar.; Antipyr.; Helleb.

OILY—Skin: Bry.; *Merc.; Nat. m.;* Plumb. m.; Psor.; Raph.; Sanic. See Seborrhœa.

PELLAGRA—*Ars.;* Ars. sul. rub.; Bov.; Cinch.; Gels.; Pedic.; Plumb. iod.; Psor.; Sec.; *Sedinha;* Sul.

Pellagra, cachexia—Ars.; Sec.

Pellagra, fissures, desquamation, skin eruptions—Graph.; *Hep.;* Ign.; Phos.; Puls.; Sep.

PEMPHIGUS—Anac.; Antipyr.; *Ars.;* Arum tr.; Bufo; Caltha; *Canth.;* Carbon. ox.; Caust.; Dulc.; *Jugl. c.; Lach.; Mancin.; Merc. c.;* Merc. pr. rub.; Merc. s.; Nat. sal.; Phos. ac.; Phos. ; *Ran. b.; Ran. sc.;* Raph.; *Rhus t.;* Sep.; Thuya.

PETICHIÆ—*Arn.;* Ars.; Calc. c.; Cur.; Mur. ac.; *Phos.;* Sec.; *Sul. ac.* See Eccl.ymosis.

PHTHIRIASIS—Bac.; Cocc.; Merc.; *Nat. m.;* Oleand.; Psor.; *Sabad.; Staph.*

PITYRIASIS (dermatitis exfoliativa)—*Ars.;* Ars. iod.; Bac.; Berb. aq.; Calc. c.; Carb. ac.; Clem.; *Colch.; Fluor. ac.; Graph.; Kali ars.;* Mang. ac.; Merc. pr. rub.; *Mez.;* Nat. ars.; Phos.; Pip. m.; *Sep.;* Staph.; *Sul.;* Sul. iod.; *Sulphur. ac.;* Tellur.; Tereb.; Thyr.

PRAIRIE ITCH—Led.; Rhus t.; Rumex; Sul.

PRURIGO—Acon.; Alnus; *Ambra;* Anthrok.; *Ars.; Ars. iod.;* Ars. sul.; Carb. ac.; *Chloral.; Dolich.;* Diosc.; Kali bich.; *Lyc.; Merc.; Mez.; Nit. ac.; Oleand.;* Oophor.; Pedic.; *Rhus t.; Rhus v.; Rumex;* Sil.; *Sul.;* Tereb.

PRURITUS (itching of skin)—Acon.; *Agar.;* Alum.; *Ambra;* Anac. oc.; *Anac.;* Anag.; *Antipyr.;* Apis; *Ars.;* Calad.; Calc. c.; Canth.; *Carb. ac.;* Chloral.; Chrysar.; *Clem.; Crot. t.; Dolich.;* Dulc.; Elaeis; *Fagop.;* Fluor. ac.; Formica; Glon.; *Graph.;* Granat.; Grind.; Guano; Hep.; *Hydrocot.;* Hyper.; Ichth.; Ign.; *Lyc.;* Kreos.; Mag. c.; Malandr.; Mang. ac.; Med.; *Merc.; Mez.; Morph.;* Niccol.; Nux v.; Oleand.; Op.; Petrol.; *Pix l.;* Prim. ob.; Psor.; Pulex; *Radium;* Ran. b.; *Rhus t.; Rhus v.; Rumex; Sep.;* Staph.; *Sul.;* Sul. ac.; Syzgium; Tar. c.; *Urt.;* Vespa; Xerophyl.

Pruritus of aged—Bar. ac.
Pruritus, of ankles—Nat. p.; Selen.; Sep.
Pruritus, of bends of elbows, knees—Selen.; Sep.
Pruritus, of chest, upper limbs—Arundo.
Pruritus, of ears, nose, arms, urethra—Sul. iod.
Pruritus, of face, hands, scalp—Clem.
Pruritus, of face, shoulders, chest—Kali br.
Pruritus, of feet, ankles—Led.
Pruritus, of feet, legs—Bov.
Pruritus, of feet, soles of—Ananth.; Hydrocot.
Pruritus, of genitals—*Ambra;* Ars. iod.; Bor.; *Calad.;* Carb. a.c.; Carbo v.; Colch.; Collins.; Crot. t.; Dulc.; Fuligo; Guano; Helon.; Kreos.; Mez.; Nit. ac.; Rhus t.; Rhus v.; *Sep.;* Sil.; Tar. c. See Female Sexual System.
Pruritus, of hands, arms—Pip. m.; Selen.
Pruritus, of joints, abdomen—Pinus sylv.
Pruritus, of knees, elbows, hairy parts—Dolich.; Fagop.
Pruritus, of nose—Morph.; Strych.
Pruritus, of orifices—Fluor. ac.

Pruritus, of thighs, bends of knees—Zinc. m.

Pruritus, of webs of fingers, bends of joints—Hep.; *Psor.*; Selen.; Sep.

Pruritus, ameliorated from cold—Berb. v.; Fagop.; Graph.; Mez.

Pruritus, ameliorated from hot water—Rhus v.

Pruritus, ameliorated from rubbing gently—Crot. t.

Pruritus, ameliorated from scratching—Asaf.; Cadm. s.; Mang. ac.; Merc. s.; *Oleand.; Rhus t.*

Pruritus, ameliorated from warmth—Ars.; Petrol.; Rumex.

Pruritus, followed by bleeding, pains, burning—Alum.; *Ars.; Crot. t.;* Murex; Pix l.; Psor.; Sep.; *Sul.*; Tilia.

Pruritus, followed by, change of site of itching—Mez.; *Staph.*

Pruritus, without eruption—Dolichos.

Pruritus, worse from contact—Ran. b.

Pruritus, worse from exposure, cold air—Dulc.; *Hep.*; Nat. s.; *Oleand.*; Petrol.; Rhus t.; *Rumex.*

Pruritus, worse from scratching—*Ars.*; Berb. v.; Crot. t.; Led.; *Mez.*; Sep.; Sul.

Pruritus, worse from undressing; warmth of bed; at P. M.—*Alum.*; Ant. c.; *Ars.*; Asimina; Bellis; Bov.; Carbo v.; Card. m.; Cistus; Dulc.; *Jugl. c.; Kali ars.;* Kreos.; Led.; Lyc.; *Menisp.; Merc.*; Merc. i. fl.; *Mez.; Nat. s.; Oleand.;* Psor.; Puls.; Rhus t.; *Rumex*; Sang.; Sep.; *Sul.*; Tub.

Pruritus, worse from washing, with cold water—Clem.; Tub.

PSORIASIS—Ant. t.; *Ars.; Ars. iod.;* Aster.; Aur. m. n.; Berb. aq.; *Bor.; Carb. ac.; Chrysar.;* Cic.; Coral.; Cupr. ac.; Fluor. ac.; *Graph.;* Hep.; Hydrocot.; Iris; *Kali ars.; Kali br.;* Kali s.; *Lyc.;* Mang. ac.; Merc. aur.; *Merc. s.;* Mur. ac.; Naph.; Nat. ars.; Nat. m.; Nit. ac.; Nit. mur. ac.; *Petrol.; Phos.;* Platanus; *Sep.;* Strych. ars.; Strych. p.; Stellar.; *Sul.;* Tereb.; Thuya; *Thyr.;* Tub.; Ustil.

Psoriasis, of palms—Calc. c.; Coral.; *Graph.; Hep.; Lyc.;* Med.; Petrol.; Phos.; Selen.

Psoriasis, of prepuce, nails—Graph.; Sep.

Psoriasis, of tongue—Graph.; Mur. ac.; *Sep.* See Tongue (Mouth).

PURPURA—Acon.; *Arn.; Ars.;* Bapt.; Bell.; Bry.; Carbo v.; Chin. s.; Chloral; *Crot.; Ham.;* Jugl. r.; Kali iod.; *Lach.;* Merc. s.; Phos. ac.; *Phos.;* Rhus t.; Rhus v.; Sec.; Sal. ac.; *Sul. ac.;* Sulphon.; Tereb.; Ver. v.

With colic—Bov.; Col.; Cupr.; Merc. c.; Thuya.

With debility—Arn.; *Ars.;* Carbo v.; Lach.; Merc. s.; *Sul. ac.*

PURPURA HÆMORRHAGICA—Alnus; *Arn.; Ars.;* Bothrops; Bry.; *Crot.;* Ferr. picr.; *Ham.;* Iod.; Ipec.; *Lach.;* Led.; Merc. c.; Merc. s.; Millef.; Naja; Nat. nit.; *Phos. ac.; Phos.;* Rhus v.; Sec.; *Sul. ac.; Tereb.;* Thlaspi.

PURPURA RHEUMATICA—Acon.; Ars.; *Bry.;* Merc. s.; *Rhus t.;* Rhus v.

RAYNAUD'S DISEASE—See Gangrene.

RHINO-SCLERMA—Aur. m. n.; *Calc. p.;* Guarana; Rhus r.

ROSEOLA (rose-rash)—*Acon.;* Bell.; Cub.

RUPIA—Æthiops; Ant. t.; *Ars.;* Berb. aq.; Clem.; Graph.; Hydr.; *Kali iod.;* Lach.; Merc. i. r.; Nit. ac.; *Phyt.;* Sec.; Syph.; Thyr. See Syphilis (Male Sexual System).

SARCOMA CUTIS—Calc. p.; *Condur.;* Nit. ac.; Sil.

SCABIES (itch)—Aloe; Anthrok.; Caust.; *Crot. t.; Hep.;* Lyc.; Merc.; Nux v.; *Psor.;* Rhus v.; Selen.; *Sep.; Sul.*

SCLERODERMA—**scleriasis (hidebound skin)**: Alum.; *Ant. c.;* Arg. n.; Ars.; Berb. aq.; *Bry.;* Caust.; *Crot. t.;* Echin.; *Elaeis; Hydrocot.;* Lyc.; Petrol.; Phos.; Ran. b.; Rhus r.; Sars.; Sil.; Still.; Sul.; Thiosin.; *Thyr.*

SCROFULODERMA—Calc. iod.; *Calc. s.;* Petrol.; Scroful.; Ther. See Separate Diseases.

SEBACEOUS CYSTS (wen)—*Bar. c.; Benz. ac.;* Brom.; Calc. sil.; *Con.;* Graph.; Hep.; Kali br.; *Kali iod.;* Nit. ac.; Phyt.; Thuya. See Scalp (Head).

SEBORRHŒA—*Am. m.; Ars.; Bry.;* Bufo; *Calc. c.;* Cinch.; Graph.; *Iod.;* Kali br.; *Kali c.;* Kali s.; Lyc.; Merc. s.; Mez.; *Nat. m.; Phos.; Plumb. m.;* Psor.; *Raph.;* Rhus t.; Sars.; *Selen.;* Sep.; Staph.; Sul.; Thuya; *Vinea.* See Scalp (Head).

SENSIBILITY OF SKIN—**Diminished, or lost (analgesia, anæsthesia)**: Acet. ac.; *Acon.;* Ars.; Aur.; Bufo; *Can. ind.; Carbon. ox.;* Carbon. s.; Elaeis; Hyos.; *Ign.;* Kali br.; Merc.; *Nux v.; Plumb. m.;* Pop. c.; Sec.; *Zinc. m.*

Sensibility of skin increased to atmospheric changes—Dulc.; Hep.; Kali c.; Psor.; *Sul.*

SPOTS—**Blue**:Ars.; Led.; Sul. ac.

Spots, brown—Bac.; Card. m.; Con.; Iod.; Phos.; *Sep.;* Thuya.

Spots, circumscribed pigmentation following eczematous inflammation—Berb. v.; Lach.; *Lyc.;* Med.; Merc. d.; Merc.; *Nit. ac.;* Sil.; Sul.; Ustil.

Spots, copper-colored—*Carbo an.;* Carbo v.; *Coral.;* Syph.

Spots, livid—Agave; *Ail.; Bapt.;* Bothrops; *Morph.;* Ox. ac.; Sec.; *Sul. ac.*

Spots, red—Agar.; Bell.; Calc. c.; Con.; Kali c.; Sul.; Veronal.

Spots, white—Graph.; Sul.

Spots, yellow—Nat. p.; Phos.; Plumb. m.; Sep.; Sul.

Spots, yellow turning green—Con.

STROPHULUS (tooth rash)—Apis; *Bor.;* Calc. c.; *Cham.;* Cic.; Led.; Rhus v.; *Spiranth.;* Sumb.

SUDAMINÆ—Am. m.; Bry.; Urt.

SYCOSIS (barber's itch)—Anthrok.; *Ant. t.;* Ars.; Aur. m.; *Calc. c.;* Calc. s.; Chrysar.; *Cic.;* Cinnab.; Cocc.; Cypressus; *Graph.; Kali bich.;* Kali m.; Lith. c.; *Lyc.;* Med.; *Merc. pr. rub.;* Nat. s.; *Nit. ac.;* Petrol.; Plant.; *Plat.;* Sab.; Sep.; Sil.; *Staph.;* Stront. c.; Sul.; *Sul. iod.;* Tellur.; *Thuya.*

SYPHILIDÆ—See Syphilis (Male Sexual System).

TINEA FAVOSA—favus: Agar.; Ars. iod.; *Brom.*; Calc. c.; Dulc.; Graph.; Hep.; Jugl. r.; *Kali c.*; Lappa; *Lyc.*; Med.; *Mez.*; Oleand.; Phos.; *Sep.*; Sulphur. ac.; Sul.; Ustil.; Vinca; *Viola tr.* See Scalp (Head).

TINEA VERSICOLOR (chromophytosis)—Bac.; Chrysar.; Mez.; *Nat. ars.*; *Sep.*; Sul.; Tellur.

TRICHOPHYTOSIS—ringworm: Ant. c.; Ant. t.; *Ars.*; *Bac.*; Calc. c.; Calc. iod.; *Chrysar.*; *Graph.*; Hep.; Jugl. c.; Jugl. r.; Kali s.; Lyc.; Mez.; Psor.; Rhus t.; Semperv. t.; *Sep.*; Sul.; *Tellur.*; Tub.; Viola tr. See Scalp (Head).

Trichophytosis, in intersecting rings over great portion of body; fever; great constitutional disturbances—Tellur.

Trichophytosis, in isolated spots on upper part of body—Sep.

ULCERS—Anac. oc.; *Ananth.*; *Anthrac.*; Arn.; *Ars.*; Aster.; Bals. per.; Bell.; *Calc. c.*; *Calc. p.*; *Calc. sil.*; *Calc. s.*; Calend.; *Carb. ac.*; *Carbo an.*; *Carbo v.*; Carbon. s.; Caust.; Cistus; *Clem.*; Commocl.; Con.; Crot.; Cupr. ars.; *Echin.*; *Fluor. ac.*; Galium ap.; *Geran.*; Graph.; Ham.; *Hep.*; Hippoz.; *Hydr.*; Iod.; Jugl. r.; Kali ars.; *Kali bich.*; Kali iod.; *Lach.*; Merc. c.; *Merc. s.*; *Mez.*; Nat. s.; *Nit. ac.*; *Pæonia*; Petrol.; Phos. ac.; Phos.; *Phyt.*; Psor.; Radium; Ran. ac.; Scrophul.; Sep.; *Sil.*; Sul. ac.; Sul.; *Syph.*; Tar. c.; Thuya; Trychnos.

Bleeding, easily, when touched—Ars.; *Carbo v.*; Dulc.; Hep.; Kreos.; *Lach.*; Merc.; Mez.; *Nit. ac.*; *Petrol.*; Phos.

Burning—Alumen; *Anthrac.*; *Ars.*; *Carbo v.*; Hep.; Kreos.; Mez.; Thuya.

Cancerous, malignant—Anthrac.; *Ars.*; *Aster.*; Carbo an.; Chimaph.; Clem.; Condur.; Fuligo; *Galium ap.*; Hydr.; Kreos.; Lach.; Tar. c.; Thuya.

Deep—Asaf.; Commocl.; *Kali bich.*; Kali iod.; Mur. ac.; *Nit. ac.*; Tar. c.

Eroding, of face—Con.

Fistulous—*Calc. fl.*; Calend.; Kali iod.; Nit. ac.; Phyt.; *Sil.*; Thuya.

Indolent, torpid—*Anag.*; Aster.; Bar. c.; Calc. fl.; *Calc. iod.*; *Calc. p.*; Carbo v.; Chel.; Con.; Cupr.; Eucal.; Euphorb.; Fluor. ac.; Fuligo; *Geran.*; Graph.; Hydr.; Kali bich.; *Kali iod.*; Lach.; Lyc.; *Merc. s.*; Nit. ac.; Pæonia; Phyt.; *Psor.*; Pyr.; *Sil.*; *Sul.*; Syph.; Syzyg.

Inflamed—*Ars.*; *Bell.*; Calend.; Carbo an.; Phyt. See Sensitive.

Phagedenic—*Ars.*; Carbo v.; *Crot.*; Kali ars.; Merc. c.; Merc. d.; Merc.; *Nit. ac.* See Gangrenous.

Scrofulous—*Calcareas*; Cinch.; Hep.; Iodides; Mercuries; Nit. ac.; *Sil.*; Sul.

Sensitive—Angust.; Arn.; *Ars.*; *Asaf.*; *Calend.*; Dulc.; Graph.; *Hep.*; *Lach.*; Mez.; *Nit. ac.*; Pæonia; Sil.; Tar. c.

Smooth, pale, shallow, on scalp, penis—Merc.

Superficial, flat—Ars.; Coral.; Lach.; Nit. ac.; Thuya.

Superficial, serpiginous—Chel.; Merc. c.; *Merc. s.*; Phos. ac.

Syphilitic—Ars.; *Asaf.*; Carbo v.; *Cinnab.*; Cistus; Coral.; *Fluor. ac.*; Graph.; Hep.; *Iod.*; *Kali bich.*; Kali iod.; Lach.; Lyc.; *Merc. c.*; *Merc. i. r.*; Merc. s.; *Nit. ac.*; Phyt.; Sars.; Still.

Traumatic—Arn.; Con.

Varicose—Calc. fl.; Calend.; *Card. m.; Carbo v.;* Clem. vit.; Condur.; Eucal.; *Fluor. ac.; Ham.;* Lach.; Phyt.; Psor.; Pyr.; *Sec.*

Verrucous, on cheek—Ars.

Ulcers, from pemphigus blisters on toes, with ulcerated borders, moist, red, flat surface—Petrol.

Ulcers, from scarlet fever—Cham.

Ulcers, with base, blue or black—*Ars.;* Calc. fl.; Carbo an.; Lach.; Mur. ac.; Tar. c.

With base, dry, lardaceous—Phyt.

With base, indurated—*Alumen; Calc. fl.;* Commocl.; Con.

With base, lardaceous, surrounded with dark halo; dirty, unhealthy look; apt to coalesce—Merc. v.

With base, like raw flesh—Ars.; Merc. s.; *Nit. ac.*

With discharge, fetid, purulent, sloughing—*Ananth.; Anthrac.;* Ars.; Asaf.; Bapt.; Calc. fl.; *Calend.; Carb. ac.; Carbo v.;* Con.; Crot. t.; *Echin.;* Eucal.; Fluor. ac.; Gels.; *Geran.; Hep.;* Lach.; Merc. c.; *Merc. s.; Mez.;* Mur. ac.; *Nit. ac.;* Pæonia; Phos. ac.; Psor.; Pyr.; Puls.; Sil.; Sul.; *Thuya.*

With discharge, glutinous—*Graph.;* Kali bich.

With discharge, ichorous—Aster.; Carbo v.; *Carb. ac.;* Coral.; *Mez.*

With discharge, ichorous, foul—Anthrac.; *Ars.;* Asaf.; Mez.

With discharge, thin, acrid, foul—*Ars.;* Asaf.; Kali iod.; Nit. ac.

With edges, deep, regular, "punched out"—Kali bich.; Phos.

With edges, eczematous, copper-colored—Kali bich.

With edges, gangrenous—Anthrac.; *Ars.; Carbo v.;* Kreos.; Lach.; Nit. ac.; Sec.; *Sul. ac.;* Tar. c.

With edges, indurated—Calc. fl.; *Carbo an.;* Commocl.; Nit. ac.; Pæonia; Phos. ac.

With edges, irregular, undefined—*Merc. s.;* Nit. ac.

With edges, raised—Ars.; Calend.; Nit. ac.; Phos. ac.; *Sil.* See Granulations.

With fungous growths—Mur. ac.

With glazed, shining appearance—Lac c.

With granulations, exuberant—Apium gr.; *Ars.;* Carbo an.; *Caust.;* Fluor. ac.; *Nit. ac.;* Petrol.; Phos. ac.; *Sil.;* Thuya.

With itching—Mez.; Phos. ac.; Sil.

Without pain or redness; uneven, jagged base, dirty pus—Phos. ac.

With pain, in small spot, lightning-like; worse from warmth—Fluor. ac.

With pain, splinter-like—Ham.; Hep.; *Nit. ac.*

With pimples surrounding it—Grind.; *Hep.;* Lach.; Merc. s.

With small ulcers, surrounding it—Phos.; Sil.

With stupor, low delirium, prostration—Bapt.

With vesicles, surrounding it; red shining areolæ—Fluor. ac.; Hep.; *Mez.*

UNHEALTHY SKIN—Every scratch festers, or heals with difficulty—*Bor.;* Bufo; Calc. c.; Calc. s.; Calend.; Carbon. s.; Cham.; *Graph.; Hep.;* Hydr.; Lyc.; *Merc. s.; Petrol.;* Pip. m.; Psor.; *Pyr.; Sil.; Sul.*

URTICARIA (hives, nettle rash)—Acon.; Anac.; Anthrok.; *Ant. c.; Antipyr.;* Apium gr.; *Apis; Ars.; Astac.;* Berb. v.; *Bombyx; Bov.;* Calc. c.;

Camph.; Chin. s.; *Chloral; Cim.;* Cina; Condur.; Con.; *Cop.;* Crot. t.; *Dulc.;* Fagop.; *Fragar.;* Hep.; Homar. fl.; *Ichth.;* Ign.; Ipec.; Kali c.; Kali chlor.; Medusa; Nat. m.; *Nat. p.;* Nit. ac.; Nux v.; Petrol.; *Puls.; Rhus t.;* Rhus v.; Robin.; Sanic.; Sep.; Stann.; Stroph.; Strych. p.; *Sul.;* Tereb.; Tetradyn.; *Triost.; Urt.;* Ustil.; Vespa.

Chronic—*Anac.; Ant. c.;* Antipyr.; *Ars.; Astac.; Bov.;* Calc. c.; *Chloral;* Condur.; *Cop.; Dulc.;* Hep.; Ichth.; *Lyc.;* Nat. m.; *Rhus t.;* Sep.; Stroph.; *Sul.; Urt.*

Nodosa—Bov.; Urt.

Tuberosa—*Anac.;* Bolet. lur.

CAUSE—CONCOMITANTS—From emotion: Anac.; Bov.; Ign.; Kali br.
From exertion, excessive—Con.; Nat. m.
From exposure—Chloral.; *Dulc.;* Rhus t.
From gastric derangement—*Ant. c.;* Ars.; Carbo v.; Cop.; Dulc.; Nux v.; *Puls.;* Robin.; Triost.
From menstrual conditions—Bell.; *Cim.; Dulc.;* Kali c.; Mag. c.; Puls.; Ustil.
From shellfish, roe—Camph.
From suppressed malaria—Elat.
From sweat—Apis.
With catarrh—Cepa; Dulc.
With chill, of intermittents—Ign.; Nat. m.
With constipation, fever—Cop.
With croup, alternating—Ars.
With diarrhœa—Apis; Bov.; *Puls.*
With edema—*Apis;* Vespa.
With erosion, on toes—Sul.
With itching, burning after scratching; no fever—Dulc.
With liver disturbance—Astac.
With petechial disturbance, or erysipelatous eruption—Fragar.
With rheumatic lameness, palpitation, diarrhœa—*Bov.;* Dulc.
With rheumatism, alternating—Urt.
With sequelæ, from suppressed hives—Apis; Urt.
With sudden coming and going—Antipyr.
With sudden, violent onset; syncope—Camph.

MODALITIES-AGGRAVATIONS: At climacteric: Morph.; Ustil.
At menstrual period—*Cim.; Dulc.;* Kali c.; Mag. c.
At night—Ant. c.; Ars.
From bathing, walking in A. M.—Bov.
From cold—Ars.; Dulc.; Rhus t.; Rumex; Sep.
From exertion, exercise—Apis; Calc. c.; Hep.; Nat. m.; Psor.; Sanic.; Urt.
From fruit, pork, buckwheat—Puls.
From open air—Nit. ac.; Sep.
From spirituous drinks—Chloral.
From warmth—Apis; Dulc.; Kali c.; Lyc.; Sul.
In children—Cop.
Periodically, every year—Urt.

AMELIORATIONS—From cold water: Apis; Dulc.

From hot drinks—Chloral.

From open air—Calc. c.

From warmth—Ars.; Chloral; Sep.

VACCINIA—*Acon.*; Ant. t.; Apis; *Bell.;* Merc. s.; Phos.; *Sil.;* Sul.; *Thuya;* Vac.

VERUCCA (warts)—Acet. ac.; Am. c.; Anac. oc.; Anag.; *Ant. c.;* Ant. t.; Ars. br.; Aur. m. n.; Bar. c.; *Calc. c.;* Castorea; Cast. eq.; *Caust.;* Chrom. oxy.; Cinnab.; *Dulc.; Ferr. picr.;* Kali m.; Kali perm.; Lyc.; *Mag. s.; Nat. c.;* Nat. m.: Nat. s.; *Nit. ac.;* Ran. b.; Semperv. t.; Sep.; *Sil.;* Staph.; Sul.; Sul. ac.; *Thuya;* X-ray.

Bleed easily—Cinnab.

Bleed easily, jagged, large—Caust.; *Nit. ac.*

Condylomata, fig warts—Calc. c.; *Cinnab.;* Euphras.; Kali iod.; *Lyc.;* Med.; Merc. c.; Merc. s.; Nat. s.; *Nit. ac.;* Phos. ac.; *Sab.;* Sep.; Sil.; *Staph.; Thuya.*

Cracked, ragged, with furfuraceous areola—Lyc.

Flat, smooth, sore—Ruta.

Horny, broad—Rhus t.

Large, seedy—Thuya.

Large, smooth, fleshy, on back of hands—Dulc.

Lupoid—Ferr. picr.

Moist, itching, flat, broad—Thuya.

Moist, oozing—Nit. ac.

Painful, hard, stiff, shining—Sil.

Painful, sticking—*Nit. ac.;* Staph.; Thuya.

Pedunculated—Caust.; Lyc.; *Nit. ac.;* Sab.; Staph.; *Thuya.*

Situated, on body, general—Nat. s.; Sep.

Situated, on breast—Castor.

Situated, on face, hands—Calc. c.; Caust.; Carbo an.; Dulc.; Kali c.

Situated, on forehead—Castorea.

Situated, on genito-anal surface—Nit. ac.; Thuya.

Situated, on hands—Anac.; *Bufo;* Ferr. magnet.; Kali m.; Lach.; Nat c.; *Nat. m.;* Rhus t.; Ruta.

Situated, on neck, arms, hands, soft, smooth—Ant. c.

Situated, on nose, finger tips, eye brows—Caust.

Situated, on prepuce—Cinnab.; Phos. ac.; Sab.

Small, all over body—Caust.

Smooth—Calc. c.; Ruta.

Sycotic, syphilitic—Nit. ac.

WHITLOW—felon, panaritium: Alum.; Am. c.; *Anthrac.;* Apis; Bell.; *Bry.;* Bufo; Calc. fl.; Calc. s.; Calend.; Cepa; Crot.; *Diosc.; Fluor. ac.; Hep.;* Hyper.; Led.; Merc. s.; Myrist. seb.; Nat. s.; Ol. myrist., Phos.; *Sil.;* Tar. c.

Malignant tendency—Anthrac.; *Ars.;* Carb. ac.; *Lach.*

Predisposition to—Diosc.; Hep.

Recurrence—Sil.

Traumatic—Led.

FEVER

CHILLINESS, coldness—Abies c.; *Acon.*; Æth.; *Agar.*; Alum.; *Ant. t.*;
Apis; *Aran.*; Arn.; *Ars.*; *Ars. iod.*; Asar.; Astac.; Bapt.; Berb. v.;
Bry.; *Calc. ars.*; *Calc. c.*; *Calc. sil.*; Calend.; *Camph.*; Canth.; *Caps.*;
Carbo v.; Castor.; Caust.; Ced.; Cimex; Cocaine; *Colch.*; Corn. fl.;
Crat.; Dulc.; *Echin.*; Eup. purp.; *Ferr. m.*; *Gels.*; Graph.; *Helod.*;
Hep.; Ipec.; Jatropha; *Kali c.*; Lac d.; *Laur.*; *Led.*; Lob. purp.; Lyc.;
Mag. p.; *Menyanth.*; *Merc. s.*; Morph.; Mosch.; *Nat. m.*; *Nux v.*;
Op.; Phos.; Pimpin.; Plat.; *Puls.*; Pyrus; Radium; Sabad.; *Sec.*;
Sil.; Sul.; *Tab.*; *Tela ar.*; Val.; *Ver. a.*

Chilliness, after epileptic fit—Cupr. m.

Chilliness, in abdomen, legs—Menyanth.

Chilliness, in arms—Raph.

Chilliness, in back and feet—Bell.; Canth.

Chilliness, in back, between shoulder blades—*Am. m.*; Castor.; *Lachnanth.*;
Pyr.; Tub.

Chilliness, in back, hips, to legs—Ham.

Chilliness, in body and feet, head and face hot—Arn.

Chilliness, in body, with face and breath hot—Cham.

Chilliness, in bones, extremities; severe, general—Pyr.

Chilliness, in chest, on walking in open air—Ran. b.

Chilliness, in forearms—Carbo v.; Med.

Chilliness, in hands—Dros.

Chilliness, in hands and back—Cact.

Chilliness, in hands, back, feet and knees—Benz. ac.; *Chin. ars.*

Chilliness, in hands, body warm—Tab.

Chilliness, in head and limbs—Calc. c.; Ferr. m.

Chilliness, in knees—*Carbo v.*; Cimex; Phos.

Chilliness, in lower limbs—Calc. c.; Cocc.

Chilliness, in lumbar region—Agar.

Chilliness, in single parts—*Asar.*; Calad.; *Calc. c.*; Kali bich.; Paris; Puls.

Chilliness, in waves, along spine—*Abies c.*; *Acon.*; Æsc.; *Ars.*· Bolet.;
Calend.; Conv.; Dulc.; Echin.; Frax. am.; *Gels.*; Helod.; *Mag. p.*;
Med.; Raph.; Strych.; Tub.; *Zinc. m.*

**Chilliness, with aching in shoulders, joints, small of back; yawning, stretch-
ing**—Bolet.

Chilliness, with catarrh—Merc. s.

Chilliness, with cough, dry, fatiguing—Rhus t.

Chilliness, with deficient, animal heat—*Alum.*; Bar. c.; Calc. c.; Calc. p.;
Calc. sil.; *Led.*; Lyc.; Psor.; *Sep.*; Sil.; Staph.; Thuya; Ver. a.

Chilliness, with desire to uncover abdomen—Tab.

Chilliness, with evening pains of whatever kind; in warm room—Puls.

Chilliness, with face, head, palms hot—Ferr. m.

Chilliness, with face hot—Dros.; Ign.

**Chilliness, with flatulent colic, nausea, vertigo, hot skin, sweat, heat of
head**—Cocc.

Chilliness, with headache—Conv.

Chilliness, with headache, extending to parietal region, red eyes—Ced.

Chilliness, with heat and desire to stretch—Rhus t.

Chilliness, with heat, alternately—Abies n.; Acon.; *Apis; Ars.;* Bapt.; Bell.; Bolet.; Bry.; *Cham.;* Dig.; Laur.; Mag. s.; Merc. c.; *Merc. s.;* Phyt.; Puls.; Solan. n.; Solid.

Chilliness, with ill humor—Caps.

Chilliness, with loquacity—Pod.

Chilliness, with nausea—Echin.; *Ipec.*

Chilliness, with nervousness—*Asar.;* Cim.; Croc.; *Gels.;* Gossyp.; Nat. m.

Chilliness, with no relief from warmth—Aran.; *Cadm. s.;* Caust.; Chin. s.; Dros.; Laur.; Mag. p.; *Merc. s.;* Pulex; Puls.; Sil.

Chilliness, with pain—Coff.; Dulc.; *Puls.;* Sil.

Chilliness, with pain, racking in limbs, anxious restlessness—Ars.

Chilliness, with pallor—Cocaine.

Chilliness, with pruritus—Mez.

Chilliness, with rheumatic pain, and soreness—Bapt.; Homar.; Rhus t.

Chilliness, with septic symptoms—*Pyr.;* Tar. c.

Chilliness, with suffocative feeling—Arg. n.; Mag. p.

Chilliness, with thirst—Acon.; *Ars.;* Caps.; Carbo v.; Conv.; Dulc.; *Ign.; Sec.;* Sep.; *Ver. a.*

Chilliness, with thirstlessness—Dros.; Gels.; Nux m.; *Puls.*

Chilliness, worse after anger—Aur.; *Bry.;* Cham.

Chilliness, worse after dinner—Mag. p.

Chilliness, worse after drinking—Caps.

Chilliness, worse after eating A. M.—Puls.

Chilliness, worse from dampness, rain, not relieved by warmth—Aran.

Chilliness, worse from least exposure, "air goes right through"—*Acon.;* Agar.; Agraph.; Am. phos.; Arg. n.; *Ars.;* Ars. iod.; Astac.; *Calc. c.; Calc. p.;* Calend.; Canchal.; Caps.; Cinch.; *Hep.; Kali c.;* Merc. c.; *Merc. s.;* Mez.; *Nux v.; Psor.;* Sep.; *Sil.;* Tub.

Chilliness, worse from least motion—Ars.; *Nux v.; Spig.*

Chilliness, worse from touch—Acon.; *Kali c.; Sil.;* Spig.

Chilliness, worse from warmth, covering—*Camph.;* Hep.; Med.; Sanic.; *Sec.;* Sul.

Chilliness, worse in morning—Calc. c.

Chilliness, worse toward evening and night—Acon.; Alum.; Am. c.; Ars.; Ced.; Dulc.; Mag. c.; Mag. p.; Menthol; *Merc. s.;* Ol. j. as.; *Phos.; Puls.;* Sep.

FEBRILE HEAT—Abies n.; Acet. ac.; *Acon.; Æsc.;* Æth.; *Agar.; Agrost.;* Allium s.; Ant. c.; Arn.; *Bapt.; Bell.; Bry.;* Calop.; Camph.; *Canth.;* Carbo v.; *Cham.;* Chin. ars.; *Cim.;* Cinch.; Dulc.; Eucal.; *Ferr. p.; Gels.;* Glon.; Ign.; Iod.; *Merc.;* Millef.; Morph.; Nit. ac.; Nux m.; *Nux v.;* Op.; Phyt.; Pulex; *Puls.; Rhus t.; Samb.;* Sep.; Sil.; Spiræa; *Spiranth.;* Stram.; Tereb.; Val.; *Ver. v.*

Febrile heat, ascends from pelvic organs—Sep.

Febrile heat, from anger—Cham.; Cocc.; Sep.

Febrile heat, in evening; falls asleep during, awakens when it ceases— Calad.

Febrile heat, in flashes, ebullitions—Acet. ac.; *Amyl;* Antipyr.; *Ars.;*
Ars. iod.; Bolet.; Calc. c.; *Carls.;* Chimaph.; *Dig.;* Erech.; Fer. red.;
Frax. am.; Hep.; Ign.; Indigo; Iod.; Jabor.; *Kali c.;* Lach.; Lyc.;
Med.; Merc. s.; *Niccol.;* Petrol.; *Phos.;* Puls.; *Sang.;* Sep.; *Sul.;*
Sul. ac.; Urt.; Val.; Viscum; Yohimb.

Febrile heat, in lower part of back, hip, thighs—Berb. v.

Febrile heat, in palms of hands—Chenop. gl.

Febrile heat, in soles of feet—Canth.

Febrile heat, in spots—Agar.; Apis.

Febrile heat, in whole body, face red, hot; yet chilly from least motion or
uncovering—Nux v.

Febrile heat, with chill predominant—Bry.

Febrile heat, with colic—Ver. a.

Febrile heat, with decline towards A. M., without sweat—Gels.

Febrile heat, with delirium; headache—Agar.; Bell.

Febrile heat, with drowsy stupefaction; agonized tossing about, in search
of a cool place; must be uncovered; vomiting, diarrhœa; convulsions—
Op.

Febrile heat, with dryness, during sleep or on falling asleep; deep, dry,
cough—Samb.

Febrile heat, with dryness, no sweat—Alum.; *Nux m.*

Febrile heat, with excitement, nervous agitation—*Acon.;* Tela ar.

Febrile heat, with external coldness—Ars.; Canth.

Febrile heat, with faintness, sweat—*Dig.;* Sep.; *Sul.;* Sul. ac.

Febrile heat, with flatulence, bowel movement—Radium.

Febrile heat, with headache—Astac.

Febrile heat, with headache as from thousand hammers—Nat. m.

Febrile heat, with hot face, back chilly, feet cold—Puls.

Febrile heat, with hot face, cold hands and feet—Stram.

Febrile heat, with hot face, cool body, asthenic states—Arn.; Phyt.

Febrile heat, with hot face, unquenchable thirst, taste of bile, nausea, anxiety, restlessness, dry tongue; after anger—Cham.

Febrile heat, with hunger, for days preceding—Staph.

Febrile heat, with itching eyes, tearing in limbs, numbness of body, headache
—Ced.

Febrile heat, with lassitude, in afternoon; throbs all over—Lil. t.

Febrile heat, with night sweats—*Acet. ac.;* Hep.

Febrile heat, with palpitation, precordial anguish—Calc. c.

Febrile heat, with prostration—Ant. t.; *Chin. ars.;* Phyt.

Febrile heat, with pulsations—*Bell.; Lil. t.;* Puls.; Thuya.

Febrile heat, with pulsations, and distended veins—*Puls.;* Thuya.

Febrile heat, with red spot on left cheek—Acet. ac.

Febrile heat, with restlessness, cheeks red, apathy—Iod.

Febrile heat, with restless sleep—Calc. c.

Febrile heat, with skin dry, hot; face red or red and pale alternately; arterial
excitement; anguish, restlessness, tossing about—Acon.

Febrile heat, with skin dry, pungent; arterial excitement; distended, superficial vessels—Bell.

Febrile heat, with slow, nervous, insidious course; vertigo—Cocc.

Febrile heat, smothered feeling, if covered—Arg. n.

Febrile heat, with soreness of body—*Arn.;* Franc.; Phyt.; *Rhus t.*

Febrile heat, with spasms—Acetan.; *Bell.*

Febrile heat, with stretching of limbs—Rhus t.

Febrile heat, with sudden onset; dry, burning skin; rapid, small, wiry pulse—Pyr.

Febrile heat, with tendency to cover up—Ign.; *Nux v.;* Samb.; Stann.

Febrile heat, with thirst—*Acon.;* Ant. c.; Bry.; Laur.; Puls.; Tereb.

Febrile heat, with thirstlessness—*Acet. ac.;* Æth.; Bell.; Gels.; *Ign.;* Mur. ac.; *Nux m.; Puls.;* Samb.

Febrile heat, worse at night—Acon.; Æsc.; Ant. c.; Ars.; Bell.; Calad.; *Calc. c.;* Gels.; *Hep.;* Kali s.; Mag. c.; *Petrol.;* Phos.; *Puls.;* Sil.; Stann.; Urt.

Febrile heat, worse during menses—Calc. c.; Thuya.

Febrile heat, worse during sleep—Acon.; Calad.; *Samb.*

Febrile heat, worse covering up—Ign.

Febrile heat, worse from motion, then chilly—Nux v.

Febrile heat, worse from uncovering—*Merc. s.; Nux v.;* Samb.; Stront.

Febrile heat, worse in afternoon—Azadir.; Bell.; Ferr.

Febrile heat, worse in morning in bed—Kali c.

Febrile heat, worse on awaking—Laur.

Febrile heat, worse when sitting, walking in open air—Sep.

SWEAT: TYPE—Bloody: *Crot.;* Lach.; Lyc.; Nux m.; Nux v.

Cold, clammy—Abies c.; *Acet. ac.;* Æth.; *Amyl;* Ant. ars.; *Ant. t.; Ars.;* Benz. ac.; Cact.; *Calc. c.;* Calc. p.; *Camph.;* Canth.; *Carbo v.;* Cinch.; Corn. fl.; Crot.; *Cupr. ars.;* Dig.; Dulc.; Elaps; Euphorb. d.; Formal.; Ign.; Ipec.; Lach.; Laur.; Lob. infl.; Lupul.; Lyc.; Med.; Merc. c.; Merc. cy.; *Merc. s.;* Nat. c.; Pyr.; *Sanic.; Sec.;* Sul. ac.; *Tab.;* Tela ar.; *Tereb.; Ver a.;* Ver. v.

Greasy, oily—Bry.; Carbo v.; Cinch.; Lupul.; Mag. c.; *Merc. s.*

Hot—Æsc.; Carbo v.; *Cham.;* Chenop. gl.; *Lach.; Op.;* Tilia; Ver. v.

LOCALIZED, in general—Bry.; *Calc. c.;* Cinch.; *Fluor. ac.;* Hep.; *Petrol.;* Phos.; Plectranth.; *Puls.;* Selen.; *Sil.;* Sul.

Localized, in anterior part of body—Selen.

Localized, in axillæ—Calc. c.; Nit. ac.; Osm.; Petrol.; Sep.; Sil. See Locomotor System.

Localized, on chest—*Calc. c.;* Cocc.; Euphras.; *Phos.;* Stann.; Strych.

Localized, on covered parts—Bell.

Localized, on extremities, upper right—Formal.

Localized, on face, forehead—*Acet. ac.;* Benz. ac.; Calc. c.; Cina; Euphorb. d.; *Lob. infl.;* Phos.; Rheum; Sinap.; Stann.; Sul.; Val.; *Ver. a.*

Localized, on feet—Calc. c.; *Graph.;* Lact. ac.; Merc. s.; *Petrol.;* Phos.; Sep.; Sil. See Feet (Locomotor System).

Localized, on genitals—Calc. c.; Petrol.; Phos. ac.; Thuya. See Male Sexual System.

Localized, on hands—Calc. c.; Cina; Con.; Fluor. ac.; Nit. ac.; *Phos.;* Sil. See Locomotor System.

Localized, on head, nape of neck—Bell.; *Calc. c.;* Phos.; Puls.; Rheum; *Samb.; Sanic.; Sil.;* Stann.; Strych.; *Ver. a.*

Localized, on lower body—Croc.; Ran. ac.; Sanic.

Localized, on part lain on—Acon.

Localized, on parts in contact with each other—Niccol. s.

Localized, on posterior part of body—Sep.

Localized, on side not reclined upon—Benz.; Thuya.

Localized, on uncovered parts—Thuya.

Localized, on upper body—Azadir.; Calc. c.; Cham.; Kali c.; Nux v.; Sil.

Localized, unilaterally—Jabor.; Nux v.; Puls.

ODOR—Fetid, offensive: Art. v.; Bapt.; *But. ac.;* Calc. c.; *Carbo an.;* Cimex; Con.; Daphne; Fluor. ac.; *Hep.;* Kali iod.; *Lyc.; Merc. s.; Nit. ac.;* Ol. an.; Osm.; *Petrol.;* Phos.; *Psor.;* Puls.; *Sep.; Sil.;* Solan. t.; Stann.; *Staph.;* Sul.; *Taxus; Thuya;* Variol. See Bromidrosis (Skin).

Odor, musty, mouldy—Stann.

Odor, sour, acid—Arn.; Bry.; *Calc. c.; Cham.;* Fluor. ac.; Graph.; *Hep.;* Kreos.; Lac d.; *Mag. c.;* Merc.; Nux v.; Pyr.; *Rheum;* Robin.; Sanic.; Sep.; *Sil.; Sul.; Sul. ac.;* Thuya.

Odor, sweetish—*Calad.;* Thuya.

Odor, urinous—Eryng. aq.; Nit. ac.

PROFUSE sweat (hyperidrosis)—*Acet. ac.;* Acon.; Æsc.; *Agaricin;* Am. acet.; Ant. t.; Ars.; *Ars. iod.; Bapt.; Bell.;* Bolet.; Bry.; *Calc. c.;* Canth.; Cham.; *Cinch.;* Cocc.; Con.; Croc.; Eser.; *Ferr. iod.;* Ferr. m.; Fluor. ac.; Graph.; *Hep.;* Hyper.; *Iod.; Jabor.; Kali c.;* Lact. ac.; Lob. infl.; *Merc. s.;* Morph.; *Nit. ac.;* Nux v.; Op.; *Phos. ac.;* Phos.; *Piloc.;* Polyp.; *Psor.;* Puls.; Sal. ac.; *Samb.;* Sanic.; *Selen.; Sep.; Sil.;* Stann.; Sul.; Sul. ac.; Thuya; Tilia; *Ver. a.;* Zinc. m.

Profuse, debilitating (colliquative)—*Acet. ac.;* Camph.; Carbo an.; *Carbo v.;* Castor.; Chrysanth.; *Cinch.;* Eup. perf.; Ferr. m.; Gels.; *Merc. v.;* Nit. ac.; Nitrum; Op.; Phell.; *Phos. ac.;* Phos.; Pyr.; Rhus gl.; *Salvia; Samb.;* Stann.; Sul. ac.

SCANTY—Apis; Conv.; Lach.; *Nux m.*

Viscid—Abies c.; Fluor. ac.; Hep.; *Lyc.; Merc. s.;* Phallus; Phos.

Yellow, staining—Ars.; Carbo an.; Lach.; Lyc.; *Merc. s.*

OCCURRENCE—After acute diseases: Psor.

After eating, drinking—Carbo v.; Cham.; Kali c.

At end of fever, or only at beginning of sleep—Ars.

During climacteric—Hep.; *Jabor.;* Tilia. See Female Sexual System.

During exertion, motion—Asar.; But. ac.; *Calc. c.;* Carbo an.; *Cinch.;* Eup. purp.; *Eupion;* Graph.; *Hep.; Iod.;* Kali c.; Lyc.; Merc. c.; *Merc. s.;* Nat. c.; Nat. m.; *Phos. ac.; Psor.;* Sep.; *Sil.;* Sul.

During morning, day time—Bry.; Carbo an.; Carbo v.; Hep.; Lyc.; Nat. m.; Nux v.; Phos.; Sep.; Sil.; Sul.; Zinc. m.

During morning, early—Stann.

During sleep (night sweats)—*Acet. ac.;* Agar.; *Agaricin;* Aral.; *Ars. iod.;* Bar. c.; Bell.; Bolet.; *Calc. c.;* Carbo an.; Carbo v.; Cham.; Chrysanth.; *Cinch.;* Con.; Corn. fl.; Euphras.; Ferr. p.; *Hep.; Iod.;* Ipec.; *Jabor.;* Kali c.; Kali iod.; Lyc.; *Merc. s.;* Myos.; Nat. tell.; Nit. ac.; Nux v.; Op.; Petrol.; *Phos. ac.;* Phos.; Phyt.; Picrot.; *Piloc.; Pop. tr.;* Psor.;

Salvia; Sang.; Sanic.; Sep.; *Sil.;* Stann.; Staph.; Stront. c.; Sul.; Tarax.; Thall.; *Thuya;* Tilia; Zinc. m.

During waking hours—Con.; Hep.; Merc.; Phos. a*..* Phos.; *Samb.*

From nervous depression, phthisis; convalescence, from acute disease—Jabor.

From nervous shock; sitting quietly—Anac.; Sep.

Sweat, affords no relief, or aggravates symptoms—Ant. t.; Bell.; Bolet.; Chin. s.; Ferr. m.; Formica; *Hep.; Merc. s.;* Phos. ac.; Pyr.; Sep.; Stram.

Sweat, affords relief, to symptoms—*Acon.; Ars.; Calad.;* Cupr. m.; Eup. perf.; Franc.; *Nat. m.; Psor.;* Senega; *Ver. a.*

TYPE OF FEVER: BILIOUS—*Bapt.;* Bry.; *Cham.;* Cinch.; Col.; Crot.; Euonym.; *Eup. perf.;* Gels.; Ipec.; Lept.; *Merc. c.; Merc. s.;* Nux v.; Nyct.; Pod.; Rhus t.; Tarax.

CATHETER—*Acon.;* Camph. ac.; Petros.

DENGUE—*Acon.;* Ars.; Bell.; Bry.; Canth.; Cinch.; *Eup. perf.; Gels.;* Ipec.; Nux v.; *Rhus t.;* Rhus v.

DYSENTERIC—Nux v.

ENTERIC—TYPHOID FEVER—Agar.; Agaricin; *Ail.; Apis;* Arg. n.; *Arn.; Ars.;* Arum tr.; *Bapt.; Bell.;* Bry.; Calc. c.; *Carbo v.;* Cina; Cinch.; Colch.; Crot.; Cupr. ars.; Echin.; *Eucal.; Gels.;* Glon.; *Helleb.;* Hydr.; *Hyos.;* Hyosc. hydrobr.; Iod.; Ipec.; Kali p.; *Lach.;* Laur.; *Lyc.;* Merc. cy.; *Merc. s.;* Methyl. bl.; Mosch.; *Mur. ac.; Nit. ac.; Nux m.; Op.; Phos. ac.; Phos.; Pyr.; Rhus t.;* Selen.; *Stram.;* Strych.; Sul. ac.; Sumb.; *Tereb.;* Vaccin. myr.; Val.; Ver. a.; Xerophyl.; Zinc. m.

CONCOMITANTS—Biliousness: *Bry.;* Chel.; Hydr.; Lept.; *Merc. s.;* Nux v.

Carriers; after inoculation with anti-typhoid serum—Bapt.

Constipation—*Bry.;* Hydr.; Nux v.; Op.

Decubitus—Arn.; *Ars.;* Bapt.; Carbo v.; *Lach.;* Mur. ac.; Pyr.; *Sec.*

Delirium—Agar.; *Agaricin;* Ars.; Bapt.; *Bell.;* Can. ind.; *Hyos.; Hyosc. hydrobr.;* Lach.; Methyl. bl.; Op.; Phos. ac.; Phos.; Rhus t.; *Stram.;* Tereb.; Val.

Diarrhœa—Arn.; *Ars.;* Bapt.; Crot.; *Cupr. ars.; Epilob.;* Lach.; *Merc. s.;* Phos. ac.; Rhus t.

Diarrhœa, involuntary—Apis; *Arn.;* Ars.; Hyos.; Mur. ac.; *Phos. ac.*

Ecchymoses—*Arn.; Ars.;* Carbo v.; Mur. ac.

Epistaxis—*Acon.; Bry.;* Croc.; *Ham.; Ipec.;* Meli.; Phos. ac.; Rhus t.

Fever—Ars.; *Bapt.; Bell.;* Gels.; Methyl. bl.; Rhus t.; Stram.

Gastric symptoms—*Bry.;* Canth.; Carbo v.; *Hydr.;* Merc. s.; Nux v.; Puls.

Headache—Acetan.; *Bell.; Bry.;* Gels.; Hyos.; Nux v.; Rhus t.

Hæmorrhage—*Alumen;* Alum.; Ars.; *Bapt.;* Carbo v.; Cinch.; *Crot.;* Elaps; *Ham.;* Hydrastin. sul.; Ipec.; Kreos.; Lach.; *Millef.; Mur. a..; Nit. ac.;* Nux m.; *Phos. ac.;* Sec.; *Tereb.*

Insomnia—Bell.; *Coff.;* Gels.; *Hyosc. hydrobr.; Hyos.;* Op.; Rhus t.

Laryngeal affections—Apis; Merc. c.

Multiple abscesses—Ars.; Hep.; Sil.

Myocarditis—Pineal gland ext.

Nervous symptoms, adynamia—Agar.; *Agaricin;* Apis; *Ars.;* Bapt.; *Bell.;* Bry.; Cocc.; Colch.; Gels.; Helleb.; *Hyos.; Hyosc. hydrobr.; Ign.;* Lach.; Lyc.; *Mur. ac.; Phos. ac.; Phos.;* Rhus t.; *Stram.;* Sumb.; Val.; Zinc. m.

Nervous symptoms, collapse—*Ars.; Camph.;* Carbo v.; Cinch.; Hyosc. hydrobr.; *Laur.;* Mur. ac.; Sec.; Ver. a.

Peritonitis—Ars.; *Bell.;* Carbo v.; Col.; *Merc. c.;* Rhus t.; Tereb.

Pneumonia, bronchial symptoms—*Ant. t.;* Ars.; Bell.; *Bry.;* Hyos.; *Ipec.;* Lach.; *Phos.;* Puls.; Rhus t.; *Sang.;* Sul.; Tereb.

Putrescent pneumonia—Ars.; Mur. ac.

Soreness, muscular—*Arn.;* Bapt.; Bry.; Gels.; *Rhus t.*

Stage of convalescence—Ars. iod.; Carbo v.; *Cinch.;* Cocc.; Hydr.; Kali p.; Nux v.; *Psor.;* Sul.; Tarax.

Tympanites—*Asaf.; Ars.;* Bapt.; *Carbo v.;* Cinch.; Cocc.; Colch.; Lyc.; Mehtyl bl.; Millef.; Mur. ac.; *Nux m.; Phos. ac.;* Rhus t.; *Tereb.*

Ulcer, corneal—Apis; Ipec.

Urination, profuse—Gels.; Mur. ac.; *Phos. ac.*

Urination, scanty, painful—Apis; Ars.; *Canth.*

EXANTHEMATA: ERUPTIVE FEVER: RUBELLA—(rotheln, German measles): Acon.; Bell.; Cop. See Rubeola (Measles).

RUBEOLA—MEASLES—*Acon.;* Ail.; Ant. t.; *Ars.; Ars. iod.;* Bell.; *Bry.;* Camph.; Coff.; Dulc.; Eup. perf.; *Euphras.;* Ferr. p.; *Gels.;* Ipec.; *Kali bich.;* Kali m.; Lach.; Merc. c.; Merc. pr. rub.; Merc. s.; Op.; *Puls.;* Rhus t.; Scilla; Spong.; *Sticta;* Stram.; Sul.; Ver. v.; Viola od.

CONCOMITANTS: Adenitis—Kali bich.; Merc. i. r.

Bronchial and pulmonary symptoms—*Ant. t.;* Bell.; *Bry.;* Chel.; Ferr. p.; *Ipec.;* Kali bich.; *Phos.;* Rumex; *Sticta;* Ver. v.; Viola iod.

Bronchial and pulmonary symptoms persisting—Calc. c.; Iod.; Kali c.; Sil.; Sul.

Catarrhal symptoms—Ars.; Cepa; Dulc.; *Euphras.;* Gels.; Kali bich.; Merc. s.; *Puls.;* Sabad.; *Sticta.*

Cerebral and convulsive symptoms—Æth.; Apis; *Bell.;* Camph.; Coff.; *Cupr. ac.;* Stram.; Ver. v.; Viola od.; Zinc. m.

Cough, croupy—Acon.; Coff.; Dros.; Euphras.; Gels.; *Hep.;* Kali bich.; *Spong.;* Sticta.

Diarrhœa—Ars.; Cinch.; *Ipec.;* Merc. s.; *Puls.;* Ver. a.

Diphtheritic symptoms—Lach.; Merc. cy.

Epistaxis—Acon.; Bry.; Ipec.

Eye symptoms—Ars.; *Euphras.;* Kali bich.; Puls.

Gangrene of mouth, vulva—Ars.; Kali chlor.; Lach.

Insomnia, cough—Calc. c.; Coff.

Laryngitis—Dros.; Gels.; *Kali bich.;* Viola od.

Low fever, toxemia—*Ail.; Ars.;* Bapt.; Carbo v.; Crot.; *Lach.; Mur. ac.; Rhus t.;* Sul.

Malignant types (black or epidemic)—Ail.; *Ars.;* Crot.; Lach.

Otalgia, rheumatoid symptoms—Puls.

Rash, retrocedent, or suppressed—Ant. t.; Apis; *Bry.*; Camph.; *Cupr. ac.*; *Ipec.*; *Lach.*; *Stram.*

Rash, tardy development—Ant. t.; Apis; *Bry.*; Cupr. m.; Dulc.; Gels.; Ipec.; *Stram.*; Sul.; Tub.; Ver. v.; *Zinc. m.*

Sequelæ—Am. c.; *Ars.*; Bry.; Camph.; Coff.; *Cupr. ac.*; Dros.; Kali c.; Merc. c.; Merc. s.; Op.; *Puls.*; Sang.; Sticta; *Sul.*; *Tub.*; Zinc. m.

SCARLET FEVER—*Acon.*; *Ail.*; Am. c.; *Apis*; *Ars.*; Arum; *Asimina*; *Bell.*; Bry.; Canth.; *Carb. ac.*; Chin. ars.; Commocl.; *Crot.*; Cupr. ac.; Cupr. m.; Dub.; Echin.; Eucal.; *Gels.*; Hep.; Hyos.; Ipec.; Kali chlor.; Kali s.; Lac c.; *Lach.*; Lyc.; Merc. s.; Merc. i. r.; *Mur. ac.*; Op.; Phyt.; *Rhus t.*; Sang.; Sil.; Solan. n.; Spig.; *Stram.*; Tereb.; Zinc. m.

CONCOMITANTS: Adenitis, cervical—Ail.; Am. c.; Asimina; *Bell.*; Carb. ac.; Crot.; Hep.; Lach.; *Merc. i. r.*; Merc. s.; *Rhus t.*

Adenitis, parotid—Am. c.; Phyt.; Rhus t.

Albuminuria and dropsy—Acon.; Am. c.; *Apis*; Apoc.; *Ars.*; *Canth.*; Colch.; *Dig.*; *Helleb.*; Hep.; Kali chlor.; Lach.; Nat. s.; *Tereb.* See Nephritis (Urinary System).

Anginosa (sore throat)—Acon.; *Ail.*; *Apis*; Ars.; *Asimina*; *Bar. c.*; *Bell.*; Brom.; Kali perm.; Lac c.; *Lach.*; Merc.; Mur. ac.; *Phyt.*; Rhus t.

Anginosa, ulcerativa—*Am. c.*; Apis; *Ars.*; ʻArum; Bar. c.; Crot.; Hep.; *Lach.*; *Merc. cy.*; Merc. i. r.; *Mur. ac.*; Nit. ac.

Cellulitis—Ail.; Am. c.; *Apis*; Lach.; *Rhus t.*

Chronic tendencies aroused—Calc. c.; Hep.; Rhus t.

Diarrhœa—Ail.; Ars.; Asimina; Phos.; Rhus t.

Edema of glottis—*Apis*; Apium v.; Chin. s.; Merc. c.

Edema of lungs—*Ant. t.*; Can. s.; Phos.; Scilla.

Fever—Acon.; *Apis*; Asimina; Bapt.; *Bell.*; Gels.; Rhus t.

Laryngitis—Brom.; Spong.

Malignant tendency, adynamia—Ail.; Am. c.; *Apis*; *Ars.*; Arum; Bapt.; *Carb. ac.*; Carbo v.; *Crot.*; Cupr. ac.; Echin.; Hydroc. ac.; *Lach.*; Merc. cy.; *Mur. ac.*; Phos.; *Rhus t.*; Tab.; Zinc. m.

Miliary type—*Acon.*; Ail.; Am. c.; Apis; Ars.; Bry.; *Coff.*; Kali ars.; Lach.; Rhus t.

Nervous, convulsive, cerebral symptoms—Æth.; Ail.; Am. c.; Apis; Ars.; *Bell.*; Camph.; *Cupr. ac.*; Cupr. m.; *Hyos.*; Rhus t.; *Stram.*; Sul.; Zinc. m.

Rash, delayed development—Apis; Ars.; *Bry.*; Lach.; Rhus t.; Zinc. m.

Rash, hæmorrhage in—Crot.; *Lach.*; Mur. ac.; Phos.

Rash, livid—*Ail.*; *Lach.*; Mur. ac.; Solan. n.

Rash, livid, partial, patchy—Ail.

Rash, retrocedent, threatened brain paralysis—*Ail.*; Am. c.; Cupr. ac.; Sul.; Tub.; *Zinc. m.*

Rash, retrocession of—Am. c.; *Apis*; Ars.; Bry.; Calc. c.; *Camph.*; *Cupr. ac.*; Cupr. m.; *Stram.*; Sul.; Ver. a.; *Zinc. m.*

Raw, bloody, itching, painful, surfaces; must pick and bore into them—Arum.

Rheumatic symptoms—Bry.; *Rhus t.*; Spig.

SEQUELAE: Adenitis—Brom.; Hep.; Lach.; *Merc. i. r.;* Phyt.
Deafness; sore, bleeding nose—Mur. ac.
Desquamation, in large flakes, several times—Arum.
Ear disorders—Bell.; Carb. ac.; Carbo v.; Gels.; *Hep.; Merc. s.;* Sil.; Sul.
Nephritis (post-scarlatinal)—Apis; Ars.; Arum; Canth.; Helleb. See Urinary System.
Nose disorders—Arum; Aur. mur.; Mur. ac.; Sul.
Stomatitis ulcerative—Arum; Mur. ac.
Typhoidal symptoms—Ail.; Arum; *Hyos.;* Lach.; *Rhus t.;* Stram. See Malignant.
Vomiting—Ail.; Asimina; *Bell.;* Cupr. m.

VARICELLA—CHICKENPOX—*Acon.; Ant. t.;* Apis; Bry.; *Dulc.;* Kali m.; Led.; *Merc. s.;* Rhus d.; *Rhus t.;* Urt.; Variol.

VARIOLA—SMALLPOX—Acon.; Am. c.; Anac.; *Ant. t.;* Apis; Ars.; *Bapt.; Bry.; Carb. ac.;* Chin. s.; Cim.; Crot.; Cupr. ac.; Gels.; *Hep.;* Hydr.; *Kali bich.;* Lach.; *Merc. s.;* Millef.; Op.; Phos.; *Rhus t.; Sarrac.;* Sinap.; Sul.; Thuya; *Variol.;* Ver. v.

TYPE—Confluent: Ars.; Hippoz.; *Merc. s.;* Phos.; Sul.; Variol.
Discrete—*Ant. t.; Bapt.;* Bell.; Gels.; Sul.
Hæmorrhage—Ars.; Crot.; Ham.; Lach.; Phos.; Nat. nit.; *Sec.;* Sul.
Malignant—Am. c.; Ant. t.; *Ars.;* Bapt.; *Carb. ac.; Crot.; Lach.; Mur. ac.;* Phos. ac.; Phos.; *Rhus t.;* Sec.; Sul.; Variol.

COMPLICATIONS—Adenitis: *Merc. i. r.;* Rhus t.
Boils—*Hep.;* Phos.; Sul.
Collapsic symptoms—Ars.; Carbo v.; Lach.; *Mur. ac.;* Phos. ac.
Delirium—*Bell.;* Stram.; Ver. v.
Dropsical swellings—*Apis;* Ars.; Canth.
Fever, initial—*Acon.;* Ant. t.; *Bapt.; Bell.;* Gels.; Variol.; *Ver. v.*
Fever, suppurative—Acon.; Bell.; Merc.; *Rhus t.*
Ophthalmia—Merc. s.; Sul.
Pulmonary symptoms—Acon.; *Ant. t.;* Bry.; *Phos.;* Sul.; Ver. v.
Repercussion of eruption—Ars.; *Camph.;* Cupr. m.; Sul.; Zinc. m.

FEBRICULA (simple, continued fever)—*Acon.;* Arn.; *Ars.; Bapt.;* Bell.; Bry.; Camph.; *Ferr. p.;* Gels.; Ipec.; Kal.; Merc. s.; Nux v.; Puls.; *Rhus t.*

GASTRIC—Acon.; *Ant. c.; Ars.; Bapt.; Bry.;* Calc. c.; Cinch.; Hydr.; *Ipec.;* Lyc.; Merc. s.; Nux v.; Phos. ac.; *Puls.;* Rhus t.; Santon.

HECTIC—Abrot.; *Acet. ac.;* Acon.; Arg. m.; *Ars.;* Ars. iod.; *Bals. per.; Bapt.;* Calc. c.; Calc. iod.; Calc. s.; Carbo v.; *Chin. ars.; Cinch.; Ferr. m.;* Gels.; *Hep.;* Iod.; Lyc.; Med.; *Merc. s.;* Nit. ac.; Ol. j. as.; Phell.; Phos. ac.; *Phos.;* Pyr.; *Sang.;* Sil.; Stann.; Sul.

INFLAMMATORY—Acon.; Bell.; Bry.

INFLUENZA (grippe)—*Acon.;* Æsc.; Ant. ars.; Ant. iod.; Ant. t.; Arn.; *Ars.; Ars. iod.;* Ars. s. r.; Asclep. t.; *Bapt.; Bell.;* Brom.; *Bry.;* Calc. c.; Camph.; Canchal.; *Carb. ac.;* Card. m.; Caust.; *Cepa; Chin. s.;* Cinch.; Cupr. ars.; Cycl.; Dros.; *Dulc.;* Eryng.; *Eucal.; Eup. perf.;* Euphorbia; Euphras.; Ferr. p.; *Gels.;* Glon.; Glycerin; Gymnocl.;

Influenzin; Iod.; Ipec.; Kali bich.; Kali c.; Kali iod.; Kali s.; Lach.; Lob. cer.; *Lob. purp.;* Lyc.; Merc. s.; *Nat. sal.; Nux v.; Phos.;* Phyt.; Pod.; Psor.; Puls.; Pyr.; Rhus r.; *Rhus t.;* Rumex; *Sabad.;* Sal. ac.; Sang.; *Sang. n.;* Sarcol. ac.; Senega; Silph.; Spig.; Spong.; *Sticta;* Sul.; *Sul. rub.;* Triost.; Ver. a.

Influenza, debility of—Abrot.; Adon. v.; *Ars. iod.; Avena;* Carb. ac.; *Chin. ars.;* Chin. s.; *Cinch.;* Con.; Eup. perf.; Gels.; *Iberis;* Lac c.; Lathyr.; Phos.; Psor.; Sal. ac.; Sarcol. ac.

Influenza, pain remaining—Lycopers.

INTERMITTENT FEVER (ague, malarial)—Acon.; *Alston.;* Am. m.; *Am. picr.; Amyl;* Ant. c.; Ant. t.; *Apis; Aran.;* Arn.; *Ars.;* Ars. br.; Azadir.; Baja; Bapt.; Bell.; Bolet.; Bry.; Cact.; *Camph. monobr.;* Canchal.; *Caps.;* Carb. ac.; *Carbo v.;* Ceanoth.; *Ced.;* Centaur.; *Chin. ars.; Chin. mur.; Chin. s.;* Chionanth.; Cimex; *Cina; Cinch.; Corn. fl.;* Crot.; *Echin.;* Elat.; Eucal.; *Eup. perf.; Eup. purp.;* Ferr. m.; Ferr. p.; *Gels.; Helianth.;* Hep.; Hydr.; *Ign.; Ipec.; Lach.;* Laur.; Lyc.; Malland.; *Menyanth.;* Methyl. bl.; *Nat. m.;* Nat. s.; Nitrum; *Nux v.;* Op.; Ostrya; Pambot.; Parth.; Petros.; Phell.; *Phos. ac.;* Pod.; Polyp.; Puls.; Rhus t.; Sabad.; Spig.; Sul.; Tarax.; *Tela ar.;* Thuya; Urt.; Verb.; *Ver. a.;* Ver. v.

TYPE—Abuse of quinine, cachexia: Am. m.; Aran.; Arn.; *Ars.;* Ars. iod.; *Calc. ars.;* Carbo v.; Ceanoth.; Chelone; *Chin. ars.;* Eucal.; Eup. perf.; Ferr. m.; *Hydr.; Ipec.; Lach.;* Malar. off.; Malland.; *Nat. m.; Polymia;* Puls.; Sul.; Ver. a.

Chronic, inveterate cases—Abies n.; Am. m.; Aran.; *Ars.;* Ars. br.; Calc. ars.; Canchal.; Carbo v.; Corn. c.; Corn. fl.; *Helianth.;* Ign.; *Nat. m.; Puls.;* Pyr.; Querc.; Tela ar.   See Abuse of Quinine.

Congestive—Camph.; *Op.; Ver. a.*

Dumb ague—*Ars.;* Ced.; Chelone; Chin. s.; *Gels.; Ipec.;* Malland.; *Nux v.*

Impure cases, in non-malarial regions—Ipec.; Nux v.

Nervo-hysterical persons—Aran.; Cocc.; Ign.; Tar. h.

Pernicious cases—*Ars.;* Camph.; Chin. hydrobr.; *Chin. s.;* Crot.; *Ver. a.*

Recent cases—Acon.; Aran.; Ars.; Chin. s.; Cinch.; Ipec.; Tar. h.

Stages, partial, irregular—Aran.; *Ars.;* Cact.; *Carbo v.;* Eup. perf.; Eup. purp.; *Ipec.;* Nat. m.

Stages, regular, well defined—*Chin. s.;* Cinch.

CHILL: OCCURRENCE—TYPE—Afternoon: 1 P. M. daily: Ferr. p.

Afternoon, 2 P. M.—Calc. c.; Lach.

Afternoon, 3 P. M.—Apis; Chin. s.

Afternoon, 3-4 P. M.—Lyc.; Thuya.

Afternoon, 4-8 P. M.—Lyc.

Afternoon, 4 P. M.—Æsc.

Afternoon, 5 P. M.—Cinch.

Afternoon, late, evening, night—Aran.; Bolet.; Ced.; Ipec.; Petrol.; Tar. h.

Anticipating—*Chin. s.;* Cinch.; Nux v.

Forenoon—Cinch.; Formal.; Nux v.

Hebdomadal—Cinch.

Midday—Gels.

Midnight—Ars.; Nux v.

Mingled, with heat—Ant. t.; Apis; *Ars.;* Cinch.; *Nux v.;* Tar. h.; Ver.
a. See Chilliness.

Morning—Chin. s.

Morning, 1-2 A. M.—Ars.

3 A. M.—Thuya.

4 A. M.—Ferr. m.

5 A. M.—Cinch.

6-7 A. M.—Pod.

7-9 A. M.; at noon following day—Eup. perf.

9-11 A. M.—Bapt.; Bolet.; Mag. s.; *Nat. m.;* Wyeth.

11 A. M. and 11 P. M.—Cact.

Periodical—*Aran.;* Ars.; Bolet.; Cact.; *Ced.; Chin. s.;* Cina; Cinch.;
Eucal.; Ipec.

Periodical, every 7 or 14 days; never at night—Cinch.

Periodical, every spring—Carbo v.; *Lach.;* Sul.

Prolonged—Aran.; Bolet.; Cact.; Canchal.; *Caps.; Chin. s.;* Eup. purp.;
Ipec.; Menyanth.; Nat. m.; *Nux v.;* Plumb.; Pod.; Puls.; Pyr.; *Sabad.;*
Ver. a.; Ver. v.

Quartan—Baja; *Chin. s.;* Cinch.; Helleb.

Quotidian—Ars.; Bolet.; Chin. s.; Ign.; Lob. infl.; Nitrum; Nux v.;
Plumb.; Tar. h.

Slight—*Ars.;* Azar.; Carbo v.; Cina; Cinch.; Eup. perf.; Eup. purp.;
Ipec.

Tertian—Calc. c.; *Chin. s.;* Cinch.; Ipec.; Lyc.

LOCATION—Abdomen:—*Apis; Calc. c.;* Menyanth.

Back—Apis; Bolet.; Conv.; Dulc.; *Eup. perf.;* Eup. purp.; *Gels.; Lach.;*
Mag. s.; *Nat. m.;* Pyr.

Back, between scapulæ—Am. m.; *Caps.;* Pyr.; Sep.

Back, dorsal region—Eup. perf.; Lach.

Back, lumbar region—Eup. perf.; Nat. m.

Breast—Cinch.

Feet—Gels.; Lach.; Nat. m.; Sabad.

Hand, left—Carbo v.; Nux m.

Nose, tip of—Menyanth.

Thigh—Rhus t.; *Thuya.*

CONCOMITANTS—Anxiety, exhaustion, hypochrondriacal ideas, mental confusion, vertigo, tension of stomach, no relief from warmth—Nux. v.

Anxiety, palpitation, nausea, canine hunger, pressing pain in hypogastrium,
congestive headache, distended painful veins—Chin. s.; Cinch.

Blue lips, nails—Eup. perf.; Eup. purp.; Menyanth.; Nat. m.; *Nux v.;*
Ver. a.

Cardiac region, pain in—Cact.; Tar. h.

Collapsic symptoms; skin icy cold; pallor, cold sweat on forehead—Ver. a.

Cough, dry, teasing—Rhus t.

Diarrhœa—Caps.; Elat.; Ver. a.

Face and hands bloated—Lyc.

Face red—Ferr. m.; Ign.; Nux v.

Forehead, cold sweat on—Ipec.; Ver. a.

Gastric symptoms—*Ant. c.;* Arg. n.; Ars.; Bolet.; Canchal.; Euo. perf.; *Ipec.;* Lyc.; *Nux v.;* Puls.

Hands, feel dead—Apis; Nux v.

Headache—Bolet.; Chin. s.; Cinch.; Conv.; *Eup. perf.;* Eup. purp.; Nat. m.; Nux v.

Headache, vertigo, yawning, stretching, general discomfort—Ars.

Heart symptoms, enterrhagia—Cact.

Hæmorrhoidal symptoms—Caps.

Hyperæsthesia—Ign.

Hyperæsthesia of spine—Chin. s.

Loquacity—Pod.

Nausea before chill—Ipec.

No two chills alike—Puls.

Pain in bones, limbs, soreness—Aran.; Bolet.; Canchal.; *Caps.;* Chin. s.; Cinch.; *Eup. perf.;* Eup. purp.; Formal.; *Gels.;* Nat. m.; Nux v.; Phell.

Pains, in joints—Cinch.

Pains, in knees, ankles, wrists, hypogastrium—Pod.

Restlessness—Ars.; Eup. perf.; Rhus t.

Sighing—Ign.

Thirst—*Apis; Ars.; Caps.;* Carbo v.; Cina; Cinch.; Conv.; Dulc.; *Eup. perf.; Ign.; Nat. m.;* Nux v.; Nyctanth.; Ver. a.; Wyeth.

Thirst, after chill—Ars.

Thirst, before chill—Chin. s.; Cinch.; *Eup. perf.;* Gels.; Menyanth.; Nyctanth.

Thirstlessness—Chin. s.; Cimex; Cinch.; *Eup. purp.;* Gels.; Nat. m.

Vehemence, rage, preceding—Cimex.

Vomiting, bilious—*Eup. perf.;* Ipec.; Lyc.; Nat. m.; Nux v.; Nyxtanth.

Yawning, somnolency, accelerated breathing—Nat. m.

Yawning, stretching—Ars.; Elat.; Lyc.; Nux v.

MODALITIES—Aggravated from acids: Lach.

Aggravated, from drink—Caps.

Aggravated, from exposure—Nux v.

Aggravated, from exposure, lying down—Cimex.

Aggravated, from motion—Apis.

Aggravated, from warmth—Apis; Canchal.; Chin. s.; Cinch.; Nux v.

Ameliorated from warmth—Caps.; Ign.

FEVER PAROXYSM—Afternoon, glowing heat, in face, hands, feet—Azadir.

Anxiety, restlessness, lipothymia, oppression—Ars.

Backache—Eup. perf.; Nat. m.

Chill, intermingled—Ars.; Chin. s.; Cinch.; Nux v.; Tar. h

Chilliness, after heat of face—Calc. c.

Congestion of head, drowsiness, costiveness, rectal and vesical tenesmus; chilled from uncovering—Nux v.

Delirium—Ars.; Pod.; Sabad.

Desire to be covered—Nux v.

Desire to be uncovered—Ign.; Ipec.

Diarrhœa—Ant. c.; Ipec.; Ver. a.

Dyspnœa—Apis; Ars.; Conv.; Ipec.

Face, hot, feet cold—Cinch.; Petrol.

Face pale, insomnia—Ant. t.

Gastric symptoms—Ars.; Eup. perf.; *Ipec.;* Nux v.; Puls.

Hands warm, face cold—Cina.

Headache—Apis; Ars.; *Bell.;* Ced.; Cinch.; Eup. perf.; *Nat. m.;* Nux v.; Wyeth.

Headache, yellowish tongue, nausea, faintness in epigastrium, costiveness—Polyp.

Heat, burning—Apis; *Ars.;* Caps.; *Eup. perf.;* Formal.; *Ipec.;* Lach.; *Nux v.*

Hunger—Cina; Cinch.

Hydroa—Hep.; *Nat. m.;* Rhus t.

Lachrymation—Sabad.

Loquacity—Pod.

Mental confusion—Formal.

Nettle rash—Apis; Ign.; Rhus t.

Night—Ars.

Pain, colicky—Cina.

Pain, in head, back, limbs—Nux v.

Pain in the vertebræ, dorsal—Chin. s.

Pain, spasms, paralysis—Ars.

Paroysms, frequent, transient—Carbo v.

Prolonged heat—Ars.; Bolet.; Ign.

Prostration, fainting, cold sweat—Ver. a.

Pupils, immobile, pain in abdomen, sopor, tension throughout body—Op.

Sighing—Ign.

Sleepiness—Ant. t.; Apis; Corn. fl.; Gels.; Op.

Thirst—*Ars.;* Chin. s.; Cinch.; *Eup. perf.;* Nat. m.; Nux v.; Nyxtanth.; Op.; Ver. a.

Thirstlessness—Apis; Caps.; Chin. s.; Cimex; Cinch.; *Ign.;* Nat. m.; Puls.; Sabad.; Wyeth.

Tongue clean—Ars.; Cina.

Trembling of limbs, slow pulse—Chin. s.; Op.

Unconsciousness—Nat. m.

Vomiting—Ars.; Cim.; Cina; Eup. perf.; *Ipec.;* Ver. a.

Sweat—Ant. c.; Aran.; Azadir.; Bolet.; Bry.; *Chin. s.;* Cimex.; Cina; *Cinch.;* Conv.; Eup. perf.; Lyc.; Nat. m.; Nux v.; Op.; *Phos. ac.;* Ver. a.; Wyeth. See Sweat.

Sweat scanty or absent—*Apis;* Ars.; Carbo v.; Eup. perf.; Nux v.

Sweat, with coldness—Plumb.

Sweat, with covering up—Cinch.; Hep.

Sweat, with relief of pains—Nat. m.

Sweat, with sleep—Cinch.; Con.; Pod.; Thuya.

Sweat, with thirst—Ars.; *Chin. s.;* Nux v.

APYREXIA—Adynamia, gastro-intestinal pains, sallow face, dropsical swellings, enlarged liver and spleen, restlessness, sleeplessness, spams, diarrhœa, albur inaria—Ars.

Adynamia hydræmia, chlorosis—Cinch.; Puls.

Adynamia, morning headache, depression, costiveness, amenorrhœa, enlarged liver, desire for quiet, sallow face—Nat. m.

Gastro-enteric symptoms—Cinch.; Hydr.; *Ipec.*; *Nux v.*; Puls.

Jaundice—Ars.; Bolet.; Card. m.; Nux v.; Pod.

Nervous symptoms—Gels.

Pains—Led.

Relapses from dietetic errors—Ipec.

Spleen enlarged—Ars.; *Ceanoth.*; Chin. s.; Cinch.; Ferr. m.; Nat. m.

Thirst—Ars.; Cimex; Ign.

Vomiting—Ipec.

Vomiting, abdominal griping, pain in back, loins—Ver. a.

LOW FEVERS—*Ail.*; *Arn.*; *Ars.*; Bapt.; Camph.; Cocc.; Crot.; Eup. ar.; *Lach.*; *Mur. ac.*; Nit. sp. d.; *Phos. ac.*; Phos.; Pyr.; *Rhus t.*; Tereb.; *Urt.* See Typhus.

MEDITERRANEAN FEVER—Bapt.; Bry.; *Colch.*; Merc. s.; Rhus t.

PUERPERAL FEVER—Acon.; Pyr.; Ver. a. See Female Sexual System.

REFLEX, from local irritation—*Cham.*; *Cina*; Gels.; Ign.; Ipec.; Merc.; Nux v.; Sang.; Sul.; Ver. v.

RELAPSING FEVER—*Acon.*; Ars.; *Bapt.*; *Bry.*; Cim.; *Eucal.*; Eup. perf.; Rhus t.

REMITTENT FEVER—Acon.; Ant. c.; *Ars.*; Bell.; Bry.; *Chin. s.*; *Cina*; Cinch.; Crot.; *Gels.*; Hyos.; *Ipec.*; Merc. s.; Nit. ac.; Nux v.; Nyctanth.; Puls.; Rhus t.; Sul.

Remittent, bilious, low—Bry.; *Crot.*; *Eup. perf.*; Gels.; Ipec.; Merc. d.; Nyctanth.; Pod.

Remittent, in children—Ant. c.; Cina; *Gels.*; Lept.; Puls.; Santon.

SEPTIC FEVER—Ail.; Anthrac.; *Ars.*; Crot.; Echin.; *Pyr.*; Ver. v. See Pyemia (Generalities).

SYNOCHAL FEVER—*Acon.*; Bapt.; Bell.

TRAUMATIC FEVER—Acon.; *Arn.*; Ars.; Cinch.; Lach. See Injuries (Generalities).

TYPHUS FEVER—Acet. ac.; Agar.; *Ail.*; Apis; *Ars.*; Arum; *Bapt.*; *Bell.*; Calc. c.; *Camph.*; Chin. s.; Cinch.; Crot.; Helleb.; *Hyos.*; Kreos.; *Lach.*; Merc. i. r.; Merc. s.; Merc. v.; Mur. ac.; Nit. ac.; *Op.*; *Phos. ac.*; Phos.; Pyr.; *Rhus t.*; Stram.; Ver. a.

Cellulitis, adenitis (salivary)—Bell.; Chin. s.; *Merc. i. r.*

Nervous symptoms—Agar.; *Bell.*; *Hyos.*; Lach.; Op.; Phos. ac.; Phos.; *Stram.*

Toxemia—*Ars.*; *Mur. ac.*; Pyr.; Rhus t. See Typhoid.

URETHRAL FEVER—*Acon.*; Ars.; *Chin. ars.*; Cinch.; *Gels.*; Hep.; Lach.; Phos.; Rhus t.; Sil.

WORM FEVER—Bell.; *Cina*; *Merc. s.*; Santon.; Sil.; Spig.; Stann.

YELLOW FEVER—*Acon.*; Ant. t.; Apis; *Arg. n.*; *Ars.*; Bell.; *Bry.*; *Cadm. s.*; Camph.; Canth.; Carb. ac.; *Carbo v.*; Chin. s.; Cinch.; Coff.; Crot. casc.; *Crot.*; Cupr.; Gels.; Guaco; *Hyos.*; Ipec.; *Lach.*; Merc.; Op.; *Phos.*; Plumb.; Sab.; Sul. ac.; Tereb.; Ver. a.

NERVOUS SYSTEM

BRAIN: EPILEPSY—(grand mal): *Absinth.;* Æth.; *Agar.;* Am. br.; Amyl; *Arg. n.; Art. v.;* Ars.; Aster.; Atrop.; Aur. br.; Avena; *Bell.;* Bor.; *Bufo;* Calc. ars.; *Calc. c.;* Calc. p.; Camph.; Can. ind.; *Caust.;* Cic. mac.; *Cic.;* Cim.; *Cocc.;* Con.; Cupr. ac.; *Cupr. m.; Ferr. cy.;* Ferr. p.; Gels.; Glon.; Hep.; *Hydroc. ac.; Hyos.; Ign.;* Illic.; Indigo; Irid.; *Kali br.;* Kali cy.; Kali m.; Kali p.; *Lach.;* Mag. c.; Mag. p.; Meli.; Methyl. bl.; Nit. ac.; *Nux v.; Ænanthe;* Op.; Œstrus; Passifl.; Phos.; Picrot.; Plumb. m.; Psor.; *Salam.;* Santon.; Sec.; *Sil.; Solan. c.;* Spiræa; *Stram.;* Strych.; *Sul.;* Sumb.; Tar. h.; Tub.; Val.; *Verb.;* Viscum; Zinc. cy.; Zinc. v.; *Ziʰia.*

CAUSE—CONCOMITANTS—Aura absent: Zinc. v.
  Aura absent; several fits, close together—Art. v.
  Aura begins, as painful spot, between shoulders, or dizziness, flashes of heat, from abdomen to head—Indigo.
  Aura begins, as sensation of mouse running up limb; heat from stomach; visual or aural disturbance—*Bell.;* Calc. c.; Sul.
  Aura begins, in brain, as a wavy sensation—Cim.
  Aura begins, in knees, ascends to hypogastrium—Cupr. m.
  Aura begins, in left arm—Sil.
  Aura begins, in solar plexus—Bufo; Calc. c.; Nux v.; Sil.
  Aura begins, in stomach or genitals—Bufo.
  Aura begins, in upper or lower limbs—Lyc.
  Aura descends—Calc. c.
  Aura felt, in heart region—Calc. ars.
  During full moon; nocturnal—Calc. c.
  During new moon; nocturnal—Caust.; Cupr. m.; Kali br.; Sil.
  During sleep—Bufo; Cupr.; Lach.; *Op.;* Sil.
  Followed by deep sleep—Æth.; Hyos.; Kali br.; Lach.; *Op.*
  Followed by hiccough—Cic.
  Followed by nausea, vomiting—Bell.
  Followed by prostration—Æth.; *Chin. ars.; Cic.;* Hydroc. ac.; Sec.; Sil.; *Strych.;* Sul.
  Followed by rage, automatic impulse—Op.
  Followed by restlessness—Cupr. m.
  Followed by tumor—Arg. n.; Cic.
  From eruptions, suppressed—Agar.; Calc. c.; Cupr. m.; Psor.; *Sul.*
  From fright, emotional causes—*Arg. n.;* Art. v.; Bufo; Calc. c.; Cham.; Hyos.; *Ign.;* Sil.; Stram.
  From hysteria—Asaf.; Cocc.; Cupr. m.; Hyos.; *Ign.;* Mosch.; Œnanthe; *Solan. c.;* Sumb.; Tar. h.; *Zinc. v.*
  From injury—Con.; Cupr. m.; Meli.; Nat. s.
  From jealousy—Lach.
  From menstrual disturbances—Arg. n.; Bufo; Caul.; Caust.; Ced.; *Cim.;* Cupr. m.; Kali br.; *Millef.;* Œnanthe; Puls.; Solan. c.
  From pregnancy—Œnanthe.

From scleroses; brain tumors—Plumb. m.
From sexual disturbances—Art. v.; *Bufo;* Calc. c.; Plat.; Stann.; Sul.
From syphilis, tubercular—Kali br.
From taking cold; nocturnal; worse right side—Caust.
From valvular disease—Calc. ars.
From vital drains; onanism—Lach.
From wet exposure—Cupr. m.
From worms—Cic.; Cina; Indigo; Sant.; Sil.; Stann.; Sul.; Teucr.
In children—Æth.; Art. v.; *Bell.;* Bufo; Calc. c.; Cham.; Cupr. m.; Ign.; Sil.; Sul.

Periodical seizures—Ars.; Cupr. m.
Preceded, by cold on left side of body—Sil.
Preceded, by dilated pupils—Arg. n.
Preceded, by gastric flatulency—*Arg. n.;* Nux v.; Psor.; Sul.
Preceded, by irritability, rambling—Bufo.
Preceded, by malaise—Cic.
Preceded, by memory, confused—Lach.
Preceded, by palpitation, vertigo—Lach.
Preceded, by sudden cry—Cupr. m.; Hydroc. ac.
Preceded, by tremblings, twitchings—Absinth.; Aster.
Preceded, by vesicular eruption—Cic.
Recent cases—*Bell.;* Caust.; Cupr. m.; *Hydroc. ac.; Ign.;* Op.; Plumb. m.; Stram.

Recurrent, several times daily—Art. v.; Cic.
Status epilepticus—*Acon.;* Æth.; *Bell.;* Cocc.; Œnanthe; Plumb.; Zinc. m.
With consciousness—Ign.
With face red, thumbs clenched, jaws locked, foam at mouth, eyes turned downwards, pupils fixed, dilated, pulse small, quick, hard—Æth.
With paralysis following—*Caust.;* Plumb. m.; Sec.
With swelling of stomach, screaming, unconsciousness, trismus, distorted limbs; frequent during night; recurrent tendency—Cic.
With vertigo (epileptic)—Arg. n.; Bell.; Calc. c.; Caust.; Cocc.; Cupr.; Hydroc. ac.; Nit. ac.; Op.; Sil.; Stram.

PARALYSIS—Remedies in general: Absinth.; *Acon.;* Agar.; Alum.; Angust.; Aragal.; Arg. iod.; *Arg. n.;* Ars. iod.; Asaf.; Astrag.; Aur.; Bar. ac.; Bar. c.; *Bar. m.; Bell.;* Calc. caust.; Calend.; *Can. ind.;* Carbon. oxy.; Carbon. s.; *Caust.;* Chin. s.; Cic.; *Cocc.;* Colch.; *Con.; Cupr. m.; Dulc.; Gels.;* Graph.; Grind.; *Guaco;* Helod.; Hydroc. ac.; Hyos.; *Hyper.;* Ign.; Iris fl.; Kali br.; *Kali c.;* Kali iod.; Kali p.; Lach.; Latrod. has.; Lol. tem.; Merc. c.; Nat. m.; Nux v.; *Oleand.;* Op.; Ox. ac.; Oxytr.; *Phos.;* Physal.; *Physost.;* Picr. ac.; Plat.; Plectranth.; *Plumb. ac.; Plumb. iod.; Plumb. m.; Rhus t.;* Stann.; Staph.; Sec.; Strych. ferr. cit.; Sul.; Tab.; *Thall.;* Ver. a.; Xanth.; Zinc. m.; Zinc. p.

TYPE—Agitans:—*Agar.;* Ars.; Aur. sul.; Avena; Bufo; Camph. monobr.; Can. ind.; Cocaine; Cocc.; *Con.; Dub.;* Gels.; Helod.; *Hyos.;* Hyosc. hydrobr.; Kali br.; Lathyr.; Lolium; Mag. p.; Mang. ac.; Merc. s.; *Merc.;* Nicotine; Phos.; Physos.; *Plumb.;* Scutel.; Tab.; Tar. h.; Zinc cy.; *Zinc. picr.*

Ascending spinal—Alum.; Bar. ac.; *Con.;* Gels.; Lathyr.; Led.; *Ox. ac.; Phos.;* Picr. ac.; Sec. See Spine.

Bulbar—Guaco; Mang. ox.; Plumb. m.

General of insane—Ant. c.; Ars.; Aur.; Bell.; *Can. ind.;* Caust.; Hyos.; Kali br.; Kali iod.; Merc. c.; Nat. iod.; Nux v.; Op.; *Phos.;* Physost.; Plumb.; Stram.; Sul.; Ver. a.

Gradually appearing—Caust.

HEMIPLEGIA—Ambra; *Arn.;* Ars.; *Aur. m.;* Bapt.; *Bar. c.; Bothrops;* Carbon. s.; *Caust.;* Chenop.; *Cocc.;* Cur.; Elaps; Hydroc. ac.; Irid.; *Lach.; Nux v.; Oleand.;* Phos.; Physost.; Picr. ac.; *Rhus t.; Sec.;* Stann.; Strych.; Ver. v.; Vipera; Xanth.

Hemiplegia, left—Ambra; *Arn.;* Bapt.; Bell.; Cocc.; Cupr. ars.; *Lach.;* Lyc.; Physost.; Ver. v.; Xanth.

Hemiplegia, right—Bell.; *Caust.;* Chenop.; Cur.; Elaps; Irid.

Hysterical—Acon.; Arg. n.; Asaf.; Cocc.; *Ign.;* Phos.; *Tar. h.*

Infantile (poliomyelitis anterior)—*Acon.;* Æth.; Bell.; *Calc. c.; Caust.;* Chrom. s.; *Gels.;* Lathyrus; Nux v.; Phos.; *Plumb. m.;* Rhus t.; Sec.; Sul. See Spine.

Labio-glosso-pharyngeal—Anac.; Bar. c.; *Bell.;* Caust.; Cocc.; Con.; Gels.; Mang. binox.; Nux v.; Oleand.; *Plumb.*

Landry's paralysis—Aconitin.; Con.; Lyssin.

Lead—*Alumen;* Caust.; Cupr.; Kali iod.; Nux v.; Op.; Plumb.; Sul. ac.

LOCALIZED, in ankles, in afternoon—Cham.

Localized, in arms, hands—Cupr. m.; Thyr.

Localized, in bladder—Caust.; Nux v.

Localized, in chest—Gels.

Localized, in eye muscles—Caust.; Con.; *Gels.;* Phos.; Physost.; Rhus t.

Localized, in face (Bell's palsy)—Acon.; *Am. phos.;* Bar. c.; Bell.; Caust.; Cur.; Gels.; Graph.; *Kali chlor.;* Nat. m.; Rhus t.; Solan. ves.; *Zinc. picr.*

Localized, in feet at night—Cham.

Localized, in forearm (wrist drop)—Cur.; Ferr. ac.; Plumb. ac.; Plumb. m.; Ruta; Sil.

Localized, in motor nerves—Cur.; Cystisin; *Gels.; Ox. ac.; Phos.; Physost.;* Xanth.

Localized, in neck—Cocc.

Localized, in sensory nerves—*Cocaine;* Laburn.; Plat.

Localized, in sphincters—Ars.; *Caust.;* Gels.; Naja; Nux v.; Phos.; Physost.

Localized, in throat, vocal cords—Bell.; Bothrops; Canth.; *Caust.;* Cocaine; Cocc.; *Gels.;* Kali p.; Ox. ac.; Plumb.

PARAPLEGIA—Acon.; Alum.; Anhal.; *Arg. n.;* Arn.; Ars.; *Bell.;* Caul.; *Caust.; Cocc.;* Con.; *Cupr. m.;* Cur.; Dulc.; Formica; *Gels.; Hyper.;* Kali iod.; *Kali tart.;* Kal.; Lach.; *Lathyr.;* Latrod. has.; Mang. ac.; Merc. c.; *Nux v.; Ox. ac.;* Phos.; Physost.; Picr. ac.; *Plumb. ac.; Rhus t.; Sec.;* Strych.; *Thall.;* Thyr.

Paraplegia, hysterical—*Cocc.;* Con.; Cupr.; *Ign.;* Nux v.; Plumb.; *Tar. h.*

Paraplegia, spastic—Gels.; Hyper.; *Lathyr.;* Nux v.; **Plectranth.; Sec.** See Sclerosis (Spine).

POST-DIPHTHERITIC—*Arg. n.;* Aur. mur.; Avena; Botul.; *Caust.; Cocc.;* Con.; *Diph.; Gels.;* Kali iod.; *Lach.;* Nat. m.; Nux v.; Phos.; Phyt.; Plumb. ac.; Plumb. m.; Rhod.; Rhus t.; Sec.

Pseudo-hypertrophic—Cur.; *Phos.;* Thyr.

Rheumatic—*Caust.;* Dulc.; Lathyr.; Phos.; *Rhus t.;* Sul.

Spinal origin—Alum.; Bell.; Can. ind.; *Con.;* Irid.; *Lathyr.; Phos.;* Physost.; *Picr. ac.;* Plumb.; Xanth.

PETIT MAL—*Art. v.;* Bell.; Caust.; Phos.; *Zinc. cy.*

SLEEP—DROWSINESS: Æth.; Am. c.; Ant. c.; *Ant. t.; Apis;* Apoc.; Arn.; Aur.; *Aur. mur.;* Bapt.; Bar. mur.; Can. ind.; *Carbon. ox.;* Carbon. s.; Caust.; *Cinch.; Clem.;* Coca; Cocc.; Cornus fl.; *Cycl.;* Dub.; Ferr. p.; *Gels.; Helleb.;* Helon.; Hydroc. ac.; Hyper.; *Indol;* Kali br.; Kali c.; Laburn.; Lathyrus; Linar.; Lob. purp.; *Lupul.; Morph.;* Naja; *Nux m.; Op.;* Phos. ac.; Phos.; Pyr.; Rhus t.; Rosmar.; Sarcol. ac.; *Scrophul.;* Selen.; Senec.; Sulphon.; Thea; Zinc. m.

Drowsiness, after meals—Bism.; *Cinch.;* Graph.; Kali c.; *Lyc.;* Nux m.; Nux v.; Paul.; *Phos.;* Puls.; Scrophul. See Indigestion (Stomach).

Drowsiness, during day—*Agar.;* Alum.; *Am. c.;* Anac.; *Ant. c.; Calc. c.;* Calc. p.; Can. s.; Carbo v.; *Cinch.;* Cinnab.; *Colch.;* Euphras.; Graph.; Indol; Kali c.; Lupul.; *Lyc.;* Mag. m.; Merc. c.; Merc.; *Nat. c.;* Nat. m.; Nux m.; *Op.; Phos.; Sep.;* Sil.; Spong.; Staph.; *Sul.;* Tub.

Drowsiness, during day, wakeful at P. M.—*Abies n.;* Cinnab.; Colch.; Graph.; Lach.; *Lyc.;* Merc.; Phos. ac.; Sil.; Staph.; Thea. See Insomnia.

Drowsiness, in A. M. and forenoon—Alum.; Anac.; *Am. c.;* Bism.; Carbo v.; Nat. m.; *Nux v.;* Petrol.; Zinc. m.

Drowsiness, in early evening—Calc. c.; Mang. ac.; *Nux v.;* Phos.; Puls.; Sep.; *Sul.*

Drowsiness, in evening, while sitting reading—Nux v.

Drowsiness, yet cannot sleep—Ambra; *Apis; Bell.;* Can. ind.; Caust.; *Cham.;* Coca; Coff.; Cupr. m.; Ferr. m.; *Gels.;* Lach.; Morph.; *Op.;* Sil.; Stram.

INCUBUS (nightmare)—Acon.; Am. c.; Arn.; *Aur. br.;* Bapt.; *Can. ind.;* Chloral; *Cina;* Cyprip.; Daphne; *Kali br.;* Kali p.; Op.; *Nux v.;* Nit. ac.; Pæonia; Pariet.; Phos.; Ptel.; Scutel.; Solan. n.; Sul.

INSOMNIA (sleeplessness)—Remedies in general: Absinth.; Acon.; Agar.; Alfal.; Alum.; Ambra; Am. c.; *Anac.;* Ant. c.; Apis; Apomorph.; Aquil.; Arn.; Arg. n.; *Ars.;* Aur.; *Avena;* Bept.; *Bell.;* But. ac.; Cact.; Caffeine; *Calc. c.; Camph.; Camph. monobr.; Can. ind.;* Caul.; *Cham.;* Chin. s.; Chloral; Chrysanth.; *Cim.; Cinch.;* Coca; *Cocaine; Cocc.; Coff.;* Col.; *Cyprip.;* Daphne; Dipod.; *Gels.; Hyos.; Hyosc. hydrobr.; Ign.;* Iod.; *Kali br.;* Kali p.; Lecith.; Lil. t.; *Lupul.;* Lyssin; Mag. p.; Merc.; *Nux v.; Op.; Passifl.;* Phos.; Picr. ac.; *Puls.;* Selen.; *Scutel.;* Stann.; Staph.; Sulphon.; *Sul.; Sumb.;* Stram.; Tela ar.; Thea; Val.; Xanth.; Yohimb.; Zinc. p.; Zinc. v.

CAUSES—OCCURRENCE—Abdominal disturbances:—Ant. t.; Cupr. **m.**

Aching in bones—Daphne.

Aching in legs, yet cannot keep them still—Med.

Aching in muscles, too much exhausted, tired out—Helon.

Alcoholic, drug, habits—Ars.; Avena; Can. ind.; *Cim.; Gels.; Hyos.; Nux v.;* Op.; Sec.; Stram.; *Sumb.*

Anxiety, driving him out of bed, aggravated after midnight—Ars.

Aortic disease—Crat.

Arterial pulsations—Acon.; *Bell.; Cact.; Glon.;* Sec.; Selen.; Sul.; **Thea.**

Banqueting, late suppers—Puls.

Bed feels too hard, cannot lie on it—Arn.; Bry.; *Pyr.*

Bed feels to hot, unable to lie on it—Op.

Chest oppression—Physal.

Chronic nicotinism—Plant.

Coffee, abuse—Cham.; *Nux v.*

Coldness of body—*Acon.;* Ambra; Camph.; *Carbo v.;* Cistus; *Ver. a.*

Coldness of knees—Apis; *Carbo v.*

Cramps—Argen. mex.; Col.; Cupr. m.

Delirium—Acon.; *Bell.*: Cact.; Calc. c.; *Can. ind.;* Gels.; *Hyos.;* Kali br.; Phos.; *Stram.;* Ver. a. See Mind.

Dentition—Bell.; Bor.; *Cham.;* Coff.; Cyprip. See Teeth.

Menopause; women with prolapsus uteri or uterine irritation—Senec.

Mouth and throat sore—Arum; Merc.

Multiple neuritis—Con.

Weaning of child—Bell.

DREAMS—Accidents, falling from height, etc.: Arn.; Bell.; Calc. c.; *Dig.;* Lyc.; Nit. ac.; Sil.; Ver. a.

Animals, snakes—Arg. n.; Daphne; Lac c.; Op.; Ran. sc.

Anxious—Abies n.; *Acon.;* Ambra; Anac.; *Apis; Arg. n.;* Arn.; *Ars.; Bell.; Bry.;* Calc. c.; Caust.; Can. ind.; Canth.; *Cham.;* Cinch.; Euphorb. dath.; Ferr. p.; Graph.; Ign.; Kali c.; Lyc.; Nat. m.; Nit. ac.; Nux v.; Oxytr.; Puls.; *Rhus t.;* Sec.; Sep.; *Sil.;* Staph.; *Sul.;* Zinc. m.

Business matters he forgets during day—Selen.

Confused—Alum.; Cinch.; Glon.; Helleb.; Hydroc. ac.; Phos.

Continues, after being apparently awake—Calc. c.; Cinch.; Nat. m.

Death, or dead persons—Arn.; *Ars.;* Calc. c.; Can. ind.; Crot. casc.; Crot.; Elaps; *Lach.;* Nit. ac.; Ran. sc.

Dreamful—Alum.; Brom.; Con.; Hyos.; Ign.; Lyc.; Nit. ac.; Phos.; Sep.

Drinking—Ars.; Med.; Nat. m.; Phos.

Exertion of body, toil, business—Apis; Ars.; Bapt.; *Bry.;* Nat. m.; Nux v.; Phos.; Puls.; *Rhus t.;* Selen.; Staph.

Fantastic, pleasant—Op.

Fires, flames, lightning—Bell.; Euphras.; Lach.; Phos.

Flying through air—Apis; *Rhus gl.;* Sticta.

Forgotten matters—Selen.

Happy dreams—Sul.

Hæmorrhage—Phos.

Horrible—Adon. v.; *Arg. n.; Aur.;* Bapt.; *Bell.; Cact.;* Calc. c.; Can. ind.; Castor.; *Cham.; Cinch.; Colch.;* Eupion; Graph.; *Hyos.;* Kali br.; Kali c.; *Lil. t.;* Lyc.; *Merc. c.;* Nux v.; Op.; Phos.; Psor.; Puls.; Ran. sc.; *Rhus t.;* Sec.; Sep.; Stram.; *Sul.;* Thea; *Zinc. m.*

Images bewildering, figures—Bell.; Hyos.

Lascivious—Arg. n.; Ars.; *Can. ind.;* Canth.; *Cob.; Diosc.;* Ham.; *Hyos.;* Ign.; Nat. m.; Nit. ac.; Op.; Phos. ac.; *Phos.;* Sil.; *Staph.;* Thuya; Ustil.; Ver. v.   See Emissions (Male Sexual System).

Laughs, during—Alum.; Caust.; Hyos.; Lyc.

Robbers—Bell.; *Nat. m.;* Psor.; Ver. a.

Vivid—Agar.; *Arg. n.;* Brom.; *Can. ind.;* Cenchris; Cham.; Coff.; Daphne; Diosc.; Hydroc. ac.; *Hyos.;* Indol; Iod.; Mang. ac.; Nat. m.; Petrol.; Phos.; Puls.; Pyr.; *Sul.;* Tub.; Ver. v.   See Anxious.

Dry mouth—Apis; Calc. c.; Caust.; Lach.; *Nux m.; Paris;* Puls.; Tar. h.

Emotional causes (grief, worry, anxiety, over-excitement, nervousness)— Absinth.; *Acon.; Alfal.; Ambra;* Am. val.; Aur.; Bry.; *Can. ind.;* Cham.; Chin. ars.; Chloral; *Cim.;* Coca; *Coff.;* Col.; *Gels.; Hyos.;* Hyosc. hydrobr.; *Ign.; Kali br.;* Mosch.; Nat. m.; *Nux v.; Op.;* Passifl.; Phos. ac.; Plat.; Senec.; *Sep.; Stram.;* Sul.; Thea; Val.; Zinc. v.

Exhaustion, debility, over-exertion of mind or body—*Arn.; Ars.;* Avena; Can. ind.; Chin. s.; Chloral; *Cim.; Cinch.;* Coca; *Cocc.; Colch.;* Dipod.; *Gels.;* Hyos.; Kali br.; *Nux v.;* Passifl.; Piscidia; *Phos.*

Eyes, half open, during—Bell.; *Cham.;* Hyos.; Ipec.; *Op.;* Pod.; *Zinc. m.* See Eyes.

Every second night—Cinch.; Lach.

Fears suffering from mental and physical exhaustion on waking—Lach.; Syph.

Formication in calves and feet—Sul.

Grinding of teeth—*Bell.;* Cic.; *Cina;* Helleb.; Kali br.; *Pod.; Santon.;* Spig.; Zinc. m.

Heat in general—Acon.; Arn.; Bar. c.; *Bell.;* Bor.; Caust.; Cham.; *Hep.;* Kali br.; Mag. m.; Meph.; Op.; *Sanic.;* Sil.; *Sul.*

Hunger—*Abies n.;* Apium gr.; *Cina;* Ign.; Lyc.; *Psor.;* Sul.

Hyperacute senses—Asar.; *Bell.;* Calad.; Calc. br.; Cham.; Cocc.; *Coff.;* Ign.; Nux v.; *Op.;* Tar. h.; Val.; Zinc. v.

In aged—*Acon.;* Ars.; Op.; Passifl.; *Phos.*

In children—*Absinth.; Acon.;* Ars.; *Bell.;* Calc. br.; *Cham.; Cina; Cyprip.;* Hyos.; Kali br.; *Passifl.;* Phos.; Puls.; Sul.

Itching—Acon.; *Agar.;* Alum.; Psor.; Teucr.; Sul.; Val.

Itching of anus—*Aloe;* Alum.; Coff.; Ign.; *Indigo.*

Itching of scrotum—Urt.

Mental activity, flow of ideas—Acon.; Apium gr.; Apis; Bry.; Calc. c.; *Cinch.; Cocc.; Coff.;* Gels.; Hep.; *Hyos.;* Lyc.; Meph.; *Nux v.;* Puls.; Sep.; Ver. a.; Yohimb.

Moaning, whining, during—Ant. t.; Arn.; Ars.; Aur.; *Bapt.; Bell.;* Carbo v.; *Cham.;* Cic.; Cupr. ac.; *Gels.; Helleb.;* Hyos.; Kali br.; Lach.; Lyc.; *Mur. ac.;* Nat. m.; Nit. ac.; *Op.; Pod.;* Puls.; Rhus t.; Ver. a.

Mouth, open—Merc.; Rhus t.; Samb.

Nose stopped up must breathe per orem—Am. c.; Lyc.; Nux v.; Samb.

Pains—Ars.; Can. ind.; *Cham.;* Col.; Mag. m.; Merc.; Passifl.; Puls.; Sinap. n.

Palpitation—Acon.; Alum.; Am. c.; *Cact.; Icd.;* Lil. t.; Lycop.; Rhus t.; Sep.

Picks at bed clothes, during—Op.

POSITION—Must lie in knee-chest position: Med.

Must lie on back—Am. c.; *Ars.;* Cina.

Must lie on back with thighs drawn upon abdomen, hands above head; disposition to uncover lower limbs—Plat.

Must lie on belly—Acet. ac.; Am. c.

Must lie on hands and knees—Cina.

Must lie with hands over head—Ars.; Nux v.; Plat.; Puls.; Sul.; Ver. a.

Must lie with hands under head—Acon.; Ars.; Bell.; Cinch.; Col.; Plat.

Must lie with legs apart—Cham.; Plat.

Must lie with legs crossed—Rhod.

Must lie with one leg drawn up, other stretched out—Stann.

Must move or fidget feet constantly—Zinc. m.

Must stretch violently for hours—Amyl; Plumb. m.

RESTLESSNESS, awakens frequently (catnaps)—Bar. c.; *Calc. c.;* Dig.; Ferr. m.; *Ign.;* Lyc.; Nit. ac.; Nux v.; *Phos.;* Plat.; Sarcol. ac.; *Selen.;* Sil.; Stram.; *Sul.*

Restlessness, during—*Acon.; Agar.;* Alum.; Ambra; Apis; Apoc.; Arg. n.; Arn.; *Ars.; Bapt.; Bell.;* Bry.; Calc. c.; *Can. ind.;* Castor.; Caust.; *Cham.;* Cina; *Cim.;* Cinch.; Coca; Cocaine; *Coff.;* Eup. perf.; Gels.; Glon.; Graph.; *Hyos.; Ign.; Jal.;* Kali br.; Lac d.; Lyc.; Menthol; Nit. ac.; Nux v.; Passifl.; Psor.; Ptel.; Puls.; Radium; *Rhus t.;* Ruta; Santon.; Sarcol. ac.; *Scutel.; Stram.;* Stront. c.; Sulphon.; *Sul.;* Tar. h.; Thea; Zinc. m.

Restlessness, kicks off clothes—Hep.; Op.; Sanic.; *Sul.*

Restlessness, rolling head—Apis; *Bell.;* Helleb.; *Pod.;* Zinc. m.

Sexual causes—Can. ind.; *Canth.; Kali br.; Raph.* See Sexual System.

Shocks, electric-like, on falling asleep—Ant. t.; *Cupr. m.;* Ign.; Ipec.

Shrieks, screams, awakens frightened—Ant. c.; Ant. t.; *Apis;* Aur.; *Bell.;* Bor.; *Bry.;* Cham.; *Cic.; Cina;* Cinch.; *Cupr. ac.;* Cyprip.; Dig.; *Helleb.; Hyos.;* Ign.; Iodof.; Kali br.; Lyc.; Nux m.; Phos.; Psor.; Puls.; Spong.; *Stram.;* Tub.; *Zinc. m.*

Singing, during—Bell.; Croc.; Phos. ac.

Singing on awakening—Sul.

Skin dry—Thea.

Sleepless, in evening, before midnight—*Ars.;* Lach.; *Lil. t.;* Nat. m.; Nux v.; Phos. ac.; Phos.; *Puls.; Rhus t.;* Selen.; Thuya.

Sleepless, after 2-3 A. M.—Apium gr.; Bapt.; Bellis; Bry.; *Calc. c.;* Cinch.; *Coff.;* Gels.; *Kali c.;* Kal.; Nat. c.; Nat. m.; Nit. ac.; *Nux v.; Selen.;* Sep.

Snoring, during—Cinch.; Laur.; *Op.;* Sil.; Stram.; Tub.; *Zinc. m.*

Soporous, deep, heavy sleep—Am. c.; Ant. c.; *Apis;* Arn.; Cinch.; *Cupr. m.; Helleb.;* Hyos.; Kali br.; Lact. v.; Laur.; Lonic.; Lupul.; *Morph.;* Naja; Nux m.; *Op.; Phos. ac.;* Piscidia; Pod.; Rhus t.; Sec.; *Stram.; Sul.*

Spasmodic symptoms, during (jerkings, twitchings, startings)—Acon.; *Æth.*; *Agar.*; Ambra; Ant. c.; *Apis;* Ars.; *Bell.;* Bor.; Brom.; Bry.; Calc. c.; Carbo v.; Castor.; Caust.; *Cham.; Cina;* Cinch.; *Cupr. ac.;* Daphne; Helleb.; *Hyos.; Ign.;* Kali c.; *Lyc.;* Morph.; Nit. ac.; Nux v.; Passifl.; Phos.; Samb.; Sil.; *Stram.; Sul.;* Tar. h.; Val.; *Zinc. m.;* Zizia.

Suddenly wide awake—Sul.

Suffocation, loss of breath, on falling asleep—*Am. c.;* Ars.; *Cur.;* Graph.; *Grind.;* Kali iod.; *Lach.;* Lac c.; *Merc. pr. rub.;* Morph.; Naja; Op.; Samb.; *Spong.;* Stront. c.; Sul.; Teucr.

Sweating, during—Æth.; *Calc. c.; Cham.; Cinch.;* Op.; Phos. ac.; Psor.; *Sil.;* Ver. a.   See Night Sweats (Fever).

Talking, during—Bar. c.; Bell.; Bry.; Carbo v.; *Cina;* **Graph.;** *Helleb.;* Hyos.; Kali c.; Lyc.; Sep.; Sil.; Sul.; *Zinc. m.*

Tea, abuse—Camph. monobr.; Cinch.; *Nux v.;* **Puls.**

Tobacco—Gels.

Unrefreshing, awakens wretched—Alum.; *Ant. c.;* Apium gr.; *Ars.;* Brom.; Bry.; *Cinch.;* Cob.; *Con.;* Dig.; Ferr. m.; Graph.; *Hep.; Lach.;* Lil. t.; *Lyc.;* Mag. c.; Merc. c.; Myr.; *Nux v.;* Op.; Phos.; Ptel.; *Puls.;* Rhus t.; Sarcol. ac.; Sep.; *Sul.;* Syph.; Thuya; Thymol; Tub.; Zinc. m.

Walking, during (somnambulism)—Art. v.; *Bry.; Kali br.;* Pæonia; *Sil.* See Mind.

Yawning, stretching, limbs—Acon.; *Agar.; Amyl;* Ant. t.; Arn.; Asar.; Calc. c.; Carls.; Castor.; Cepa; *Chel.; Cina;* Cinch.; Coca; Crot.; Cupr. ac.; Elat.; Euphras.; *Gels.;* Hep.; Hydroc. ac.; *Ign.;* Kali c.; Lyc.; Mang.; Morph.; *Nat. m.; Nux v.;* Plumb. m.; *Rhus t.;* Sec.; *Sil.; Sul.*

GENERALITIES—ADYNAMIA (general weakness, debility): Abies c.; *Acet. ac.;* Adren.; Æth.; *Ail.; Alet.;* Alston.; Ambra; Am. c.; *Anac.; Ant. t.; Antipyr.;* Apis; *Arg. n.;* Arn.; *Ars. iod.; A.·s.;* Asaf.; Aur.; Aur. mur.; *Avena; Bals. per.;* Bapt.; Bar. c.; Bellis; *Bry.; Calc. c.;* Calc. hypophos.; *Calc. p.;* Camph.; Can. s.; Canth.; *Carb. ac.; Carbo v.;* Caul.; *Caust.; Chin. ars.; Chin. s.; Cinch.;* Coca; *Cocc.; Colch.; Con.;* Crat.; Crot.; *Cupr. m.; Cur.; Dig.;* Dipod.; Diph.; Dulc.; *Echin.; Ferr. cit. et chin.; Ferr. m.;* Ferr. mur.; Ferr. p.; Ferr. picr.; *Gels.;* Helleb.; *Helon.;* Hep.; *Hydr.;* Hyos.; Ign.; *Iod.;* Ipec.; *Irid.;* Iris; Kali br.; *Kali c.;* Kali iod.; *Kali p.; Lac c.;* Lach.; Lact. ac.; Lil. t.; Lith. c.; Lith. chlor.; Lob. purp.; *Lyc.;* Mag. m.; Mag. p.; Meli.; Merc. c.; *Merc. cy.;* Merc. i. r.; Merc.; Murex; *Mur. ac.; Nat. c.; Nat. m.; Nat. sul.; Nit. ac.;* Nux v.; Op.; Ornithog.; Ox. ac.; *Phos. ac.; Phos.;* Physost.; Phyt.; *Picr. ac.;* Plumb. m.; *Psor.;* Rhus t.; *Ruta;* Sang.; *Sarcol. ac.;* Sec.; *Selen.;* Sep.; *Sil.;* Solid.; Spong.; *Stann.;* Stroph.; *Strych.;* Sulphon.; *Sul. ac.;* Sul.; *Tab.;* Tanac.; Tereb.; Thea; *Thuya;* Tub.; Uran. n.; Val.; *Ver. a.;* Zinc. ars.; Zinc. m.; *Zinc. p.; Zinc. picr.*

Adynamia, collapse—Acetan.; Acon.; *Ant. t.;* Arn.; Ars.; *Camph.;* Carb. ac.; *Carbo v.;* Colch.; Crat.; Crot.; Cupr. ac.; *Dig.;* Diph.; Hydroc. ac.; *Laur.;* Lob. infl.; Lob. purp.; Med.; Merc. cy.; *Morph.;* Mur. ac.; Nicot.; Op.; Pelias; Phos.; *Sec.;* Sul. ac.; *Tab.; Ver. a.;* Zinc. m.

Adynamia, afebrile—Ars.; Bapt.; Carbo v.; Cinch.

Adynamia, from acute diseases, mental strain—Abrot.; Alet.; *Alston.; Anac.;* Avena; *Calc. p.;* Carbo an.; *Carbo v.; Chin. ars.; Cinch.;* Coca; *Cocc.;* Colch.; Cupr. m.; Cur.; Dig.; Fluor. ac.; Gels.; *Helon.; Irid.;* Kali ferocy.; *Kali p.;* Lathyr.; Lob. purp.; Macroz.; Nat. sal.; Nux v.; *Phos. ac.; Phos.;* Picr. ac.; *Psor.;* Selen.; Sil.; Staph.; Strych. p.; Sul. ac.; Zinc. ars.

Adynamia, from anæsthetics; surgical shock—Acet. ac.; Hyper.

Adynamia, from depressing emotions—Calc. p.; Ign.; *Phos. ac.*

Adynamia, from diphtheria, stupor, cold limbs, low temperature, pulse rapid, weak—Diph.

Adynamia, from drugging—Carbo v.; Helon.; Nux v.

Adynamia, from excesses, vital drains—Agar.; *Anac.;* Calc. p.; *Carbo v.;* Caust.; Chin. s.; *Cinch.;* Corn. fl.; Cur.; Gins.; Kali c.; Nat. m.; *Phos. ac.; Phos.;* Selen.; Stroph.

Adynamia, from heat of summer—*Ant. c.; Gels.;* Lach.; *Nat. c.;* Selen.

Adynamia, from inebriety, bilious or remittent fevers—Eup. perf.

Adynamia, from injuries—*Acet. ac.; Arn.;* Calend.; Carbo an.; *Sul. ac.*

Adynamia, from jaundice—Ferr. picr.; Picr. ac.; Tarax.

Adynamia, from loss of sleep—*Cocc.;* Colch.; Nux v.

Adynamia, from menses; talking even fatigues—Alum.

Adynamia, from prolapsus, protracted illness, defective nutrition—Alet.; *Helon.*

Adynamia, from some deep-seated dyscrasia—Abrot.; Eup. perf.; Hydr.; Iod.; Nat. m.; Nit. ac.; *Psor.;* Sul. ac.; *Sul.;* Tub.; *Zinc. m.*

Adynamia, hysterical—Nat. m.

Adynamia, in aged—Bar. c.; Carbo v.; *Con.;* Cur.; Eup. perf.; Glycerin; Nit. ac.; Nux m.; *Phos.; Selen.*

Adynamia, nervous—Ambra; Anac.; Cur.; Gels.; Kali br.; *Phos. ac.; Phos.;* Rhus t.; Sil.; Staph.; Zinc. m.

Adynamia, with erethism—Ars.; Cinch.; Sil.

Adynamia, with frequent, faint spells during day—Murex; Nux m.; Sep.; *Sul.;* Zinc. m.

Adynamia, without erethism—Phos. ac.

Adynamia, without organic lesion or cause—Psor.

Adynamia, worse from ascending—Calc. c.; Iod.; Sarcol. ac.

Adynamia, worse from descending—Stann.

Adynamia, worse from exertion, walking—*Ars.;* Bry.; Calc. c.; Caust.; Cycl.; Ferr. m.; Lac d.; Merc. v.; Nat. c.; Nux m.; Phos. ac.; *Picr. ac.;* Sarcol. ac.; Sep.; Rhus d.; *Stann.;* Thea; Ver. a.

Adynamia, worse in A. M.—*Acal.;* Bar. m.; Bry.; Calc. c.; Con.; Corn. c.; Lac c.; Lach.; Lyc.; *Nat. m.; Nit. ac.;* Phos.; Psor.; Sep.; Stann.; Sul.; Tub.

Adynamia, worse in women worn ou. from hard mental and physical work, or, from indolence and luxury—Helon.

ALCOHOLISM—Acon.; *Agar.; Ant. t.; Apoc.;* Apomorph.; Ars.; *Asar.,* Aur.;. *Avena;* Bell.; Bism.; Calc. ars.; Calc. c.; Can. ind.; *Caps.;* Chimaph.; *Cim.; Cinch. rub.;* Cocc.; Crot.; *Cupr. ars.; Gels.;* Hydr.; *Hyos.;* Ichthy.; Kali iod.; Lach.; Led.; Lob. infl.; Lupul.; *Nux v.; Op.;* Phos.; Psor.; *Querc.; Ran. b.;* Stercul.; Stram.; Stroph.; *Strych.*

m.; Sul. ac.; Sul.; Syph.; Tub.; Zinc. m. See Chronic Gastritis (Stomach).

Alcoholism, hereditary tendency—Asar.; Psor.; Sul.; Sul. ac.; Syph.; Tub.

Alcoholism: to overcome habit—Angel.; Bufo; *Cinch. rub.; Querc.;* Stercul.; Sul. ac.; Sul.

ATHETOSES—Lathyr.; Strych.

BERI-BERI—*Elat.;* Lathyr.; Rhus t.

CHOREA (St. Vitus dance)—Absinth.; *Agar.; Agaricin; Arg. n.; Ars.;* Art. v.; Asaf.; Aster.; Avena; *Bell.;* Bufo; *Calc. c.;* Calc. p.; *Caust.;* Cham.; Chloral; Cic.; *Cim.; Cina;* Cocaine; *Cocc.;* Con.; Croc.; *Cupr. ac.;* Cupr. m.; Eup. ar.; Ferr. cy.; *Ferr. red.;* Hippom.; *Hyos.; Ign.; Iod.;* Kali br.; Latrod.; *Mag. p.; Myg.; Nat. m.; Nux v.; Op.;* Phos.; Physost.; Pictrox.; Psor.; Puls.; *Santon.; Scutel.;* Sep.; Solan.; *Spig.; Stram.; Strych.;* Strych. p.; Sulphon.; Sul.; *Sumb.;* Tanac.; *Tar. h.;* Thasp.; Thuya; *Ver. v.; Viscum;* Zinc. ars.; *Zinc. br.;* Zinc. cy.; *Zinc. m.;* Zinc. v.

CAUSE—OCCURRENCE—Anemia: Ars.; Cinch.; *Ferr. red.;* Hyos.

Corybantism—Bell.; Hyos.; Stram.

Eruptions, suppressed—Zinc. m.

Fright—Calc. c.; Cim.; Cupr.; *Ign.;* Laur.; Nat. m.; Stram.; Tar. h.; Zinc. m.

Nervous disturbances—*Asaf.;* Bell.; *Cim.; Cocc.;* Croc.; Gels.; Hyos.; *Ign.;* Kali br.; Op.; Sticta; Stram.

Onanism—Agar.; Calc. c.; Cinch.

Pubertic—Asaf.; Caul.; *Cim.;* Ign.; Puls.

Reflex, from dentition, pregnancy—Bell.

Relief, from music, sight of bright colors—Tar. h.

Relief, from sleep—*Agar.;* Cupr. m.

Rheumatism—Caust.; *Cim.;* Spig.

Rhythmical motions—Agar.; Caust.; Cham.; Cim.; Lyc.; *Tar. h.*

Scrofulous, tubercular—Calc. c.; *Calc. p.;* Caust.; *Iod.;* Phos.; Psor.

Worms—Asaf.; Calc. c.; *Cina;* Santon.; *Spig.*

Worse, at approach of thunder storm—*Agar.*

Worse, during sleep—Tar. h.; *Zizia.*

Worse, face—*Caust.;* Cic.; Cupr.; Hyos.; *Myg.;* Nat. m.; Zinc. m.

Worse, from cold, noise, light, emotions—Ign.

Worse, in spasms, partial, changing constantly—Stram.

Worse, left arm, right leg—Agar.; Cim.

Worse, right arm, left leg—Tar. h.

Worse, right side, tongue affected, staccato speech—Caust.

Worse unilaterally—Calc. c.

CONVULSIONS—Remedies in general: *Absinth.;* Acon.; *Æth.;* Agar.; Alum. sil.; Antipyr.; Arg. n.; Ars.; *Art. v.;* Atrop.; *Bell.; Camph.;* Can. ind.; Canth.; Carb. ac.; Castor.; *Cham.;* Chloroform; Cic. mac.; *Cic.;* Cim.; *Cina; Cocc.; Cupr. ac.; Cupr. ars.; Cupr. m.;* Dulc.; Euonym.; Gels.; *Glon.;* Helleb.; *Hydroc. ac.;* Hyper.; *Hyos.; Ign.;* Illic.; Iris fl.; *Kali br.; Laburn.;* Laur.; Lonic.; Lyssin; *Mag. p.;* Morph.; Nat. s.; Nux v.; *Œnanthe;* Op.; Ox. ac.; Passifl.; Phos.;

Physost.; Plat.; Plumb. chrom.; Plumb.; *Santon.; Sil.; Solan. c.;*
Solan. n.; *Stram.;* Strych.; Sul.; Upas art.; *Upas t.;* Ver. a.; Ver. v.;
Verbena; *Zinc. m.;* Zinc. oxy.; Zinc. s.

CAUSE AND TYPE—Anger affects mother's milk—Cham.; Nux v.

Apoplectic; in inebriates; hemorrhagic or broken down systems—Crot.

Carphopedal—Cupr. ac.; Ign.

Cataleptic—Cic.; *Mosch.*

Cerebral sclerosis or tumor—Plumb. m.

Children, infants, from reflex causes, dentition—Absinth.; Acon.; *Æth.;*
Art. v.; *Bell.;* Calc. c.; *Camph. monobr.;* Caust.; Cham.; Chloral; *Cic.;*
Cina; Cocc.; *Cupr. m.;* Cyprip.; Glon.; Helleb.; Hydroc. ac.; *Hyos.;*
Ign.; Kali br.; Kreos.; Laur.; *Mag. p.;* Meli.; Mosch.; Nux v.; *Œn-*
anthe; Op.; Santon.; Scutel.; Stann.; *Stram.; Zinc. m.;* Zinc. sul. See
Worms.

Clonic—Antipyr.; Apis; Bell.; Camph.; Carb. ac.; Cina; *Cupr. m.;*
Gels.; Hyos.; Ign.; *Nicot.;* Plumb. m.; Upas art.

Crying; approach of strangers—Op.

Exanthemata—Acon.; *Bell.;* Glon.; Thea; Ver. v.

Exanthemata, suppressed—Apis; Ars.; *Cupr. m.;* Op.; Stram.; *Zinc. m.;*
Zinc. s.

Foot sweat, suppressed—Sil.

Fright—Acon.; Cupr. m.; Hyos.; *Ign.;* Op.; Stram.

Fright, anger or emotional disturbance in nervous, plethoric persons—
Kali br.

Grief, or any emotional excitement—Ign.

Hypochondriacal—Mosch.; Stann.

Hysterical—Absinth.; Asaf.; Asar.; Castor.; Caul.; Cim.; Cocc.; *Gels.;*
Hydroc. ac.; *Hyos.; Ign.;* Kali p.; *Mosch.;* Nux m.; Plat.; Stann.;
Tar. h.

Injury—Cic.; Hyper.

Isolated groups of muscles—Acon.; *Cic.;* Cina; Cupr.; Ign.; Nux v.;
Stram.; Strych.

Labor—Acon.; Bell.; Cic.; Cupr. m.; Glon.; Hyos.; Ign.; Kali br.;
Œnanthe; Stram.; Ver. v. See Female Sexual System.

Meals followed by vomiting, shrieking, spasms—Hyos.

Menses suppressed—Gels.; Millef. See Female Sexual System.

Metastases, from other organs—Apis; Cupr.; Zinc. m.

Prodromata—Acon.; Bell.; Cham.; Ipec.; Op.

Reflected light from water, mirror—Bell.; Lyssin; *Stram.*

Sleep, loss of—Cocc.

Spinal origin—Acon.; *Cic.;* Cim.; Hydroc. ac.; *Hyper.;* Ign.; Nux v.;
Œnanthe; *Physost.*

Terminal stage—Op.; Plumb.; Zinc. m.

Tonic: Opisthotonos—Apis; *Cic.;* Cina; Cupr. ac.; Cupr. m.; *Hydroc.*
ac.; Ign.; Ipec.; Mag. p.; Mosch.; Nicot.; *Nux v.;* Physost.; Plat.;
Plumb. m.; Solan. c.; Solan. n.; Stram.; *Strych.; Upas;* Ver. v.

Uremic—*Carb. ac.;* Cic.; *Cupr. ars.;* Glon.; Helleb.; *Hydroc. ac.;* Kali
br.; Merc. c.; Œnanthe; *Op.;* Plumb.; Piloc.; Urt. See Urinary System.

Uterine disease—Cim.

Vaccination—Sil.; Thuya.

Whooping cough—Cupr. m.; Kali br.

Worms—Cic.; *Cina; Hyos.; Indigo;* Kali br.; Sabad.; *Santon.;* Spig.; Tanac.

CONCOMITANTS—Beginning in face; unilateral; shallow breathing—Cina.

Beginning in fingers, toes, radiates all over—Cupr. m.

Bladder, chest, intestines, striated muscles, cheifly involved; drowsiness, rigid limbs; sudden onset; head hot, feet cold—Bell.

Calves of legs; clenched thumbs; cyanosis—Cupr. m.

Chorea-like—Sticta.

Convulsive jerkings, of limbs and head—Bufo; Cham.; *Cic.;* Hyos.

Cyanosis—Cupr. ac.; Hydroc. ac.

Extremities cold—Bell.; Helleb.; Hydroc. ac.; *Nicot.;* Œnanthe.

Eyes half open, upturned; breathing, deep, stertorous—Op.

Eyes turned downward—Æth.

Fever; skin hot, dry; child frets, screams, gnaws its fists; twitching of single muscles—Acon.

Followed by collapse—Nicot.

Followed by deep sleep—Cupr. ac.; *Op.;* Zinc. m.

Followed by paresis—Acon.; *Elaps;* Lonic.; Plumb. m.

Followed by restlessness—Cupr. m.

No cerebral congestion—Ign.

No fever—Ign.; *Mag. p.; Zinc. m.*

Pale face; rolling eyes; gnashing teeth—Zinc. m.

Preceded, by gastro-intestinal symptoms—Æth.; Cupr. ars.

Preceded, by restlessness—Arg. n.; Hyos.

Shrieks, screams, before, and during—*Apis;* Cina; Cupr. m.; *Helleb.;* Op.

Terrible pains—Plumb. chrom.

Tremor, spasm of glottis, febrile paroxysm—Ign.

Twitchings, cramps, gastro-enteric symptoms—Nux v.

Twitchings of single muscles or groups, especially of upper body—Stram.

Twitchings over entire body—Cic.; Hyos.

Twitchings worse upper body, continue after delivery—·Cic.

Violent vomiting—Æth.; Upas.

With consciousness—Cina; Nux v.; Plat.; *Stram.; Strych.*

Without consciousness—Bell.; Calc. c.; *Cic.;* Cupr. ac.; Cupr. ars.; *Cupr. m.;* Glon.; Hydroc. ac.; *Hyos.; Mosch.;* Œnanthe; *Op.;* Stram.

Worse from touch, motion, noise—Cic.; Ign.; Lyssin; Nux v.; Stram.; Strych.

DEFICIENT REACTION—Ambra; Am. c.; Calc. c.; Camph.; Caps.; *Carbo v.;* Carbon. s.; Caust.; Cic.; Cupr. m.; Helleb.; Iod.; *Laur.;* Nat. ars.; Nat. s.; *Op.;* Psor.; Radium; *Sul.; Tub.;* Val.; X-ray.; *Zinc. m.*

EXOPHTHALMIC GOITRE (Basedow's disease)—Amyl; Antipyr.; Ars.; Ars. iod.; Aur.; *Bell.;* Brom.; *Cact.;* Calc. c.; Colch.; Ephedra; Ferr. iod.; *Ferr. m.;* Ferr. p.; Fucus; *Glon.; Iod.;* Lycop.; Nat. m.; *Piloc.;* Pineal gl. ext.; Spart. s.; Spong.; *Thyr.*

MAL-DE-MER (seasickness)—Amyl; *Apomorph.;* Aqua mar.; Arn.; Cereum ox.; Chloral; *Cocc.;* Cucurb.; Glon.; Kali br.; Kali p.; Morph.; Nicot.; *Nux v.; Petrol.; Staph.; Tab.;* Thea; *Ther.* See Vomiting (Stomach).

MORPHINISM—Apomorph.; *Avena;* Can. ind.; Cim.; Ipec.; Lob. infl.; *Macrot.;* Nat. p.; Passifl.

MORVAN'S DISEASE—Aur.; *Aur. mur.;* Bar. mur.; Lach.; *Sec.;* Sil.; Thuya.

NERVOUS AFFECTIONS—Of cigar makers: Gels.

Nervous affections of girls, at puberty—Caul.; *Cim.*

Nervous affections of onanists—*Gels.;* Kali p.

Nervous affections, from excessive delicacy and sensitiveness of the senses—Cupr.

Nervous affections, from suppressed discharges, in the psoric—Asaf.; Merc. s.

Nervous affections, from tobacco, in sedentary persons; dyspepsia, right prosopalgia—Sep.

Nervous affections, from worms—*Cina;* Psor.; Sabad.

NERVOUSNESS—In general: Abies n.; Absinth.; *Acon.;* Alfal.; *Ambra;* Amyl; *Anac.;* Aquil.; Arn.; Ars.; *Asaf.; Asar.;* Avena; *Camph. mon. obr.; Cham.; Cim.; Coca;* Cocaine; *Coff.;* Cupr.; Cyprip.; Eup. ar.; *Gels.;* Glycerin; Gossyp.; Hedeoma; *Hyos.; Ign.;* Indol; *Kali br.;* Kali c.; *Kali p.; Mag. p.;* Niccol.; Nux m.; *Nux v.;* Oophor.; Op.; *Phos.;* Puls.; Santon.; Senec.; Sil.; *Stram.; Strych.;* Thea; *Ther.; Triost.; Val.;* Val. am.; Xanth.; *Zinc. m.* See Moods (Mind).

Nervousness, hypersensitiveness—*Acon.;* Ambra; Am. val.; Angust.; Ant. c.; *Apis;* Aquil.; *Asaf.; Asar.;* Arn.; Atrop.; Aur.; *Bell.; Bor.;* Bry.; Calad.; Calc. sil.; Camph.; Can. ind.; Canth.; *Cham.;* Chin. mur.; Chrysanth.; *Cim.; Cinch.; Cocc.; Coff.; Colch.;* Con.; Cupr.; Ferr. m.; Glon.; *Hep.;* Hyper.; *Ign.;* Justicia; Kali br.; Kali c.; Kali p.; Lac c.; *Lach.;* Lyssin; Mag. p.; Med.; Morph.; Nit. ac.; Nux m.; *Nux v.;* Op.; *Phos.;* Phos. hydr.; Plat.; Puls.; Sep.; *Sil.;* Spig.; Stann.; *Staph.; Strych.; Sul.; Tar. h.;* Teucr.; *Ther.; Tub.;* Zinc. m.

Nervousness, hypersensitiveness, to cold air, drafts—Acetan.; *Acon.;* Agar.; Allium s.; Ambra; Am. c.; Anac.; Ant. c.; Bac.; Bad.; *Bar. c.;* Bell.; Bor.; *Calc. c.; Calc. sil.;* Calend.; Camph.; *Caps.;* Carbo v.; Caust.; Cham.; *Cinch.; Cistus;* Con.; Cupr. m.; *Graph.;* Ham.; *Hep.; Kali c.;* Kali m.; Mag. m.; *Merc.; Mez.;* Nat. c.; *Nat. m.;* Nit .ac.; Nit. sp. d.; *Nux v.;* Physost.; *Psor.;* Ran. b.; Rhus t.; *Rumex;* Selen.; Sep.; *Sil.;* Strych.; Sul.; *Tub.*

Nervousness, hypersensitive, to least pain—*Acon.;* Arn.; Aur. m.; Aur. mur.; Cact.; *Cham.; Cinch.; Coff.; Colch.;* Hep.; Hyper.; *Ign.;* Kali p.; Latrod.; Mag. p.; Med.; Meli.; Mez.; *Morph.;* Mosch.; Nit. ac.; Nux m.; *Nux v.;* Phos.; Ran. s.; Val.; Zinc. v.

Nervousness, tremulousness, faintness—Abies c.; Ant. t.; Aquil.; *Arg. n.;* Arn.; Ars.; Asar.; *Caul.; Caust.;* Cim.; *Cinch.;* Cocc.; *Gels.; Hyos.;* Lach.; Latrod.; *Med.; Mosch.;* Murex; Nux m.; *Nux v.;* Puls.; Raph.; Sep.; Strych.; Sul.; *Sul. ac.;* Tar. h.; Val.; *Zinc. m.*

NEURASTHENIA (nervous prostration)—Remedies in general: Agn.; Alfal.;

Anac.; Anhal.; *Arg. n.;* Asaf.; Asar.; *Avena; Calc. c.; Calc. p.;* Can. ind.; *Cinch.;* Cob.; Coca; *Cocc.;* Cupr. m.; Cur.; *Fluor. ac.; Gels.;* Glycerin; Graph.; *Helon.;* Hyper.; Ign.; *Kali hypoph.; Kali p.;* Lach.; Lathyrus; *Lecith.;* Lob. purp; Mosch.; *Nat. m.; Nux v.; Onosm.; Ox. ac.; Phos.;* Physost.; *Picr. ac.;* Pip. m.; Plumb.; Puls.; Sacchar. of.; Sarcol. ac.; *Scutel.; Sil.;* Stann.; Staph.; *Strych. p.;* Tar. h.; Tub.; Turnera; Verbena; Xanth.; *Zinc. m.; Zinc. p.; Zino. picr.* See Adynamia.

Cerebral symptoms, unable to apply mind—*Anac.;* Aur.; Calc. c.; *Gels.; Kali p.;* Nux v.; *Phos. ac.;* Phos.; *Picr. ac.;* Sil.; Scutel. See Brain Fag (Mind).

From long, concentrated grief—Ign.

Gastric form—*Anac.;* Gent.; Nux v.; Strych. p.

Hypochondriacal tendency—*Aur.;* Coca; Con.; Kali br.; Nat. m.; Sul.

In females—Alet.; Aloe; Ambra; Ars.; Aur.; Bellis; Calc. c.; Cinch.; *Cocc.; Epiph.;* Ferr.; *Helon.;* Hyos.; *Ign.;* Iod.; Kali p.; *Lach.;* Lyc.; *Mag. c.;* Mag. p.; Phos. ac.; *Picr. ac.;* Puls.; *Sep.;* Sil.; Sul.; Zinc. v.

Insomnia—Ambra; Ars.; Aur.; *Cim.;* Coff.; Nux v.; Zinc. p. See Sleep.

Sexual origin—Agar.; *Agn.; Anac.;* Calad.; *Cinch.;* Coca; Gels.; *Graph.* Lecith.; Lyc.; Nat. m.; Nux v.; Onosm.; *Phos. ac.; Phos.; Picr. ac.;* Plat.; *Sabal;* Selen.; Sep.; *Staph.;* Thymol; Turnera; Zinc. picr. See Female Sexual System.

NEUROSES—Of children: Passifl.

Neuroses of professional men—Gels.

TREMORS—Twitchings, trembling: *Absinth.; Agar.;* Agaricin; Anac.; *Ant. t.;* Apis; *Arg. n.;* Ars.; Bell.; Camph.; Can. ind.; *Caust.;* Cham.; Cic.; *Cim.;* Cinch.; *Cocc.;* Cod.; Ferr. p.; *Gels.;* Hep.; *Hyos.; Hyosc. hydrobr.; Ign.;* Iod.; Kali br.; Kali p.; *Lach.;* Latrod.; Lith. chlor.; Lyc.; *Med.; Merc. s.;* Morph.; Mosch.; Nat. m.; *Nux v.;* Op.; Oxytr.; *Phos. ac.; Phos.;* Physost.; Plumb.; Rhus t.; Sabad.; Scutel.; Sil.; *Stram.;* Sul.; Tar. h.; Tub.; Val.; Veratrin; Ver. v.; Viscum alb.; *Zinc. m.;* Zinc. p.

Alcoholic—*Ant. t.;* Cocaine; Cocc.; *Nux v.*

Disseminated sclerosis—Acet. ac.; Ars.; *Hyos. hydrobr.*

From smoking—Kali c.; Nit. ac.; Sep.

Senile—Avena; Can. ind.; Cocaine; *Phos.*

NERVES: NEURITIS (Inflammation)—*Acon.; Æsc.;* Ananth.; Arg. n.; *Arn.; Ars.; Bell.;* Bellis; Benzin. din.; Berb. v.; *Carbon. s.;* Caust.; *Ced.; Cepa;* Cim.; Con.; Ferr. p.; *Gels.; Hyper.;* Merc.; Nux v.; Pareira; Phos. ac.; Phos.; *Plumb.;* Plumb. phos.; Rhus t.; Sang.; *Stann.;* Stront. c.; Strych.; *Thall.;* Urt.; Zinc. p.

TYPE—Alcoholic: Nux v.; Strych.

Diphtheritic—Gels.

Of anterior crural—Pareira.

Of circumflex—Sang.

Of lesser sciatic—Æsc.

Of lumbo-sacral plexus—Berb. v.

Of upper dorsal roots—Ananth.

Injuries of nerves—Bellis; Cepa; *Hyper.;* Phos. ac.

Multiple—Bov.; Con.; Morph.; Thallium.

Retro-bulbar, with sudden loss of sight—Chin. s.

Traumatic—Arn.; Calend.; *Cepa; Hyper.*

NEURALGIA—Remedies in general: Acetan.; *Aconitin; Acon.;* Agar.; Am picr.; Am. val.; Amyl; Aran.; *Arg. n.; Arn.; Ars.;* Atrop.; *Bell.;* *Bry.;* Cajup.; *Can. ind.;* Caust.; Cepa; *Cham.; Chel.; Chin. ars.;* *Chin. s.;* Ced.; *Cim.; Cinch.; Coff.; Col.;* Commocl.; Con.; Cornu; fl.; Diosc.; *Gels.;* Glon.; *Gnaph.;* Hyper.; *Ign.;* Ipec.; Kali ars.; *Kali bich.;* Kali ferrocy.; Kali iod.; *Kal.;* Lach.; Mag. c.; *Mag. p.;* Menyanth.; *Mez.; Morph.;* Nat. m.; Niccol. s.; Nux v.; Onosm.; Ox. ac.- Paris; *Phos.; Phyt.;* Plant.; Plat.; Prun. sp.; *Puls.;* Ran. b.; *Rhod.;* Sil.; *Spig.; Stann.;* Staph.; *Sul.;* Sumb.; Thea; Ther.; Thuya; Tub.; Val.; *Ver. a.; Verbasc.;* Xanth.; Zinc. p.; *Zinc. v.*

CAUSE—TYPE—Anemia: *Ars.;* Cinch.; *Ferr.;* Kali ferrocy.; Puls.

Chronic cases, or later life—*Arn.;* Kreos.; *Phos.;* Sul.; Thuya.

Climacteric—Lach.

Gout, rheumatism—Cim.; *Colch.;* Col.; Kal.; Phyt.; Ran. b.; *Rhod.;* Rhus t.; Sul.

Idiopathic cases—Acon.; Ars.

Influenza, debility—Ars.

Malaria—Aran.; *Ars.;* Ced.; *Chin. s.;* Cinch.; Menyanth.; Nat. m.; *Niccol. s.;* Stann.; Sul.

Recent origin, occurring in young—*Acon.; Bell.;* Col.; *Gels.;* Kal.; Spig.

Syphilis—*Kali iod.;* Mez.; Phyt.

Traumatic, in amputated limbs—Am. m.; Arn.; *Cepa; Hyper.;* Kal.; *Phos. ac.;* Symphyt.

Zoster, after—*Mez.;* Morph.

LOCATION—Brachial plexus, cervico-brachial: *Acon.r.; Bry.;* Cepa; Cham.; Coccus; Corn. fl.; Hyper.; *Kal.; Merc.; Nux v.;* Paris; *Rhus t.; Sul.;* Tereb.; *Ver. a.*

Cervico-occipital—Bell.; Bry.; Chin. s.; Cinch.; Nux v.; Puls.; Zinc. p.

Ciliary—*Cim.;* Gels.; Mez.; Nat. m.; *Spig.* See Ciliary Neuralgia (Eye).

Crural anterior—Am. m.; Coff.; *Col.;* Gels.; *Gnaph.; Limul.;* Nat. ars.; Œnanthe; Solan. lyc.; Spig.; *Staph.;* Sul.; *Xanth.*

Infra-orbital—*Arg. n.;* Bell.; Mag. p.; Mez.; Nux v.; Phos. See Trifacial.

Intercostal—Acon.; Aran.; *Arn.; Ars.;* Ars. iod.; *Asclep. t.;* Aster.; Bell.; Brom.; *Bry.; Chel.; Cim.;* Gaulth.; Mag. p.; Menthol; *Mez.;* Morph.; Nux v.; Paris; Phos.; Puls.; *Ran. b.;* Rhod.; Samb.; Zinc. m.

Lumbo-abdominal—Aran.; Bell.; Clem.; Col.; Cupr. ars.; Ham.; Mag. p.; Nux v.

Phrenic—Bell.

SCIATICA—Acetan.; *Acon.; Am. m.;* Apoc.; Arn.; *Ars.;* Ars. met.; Ars. s. r.; *Bell.;* Bry.; Caps.; Carbon. oxy.; Carbon. s.; *Cham.;* Cinch.; *Col.;* Cotyled.; Diosc.; Gaulth.; Gels.; *Gins.; Gnaph.;* Hymosa; Hyper.; *Ign.; Indigo; Iris;* Kali c.; *Kali iod.;* Kali p.; Lac c.; Lyc.; Mag. p.; Nat. s.; Nyctanth.; Nux v.: Pall.; *Phyt.; Plumb.;* Polyg.; Ran. b

Rhus t.; Ruta; Sal. ac.; Sep.; Staph.; Strych.; *Sul.;* Sul. rub.; Syph.; Tellur.; Tereb.; Theine; Thuya; Val. ; Ver. a.; *Viscum;* Xanth.; Zinc. v.

Sciatica, acute cases—*Acon.;* Bry.; Cham.; *Col.;* Ign.

Sciatica, chronic cases—*Ars.;* Calc. c.; Kali iod.; Lyc.; Phos.; *Plumb.;* Ran. b.; *Rhus t.;* Sul.; Zinc. m.

Sciatica. in summer, croupy cough in winter—Staph.

Sciatica, rheumatic—Acon.; Bry.; *Cim.;* Guaiac.; Hymosa; Led.; *Rhus t.*

Sciatica, syphilitic— *Kali iod.;* Merc. c.; Phyt.

Sciatica, uterine—Bell.; Ferr.; Graph.; Merc.; *Puls.;* Sep.; Sul.

Sciatica, vertebral origin—Lac c.; Nat. m.; Phos.; Sil.; Sul.; Tellur.

Spermatic cord—*Clem.;* Col.· Ham.; *Ol. an.;* Ox. ac.; Rhod.; Spong. See Male Sexual System.

Spine—Paris. See Spine.

Sub-orbital—Caust.; Colch.; Con.; Kali c.; Phos. See Trifacial.

Supra-orbital—Arg. n.; Asaf.; *Ced.;* Chel.; *Chin. s.;* Cim.; *Kali bich.;* Mag. p.; Morph.; *Nux v.;* Ran. b.; *Spig.;* Stann.; Theine; Tongo; Viola od. See Prosopalgia (Face).

Teeth—Kreos.; Merc.; Mez.; Plant.; Staph.; Verbasc. See Odontalgia (Teeth).

Trifacial—*Acon.;* Amyl; *Aran.;* *Arg. n.;* *Ars.;* Arundo; *Bell.;* Cact.; Ced.; Cepa; *Cham.;* *Chel.;* *Cim.;* Cinch.; Colch.; Col.; Ferr.; *Gels.;* Glon.; *Kal.;* Mag. p.; Merc.; *Mez.;* Nat. s.; *Nux v.;* Phos.; Puls.; Rhus t.; Sabal; Sang.; *Spig.;* Stann.; Thuya; Tongo; Ver. a.; *Verbasc.;* Zinc. m.; *Zinc. v.* See Prosopalgia (Face).

Ulnar—Hyper.; Kal.; Lycopers.; Oxytr.; Rhus t.

TYPE OF PAIN—**Bruised:** Apis; Arn.; Bellis; Corn. fl.; Phyt.; Ruta.

Burning—Acon.; Anthrac.; Apis; *Ars.;* Caps.; Cepa; Sal. ac.; Spig.

Cramp-like, constrictive—Am. m.; *Cact.;* Caul.; Cim.; *Col.;* Con.; Cupr. m.; Gnaph.; Iris; *Mag. p.;* Nux v.; *Plat.;* Plumb.; Stann.; Sul.; Thuya; *Verbasc.*

Drawing—*Cham.;* Cinch.; Col.; Phos. ac.; Phos.; *Puls.;* Spig.; *Stann.;* Sul.; Verbasc. See Tearing.

Intermittent—*Ars.;* Chin. s.; *Cinch.;* *Col.;* Cupr. m.; *Ign.;* Mag. p.; Nux v.; *Spig.;* Sul. See Periodical.

Lancinating, electric shock like—Acon.; *Bell.;* Cact.; Caust.; Cim.; Col.; Daphne; Gels.; Mag. c.; *Mag. p.;* *Nux v.;* Phyt.; Plumb.; *Strych.;* Sul. ac.; Ver. a.; *Verbasc.;* Xanth.; Zinc. p.

Localized, in spots—Ign.; Kali bich.; Lil. t.; Ox. ac.

Onset gradual, cessation gradual—Arg. n.; Plat.; *Stann.;* Sul.; Ver. a.

Onset sudden, cessation sudden—*Bell.;* Carb. ac.; Chrom. ac.; Col.; Kali bich.; *Mag. p.;* Ovig. p.; Oxytr.

Periodical—*Aran.;* Ars.; *Ced.;* Chin. s.; Chrom. ac.; Kali bich.; *Niccol. s.;* Nux v.; Ox. ac.; Parth.; Sal. ac.; *Spig.;* Sul.; Toxicophis; *Verbasc.*

Plug-like—Anac.

Severe, drives him frantic—*Acon.;* Arg. n.; Ars.; *Bell.;* *Cham.;* Carb. ac.; Cinch.; Coff.; Colch.; *Col.;* Kreos.; *Mag. p.;* Morph.; Nux v.; Ox. ac.; *Spig.;* Ver. a.

Splinter-like—Ign.; Rhus t.

Tearing, shifting, darting, shooting—Æsc.; Arg. n.; *Ars.;* *Bell.;* Bry.;
Caust.; *Cham.;* Cinch.; *Col.;* Diosc.; Gels.; Gnaph.; Ign.; Kal.; *Mag.
p.;* Mez.; Nux v.; Paraf.; Phos.; Phyt.; Puls.; Rhus t.; Ruta; Sang.;
Spig.; Tereb.

Tearing, shooting, along tracts, of large nerves—Gels.

Tearing, shooting, darting like chain lightning, ending in sharp, vice-like
grip—Cact.

Tearing, shooting, to chest, trunk—Corn. fl.

Tearing, shooting, to extremities—Col.; Gnaph.; Graph.; Kal.; Pall.

Tearing, shooting, to face, shoulder, pelvis—Arundo.

Tearing, shooting, upwards—Kal.

CONCOMITANTS—Alternates with pain elsewhere; not deeply rooted cases—
Ign.

Anesthesia—*Acon.;* Ars.; Kal.

Anguish, restlessness—Acon.; Ars.

Arms feel cold, swollen, paralyzed—Ver. a.

Beginning, in pneumogastric nerve disorders—Arn.

Cardiac anxiety—Spig.

Coldness—Agar.; Ars.; *Menyanth.;* Mez.; Nat. m.; Nux v.; Plat.; Puls.;
Rhus t.; Sep.; Spig.; Ver. a.

Congestive symptoms—Acon.; Bell.; Gels.

Eructations, gastric symptoms—Ver. a.; Verbasc.

Face pale, restlessness, sweat—Spig.

Face red—Acon.; *Bell.;* Cham.; Verbasc.

Fainting, sudden—Cham.; Hep.; Morph.

Heat of one part, coldness of other—Pimenta.

Hyperesthesia—*Bell.;* Coff.; Ign.; Kali iod.; Tereb.

Lachrymation—Chel.; Mez.; *Puls.;* Rhus t.

Mania following—Cim.

Muscular contraction, spasmodic—Am. m.; *Bell.;* Gels.; Mag. p.; *Nux v.;*
Plat.; Plumb. m.; Zinc. m.

Nervous agitation—*Acon.;* Am. val.; Ars.; *Cham.;* *Coff.;* Gels.; *Mag. p.;*
Spig.

Numbness—*Acon.;* Agar.; Caust.; *Cham.;* Col.; Glon.; *Gnaph.;* Graph.;
Kal.; Lac c.; Led.; Lith. c.; Merc.; Mez.; *Plat.;* *Rhus t.;* Sep.; Spig.

Salivation, stiff neck—Mez.

Skin, feels pinched—Sul. ac.

Torpor—Plat.

Weakness—*Ars.;* Cinch.; Colch.; Gels.; Kal.; *Ver. a.*

MODALITIES—AGGRAVATION: Bending back—Caps.

Cold—*Ars.;* Bell.; Caps.; Cinch.; Col.; Kali bich.; *Mag. p.;* Rhus t.;
Ruta.

Exertion, mental—Kal.

Jar, concussion—*Bell.;* Caps.; *Spig.;* *Tellur.*

Left side—Acon.; *Ars.;* Caust.; Ced.; Colch.; *Col.;* Iris; Kali bich.; Mag.
c.; *Mez.;* Morph.; Nux v.; Rhus t.; *Spig.;* Sumb.

Lying down—Am. m.; Gnaph.

Lying, on affected side—Col.; Kali iod.

Midnight—Ars.; Bell.; Mez.; Sul.

Morning—Acon.; Chin. s.; Nux v.

Morning, 9 A. M.-4 P. M.—Verbasc.

Motion—Acon.; Ars.; Bell.; *Bry.;* Cinch.; Coff.; Colch.; Col.; Gnaph.; Nux v.; Phyt.; Ran. b.; *Spig.; Verbasc.*

Night—Acon.; *Ars.;* Bell.; *Cham.;* Cim.; Coff.; Ginseng; Ign.; *Kali iod.; Mag. p.; Merc.;* Mez.; Plat.; Phyt.; Puls.; *Rhus t.;* Ruta; Sal. ac.; *Syph.;* Tellur.

Noon (12-1)—Nat. m.; Sul.

Pressure—Ars.; Gels.; Plumb.; Verbasc.; Zinc. m.

Rest, first beginning to move—Lac c.; Rhus t.

Rest, sitting—Am. m.; Ars.; Mag. c.; *Rhus t.; Val.*

Right side—*Bell.;* Chel.; Diosc.; Gnaph.; *Kal.; Lyc.; Mag. p.;* Morph.; Puls.; Ran. b.; Sul. ac.; Tellur.

Standing, resting foot on floor—Bell.; *Val.*

Stooping or straightening limb after previous exertion—Spig.

Talking, sneezing, change of temperature—Verbasc.

Touch—Ars.; *Bell.;* Bry.; *Cinch.;* Col.; *Lach.;* Mag. p.; Mez.; *Nux v.;* Plumb.; *Spig.*

Touching or closing teeth—Verbasc.

Warmth—Cham.; Mez.; Plumb.; *Puls.;* Xanth.

AMELIORATION—Bending backward: Diosc.

Bending forward—Col.

Closing eyes—Bry.

Cold—Ars.; Puls.

Daybreak—Syph.

Flexing thigh, on abdomen—Gnaph.

Kneeling down, pressing head firmly against floor—Sang.

Lying still, rest—Am. m.; Bry.; Diosc.; Kreos.; *Mag. p.;* Nux v.

Motion, walking—Am. m.; *Ars.; Diosc.; Ign.;* Kali bich.; Kali iod.; Mag. c.; Ox. ac.; *Puls.; Rhus t.;* Sep.; Sul.; Val.

Pressure—Ars.; Bell.; *Bry.;* Coff.; *Col.; Mag. p.;* Menyanth.; *Mez.;* Nux v.; Plumb.; Spig.

Rubbing—Acon.

Sitting—Bell.; Gnaph.

Warmth—*Ars.;* Bell.; Col.; *Mag. p.;* Morph.; Nux v.; Phos.; Rhus t.

SLEEPING SICKNESS—Ars.; Atoxyl.

SPINAL CORD—Anemia: Agar.; *Plumb.; Sec.;* Strych. p.; Tar. h.

Burning—Agar.; *Alum.;* Alum. sil.; Ars.; Bell.; Gels.; *Guaco;* Kali c.; Kali ferrocy.; Kali p.; Med.; Nux v.; Phos. ac.; *Phos.;* Physost.; *Pict ac.;* Strych. p.; Sul.; *Zinc. m.*

Coldness—Cim.; Strych.

Concussion—*Arn.;* Bellis; Cic.; Con.; *Hyper.;* Physost.

Congestion—Absinth.; *Acon.; Agar.;* Arn.; Bell.; *Gels.;* Hyper.; *Nux v.;* Onosm.; Oxytr.; Phos.; Physost.; Sec.; Sil.; *Strych.;* Tab.; Ver. v.

DEGENERATION (Softening, sclerosis, etc.)—Alum.; Alum. sil.; Arg. n.; Aur.; *Aur. mur.;* Bar. mur.; Carbon. s.; Naja; Ox. ac.; *Phos.;* Physost.; Picr. ac.; *Plumb. iod.;* Plumb. m.; Zinc. See Locomotor Ataxia.

Degeneration, lateral sclerosis—*Arg. n.;* Cupr.; Hyper.; Lathyrus; Plumb.

Degeneration, multiple sclerosis—*Arg. n.; Atrop.; Aur.;* Bar. c.; Bell.; Calc.; Caust.; Chel.; *Crot.;* Gels.; *Lathyr.;* Lyc.; *Nux v.;* Ox. ac.; Phos.; Physost.; Plumb.; Sil.; *Strych.;* Sul.; Tar. h.; Thuya.

Hemorrhage in—Acon.; *Arn.; Bell.;* Lach.; Nux v.; Sec.

HYPERESTHESIA—Abrot.; Acon.; *Agar.;* Apis; Arg. n.; *Ars.; Bell.;* Bry.; *Chin. ars.;* Chin. s.; *Cim.; Cocc.;* Crot.; *Hep.; Hyper.; Lach.; Lac c.;* Lob. infl.; *Ign.;* Med ; Menisp.; Nat. m.; *Ox. ac.;* Phos. ac.; Phos.; Physost.; Pod.; Ran. b.; Rhus t.; Sec.; Senec. jac.; *Sil.; Strych. p.;* Sul.; *Tar. h.;* Tellur.; *Ther.;* Viscum; *Zinc. m.*

Hyperesthesia, between vertebræ—Chin. s.; Nat. m.; Ther.

Hyperesthesia from using arms in sewing, typewriting, piano playing—Agar.; *Cim.;* Ran. b.

Hyperesthesia, middorsal—Strych. p.; Tellur.

Hyperesthesia, sacral—Lob. infl.

Hyperesthesia, sits sideways to prevent pressure on spine—Chin. s.; Ther.; Zinc. m.

Hyperesthesia, spasmodic pain in chest and cardiac region from touch—Tar. h.

Hyperesthesia, worse from least jar or noise—Ther.

INFLAMMATION (meningitis)—Acon.; *Bell.; Bry.;* Kali iod.; Merc.; Nat. s.; Ox. ac.; Ver. v. See Myelitis.

Inflammation (myelitis)—*Acon.;* Arg. n.; *Arn.; Ars.; Bell.;* Bellis; Bry.; Chel.; *Cic.;* Con.; Crot.; Dulc.; Gels.; Hyos.; Hyper.; Kali iod.; Lach.; *Lathyr.; Merc.;* Naja; Nat. s.; *Nux v.; Ox. ac.; Phos.;* Physost.; Picr. ac.; *Plumb. m.;* Rhus t.; *Sec.;* Stram.; *Strych.;* Ver. a.; *Zinc. p.*

Inflammation, chronic (myelitis)—*Ars.; Crot.;* Lathyr.; *Ox. ac.; Plumb. m.;* Strych.; Thallium.

Inflammation, spasmodic form—Arg. n.; Ars.; Chel.; Merc.; Ver. a.

IRRITATION—*Agar.;* Ambra; *Arg. n.;* Arn.; Bell.; *Bellis;* Chin. ars.; Chin. s.; *Cim.;* Cob.; *Cocc.;* Cupr.; Gels.; *Guaco; Hyper.; Ign.;* Kali c.; Kali p.; Naja; *Nat. m.; Nux v.;* Ox. ac.; Phos.; *Physost.; Picr. ac.;* Plat.; Puls.; Ran. b.; *Sec.;* Sep.; *Sil.;* Staph.; Strych. p.; Sul.; *Tar. h.; Tellur.;* Ther.; Tub.; *Zinc. m.;* Zinc. v. See Hyperesthesia.

Irritation, from sexual excesses—Agar.; Kali p.; Nat. m.

LOCOMOTOR ATAXIA—Agar.; *Alumen;* Alum. chlor.; *Alum.;* Am. m.; Angust.; Arag.; *Arg. n.;* Ars.; Ars. br.; *Atrop.; Aur. mur.; Bell.;* Can. ind.; Carbon. s.; Carbo v.; Caust.; Chrom s.; Condur.; *Con.;* Cur.; Dub.; *Ferr. picr.; Fluor. ac.;* Gels.; Hyos.; *Ign.;* Kali br.; *Kali iod.;* Lathyr.; Lyc.; *Mag. p.;* Merc. b.; Nat. iod.; Nit. ac.; *Nux v.;* Onosm.; *Ox. ac.;* Pedic.; *Phos.;* Phos. hydr.; *Physost.; Picr. ac.;* Picrot.; *Plumb. m.; Plumb. phos.;* Rhus t.; Ruta; Sabad.; *Sec.; Sil.;* Stram.; *Strych.;* Tar. h.; Thall.; Thiosin.; *Zinc. p.;* Zinc. s.

CONCOMITANTS—Early stage: Angust.; Atrop.; *Bell.;* Con.; Ign.; Nux v.; Sec.; Strych.; Tar. h.; Zinc. m.; Zinc. s.

Enuresis and urinary symptoms—Bell.; Berb. v.; Equis.; Ferr. p. See Urinary System.

Fulgurating pains—*Acetan.;* Æsc.; Agar.; Alum.; *Am. m.;* Angust.; Arg. n.; *Ars.;* Ars. iod.; *Atrop.;* Bar. m.; *Bell.;* Berb. v.; Dig.; *Fluor. ac.;* Guaiac.; Hyos.; Ign.; *Kal.;* Lyc.; Merc. c.; Nit. ac.; Nux m.; *Nux v.;* Phos.; *Physost.;* Piloc.; Plumb. iod.; Plumb. m.; Sabad.; Sant.; *Sec.;* Sil.; *Stront. c.;* Strych.; Thall.; Thiosin.; Zinc. m.; *Zinc. p.; Zinc. s.*

Gastric symptoms—*Arg. n.;* Bell.; Carbo v.; Ign.; Lyc.; *Nux v.;* Thiosin.

Muscular weakness, anæsthesia of skin, and muscular sense—Can. ind.

Ocular symptoms—Bell.; Con.; Ferr. picr.; Phos. See Eye.

Sexual excitement—Kali br.; Picr. ac.; Phos.

Syphilitic cases— *Kali iod.;* Merc. c.; Nit. ac.; Sec.

Ulcer of heel—Sil.

Vesical and anal symptoms—Alum.; Fluor. ac.; Ign.; Nux v.; Strych.; Tar. h.; Thiosin.

PAIN IN SPINE—Abrot.; Acon.; Adon. v.; *Agar.; Arg. n.;* Cact.; Cim.; Gels.; *Hyper.;* Lact. v.; Lob. syph.; Menisp.; Niccol. s.; *Ox. ac.;* Paraf.; Physost.; Strych.; Sec.; Tar. h.; Ther.; *Zinc. m.* See Backache (Locomotor System).

PARESIS—Cocc.; Con.; *Irid.;* Plectranth.; Plumb. iod.; Sec.; *Strych.* See Paralysis.

TETANY—Acon.; Cocc.; Graph.; Lyc.; Merc.; Plumb.; Sec.; *Solan. n.*

TETANUS—Aconitin; *Acon.;* Amyl; *Angust.;* Arn.; Bell.; Calend.; Camph.; Carbon. s.; Chloral; *Cic.; Cocc.;* Con.; Cupr.; *Cur.;* Gels.; Hydroc. ac.; *Hyos.; Hyper.;* Ign.; *Ipec.;* Kali br.; Lach.; Laur.; Led.; Lyssin; Mag. p.; Morph.; Mosch.; Nicot.; *Nux v.;* Œnanthe; *Op.;* Ox. ac.; *Passifl.; Physost.;* Phyt.; Plat.; Scorpio; *Stram.; Strych.;* Tab.; Tereb.; Thebain; *Upas;* Ver. a.; Zinc. m. See Trismus (Face).

TIC CONVULSIF—Arg. n.; Hyos.; Laur.; Lyc.; Sep.; Tar. h.; Zinc.

WEAKNESS OF SPINE—*Æsc.;* Alum. sil.; Arg. n.; Bar. c.; *Calc. p.;* Cocc.; *Con.;* Nat. m.; Phos.; Picr. ac.; Selen.; Sil.; *Strych.;* Zinc. picr. See Back (Locomotor System).

GENERALITIES

ABSCESS—Acute: Acon.; *Ananth.;* Anthrac.; Apis; *Arn.;* Ars.; *Bell.;* Calc. hypoph.; *Calc. s.;* Calend.; *Carb. ac.;* Chin. s.; Cinch.; Crot.; Fluor. ac.; *Hep.;* Hippoz.; *Lach.;* Lapis alb.; Lyc.; *Merc. s.; Myrist. seb.; Nit. ac.;* Phos. ac.; Phos.; *Rhus t.; Sil.;* Sil. mar.; Syph.; *Sul.; Tar. c.;* Vespa.

About bones—Asaf.; *Aur.;* Calc. fl.; Calc. hypoph.; Calc. p.; Fluor. ac.; Mang.; *Phos.;* Puls.; *Sil.;* Symphyt.

About joints—Calc. hypoph.; Sil.

Chronic—Arn.; Calc. c.; *Calc. fl.;* Calc. iod.; Calc. p.; Carbo v.; Cham.; Cinch.; Fluor. ac.; Graph.; Hep.; *Iod.;* Iodof.; Kali iod.; Merc. i. r.; *Merc. s.;* Ol. j. as.; Phos.; *Sil.;* Sul.

Muscles, deep-Calc. c.

Psoas abscess—Sil.; Symphyt.

To abort—Apis; Bell.; Bry.; *Hep.; Merc. s.*

To hasten suppuration—Guaiac.; *Hep.;* Lach.; Merc. s.; Operc.; Phos.; Phyt.; *Sil.*

ACROMEGALY—Pituit. ext.; Thyr.

ADDISON'S DISEASE—*Adren.;* Ant. c.; Apomorph.; *Arg. n.; Ars.;* Ars. iod.; Bac.; Bell.; Calc. ars.; Calc. c.; Hydroc. ac.; *Iod.;* Kreos.; Nat. m.; Nit. ac.; Phos.; Sec.; *Sil.;* Spig.; Sul.; *Suprarenal ext.;* Thuya; *Tub.;* Vanad.

ANEMIA—Chlorosis: Acet. ac.; *Alet.;* Alum.; *Arg. n.; Arg. oxy.;* Arn.; *Ars.;* Aur. ars.; Bism.; Calc. ars.; *Calc. c.;* Calc. lact.; *Calc. p.;* Calop.; Carbo v.; Chin. ars.; *Chin. s.;* Cic.; *Cinch.;* Con.; Crat.; Crot.; Cupr. ars.; *Cupr. m.; Cycl.;* Ferr. ars.; *Ferr. ars.;* Ferr. carb.; Ferr. et. chin.; Ferr. p.; *Ferr. iod.; Ferr. m.;* Ferr. mur.; Ferr. oxy.; *Ferr. red.;* Gossyp.; *Graph.; Helon.;* Hydr.; Iod.; *Irid.;* Kali bich.; *Kali c.;* Kali p.; Lecith.; *Lyc.; Mang. ac.;* Merc. s.; Nat. c.; *Nat. m.; Nit. ac.;* Nux v.; Petrol.; *Phos.;* Phyt.; Picr. ac.; Plat.; *Plumb. ac.; Puls.;* Rubia; Sacchar. of.; *Sec.; Sep.;* Sil.; *Strych. et ferr. cit.; Sul.;* Thyr.; Vanad.; Zinc. ars.; Zinc. mur.

From cardiac disease—Ars.; Crat.; Stroph.

From grief—Nat. m.; *Phos. ac.*

From malaria—Alston.; *Ars.; Nat. m.;* Ostrya; Robin.

From menstrual derangements—Arg. oxy.; Ars.; *Calc. c.;* Calc. p.; Crat.; *Cycl.; Ferr.; Graph.; Kali c.; Mang. ac.; Nat. m.; Puls.;* Sep.

From nutritional disturbances—Alet.; Alum.; *Calc. p.;* Ferr.; Helon.; Nux v.

From suboxidation—Picr. ac.

From syphilis—Calop.

From vital drains, exhausting disease—Acet. ac.; Alston.; *Calc. p.;* Chin. s.; *Cinch.; Ferr.;* Helon.; Kali c.; *Nat. m.; Phos. ac.;* Phos.

Hemorrhagic chlorosis—*Arg. oxy.; Ars.;* Calc. c.; Crot.; Ign.; Nat. br.

Pernicious anemia—*Ars.; Phos.;* Picr. ac.; Thyr.

Type, erythistic; worse in winter—Ferr. m.

ASPHYXIA—Am. c.; *Ant. t.; Hydroc. ac.;* Sul. hydr.; Upas.

Asphyxia neonatorum—*Ant. t.;* Laur.

BLOOD—Disorganization: Ail.; Am. c.; *Anthrac.;* Arn.; *Ars.;* Ars. hydr.;
Bapt.; Carb. ac.; *Crot.; Echin.;* Kreos.; *Lach.; Mur. ac.;* Phos.; Psor.;
Pyr.; Rhus t.; Tar. c. See Pyemia.

BONES—Club-foot: Nux v.; Phos.; Strych.

Cold feeling—Zinc. m.

Condyles, epiphyses, swollen—Conchiolin; Rhus t.

Condyles, sutures, affected—Calc. c.; Calc. p.

Cranial bones, thin, soft—Calc. c.; *Calc. p.*

Crooking—Am. c.; Calc. c.; Calc. p.; Iod.; Sil.

Development, tardy—*Calc. c.;* Calc. fl.; *Calc. p.;* Sil.

Enlargement (acromegaly)—Pituit. ext.; Thyr.

Exostoses—Arg. m.; Aur.; Calc. c.; *Calc. fl.;* Fluor. ac.; *Hekla; Kali
bich.; Kali iod.;* Lapis alb.; Malandr.; Merc. c.; *Merc. phos.;* Merc. s.;
Mez.; *Phos.; Plumb. ac.;* Ruta; *Sil.;* Still.; Sul.; Zinc. m.

Fractures, shock—Acon.; Arn.

Fractures, slow union—*Calc. p.;* Calend.; Iod.; Mang. ac.; *Mez.;* Phos.
ac.; *Ruta; Sil.; Symphyt.;* Thyr.

Inflammation (osteitis)—Asaf.; Aur. iod.; *Aur.;* Conchiol.; Hekla; Hep.;
Iod.; *Kali iod.;* Merc. s.; Mez.; *Nit. ac.;* Phos. ac.; Phos.; Staph.;
Still.; Stront. c.

Inflammation, chronic (osteitis deformans)—Aur.; Calc. p.; Hekla; Nit. ac.

Inflammation, (osteo-myelitis)—Acon.; Chin. s.; Gun powder; Phos.

NECROSIS—Angust.; *Arg. m.;* Ars.; *Asaf.;* Aur. iod.; *Aur. m.;* Calc. c.;
Calc. fl.; Calc. hypophos.; Calc. p.; Calc. sil.; Cinch.; Con.; *Fluor. ac.;*
Graph.; Hekla; *Hep.;* Iod.; Kali bich.; Kali iod.; Lach.; Med.; *Merc.
s.;* Mez.; *Nat. sil. fl.; Nit. ac.;* Phos. ac.; *Phos.;* Plat. mur.; *Sil.;*
Staph.; Sul. ac.; Symphyt.; Syph.; Sul.; Thea; Ther.; *Tub.;* Vitrum.

Facial—Hep.; Mez.; Sil.

Femur—Stront. c.

Long bones—Angust.; Asaf.; *Fluor. ac.;* Mez.; Stront. c.

Mastoid, palatine, cranial, nasal—Aur. m.

Mastoid, temporal—Calc. fl.; Caps.

Nasal—Aur.; Kali bich.

Skull—Fluor. ac.

Sternum—Con.

Tarsus—Plat. mur.

Tibiæ—Asaf.; Carb. ac.; Hep.; Lach.; Nit. ac.; Phos.

Vertebræ—Calc. c.; Nat. m.; Phos. ac.; Sil.; Sticta; Syph.

Vertebræ, inferior maxilla—Phos.

NODES—Asaf.; *Aur. mur.; Cinnab.;* Fluor. ac.; *Kali bich.; Kali iod.;*
Merc.; Mez.; Nux v.; Phyt.; *Sil.; Still.* See Syphilis (Male Sexual System).

PAIN—Agar.; Angust.; *Asaf.; Aur. m.;* Aur. mur.; Bry.; Castor eq.; Caust.;
Cinch.; Crot.; Crot. casc.; *Eup. perf.;* Euphorb.; *Fluor. ac.;* Guaiac.;
Hep.; Iod.; Ipec.; *Kali bich.; Kali iod.;* Lyc.; Lyssin; Mang. ac.;

Merc. c.; Merc. s.; *Mez.;* Phos. ac.; Phos.; *Phyt.; Rhod.;* Rhus t.; *Ruta;* Sil.; *Staph.;* Sul.; *Symphyt.;* Syph.; Ther.; Vitrum.

Burning—Aur.; Euphorb.; Fluor. ac.; Kali iod.; Phos. ac.; Sul.

Constricting, band-like—*Apis;* Carb. ac.; Hep.; Nit. ac.; Sul.

Drawing, pressing, sensitiveness—Nit. ac.

Gnawing, digging—*Aur.;* Carb. ac.; Kali iod.; Mang. ac.; Merc.; Symphyt.

Growing—Guaiac.; Mang. ac.; Phos. ac.

In coccyx—Castor eq

In face, feet—Aur. m.

In long bones—Cinnab.; Eup. perf.; Staph.; Stront.; Syph.

In shin bones—Agar.; Asaf.; Castor eq.; Carb. ac.; Dulc.; *Mez.;* Staph.; Still.; Syph.

In skull—Eup. perf.; Kali bich.

In vertebræ—Agar.

Influenzal—Eup. perf.

Localized in spots, worse, from weather changes—Rhod.

Nocturnal—*Asaf.; Aur.;* Fluor. ac.; Hep.; Iod.; *Kali iod.;* Lach.; Mang. ac.; *Merc.; Mez.;* Phos. ac.; Phyt.; Rhod.; Still.; Syph.

Pricking—Arn.; *Symphyt.*

Sore, bruised, aching—Cinch.; Conchiol.; Eup. perf.; Lyssin; Phyt.; Ruta.

Sore, bruised, as if scraped—*Ipec.;* Paris; *Phos. ac.;* Rhus t.

Sore, bruised, worse, from cold; wandering—Kali bich.

Tearing—Caust.; Colch.; Fluor. ac.; Phos. ac.

Throbbing, jerking, darting, drawing, hypersensitiveness—Asaf.

Worse, from damp weather—Merc.; Mez.; Nit. ac.; Phyt.; Rhus t.; Still.; Syph.

PERIOSTITIS—And periosteal affections: Apis; Aran.; *Asaf.; Aur. m.; Aur. mur.;* Calc. c.; Cinch.; Clem.; Colch.; Con.; Ferr. iod.; Graph.; *Guaiac.;* Hekla; Iod.; *Kali bich.; Kali iod.;* Mang. ac.; *Merc. s.; Mez.; Nit. ac.;* Phos. ac.; Phos.; *Phyt.;* Plat. mur.; Rhod.; Rhus t.; *Ruta;* Sars.; *Sil.;* Still.; Symphyt.

SOFTENING, Mollities Ossium—Calc. c.; *Calc. iod.;* Calc. p.; Guaiac.; Iod.; Merc. s.; *Phos.*

SPINAL bifida—Bry.; *Calc. p.;* Psor.; Tub.

Spinal caries (Pott's disease)—Arg. m.; Aur.; Calc. c.; Calc. iod.; *Calc. p.;* Con.; *Iod.;* Kali iod.; Merc. i. r.; *Phos. ac.; Phos.;* Pyr.; *Sil.;* Still.; Sul.; *Syph.;* Tub.; Vitrum.

Spinal curvature—Calc. c.; *Calc. p.;* Ferr. iod.; Phos.; *Sil.;* Sul.; Ther.
Wounds—Ruta; Symphyt.

BUBONIC PLAGUE—Anthrac.; Ant. t.; *Ars.;* Bapt.; Bell.; Bubon.; Carbo v.; Cinch.; *Crot.;* Ign.; Iod.; *Lach.;* Naja; Operc.; *Phos.; Pyr.;* Rhus t.; *Tar. c.*

CANCER—Remedies in general: Acet. ac.; Ananth.; *Ant. chlor.;* Apis; *Ars.;* Ars. br.; Ars. iod.; *Aster.;* Aur. ars.; Aur. m. n.; Bapt.; Bism.; Brom.; Calc. c.; Calc. iod.; Calc. ox.; Calend.; Carb. ac.; *Carbo an.;* Carbon. s.; Carcinos.; Choline; Cic.; Cinnam.; *Cistus; Condur.; Con.;*

Cupr. ac.; Eosin.; Euphorb.; Form. ac.; Formica; Fuligo; *Galium ap.*;
Guaco; Graph.; Ham.; *Hoang n.; Hydr.; Iod.*; Kali ars.; *Kali cy.*;
Kali iod.; *Kreos.; Lach.*; Lapis alb.; Lyc.; Maland.; Med.; Phos.;
Phyt.; Radium; Rumex; ac.; Sang.; *Semperv. t.*; Scirrhin.; Sedum rep.;
Sep.; Sil.; Symphyt.; Sul.; Taxus; *Thuya.*

Cancer, of antrum—Aur.; Symphyt.

Cancer, of bone—Aur. iod.; Phos.; Symphyt.

Cancer, of bowel, lower—Ruta.

Cancer, of breast—Ars. iod.; Bar. iod.; Brom.; Bufo; *Carbo an.*; Carcinos.;
Condur.; *Con.*; Form. ac.; Graph.; *Hydr.*; Phyt.; *Plumb. iod.*; Nat.
cacodyl.; Scirrhin. See Female Sexual System.

Cancer, of cæcum—Ornithog.

Cancer, of glandular structures—Hoang nan.

Cancer, of omentum—Lob. erin.

Cancer, of stomach—Acet. ac.; *Ars.*; Bism.; Cadm. s.; *Condur.*; Form. ac.;
Hydr.; Kreos.; Ornithog.; Phos.; Sec. See Stomach.

Cancer, of uterus—*Aur. m. n.*; Carbo an.; Carcinos.; Fuligo; Hydr.; Iod.;
Lapis alb.; Nat. cacodyl.; Nit. ac.; Sec. See Female Sexual System.

Cancer, to relieve pains—Alveloz.; *Apis*; Anthrac.; *Ars.*; Aster.; Bry.;
Calc. ac.; Calc. c.; Calc. ox.; Carcinos.; Ced.; Cinnam.; Condur.; Con.;
Echin.; *Euphorb.*; *Hydr.*; Mag. p.; Morph.; Op.; Ova t.; Phos. ac.;
Sil.

CARTILAGES (perichondritis)—Inflammation: Arg. m.; Bell.; Cham.; Cim.;
Oleand.; Plumb.; *Ruta.*

Cartilages, pains—Arg. m.; Ruta.

Cartilages, ulceration—Merc. c.

CELLULAR TISSUE—Indurated: *Anthrac.*; Carbo an.; Graph.; *Kali iod.*;
Kreos.; Merc.; Plumb. iod.; *Rhus t.*; Sil.

CELLULITIS—Apis; Arn.; *Ars.*; Bapt.; Crot.; *Lach.*; Mang. ac.; *Merc.
i. r.*; *Rhus t.*; Sil.; Vespa.

COMPLAINTS—ABUSE of alcoholic beverages: *Agar.*; Apomorph.; Ant.;
Ars.; Asar.; Aur.; Calc. ars.; Carbo v.; Carbon. s.; Card. m.; Coca;
Cocc.; Colch.; Eup. perf.; Hydr.; Ipec.; Lach.; Led.; *Lob. infl.*; Lyc.;
Nux v.; Querc.; *Ran. b.*; Strych.; Sul. ac.; Sul.; *Ver. a.* See Alcoholism
(Nervous System).

Abuse of aconite—Sul.

Abuse of arsenic—Carbo v.; Ferr.; Hep.; *Ipec.*; Samb.; Ver. a.

Abuse of belladonna—Hyos.; Op.

Abuse of bromide of potassium—Camph.; Helon.; Nux v.; Zinc. m.

Abuse of camphor—Canth.; Coff.; Op.

Abuse of cantharis—Apis; Camph.

Abuse of chamomilla—Cinch.; Coff.; Ign.; Nux v.; Puls.; Val.

Abuse of chloral—Can. ind.

Abuse of chlorate of potash—Hydr.

Abuse of cod liver oil—Hep.

Abuse of coffee—Cham.; Guar.; *Ign.; Nux v.*

Abuse of colchicum—Led.

Abuse of condiments—Nux v.

Abuse of digitalis—Cinch.; Nit. ac.

Abuse of drugs in general—Aloe; Hydr.; *Nux v.;* Teucr.

Abuse of ergot—Cinch.; Lach.; Nux v.; Sec.; Solan. n.

Abuse of iodides—Ars.; Bell.; *Hep.;* Hydr.; Phos.

Abuse of iron—Cinch.; *Hep.; Puls.*

Abuse of lead (plumbism)—*Alum.;* Bell.; Carbon. s.; Caust.; *Col.;* Iod.; Kali br.; *Kali iod.;* Merc.; Nux v.; *Op.;* Petrol.; Plat.; Sul. ac.

Abuse of magnesia—Nux. v.; Rheum.

Abuse of mercury—Angust.; Ant. t.; Arg. m.; Asaf.; *Aur.;* Carbo v.; Caust.; Cinch.; Clem.; Dulc.; Fluor. ac.; Guaiac.; *Hep.; Iod.; Kali iod.;* Lach.; Mez.; *Nit. ac.;* Op.; Plat. mur.; Phyt.; Pod.; Puls.; Rhus g.; Sars.; Sul.

Abuse of narcotics—Acet. ac.; Apomorph.; Avena; Camph.; Can. ind.; *Cham.;* Cim.; Ipec.; Macrot.; Mur. ac.

Abuse of nitrate of silver—Nat. m.

Abuse of phosphorus—Lach.; Nux v.

Abuse of quinine—*Ars.;* Bell.; Col.; Carbo v.; Eucal.; Ferr.; *Ipec.;* Lach.; Menyanth.; *Nat. m.;* Parth.; *Puls.;* Selen.

Abuse of salt (halophagia)—Ars.; Carbo v.; Nat. m.; *Nit. sp. d.; Phos.*

Abuse of stramonium—Acet. ac.; Nux v.; Tab.

Abuse of strychnine—Cur.; *Eucal.;* Kali br.; Physost.

Abuse of sugar—Merc. v.; Nat. p.

Abuse of sulphur—Puls.; Selen.

Abuse of tar, locally—Bov.

Abuse of tea—Abies n.; *Cinch.;* Diosc.; Ferr.; Puls.; *Selen.;* Thuya.

Abuse of tobacco—*Abies n.; Ars.;* Calad.; Calc. p.; Camph.; Chin. ars.; Cinch.; Coca; *Gels.; Ign.; Ipec.;* Kal.; Lyc.; Mur. ac.; *Nux v.; Phos.; Plant.;* Plumb.; Sep.; *Spig.;* Staph.; Tab.; Ver. a.

Abuse of tobacco, in boys—Arg. n.; Ars.; Ver. a.

Abuse of turpentine—Nux m.

Abuse of vegetable medicines—Camph.; *Nux v.*

Abuse of veratrum—Camph.; Coff.

Anæsthetic vapors, antidote—*Acet. ac.;* Am. caust.; Amyl; Hep.; Phos.

BITES of insects, snakes, dogs—Acet. ac.; Am. c.; Am. caust.; Anthrac.; *Apis;* Arn.; *Ars.;* Bell.; Calad.; Camph.; *Ced.;* Crot.; *Echin.;* Golond.; *Grind.;* Guaco; Gymnen.; Hydroc. ac.; *Hyper.;* Kali perm.; *Lach.; Led.;* Mosch.; Pyr.; Salag.; Sisyr.; Spiræa; Trychnos.

Charcoal fumes, illuminating gas, ill effects—Acet. ac.; Am. c.; Arn.; Bell.; Bov.; Coff.; Op.

CHECKED discharges, ill effects—Abrot.; Asaf.; Aur. mur.; *Bar. c.;* Bry.; *Graph.;* Lach.; *Lob. infl.;* Med.; Merc. s.; *Psor.;* Sanic.; *Sil.;* Stram.; Sul.; Zinc. m.

Checked foot sweat, ill effects—*Bar. c.;* Cupr.; Formica; Graph.; Psor.; Sanic.; *Sil.;* Zinc. m.

Checked gonorrhœa, ill effects—Graph.; Psor.; *Med.; Thuya;* X-ray.

Checked, sweats, ill effects—*Acon.;* Bellis; Dulc.; Rhus t.

CHRONIC DISEASES, to begin treatment—Calc. c.; Calc. p.; *Nux v.;* Puls.; *Sul.*

CICATRICES, affections—Calc. fl.; *Fluor. ac.;* Hyper.; Phyt.; Sil.; *Thiosin.*

Cicatrices, freshen up, reopen—*Caust.;* Fluor. ac.; *Graph.;* Mag. pol. am.; Sil.

Cicatrices, itch—Fluor. ac.

Cicatrices, pain during change of weather—Nit. ac.

Cicatrices, turn green—Led.

Cicatrices, turn red or blue—Sul. ac.

COMPLAINTS, appear, atypically—Mosch.

Complaints, appear, diagonally, upper left, lower right side—*Agar.;* Ant. t.; Stram.

Complaints, appear, diagonally, upper right, lower left side—Ambra; Brom.; Med.; Phos.; Sul. ac.

Complaints, appear, from above downwards—Cact.; *Kal.*

Complaints, appear, from below, upwards—Led.

Complaints, appear, gradually—Calc. sil.; Cinch.; Radium; Tellur.

Complaints, appear, gradually, cease gradually—Arg. n.; *Plat.; Stann.;* Stront. c.; Syph.

Complaints, appear, gradually, cease suddenly—Ign.; *Puls.;* Sul. ac.

Complaints, appear, in small spots—Coff.; *Ign.; Kali bich.;* Lil. t.; *Ox. ac.*

Complaints, appear, suddenly, cease gradually—Puls.; Sul. ac.

Complaints, appear, suddenly, cease suddenly—*Bell.;* Cact.; Carb. ac.; Eup. perf.; Eup. purp.; Ign.; Kali bich.; Lyc.; *Mag. p.;* Nit. ac.; Oxytrop.; Petrol.; Poth.; *Strych.;* Tub.

Complaints, appear, suddenly, tension acutely increases, leaves with a snap on first motion—Puls.; Rhus t.

Complaints, fatal issue; to induce "euthanasia"—Amyl; Ant. t.; *Ars.;* Carbo v.; Lach.; Tar. h.

Complaints, from chilling—*Acon.;* Coff.; Dulc.; Nux v.; Sil.

Complaints, from exposure of feet—*Calc. c.;* Cupr. m.; Nux m.; Sil.

Complaints, from exposure, to cold dry wind—*Acon.;* Bry.; Caust.; Hep.; *Rhod.*

Complaints, from living in cool, damp places—Ant. t.; *Aran.;* Ars.; Ars. iod.; Calc. c.; Calc. sil.; *Dulc.; Nat. s.;* Nux m.; *Rhus t.;* Tereb.

Complaints, from overlifting—*Arn.; Carbo an.;* Carbo v.; Kali c.; Lyc.; *Nat. c.;* Nat. m.; Phos.; *Rhus t.;* Sep.; Sul.

Complaints, from working, in clay, cold water—Calc. c.; Mag. p.

Complaints, improve, then relapse continually—Sul.

Complaints, improve, then remain stationary—Caust.; Psor.; *Sul.*

Complaints, in extremes of life—Ant. c.; *Bar. c.;* Lyc.; Millef.; Op.; *Ver. a.*

Complaints in fleshy persons—Allium s.; Am. c.; Am. m.; *Ant. c.;* Aur. m.; Bar. c.; Blatta or.; Calc. ars.; *Calc. c.; Caps.;* Carbo v.; Ferr.; *Graph.;* Kali bich.; Kali br.; *Kali c.;* Lob. infl.; Op.; Phyt.; Puls.; Thuya. See Obesity.

Complaints, in old people—Agar.; Aloe; Alumen; *Alum.; Ambra;* Ant. c.; Ars.; Aurant.; Aur. m.; *Bar. c.; Bar. m.;* Caps.; *Carbo an.;* Carbo v.; Colch.; *Con.;* Crot.; Fluor. ac.; Hydr.; Iod.; Kali c.; Lyc.; Millef.; Nit. ac.; Nux m.; *Op.;* Phos.; Sec.; Sul. ac.; *Ver. a.*

Complaints, wander, or shift about, erratic, changeable—Apis; Bell.; Benz.

ac.; Berb. v.; *Dios.*; *Ign.*; *Kali bich.*; *Kali s.*; *Lac c.*; Lil. t.; Mag. p.;
Magnolia; *Mang. ac.*; Phyt.; *Puls.*; Sanic.; Syph.; *Tub.*
Complaints, with painlessness—Op.; *Stram.*

ERUPTIONS, exanthemata, suppressed, or repercussed, ill effects—*Apis*;
Ars.; Asaf.; *Bry.*; *Camph.*; Caust.; *Cic.*; *Cupr.*; *Helleb.*; Mag. s.;
Op.; Psor.; Puls.; Stram.; *Sul.*; *Tub.*; X-ray; *Zinc. m.*

Foreign bodies, in larynx, trachea—Ant. t.; Ipec.; Sil.

Growth, too rapid, ill effects—*Calc. c.*; *Calc. p.*; Ferr. ac.; Irid.; Kreos.;
Phos. ac.; *Phos.*

Mental labor, sufferings from—*Arg. n.*; *Gels.*; Graph.; Lyc.; Nat. c.;
Nux v.; Phos. ac.; Sil.

Mining, ill effects—Card. m.; Nat. ars.

Mountain climbing, aviation, ill effects—Ars.; Coca.

Night watching, mental strain, ill effects—Bellis; Caps.; Caust.; *Cocc.*;
Colch.; Cupr.; Dipod.; *Gels.*; *Ign.*; *Lac d.*; Nit. ac.; *Nux v.*; *Phos.
ac.*; *Zinc. ac.* See Neurasthenia (Nervous System).

Nutritional disturbances, development tardy—Bac.; *Bar. c.*; *Calc. c.*; *Calc.
p.*; Caust.; Kreos.; Lac d.; Med.; Nat. m.; Pinus sylv.; *Sil.*; Thyr.

Poison oak, and rhus poisoning—Am. c.; *Anac.*; Apis; Arn.; Astac.; Cim.;
Crot. t.; Cyprip.; Echin.; Erech.; Euphorb. d.; Graph.; *Grind.*; He-
deoma; Hydrophyl.; *Led.*; Mez.; Plant.; Prim. ob.; Rhus d.; *Rhus t.*;
Sang.; Sep.; Tanac.; Urt.; Vanillin; Verb.; *Xerophyl.*

PROMAINE poisoning (decayed food)—Absinth.; Acet. ac.; *Ars.*; Camph.;
Carbo an.; Carbo v.; Cepa; Crot.; *Cupr. ars.*; Gunpowder; Kreos.;
Pyr.; Urt.; *Ver. a.*

Ptomaine poisoning (mushrooms)—Agar.; Atrop.; *Bell.*; Camph.; Pyr.

Sewer gas, or noxious effluvia, ill effects—Anthrac.; *Bapt.*; Phyt.; Pyr.

Sun exposure, ill effects: SUNSTROKE (coup-de-soleil): Acon.; *Ant. c.*;
Bell.; Bry.; Cact.; Camph.; *Gels.*; *Glon.*; Hydroc. ac.; Lach.; *Nat. c.*;
Op.; Stram.; Usnea; *Ver. v.* See Collapse (Nervous System); Modalities.

Vaccination, ill effects—Acon.; *Ant. t.*; Apis; Bell.; Crot.; Echin.; *Malandr.*; Merc. s.; *Mez.*; Sars.; Sep.; *Sil.*; Sul.; *Thuya.*

Vital drains, ill effects—Calc. p.; *Cinch.*; Ham.; *Kali c.*; *Kali p.*; Nat.
m.; *Phos. ac.*; Phos.; Psor.; Sep.; Staph.

DEGENERATION—Fatty: *Ars.*; Aur.; *Cupr.*; Kali c.; *Phos.*; Vanad.

DROPSY—Acetan.; *Acet. ac.*; Acon.; *Adon. v.*; Amelop.; Am. benz.; *Apis*;
Apoc.; Arg. phos.; *Ars.*; Ars. iod.; Asclep. s.; Asclep. vinc.; Benz. ac.;
Blatta am.; Brass.; Bry.; Cact.; Calc. ars.; Calc. c.; Caffeine; *Cahinca*;
Card. m.; *Cinch.*; Cochlear.; *Colch.*; *Conv.*; Cop.; *Crat.*; *Dig.*; Dulc.;
Elat.; Eup. purp.; Euphorb.; Ferr.; *Fluor. ac.*; Galium; *Helleb.*;
Hep.; Iod.; Iris; Iris germ.; Jatropha; *Junip.*; Kali ac.; *Kali ars.*;
Kali c.; *Kali iod.*; *Kali n.*; Lac d.; *Lach.*; Lact. v.; *Liatris*; Lyc.;
Merc. d.; Nasturt.; Nit. sp. dulc.; Onisc.; *Oxydend.*; *Phaseol.*; Phos.;
Piloc.; Prun. sp.; Psor.; Querc.; Rhus t.; *Samb. can.*; Samb.; *Scilla*;
Solan. n.; Solid.; *Stroph.*; Strych. ars.; *Tereb.*; Teucr. sc.; Thlaspi;
Toxicophis; Urium; Ur. ac.

From abuse of quinine—Apoc.

From alcoholism—Ars.; Fluor. ac.; Sul.

From eruption suppressed, sweat, rheumatism—Dulc.

From heart disease—*Adon. v.;* Apis; Apoc.; Arn.; *Ars.;* Ars. iod.; Asclep. s.; Aur. m.; *Cact.; Caffeine;* Collins.; *Conv.; Crat.; Dig.; Digitalin;* Iod.; Kal.; Liatris; Merc. d.; *Stroph.* See Heart.

From kidney disease—Ampel.; Ant. t.; *Apis;* Apoc.; Ars.; Asclep. s.; Aspar.; Chimaph.; *Dig.;* Digitalin; Eup. purp.; Helon.; Lac d.; Liatris; *Merc. c.;* Merc. d.; Plumb.; Tereb.; Uric. ac. See Urinary System.

From liver disease—*Apoc.;* Ars.; Asclep. s.; Aur.; Card. m.; Caenoth.; Chel.; Chimaph.; Lac d.; Liatris; *Lyc.;* Mur. ac.; Polymnia. See Liver (Abdomen).

From menstrual disorder at puberty, or menopause—Puls.

From spleen disease—Ceanoth.; Liatris; Querc.; Scilla. See Spleen (Abdomen).

From remittent fever—Helleb.

From scarlet fever—Acon.; *Apis;* Apoc.; *Ars.;* Asclep. s.; Colch.; Dig.; Dulc.; *Helleb.; Hep.;* Junip.; Lach.; Piloc.; Scilla; *Tereb.*

From suppressed exanthemata—Apis; Helleb.; Zinc. m.

From suppressed intermittents—Carbo v.; Cinch.; Ferr. m.; Helleb.; Lac d.

Dropsy, in newborn—Apis; Caffeine; Carbo v.; Dig.; Lach.

Dropsy, with diarrhœa—Acet. ac.

Dropsy, with serum oozing—Ars.; Lyc.; Rhus t.

Dropsy, with soreness in uterine region—Conv.

Dropsy, with suppressed urine, fever, debility—Helleb.

Dropsy, with thirst—*Acet. ac.;* Acon.; *Apoc.;* Ars.

Dropsy, without thirst—Apis; Helleb.

LOCATION—**Abdomen**—ASCITES: *Acet. ac.; Adon. v.; Apis; Apoc.; Ars.;* Aur. m.; Aur. m. n.; *Blatta am.;* Cahinca; Canth.; *Cinch.;* Cop.; *Dig.; Digitalin;* Fluor. ac.; *Helleb.;* Iod.; Kali c.; Lact. v.; Led.; *Lyc.;* Nat. chlor.; Oxydend.; *Prun. sp.;* Samb.; *Senec.;* Sep.; Tereb.; Uran. n.

Chest (hydrothorax)—*Apis;* Apoc.; *Ars.;* Ars. iod.; Colch.; *Dig.;* Helleb.; *Kali c.;* Lach.; Lact. v.; *Merc. sul.;* Scilla; *Sul.* See Chest.

Extremity, left—Cact.

General—ANASARCA:—Acetan.; Acet. ac.; Acon.; Eth.; *Apis;* Apoc.; Arn.; *Ars.;* Cahinca; *Cinch.; Conv.;* Cop.; Crat.; *Dig.;* Dulc.; Ferr. m.; *Helleb.;* Kali c.; *Liatris;* Lyc.; *Merc. c.;* Oxydend.; Picr. ac.; Prun. sp.; Tereb.; Uran. n. See Dropsy.

EFFUSION—**Threatening:** *Apis; Bry.;* Cic.; Cinch.; *Helleb.;* Iodof.; Op.; Tub.; *Zinc. m.*

GLANDERS—Acon.; Ars.; Chin. s.; *Crot.;* Hep.; Hippoz.; *Kali bich.;* Lach.; *Merc. s.;* Phos.; Sep.; Sil.; Thuya.

GLANDS—**Abscess:** Bell.; Calc. c.; Calc. iod.; Cistus; Hep.; Lapis alb.; *Merc.;* Nit. ac.; Rhus t.; *Sil.*

Affections, traumatic—Aster.; Con.

Atrophy—Iod.

Induration—Alumen; Ars.; Ars. br.; *Aster.;* Aur. mur.; Bad.; *Bar. c.; Bar. iod.;* Bar. m.; Bell.; Berb. aq.; *Brom.;* Calc. c.; Calc. chlor.; *Calc. fl.; Carbo an.;* Cinch.; *Cistus;* Clem.; *Con.;* Dulc.; Graph.; *Hekla;*

Iod.; Kali iod.; *Lapis alb.;* Merc. i. fl.; Merc. i. r.; Operc; **Phyt.;** *Rhus t.;* Spong.; Thyr.; Trifol. r.

Inflammation (ADENITIS)—Acute: Acon.; Ail.; Alumen; Ananth.; *Apis;* Ars. iod.; Bar. c.; Bar. iod.; *Bell.; Cistus;* Clem.; *Dulc.;* Graph.; *Hep.;* Iod.; *Iodof.; Kali iod.; Merc. i. r.; Merc. s.;* Operc.; *Phyt.;* Rhus t.; Sil.; *Sil. mar.*

Inflammation, chronic: GLANDULAR SWELLINGS—Acon. lyc.; *Ail.; Alnus;* Apis; Ars. br.; Ars.; *Ars. iod.;* Arum; Astacus; Aur. mur.; *Bad.; Bar. c.; Bar. iod.;* Bar. mur.; *Brom.; Calc. c.; Calc. fl.; Calc. iod.;* Calc. p.; Calend.; *Carbo an.; Cistus;* Clem.; Con.; Coryd.; Crot.; Dulc.; Ferr. iod.; Filix; Graph.; Hep.; *Iod.; Kali iod.;* Lach.; *Lapis alb.;* Lyc.; Med.; Merc. cy.; Merc. i. fl.; *Merc. i. r.;* Merc. s.; Nit. ac.; *Phyt.;* Psor.; Rhus t.; *Rumex;* Sal. mar.; Scirrhin.; *Scrophul.; Sil.;* Sil. mar.; *Spong.; Sul.;* Taxus; Thiosin.; Thuya; Tub.

LOCATION—OF GLANDULAR AFFECTION: Axillary: Acon. lyc.; *Aster.;* Bar. c.; Bell.; Calc. c.; Carbo an.; *Con.;* Elaps; Graph.; Hep.; Jugl. r.; *Lact. ac.;* Nat. s.; Nit. ac.; Phyt.; Raph.; Rhus t.; Sil.; Sul.

Bronchial—Bell.; Calc. c.; Calc. fl.; *Iod.;* Merc. c.; Tub.

Cervical—Acon. lyc.; *Am. c.;* Astac.; Bac.; *Bar. c.;* Bar. iod.; *Bell.; Brom.;* Calc. c.; Calc. chlor.; Calc. fl.; Calc. iod.; *Carbo an.;* Caust.; *Cistus;* Dulc.; Graph.; Hekla; *Hep.;* Iod.; Kali iod.; Kali m.; *Lapis alb.;* Mag. p.; *Merc. i. fl.; Merc. i. r.;* Merc.; Nit. ac.; *Rhus t.;* Rhus r.; Rhus v.; Sal. mar.; Sil.; Spong.; *Still.;* Sul.

Inguinal—Apis; Ars.; Aur.; Bac.; *Bar. c.;* Bar. m.; Bell.; *Calc. c.;* Carbo an.; Clem.; Dulc.; Graph.; Kali iod.; *Merc. i. fl.; Merc. s.; Nit. ac.;* Ocim.; Pall.; Pinus sylv.; Rhus t.; Sil.; Sul.; Xerophyl.

Mesenteric—*Ars.;* Ars. iod.; Bac.; Bar. c.; Bar. mur.; *Calc. c.;* Calc. fl.; *Calc. iod.;* Con.; Graph.; *Iod.;* Iodof.; Lapis alb.; *Merc. c.;* Mez.; Tub. See Tabes Mesenterica.

Parotid—Inflammation (Parotitis, Mumps): Acon.; Ail.; Am. c.; Anthrac.; Ant. t.; Aur. mur.; *Bar. c.;* Bar. m.; *Bell.; Brom.;* Calc. c.; Carbo an.; Cham.; Cistus; Dulc.; Euphras.; *Ferr. p.;* Hep.; *Kali bich.;* Kali m.; Lach.; Mag. p.; *Merc. c.;* Merc. cy.; Merc. i. fl.; Merc. i. r.; *Merc. s.; Phyt.;* Piloc.; *Puls.; Rhus t.; Sil.;* Sul.; Sul. iod.; Trifol.; **Trifol. r.**

Parotitis, gangrenous—Anthrac.

Parotitis, metastases to brain—Apis; Bell.

Parotitis, metastases to mammæ ovaries—Con.; Jabor. Puls.;

Parotitis, metastases to testes—Aur.; *Clem.; Ham.; Puls.;* Rhus t.

Parotitis, persistent—Bar. ac.; Bar. c.; *Con.; Iod.;* Sil.

Sebaceous glands—Lyc.; Psor.; Raph.; Sil.; Sul. See Skin.

Submaxillary—Alnus; *Arum;* Asimina; *Bar. c.;* Brom.; Calc. c.; Calend.; Cham.; Cistus; Clem.; Iod.; *Kali bich.;* Kali m.; Lyc.; Mag. p.; Merc. cy.; *Merc. i. r.;* Merc. s.; Nat. m.; Petrol.; Pinus sylv.; Phyt.; *Rhus t.;* Sil.; Staph.; Sul.; Trifol.; Trifol. r.

Thyroid (Goitre, bronchocele)—Adren.; Am. c.; Am. m.; Apis; Aur. sul.; Bad.; Bar. iod.; *Bell.; Brom.; Calc. c.;* Calc. fl.; Calc. iod.; Caust.; Chrom. s.; Cistus; *Crot. casc.;* Ferr. m.; *Fluor. ac.; Fucus;* Glon.; Hep.; **Hydr.;** Hydroc. ac.; *Iod.; Iodothyr.; Iris;* Kali c.; *Kali iod.; Lapis* *alb.;* Mag. p.; Merc. i. fl.; *Nat. m.;* Phos.; Ph*y*t.;   Pineal gl. ext.; Puls.; Sil.; *Spong.;* Sul.; *Thyr.*

Thyroid—(EXOPHTHALMIC GOITRE—Basedow's disease)—Amyl; Ars.; Ars. iod.; Aur.; Bad.; Bar. c.; *Bell.;* Brom.; *Cact.; Calc. c.;* Can. ind.; Chrom. s.; Colch.; Con.; Echin.; Ephedra; Ferr. iod.; *Ferr. m.;* Ferr. p.; *Fluor. ac.;* Fucus; *Glon.; Iod.;* Jabor.; *Lycop.;* Nat. m.; *Piloc.;* Spart. s.; Spong.; Stram.; *Thyr.*

Paroxysm—Cact.; Dig.; Glon.; Samb.

GRANULATIONS—Exuberant: Calend.; Nit. ac.; Sab.; *Sil.;* Thuya. See Ulcers.

GREASE—In horse: Thuya.

HEMOPHILIA—Small wounds, bleed profusely, or protractedly: *Adren.;* Ail.; Ars.; Bov.; Calc. lact.; Cinch.; *Crot.;* Ferr. m.; *Ham.;* Kreos.; *Lach.;* Merc.; Millef.; *Nat. sil.;* Phos.; *Sec.;* Tereb.

HEMORRHAGES—Acal.; *Acet. ac.; Achillea; Acon.; Adren.;* Alumen; Alum.; Anthrac.; *Arn.;* Ars. hyd.; Bell.; Bothrops; *Bov.; Cact.;* Canth.; Carbo v.; Chin. s.; *Cinch.; Cinnam.;* Croc.; *Crot.;* Dig.; Elaps; Erech.; Ergotin; *Erig.;* Ferr. m.; *Ferr. p.;* Ficus; Gall. ac.; Gelatin; *Geran.; Ham.; Hydrastin; Ipec.;* Kali c.; Kreos.; Lach.; Meli.; Merc. cy.; *Millef.;* Mur. ac.; Nat. sil.; *Nit. ac.;* Op.; *Phos.;* Puls.; *Sab.;* Sanguis.; *Sec.; Sul. ac.;* Sul.; *Tereb.;* Thlaspi; Tilia; *Trill.;* Ustil.; Ver. a.; Xanth.

Hemorrhage, chronic effects—Stront. c.

Hemorrhage, from traumatism—Aran.; *Arn.;* Bov.; Euphorb. pil.; Ham.; *Millef.;* Trill.

Hemorrhage, hysterical (hemosialemesis)—Bad.; Croc.; Hyos.; Ign.; Kali iod.; Merc. s.; Sticta; Sul.

Hemorrhage, with face intensely red, preceding—Meli.

Hemorrhage, with fainting tinnitus, loss of sight, general coldness, even convulsions—*Cinch.;* Ferr. m.; Phos.

Hemorrhage, with no mental anxiety—Ham.

Hemorrhage, with putrescence; tingling in limbs; debility—Sec.

Hemorrhage, without fever or pain—Millef.

Blood, bright red—*Acon.;* Bell.: Erech.; *Erig.;* Ferr. m.; *Ferr. p.; Ipec.;* Led.; *Millef.;* Nit. ac.; Phos.; Phos.; Sab.; *Trill.;* Ustil.

Blood, clotted, partly fluid—Erig.; Ferr.; Plat.; Puls.; Ratanh.; *Sab.;* Ustil.

Blood, dark, clotted—Alum.; Anthrac.; Cinch.; *Croc.;* Crot.; *Elaps;* Merc. cy.; Merc.; Mur. ac.; Plat.; *Sul. ac.;* Tereb.; *Thlaspi;* Trill.

Blood, decomposes rapidly—Acet. ac.; Am. c.; Anthrac.; *Crot.;* Lach.; Tereb.

Non-coagulable; intermittent—Phos.

Non-coagulable, thin, dark—*Crot.;* Elaps; *Lach.; Sec.;* Sul. ac.

Thin, pale, fluid—Ferr.; Tilia.

Venous, dark, clotted—Ham.; Mangif. ind.

Vicarious—Acet. ac.; Ham.

HODGKIN'S DISEASE (pseudo-leukemia)—Acon. lyc.; Acon.; *Ars.; Ars.*

iod.; Bar. iod.; Calc. fl.; Ferr. picr.; *Iod.;* Kali m.; Nat. m.; Phos.; Scrophul.

HOOK-WORM DISEASE—Carbon. tetrachl.; Chenop.; Thymol.

INFLAMMATIONS—Abrot.; *Acon.; Agrost.;* Apis; Arn.; Ars.; *Bell.; Bry.;* Canth.; Chel.; Cinch.; *Ferr. p.;* Hep.; *Iod.;* Kali bich.; Kali c.; Kali iod.; Kali m.; Kali s.; *Nat. nit.; Spiranth.;* Sul.; *Ver. v.;* Vib. op.

Inflammation, passive—*Dig.; Gels.;* Puls.; Sul.

Inflammation, surgical—Acon.; *Anthrac.;* Arn.; Ars.; Ars. iod.; *Bell.;* Bellis; Calend.; Calc. s.; Echin.; Gun powder; *Hep.;* Hyper.; Iod.; Merc. c.; Merc. i. r.; Myrtis. s.; *Pyr.;* Rhus t.; *Sil.* See Pyemia.

Inflammation, to favor absorption—Ant. t.; Apis; *Kali iod.;* Kali m.; Lyc.; Phos.; Sul.

INJURIES (traumatisms)—Acet. ac.; Acon.; Angust.; *Arn.; Bellis;* Bufo; *Calend.; Cic.;* Crot. t.; Euphras.; Glon.; *Ham.; Hyper.; Led.;* Mag. c.; Millef.; Nat. s.; Physost.; *Rhus t.;* Ruta; Stont. c.; Sul. ac.; Verb.

Bruises, contusions—Acet. ac.; *Arn.;* Bellis; *Con.;* Echin.; Euphras.; *Ham.; Hyper.;* Led.; *Rhus t.; Ruta;* Sul. ac.; *Symphyt.;* Verb.

Bruises, of bone—Arn.; Calc. p.; *Ruta; Symphyt.*

Bruises, of breast—Bellis; *Con.*

Bruises, of eye—Acon.; *Arn.;* Ham.; *Led.; Symphyt.*

Bruises, of parts, rich in sentient nerves—Bellis; *Hyper.*

Bruises, with persistence of ecchymosis—Arn.; Led.; *Sul. ac.*

Burns, scalds—Acet. ac.; Acon.; Arn.; *Ars.;* Calc. s.; Calend.; Camph.; *Canth.;* Carb. ac.; *Caust.;* Gaulth.; Grind.; Ham.; *Hep.;* Jabor.; *Kali bich.;* Kreos.; Petrol.; Rhus t.; Tereb.; *Urt.*

Burns, fail to heal, or ill effects—Carbo ac.; Caust.

Chronic effects of injuries—*Arn.;* Carbo v.; Cic.; *Con.;* Glon.; Ham.; Hyper.; Led.; *Nat. s.; Stront. c.*

Mental symptoms, from injuries—Cic.; *Glon.;* Hyper.; Mag. c.; *Nat. s.*

Post-operative disorders—Acet. ac.; Apis; *Arn.; Bellis;* Berb. v.; *Calend.;* Calc. fl.; Camph.; Croc.; Ferr. p.; *Hyper.;* Kali s.; Millef.; Naja; Nit. ac.; Raph.; Rhus t.; *Staph.;* Stront.; Ver. a.

Prostration, from injuries—*Acet. ac.;* Camph.; Hyper.; *Sul. ac.;* Ver. a.

Sprains, strains—Acet. ac.; *Acon.;* Agn.; *Arn.;* Bell.; *Bellis; Calc. c.;* Calc. fl.; Calend.; *Carbo an.;* Formica; *Hyper.;* Millef.; Nux v.; Rhod.; *Rhus t.; Ruta;* Stront.; *Symphyt.*

Sprains, tendency to—Nat. c.; Nat. m.; Psor.; *Sil.*

Tetanus prevented—Hyper.; Physost.

Wounds, bleed profusely—Arn.; *Crot.;* Ham.; Kreos.; *Lach.;* Millef.; Phos. ac.

Wounds, bleed profusely, after a fall—*Arn.;* Ham.; Millef.

Wounds, bluish, discolored—*Lach.;* Lyssin.

Wounds, bullet, from—Arn.; Calend.

Wounds, contused—*Arn.;* Ham.; Sul. ac.; Symphyt.

Wounds, dissecting, post-mortem—*Anthrac.; Apis; Ars.;* Crot.; *Echin.; Lach.; Pyr.* See Pyemia.

Wounds, incised—Arn.; Calend.; Ham.; Hyper.; Led.; *Staph.*

Wounds, involving muscles, tendons, joints—Calend.

Wounds, lacerated—Arn.; *Calend.;* Carb. ac.; Ham.; Led.; *Hyper.;* Staph.; Sul. ac.; Symphyt.

Wounds, punctured—Apis; Hyper.; *Led.;* Phaseol.

Wounds, with burning, cutting, shooting—Nat. c.

Wounds, with gangrenous tendency—Calend.; Sal. ac.; Sul. ac. See Dissecting.

LEUCOCYTHEMIA—leukemia: Aran.; *Ars.; Ars. iod.;* Bar. iod.; Benzol.; Bry.; Calc. c.; Ceanoth.; Chin. s.; Con.; *Ferr. picr.;* Ipec.; Merc.; *Nat. m.;* Nat. s.; Nux v.; Phos.; *Picr. ac.; Thuya.* See Anemia.

Leucocythemia, splenic—*Ceanoth.;* Nat. s.; Querc.; Succin.

LYMPHANGITIS—Anthrac.; *Apis;* Ars. iod.; *Bell.;* Bothrops; Bufo; Crot.; Echin.; Hippoz.; *Lach.;* Latrod. k.; Merc. i. r.; *Merc. s.;* Myg.; Pyr.; *Rhus t.*

MARASMUS (emaciation, atrophy, wasting)—*Abrot.; Acet. ac.;* Ant. iod.; Arg. m.; *Arg. n.; Ars.;* Ars. iod.; *Bar. c.; Calc. c.; Calc. p.; Calc. sil.;* Carbo an.; Carbo v.; Caust.; Cetrar.; Cinch.; Clem.; Ferr. m.; *Ferr. p.;* Fluor. ac.; Glycerin; Helon.; *Hep.; Hydr.; Iod.;* Kali iod.; Kali p.; Kreos.; Led.; *Lyc.;* Mang. ac.; *Merc. c.;* Merc. s.; Nat. c.; *Nat. m.; Ol. j. as.;* Op.; *Phos. ac.;* Phos.; Phyt.; *Plumb. ac.;* Plumb. iod.; *Plumb. m.;* Psor.; Ricin.; Rhus t.; *Samb.; Sanic.; Sars.;* Sec.; Selen.; *Sil.;* Stann.; Staph.; *Sul.; Syph.;* Tereb.; *Thuya; Tub.;* Uran.: Vanad.; *Ver. a.;* Zinc. m.

Affected parts, atrophy—Ars.; *Caust.;* Graph.; Led.; Selen.

Atrophy of children—*Abrot.;* Arg. n.; *Ars.;* Ars. sul.; Bac.; Bar. c.; *Calc. p.; Calc. sil.; Iod.; Nat. m.; Ol. j. as.;* Phos.; Pod.; Psor.; Sanic.; Sars.; *Sul.;* Thyr.; Tub.

Atrophy of face, hands, legs, feet, single parts—Selen.

Atrophy of legs—*Abrot.; Am. m.; Arg. n.; Iod.;* Pinus sylv.; Sanic.; Tub.

Atrophy of mesenteric glands (tabes mesenterica)—Ars.; Bapt.; Bar. c.; Calc. ars.; *Calc. c.;* Calc. chlor.; Calc. hypophos.; Calc. iod.; *Calc. p.;* Con.; Hep.; *Iod.;* Merc. c.; Plumb. ac.; Sacchar. of.; Sil.

Atrophy of neck, flabby, loose skin—Abrot.; Calc. p.; Iod.; *Nat. m.; Sanic.;* Sars.

Atrophy, from above, downwards—Lyc.; Nat. m.

Atrophy, from below upwards—Abrot.

Atrophy, neck so weak, unable to hold head up—*Abrot.;* Æth.; Calc. p.

Atrophy, progressive, muscular—Ars.; Carbon. s.; Hyper.; Kali hypoph.; *Phos.;* Physost.; *Plumb.;* Sec.

Atrophy, rapid—Iod.; Plumb. m.; Samb.; *Thuya; Tub.*

Atrophy, rapid, with cold sweat, debility—Ars.; *Tub.; Ver. a.*

Atrophy, with bulimia—*Abrot.;* Acet. ac.; Ars. iod.; Bar. c.; Calc. c.; Con.; *Iod.; Nat. m.;* Sanic.; Tub.; Thyr.

Atrophy, with shrivelled up look—Abrot.; *Arg. n.;* Fluor. ac.; Kreos.; Op.; Sanic.; Sars.; Sil.; *Sul.*

MUSCLES—Inflammation (myositis): Arn.; Bell.; Bry.; Hep.; Kali iod.; Merc. s.; *Mez.; Rhus t.*

Muscles, pain (myalgia)—*Acon.;* Ant. t.; *Arn.;* Ars.; Bell.; Bellis; Bry.;

Carbon. s.; Caust.; *Cim.*; Colch.; *Dulc.*; *Gels.*; Led.; *Marcot.*; Merc.;
Morph.; Nux v.; *Ran. b.*; *Rham. cal.*; *Rhus t.*; *Ruta*; Sal. ac.; Stram.;
Strych.; Val.; *Ver. a.*; Ver. v. See Rheumatism (Locomotor System).

Muscles, pain cramp-like—Ant. t.; Cholas ter.; *Cim.*; Colch.; Col.; *Cupr.
m.*; *Mag. p.*; Nux v.; Op.; Plumb. ac.; Sec.; *Sul.*; Syph.; Ver. a.

Muscles, pain, hysterical—Ign.; Nux v.; Plumb.; Puls.

Muscles, soreness, stiffness—Angust.; *Arn.*; Bad.; *Bapt.*; Bell.; *Bellis;
Bry.*; Caust.; Cic.; *Cim.*; Cupr. ac.; *Gels.*; Guaiac.; Ham.; *Helon.*;
Jacar.; *Magnol.*; Merc.; Myr.; *Phyt.*; Pyr.; *Rhus t.*; *Ruta*; Sang.

Muscles, twitchings—Acon.; *Agar.*; Angust.; Apis; Ars.; Asaf.; Atrop.;
Bell.; Bry.; Caust.; *Cham.*; Cic.; *Cim.*; Cina; *Cocc.*; Cod.; *Col.*;
Croc.; *Cupr. m.*; Ferr. red.; Gels.; Helleb.; *Hyos.*; *Ign.*; Kali br.;
Kali c.; Lupul.; Mez.; *Morph.*; *Myg.*; *Nux v.*; Op.; Phos.; Physost.;
Plumb. ac.; Puls.; *Santon.*; Sec.; Spig.; *Stram.*; *Strych.*; Tar. h.;
Ver. v.; *Zinc. m.*; Zizia.

Muscles, weakness, debility—Acet. ac.; *Alet.*; *Alumen*; Alum.; Am.
caust.; Anhal.; *Ant. t.*; Arg. n.; Ars.; Bry.; Calc. c.; Carbo v.; Caust.;
Colch.; Collin.; *Con.*; *Gels.*; *Helleb.*; Helon.; Hep.; Hydr.; Ign.;
Kali c.; Kali hypophos.; *Kali p.*; Kal.; Lob. infl.; Mag. p.; Merc. v.;
Mur. ac.; Nux v.; Onosm.; Pall.; Physal.; Physost.; *Picr. ac.*; Plumb.
ac.; Rhus t.; Sabad.; *Sarcol. ac.*; Sil.; *Strych.*; Tab.; *Ver. a.*; *Ver. v.*;
Zinc. m. See Adynamia (Nervous System).

MUTINISM of childhood—Agraph.

MYXEDEMA—Ars.; Prim. ob.; *Thyr.*

OBESITY (adiposis, corpulence)—*Am. br.*; Am. c.; Ant. c.; Ars.; *Calc. ars.;
Calc. c.*; *Calop.*; Caps.; Col.; *Fucus*; Graph.; *Iodothyr.*; Kali br.; Kali
c.; Lac d.; Mang. ac.; *Phos.*; *Phyt.*; Sabal; *Thyr.*; Tussil. fr.

Obesity, in children—*Ant. c.*; Bar. c.; *Calc. c.*; *Caps.*; *Ferr. m.*; Kali
bich.; Sacchar. of.

POLYCYTHEMIA—Phos.

PROPHYLACTICS—Catheter fever: Camph. ac.

Cholera—Ars.; Cupr. ac.; Ver. a.

Diphtheria—Apis (30); Diph. (30).

Erysipelas—Graph. (30).

Hay fever—Ars.; Psor.

Hydrophobia—Bell.; Canth.; Hyos.; Stram.

Intermittent fever—Ars.; Chin. s.

Measles—*Acon.*; Ars.; Puls.

Mumps—Trifol. rep.

Pus infection—Arn.

Quinsy—Bar. c. (30).

Scarlet fever—Bell. (30); Eucal.

Variola—Ant. t.; Hydr.; Kali cy.; *Malandr.*; Thuya; *Vaccin.*; Variol.

Whooping cough—Dros.; Vaccin.

PYEMIA, SEPTICEMIA—*Acon.*; *Anthrac.*; Apium v.; *Arn.*; *Ars.*; *Ars.*
iod.; Atrop.; *Bapt.*; Bell.; Bothrops; *Bry.*; Calend.; *Carb. ac.*; *Chin.
ars.*; *Chin. s.*; Crot.; *Echin.*; Gun powder; Hippoz.; *Hyos.*; Irid.;
Lach.; Latrod. has.; Merc. cy.; Merc. s.; Methyl. bl.; Mur. ac.; Nat.

sul. carb.; *Pyr.*; *Rhus t.*; *Sec.*; Sepsin; Sil.; Streptococcin; Tar. c.; Ver. a.

RACHITIS (rickets)—*Ars.*; Ars. iod.; Calc. ac.; *Calc. c.*; Calc. hypoph.; *Calc. p.*; Calc. sil.; Ferr. p.; Fluor. ac.; Hekla; Hep.; *Iod.*; Kali iod.; Mag. m.; Med.; Merc. s.; Nit. ac.; *Phos. ac.*; *Phos.*; Pinus sylv.; Sanic.; *Sil.*; Sul.; Supraren. ext.; Ther.; Thuya; Thyr.; *Tub.* See Scrofulosis.

SCROFULOSIS—*Æthiops;* Alnus; Alum.; Ars.; *Ars. iod.*; *Aurums;* Bac.; Bad.; *Barytas;* Brom.; *Calcareas;* Caps.; Carbo an.; *Caust.*; Cinnab.; Cistus; Clem.; Con.; Diph.; *Dulc.;* *Ferrums;* Fluor. ac.; *Graph.*; Helleb.; *Hep.*; Hydr.; *Iodides;* Iodof.; Kali bich.; Kali iod.; Kreos.; Lapis alb.; Lyc.; Mag. m.; *Mercuries;* Mez.; Nit. ac.; Ol. j. as.; Petrol.; Phos. ac.; Phos.; *Pinus sylv.*; Plumb. iod.; Psor.; Ruta; Samb.; Sedum; *Sil.*; Sil. mar.; Still.; *Sul.*; Ther.; *Tub.*; Viola tr.

SCURVY (scorbutus)—Acet. ac.; *Agave;* Alnus; *Ars.*; Bov.; Carbo v.; Chin. s.; Cinch.; *Ferr. p.*; Galium ap.; Ham.; Kali chlor.; Kali p.; Kreos.; Lach.; *Merc. s.*; *Mur. ac.*; Nat. m.; Nit. ac.; Nitro. mur. ac.; Phos. ac.; *Phos.*; Rhus t.; Staph.; Sul. ac.; Sul.; Urium.

SENILE DECAY—*Agn.*; *Arg. n.*; Ars.; *Bar. c.*; Can. ind.; *Con.*; Fluor. ac.; Iod.; *Lyc.*; *Oophor.*; Phos.; Thiosin.

SENSATION, of burning—*Acon.*; Agar.; Agrost.; Anthrac.; *Apis;* Ars.; Bell.; *Calad.;* *Canth.*; Caps.; Carbo an.; *Caust.*; *Cepa;* Cham.; *Doryph.;* Eosin; Kreos.; Ol. an.; Phos. ac.; *Phos.*; Pip. m.; Pop. c.; Rhus t.; *Sang.*; Sec.; *Sul.*; Tar. h.

Sensation, of constriction—Alum. sil.; *Anac.*; Asar.; *Cact.*; Caps.; *Carb. ac.*; Col.; Iod.; Lach.; Mag. p.; Naja; Nat. m.; *Nit. ac.*; Plumb. m.; Sec.; *Sul.*

Sensation, of numbness—*Acon.*; Agar.; Alum. sil.; *Ambra;* Ars.; Bov.; *Calc. p.;* *Ced.;* *Cham.;* Cic.; *Cocaine,* Cod.; *Con.*; Helod.; Ign.; Irid.; Kali br.; Nux v.; *Oleand.*; Onosm.; Ox. ac.; *Phos.*; *Plat.*; Plumb.; Raph.; *Rhus t.*; Sec.; Stann.; Thallium.

Sensation, of numbness, attending pains—*Acon.*; Can. ind.; *Cham.*; C3n.; *Kal.*; *Plat.*; *Rhus t.*; Stann.; Staph.

Sensation, of stitching—Acon.; *Asclep.*; *Bry.*; *Kali c.*; Mag. p.; Nat. s.; Nit. ac.; *Ran. b.*; Rumex; Scilla.

TUMORS—Ananth.; Aur. m. n.; *Bar. c.*; Bar. iod.; Bar. m.; Bellis; Calc. ars.; *Calc. c.;* *Calc. fl.*; *Cistus;* Col.; *Con.*; Eucal.; *Ferr. iod.*; Ferr. picr.; Form. ac.; Galium ap.; *Graph.*; *Hekla;* Hydr.; *Kali br.*; Kali iod.; Kreos.; Lach.; *Lapis alb.*; *Lob. erin.*; Lyc.; Malandr.; Mancin.; Med.; Merc. i. r.; Merc. per.; Nat. cacodyl.; Nat. sil.; *Phos.*; Phyt.; *Plumb. iod.*; Psor.; *Semperv. t.*; *Sil.*; Thiosin.; *Thuya;* *Thyr.*; Urea; *Uric ac.* See Cancer.

Cystic—Apis; *Bar. c.*; Calc. c.; Calc. p.; Calc. s.; *Iod.*; *Kali br.*; Platanus; Sil.; Staph. See Scalp (Head); Skin.

Bone-like, protuberances—*Calc. fl.*; *Hekla;* Lapis alb.; Malandr.; Ruta; Sil.

Enchondroma—Calc. fl.; Lapis alb.; Sil.

Epithelial—Acet. ac.; Ferr. picr. See Skin.

Epulis—Calc. c.; Plumb. ac.; *Thuya.*

Erectile—Lyc.; *Phos.*

Fibroid—*Calc. iod.;* Calc. s.; Chrom. s.; Graph.; Hydrast. m.; *Kali iod.;* Lapis alb.; Sec.; *Sil.;* Thiosin.; Thyr. See Uterus.

Fibroid, hemorrhage—*Hydrast. m.;* Lapis alb.; Sab.; Thlaspi; *Trill.;* Ustil.

Fungoid—Clem.; Mancin.; Phos.; *Thuya.*

Ganglion—Benz. ac.; Kali m.; *Ruta; Sil.*

Lipoma—*Bar. c.;* Calc. ars.; Calc. c.; Lapis alb.; Phyt.; *Thuya;* Uric ac.

Naevus on right temple, flat; in children—Fluor. ac.

Neuroma—Calend.; Cepa.

Nodulated, of tongue—Galium ap.

Papillomata—Ant. c.; Nit. ac.; Staph.; *Thuya.*

Polypi—*Calc. c.;* Cepa; *Formica;* Kali bich.; Kali s.; Lemna; Nit. ac.; *Phos.;* Psor.; Sang.; *Sang. n.;* Sil.; Teucr.; *Thuya.* See Nose, Ear, Uterus.

Ranula—Ambra; Thuya.

Sarcocele—Merc. i. r. See Male Sexual System.

Tumors of urinary passages—Analinum.

Vascular in urethra—Can. s.; *Eucal.*

Wen—Bar. c.; Benz. ac.; Calc. c.; Con.; Daphne; Graph.; Hep.; **Kali c.: Mez.**

MODALITIES

AGGRAVATION—Acids:—*Ant. c.;* Ant. t.; Ferr. m.; Lach.; Merc. c.; **Nux** v.; Phos.; *Sep.* See Stomach.

Afternoon—Æsc.; Alum.; Am. m.; Ars.; *Bell.;* Cenchris; Cocc.; Coccus; Fagop.; Kali bich.; Kali c.; Kali cy.; Kali n.; Lil. t.; Lob. infl.; *Rhus t.;* Sep.; Sil.; Still.; *Thuya;* Verbasc.; Xerophyl.; X-ray.

Afternoon, late—*Apis;* Aran.; Carbo v.; Colch.; *Col.; Helleb.; Lyc.;* Mag. p.; Med.; Meli.; Ol. an.; *Puls.;* Sabad.; Zinc. See Evening.

Air cold, dry—Abrot.; *Acon.;* Æsc.; Agar.; Alum.; *Ars.; Asar.;* Aur. m.; Bac.; *Bar. c.;* Bell.; *Bry.;* Calc. c.; *Camph.;* Caps.; Carbo an.; *Caust.; Cham.; Cinch.; Cistus;* Cupr. m.; Cur.; Euphorb. d.; *Hep.;* Ign.; *Kali c.;* Mag. p.; *Mez.;* Nat. c.; *Nux v.;* Plumb.; *Psor.; Rhod.; Rumex;* Selen.; Sep.; *Sil.; Spong.;* Tub.; Urt.; Viola od.; Viscum.

Air, open—*Acon.;* Agar.; Benz. ac.; Bry.; Cadm. s.; *Caps.;* Carbon. s.; *Cham.;* Cic.; Cocc.; Coff.; Coral.; Crot.; *Cycl.;* Epiph.; Euphras.; Ign.; Kal.; Kreos.; Linar.; Mosch.; *Nux v.;* Ran. b.; *Senega;* Solan. lyc.; Thea; X-ray. See Air, Cold.

Anger—*Bry.; Cham.;* Col.; Ign.; *Nux v.; Staph.* See Emotions (Mind).

Arms moved backward—Sanic.

Ascending stairs—Am. c.; *Ars.;* But. ac.; Cact.; *Calc. c.;* Can. s.; Coca' Glon.; *Kali c.;* Menyanth.; Spong.

Autumn; warm days, cold, damp nights—Merc. v.

Bathing—*Ant. c.;* Bellis; Calc. c.; Caust.; Formica; Mag. p.; Nux m.; Physost.; *Rhus t.;* Sep.; *Sul.* See Water.

Bed, turning in—*Con.;* Nux v.; Puls.

Beer—Bry.; *Kali bich.;* Nux m.

Bending double—Diosc.

Bending forward—*Bell.;* Kal.; Nux v.

Biting hard—Am. c.; *Verbasc.*

Breakfast, after—Cham.; *Nux v.;* Phos.; *Thuya;* Zinc. m. See Eating.

Breakfast, before—Croc.

Bright objects—*Bell.; Canth.;* Coccinel.; *Lyssin; Stram.*

Brushing teeth—Coccus; Staph.

Celibacy—Con.

Coffee—Aster.; Can. ind.; *Canth.;* Carbo v.; Caust.; *Cham.;* Ign.; Kali c.; *Nux v.;* Psor.; Thuya.

Coitus, after—Agar.; *Calad.;* Calc. s.; *Cinch.; Kali c.;* Nux v.; *Phos. ac.;* Phos.; *Selen.;* Sep.

Cold—*Acon.;* Agar.; Alumen; *Alum.;* Am. c.; Ant. c.; *Ars.;* Bad.; *Bar. c.;* Bell.; *Bry.;* Calc. c.; *Camph.;* Caps.; *Caust.; Cham.;* Collins.; Cocc.; Coff.; Con.; Crot. casc.; *Dulc.;* Formica; *Hep.;* Ign.; *Kali c.;* Kali p.; Kreos.; Lach.; Lob. infl.; *Mag. p.;* Merc.; *Mez.;* Mosch.; Nit. ac.; Nux m.; *Nux v.;* Ran. b.; *Rhod.; Rhus t.; Rumex;* Ruta; Sabad.; Selen.; *Sep.; Sil.;* Spig.; Stram.; Stront.; Sul. ac.; Tab.; Ver. a.; Xerophyl.

Concussion—Cic. See **Jar.**

Consolation—Cact.; Graph.; *Helleb.*; Ign.; Lil. t.; *Nat. m.;* Sabal; *Sep.;* Sil.

Contact, of clothing, about neck—Glon.; *Lach.;* Sep. See Touch.

Conversation—Ambra; Cocc.; *Phos. ac.; Stann.* See Talking.

Cough—Ars.; Bry.; *Cina;* Hyos.; *Phos.;* Sep.; *Tellur.* See Respiratory System.

Damp living houses—Ant. t.; *Aran.;* Ars.; *Dulc.; Nat. s.;* Tereb.

Dampness—Amphis; *Aran.; Ars. iod.;* Aster.; Bar. c.; *Calc. c.;* Calend.; Carbo v.; Chimaph.; Chin. s.; Cinch.; *Colch.;* Crot.; Cur.; *Dulc.;* Elat.; Euphras.; Formica; Gels.; Kali iod.; Lathyr.; Lemna; Magnol.; Meli.; Mur. ac.; *Nat. s.;* Nux m.; *Petrol.; Phyt.;* Radium; Rhod.; *Rhus t.;* Ruta; Sep.; Sil.; Still.; Sul.; Tub.

Dampness, cold—Am. c.; Ant. t.; Aran.; Arn.; Asclep. t.; Aster.; Bor.; *Calc. c.; Calc. p.; Dulc.;* Gels.; *Guaiac.;* Mang. ac.; *Merc.;* Nux m.; Nux v.; Physal.; Phyt.; *Rhus t.;* Sil.; Thuya; Urt.; Ver. a.

Dampness, warm—Bapt.; Brom.; Carbo v.; Carbon. s.; *Gels.;* Ham.; Phos.; Sep.

Dark—*Ars.;*' Calc. c.; Carbo an.; Phos.; *Stram.* See Emotions (Mind).

Daylight to sunset—Med.

Defecation, after—Æsc. See Stool (Abdomen).

Dentition—Æth.; *Bell.;* Bor.; Calc. c.; Calc. p.; Cham.; *Kreos.;* Phyt.; *Pod.; Rheum;* Zinc. m. See Teeth.

Dinner, after—Ars.; *Nux v.* See Stomach.

Direction, diagonally—*Agar.;* Bothrops.

Direction, diagonally, upper left, lower right—Agar.; Ant. t.; Stram.

Direction, diagonally, upper right, lower left—Ambra; Brom.; Med.; Phos.; Sul. ac.

Direction, downward—*Bor.;* Cact.; Kal.; Lyc.; *Sanic.*

Direction, outwards—Kali c.; *Sul.*

Direction, upwards—Benzin.; Eup. perf.; *Led.*

Drinking, during—Bell.

Eating—Abies n.; Æsc.; Æth.; Agar.; *Aloe;* Ant. c.; *Arg. n.; Ars.;* Bry.; *Calc. c.; Carbo v.;* Caust.; Chionanth.; Cina; *Cinch.;* Cocc.; Col.; Con.; *Crot. t.;* Dig.; *Graph.;* Hyos.; Ign.; *Ipec.;* Kali bich.; *Kali c.;* Kali p.; Kreos.; Lach.; *Lyc.;* Mag. m.; Nat. m.; Nit. ac.; *Nux v.;* Ol. an.; Petrol.; Phos.; *Puls.;* Rheum; Rumex; Samb.; *Sep.;* Sil.; *Staph.;* Strych.; Sul.; Thea; Zinc. m. See Indigestion (Stomach).

Emotional excitement—Acon.; *Ambra; Arg. n.;* Aur.; Cinch.; Cob.; *Coff.; Colch.;* Collins.; Col.; Con.; Cupr. ac.; *Gels.; Hyos.; Ign.;* Kali p.; Lyssin; Nit. sp. d.; *Nux v.;* Petrol.; Phos. ac.; *Phos.;* Sil.; *Staph.* See Mind.

Erratic, shifting, constantly changing, symptoms—Apis; Berb. v.; *Ign.; Kali bich.; Kali s.; Lac c.;* Lil. t.; *Mang. ac.;* Paraf.; Phyt.; *Puls.;* Sanic.; *Tub.*

Evening—*Acon.;* Alfal.; *Ambra;* Am. br.; Am. m.; Apis.; Ant. t.; Arn.; *Bell.;* Bry.; Cajup.; Carbo v.; Caust.; *Cepa;* Cham.; Colch.; Crot.; *Cycl.;* Diosc.; Euonym.; Euphras.; Ferr. p.; *Helleb.; Hyos.; Lyc.;* Kali s.; Merc. c.; *Merc.;* Mez.; Nit. ac.; *Phos.;* Plat.; Plumb.; *Puls.;* Ran. b.;

Rumex; Ruta; *Sep.;* Sil.; Stann.; Sul. ac.; *Syph.;* Tab.; Vib. op.; X-ray; Zinc. m.

Eyes, closing—Bry.; Sep.; Ther.

Eyes, motion of—*Bry.;* Nux v.; Spig.

Eyes, opening of—Tab.

Fasting—Croc.; Iod.

Fats—Carbo v.; *Cycl.;* Kali m.; *Puls.;* Thuya.

Feet, exposure—Con.; Cupr.; *Sil.*

Feet hanging down—Puls.

Fish—Nat. s.; Urt.

Fog—Bapt.; Gels.; Hyper. See Dampness.

Fright—*Acon.;* Gels.; *Ign.;* Op.; Ver. a.

Fruit—*Ars.;* Bry.; *Cinch.; Col.;* Ipec.; Samb.; *Ver. a.*

Gaslight—Glon.; Nat. c.

Grief—Aur.; Gels.; *Ign.; Phos. ac.;* Staph.; Ver. a. See Emotions (Mind).

Hair-cut—Acon.; *Bell.;* Glon.

Head, uncovering—Bell.; Sil. See Air, Cold.

High altitudes—Coca.

Hot drinks—Chionanth.; Lach.; Stann.

Inspiration—*Acon.; Bry.;* Phos.; Ran. b.; Spig. See Respiratory System.

Intermittently—Anac.; *Cinch.;* Strych. See Periodical.

Jar—Arn.; *Bell.;* Berb. v.; *Bry.; Cic.;* Crot.; Glon.; Ign.; Nux v.; *Spig.;* Ther.

Laughing—Arg. m.; *Dros.;* Mang. ac.; *Phos.;* Stann.; Tellur.

Laundry work—Sep.

Left side—Agar.; Arg. m.; Arg. n.; Asaf.; Aster.; *Bellis; Ceanoth.;* Chimaph.; Cim.; Colch.; Cupr. m.; Erig.; *Lach.;* Lepid.; *Lil. t.; Ox. ac.;* Pulex; Rumex; Sapon.; Sep.; Ther.; *Thuya;* Ustil.

Left side, then right side—Lac c.; *Lach.*

Light—Acon.; *Bell.;* Calc. c.; Coca; *Con.;* Colch.; Graph.; Ign.; *Lyssin; Nux v.; Phos.;* Spig.; *Stram.*

Liquors—*Agar.;* Ant. c.; *Can. ind.; Carbo v.;* Cim.; *Lach.;* Led.; *Nux v.;* Ran. b.; Stram.; *Sul. ac.; Zinc. m.* See Alcoholism (Nervous System).

Localized spots—Coff.; *Ign.; Kali bich.;* Lil. t.; Ox. ac.

Looking, downwards—Acon.; *Kal.;* Oleand.; *Spig.;* Sul.

Looking, intently, at objects—Cina; Croc.

Looking upwards—Benzoin; Calc. c.; *Puls.;* Sul.

Lower half of body—Bac. t.

Lying down—Ambra; Ant. t.; Arn.; *Ars.;* Arum; Aur.; *Bell.;* Can. s.; Caust.; Cenchris; *Con.;* Croc.; *Diosc.;* Dros.; Dulc.; *Glon.; Hyos.;* Iberis; Ipec.; Kreos.; *Lach.;* Lyc.; Menyanth.; Nat. m.; Nat. s.; Plat.; *Phos.; Puls.; Rhus t.; Rumex;* Ruta; Samb.; Sil.; Tarax.; *Trifol.;* X-ray.

Lying, on back—Acet. ac.; *Nux v.;* Puls.; Rhus t.

Lying, on left side—Arg. n.; *Cact.;* Calad.; Coccus; Iberis; *Kali c.;* Lyc.; Magnol.; *Phos.;* Plat.; *Ptel.;* Puls.; *Spig.;* Viscum.

Lying, on painful, or affected side—Acon.; Ars.; *Bar. c.;* Calad.; *Hep.; Iod.; Kali c.; Nux m.: Phos.;* Ruta; Sil.; Tellur.; Vib. op.

Lying, on painless side—*Bry.;* Cham.; Col.; Ptel.; *Puls.*

Lying, on right side—Can. ind.; *Mag. m.; Merc.; Rhus t.;* Scroph; Stann.

Lying, with head low—Ars.

Masturbation—Calc. c.; *Cinch.;* Con.; *Nux v.; Phos. ac.;* Sep.; *Staph.*

Medicines, patent, aromatic, bitter vegetable pills—Nux v.

Menses, after—Alum.; *Bor.; Graph.;* Kreos.; Lil. t.; Nat. m.; Nux v.; *Sep.; Zinc. m.*

Menses, at beginning, and close—Lach.

Menses, before—Am. c.; *Bov.; Calc. c.;* Cocc.; Con.; Cupr. m.; *Gels.; Lach.;* Lyc.; Mag. m.; *Puls.;* Sars.; *Sep.;* Ver. a.; *Zinc. m.*

Menses, during—Am. c.; Arg. n.; *Bell.;* Bov.; Cham.; *Cim.;* Con.; *Graph.;* Ham.; Hyos.; *Kali c.;* Mag. c.; *Nux v.; Puls.; Sep.;* Sil.; Sul.; Ver. a.; *Vib. op.* See Menstruation (Female Sexual System).

Mental exertion—Agar.; Aloe; Amyl; *Anac.; Arg. n.;* Aur. m.; Calc. c.; Calc. p.; *Cim.; Cocc.;* Cupr. m.; *Gels.;* Ign.; Kali p.; *Nat. c.;* Nat. m.; *Nux v.; Phos.;* Phos. ac.; *Picr. ac.;* Sabad.; Sep.; *Sil.;* Thymol. See Mind.

Midnight, after—Apis; *Ars.;* Bell.; Carbo an.; *Dros.;* Ferr. m.; *Kali c.;* Kali n.; Nit. ac.; *Nux v.;* Phos.; *Pod.;* Rhus t.; Sil.; Thuya.

Midnight, at—Aran.; *Ars.;* Mez.

Midnight, before—Arg. n.; Brom.; Carbo v.; Cham.; *Coff.;* Led.; Lyc.; *Merc.;* Mur. ac.; Nit. ac.; Phos.; *Puls.;* Ran. s.; *Rhus t.; Rumex; Spong.;* Stann.

Milk—*Æth.;* Ant. t.; Calc. c.; *Carbo v.;* Cinch.; Homar.; Mag. c.; Nit. ac.; Sep.; *Sul.*

Misdeeds of others—Colch.; *Staph.*

Moon, full—*Alum.;* Calc. c.; Graph.; Sabad.; *Sil.*

Moonlight—Ant. c.; Thuya.

Moon, new—Alum.; Caust.; Clem.; *Sil.*

Morning—*Acal.;* Alum.; Ambra; *Am. m.;* Arg. n.; Aur.; *Bry.; Calc. c.;* Can. ind.; Croc.; Crot.; Fluor. ac.; Glon.; Ign.; *Kali bich.;* Kali n.; Lac c.; *Lach.;* Lil. t.; Lith. c.; Magnol.; Med.; Myg.; *Nat. m.;* Niccol.; *Nit. ac.;* Nuph.; *Nux v.;* Onosm.; *Phos.;* Phos. ac.; Pod.; *Puls.;* Rhus t.; Rumex; Sep.; Sil.; Stellar.; Strych.; *Sul.; Verbasc.*

Morning, early (2-5 A. M.)—*Æth.;* Æsc.; *Aloe;* Am. c.; Bac.; Bell.; Chel.; Cina; Coccus; Cur.; *Kali bich.; Kali c.;* Kali cy.; Kali p.; Nat. s.; *Nux v.;* Ox. ac.; *Pod.;* Ptel.; Rhod.; *Rumex; Sul.;* Thuya; Tub.

Morning, (10-11 A. M.)—Gels.; *Nat. m.; Sep.;* Sul.

Mortification from an offense—*Col.;* Lyc.; Staph.

Motion—Æsc.; Agar.; Aloe; Am. c.; Amyl; Anhal.; Apis; *Bell.; Berb. v.;* Bism.; *But. ac.;* Cact.; Cadm. s.; *Calad.;* Calc. ars.; Camph.; Ceanoth.; *Cim.;* Cinch.; *Cocc.; Colch.;* Cupr. m.; Dig.; Equis.; Ferr. p.; *Gels.;* Gettysburg Water; Guaiac.; Helon.; *Iberis;* Ipec.; Jugl. c.; Kali m.; *Kal.;* Lac c.; *Led.;* Linar.; Lob. infl.; Mag. p.; Med.; Meli.; *Merc.;* Mez.; *Nat. m.;* Nat. s.; Nit. ac.; Nux m.; *Nux v.;* Onosm.; Pall.; Petrol.; *Phyt.;* Phos.; Picr. ac.; Plat.; Plumb.; Pulex; Puls. nut.; *Ran. b.;* Rheum; Ruta; *Sab.;* Sang.; Scilla; *Sec.;* Senega; Sil.; Solan. lyc.; *Spig.;* Still.; Strych.; Sul.; Tab.; *Tar. h.;* Thea; Thymol; Ver. a.; Viscum.

Motion, downward—*Bor.;* Gels.; Sanic.

Motion, on beginning—Puls.; *Rhus t.*; Stront. c.

Mountain climbing—*Ars.*; Coca. See Ascending.

Music—*Acon.*; Ambra; Dig.; *Graph.*; *Nat. c.*; Nux v.; Pall.; Phos. ac.; *Sab.*; Sep.; *Thuya.*

Narcotics—Bell.; *Cham.*; *Coff.*; Lach.; *Nux v.*; Thuya.

Night—*Acon.*; Ant. t.; Arg. n.; Arn.; *Ars.*; Aster.; Bac.; Bell.; Bry.; But. ac.; Cajup.; Camph.; Caust.; Cenchris; *Cham.*; Chionanth.; Cina; *Cinch.*; Clem.; *Coff.*; *Colch.*; Commocl.; *Con.*; Crot. casc.; Cupr. m.; *Cycl.*; Diosc.; Dolich.; *Dulc.*; *Ferr. m.*; Ferr. p.; Gamb.; *Graph.*; Guaiac.; *Hep.*; *Hyos.*; *Iod.*; Iris; *Kali iod.*; Lach.; Lil. t.; Mag. m.; Mag. p.; Merc. c.; *Merc.*; Mez.; Nat. m.; *Nit. ac.*; Nux m.; *Phos.*; Phyt.; Plat.; Plumb.; Psor.; *Puls.*; *Rhus t.*; Rumex; Sep.; *Sil.*; Sul.; *Syph.*; Tellur.; Thea; Thuya; Ver. a.; Vib. op.; X-ray; *Zinc. m.* See Evening.

Noise—Acon.; Asar.; *Bell.*; Bor.; *Calad.*; Cham.; *Cinch.*; Cocc.; *Coff.*; *Colch.*; Ferr.; Glon.; *Ign.*; Lyc.; Mag. m.; Med.; Nux m.; *Nux v.*; Onosm.; Phos.; Solan. lyc.; *Spig.*; Tar. h.; *Ther.*

One half of body—*Cham.*; Ign.; Mez.; *Puls.*; Sil.; Spig.; Thuya; Val.

Overeating—Ant. c.; *Nux v.*; Puls. See Eating.

Overheating—*Acon.*; *Ant. c.*; *Bell.*; Brom.; *Bry.*; Calc. c.; Carbo v.; Glon.; Lyc.; Nux m.; *Nux v.*

Pastry, rich food—Carbo v.; Kali m.; *Puls.*

Peaches—Cepa; Glon.

People, presence of—Ambra.

Periodically—Alum.; *Aran.*; *Ars.*; Ars. met.; *Cact.*; Carls.; *Ced.*; Chrom. ac.; *Cinch.*; Cupr. m.; *Eup. perf.*; Ign.; Ipec.; Kali bich.; *Nat. m.*; Niccol.; Primul. ob.; Nit. ac.; Ran. s.; Sep.; Sil.; Tar. h.; *Tela ar.*; Thuya; Urt.

Periodically, every alternate day—*Alum.*; Cinch.; Fluor. ac.; Nit. ac.; Oxytrop.

Periodically, every two weeks—Niccol.

Periodically, every 2-3 weeks—Ars. met.

Periodically, every 2-4 weeks—Carls.; Ox. ac.; Sul.

Periodically, every 3 weeks—Ars.; *Mag. c.*

Periodically, every year—Ars.; Carbo v.; Crot.; *Lach.*; Niccol.; Sul.; *Thuya*; Urt.

Periodically, 4-8 P. M.—Lyc.; Sabad.

Periodically, new and full moon—Alum.

Plants, growing near water—Nat. s.

Potatoes—Alum.

Pressure—Acon.; Agar.; *Apis*; Arg. m.; Bar. c.; Bor.; Calc. c.; Cenchris; Cina; Equis.; Guaiac.; *Hep.*; Iod.; Kali c.; *Lach.*; Led.; Lyc.; *Merc. c.*; Nat. s.; *Nux v.*; Onosm.; Ov. g. p.; Phyt.; Ran. b.; Sil.; *Ther.* See Touch.

Rest—Acon.; *Arn.*; *Ars.*; Asaf.; Aur.; Calc. fl.; Caps.; Commocl.; Con.; *Cycl.*; Dulc.; Euphorb.; *Ferr. m.*; Indigo; Iris; Kali c.; Kreos., Lith. lact.; Lyc.; Mag. c.; Menyanth.; *Merc.*; Oleand.; *Puls.*; *Rhod.*; *Rhus t.*; Sabad.; *Samb.*; Senega; *Sep.*; Stront. c.; Sul.; Tar. h.; Tarax.; Val.

Riding—Arg. m.; Berb. v.; Caust.; *Cocc.*; Lyssin; Nux m.; *Petrol.*; *Sanic.*; Ther.

Right side—*Agar.*; Am. c.; Anac.; Apis; Ars.; *Bell.*; Bothrops; *Bry.*; *Caust.*; *Chel.*; Cinnab.; Con.; Crot.; Cur.; Dolich.; Equis.; Ferr. p.; Iod.; *Kali c.*; Lith. c.; *Lyc.*; *Mag. p.*; *Merc.*; Phyt.; Pod.; Rhus t.; *Sang.*; Solan. lyc.; Tar. h.; Viola od.

Rising—*Acon.*; Am. m.; Ars.; Bell.; *Bry.*; Caps.; Carbo v.; *Cocc.*; Con.; Dig.; Ferr.; Lach.; Lyc.; *Nux v.*; Phos.; *Phyt.*; Puls.; Radium; *Rhus t.*; Sul.

Room, heated—Acon.; Alum.; Ant. c.; *Apis*; Aran. sc.; Bapt.; Brom.; Bufo; *Cepa*; Crat.; *Croc.*; Euphras.; *Glon.*; Hyper.; *Iod.*; Kali iod.; *Kali s.*; Lil. t.; *Merc.*; *Puls.*; Sab.; Vib. op. See Warmth.

Scratching—Anac.; Ars.; Caps.; *Dolich.*; *Merc.*; Mez.; *Puls.*; Rhus t.; *Staph.*; *Sul.*

Sea bathing—Ars.; Limulus; Mag. m.

Seashore—*Aqua m.*; Ars.; Brom.; *Nat. m.*; *Nat. s.*; Syph.

Sedentary habits—Acon.; Aloe; Am. c.; Anac.; Arg. n.; Bry.; Con.; *Nux q.*; Sep.

Shaving, after—Caps.; *Carbo an.*; Ox. ac.; Plumb.

Sitting—Alum.; *Bry.*; Caps.; Con.; *Cycl.*; Dig.; Diosc.; Dulc.; Equis.; Euphorb.; Ferr. m.; Hydrocot.; Lyc.; Indigo; Kali c.; Nat. c.; Nux v.; Phyt.; *Plat.*; Puls.; *Rhus t.*; *Sep.*; Sul.; Tarax.; Val.

Sitting, on cold steps—Chimaph.; *Nux v.*

Sleep, after—Ambra; *Apis*; Bufo; Cadm. s.; Calc. c.; *Cocc.*; Coccus; Crat.; Epiph.; Homar.; *Lach.*; Merc. c.; Morph.; *Op.*; Parth.; Picr. ac.; Rhus t.; Selen.; *Spong.*; Stram.; Sul.; Syph.; Thasp.; Tub.; Val.

Smoking—*Abies n.*; Bor.; Can. ind.; Chin. ars.; *Cic.*; Cocc.; *Gels.*; *Ign.*; Kal.; *Lact. ac.*; Lob. infl.; *Nux v.*; Puls.; Sec.; Spig.; Spong.; *Staph.*; Stellar.

Sneezing—*Ars.*; Bry.; Kali c.; Phos.; *Sul.*; *Verbasc.* See Jar.

Snow, melting—Calc. p.

Snow storm—Con.; Formica; Merc.; Sep.; Urt.

Solitude—*Bism.*; Kali c.; Lil. t.; Lyc.; Pall.; *Stram.* See Fears (Mind).

Soup—Alum.; Kali c. See Fats.

Spices—*Nux v.*; Phos.

Spring—Ars. br.; Aur.; Calc. p.; Cepa; Crot.; Dulc.; Gels.; Kali bich.; *Lach.*; *Nat. m.*; Nat. s.; Nit. sp. d.; Rhus t.; Sars.

Standing—Æsc.; Aloe; *Berb. v.*; Calc. c.; Con.; *Cycl.*; Lil. t.; Plat.; *Sul.*; Val.

Stimulants—Ant. c.; Cadm. s.; Chionanth.; Fluor. ac.; *Glon.*; Ign.; Lach.; Led.; Naja; *Nux v.*; Op.; *Zinc. m.*

Storm, before—*Bellis*; Meli.; *Nat. s.*; Psor.; *Rhod.*; Rhus t.

Stooping—*Æsc.*; Am. c.; Bry.; Calc. c.; Glon.; Lyssin; Merc.; Ran. b.; Spig.; *Sul.*; Val.

Straining, overlifting—Arn.; Carbo an.; *Rhus t.*; Ruta.

Stretching—Med.; Rhus t.

Sun—*Ant. c.*; *Bell.*; Bry.; Cact.; Fagop.; *Gels.*; *Glon.*; Lach.; Lyssin; *Nat. c.*; Nat. m.; Puls.; Selen. See Weather, Hot.

Sun pain—*Glon.*; Nat. m.; *Sang.*; Spig.; Tab.

Swallowing—Apis; *Bell.;* Brom.; Bry.; *Hep.;* Hyos.; *Lach.;* Merc. i. fl.; Merc. i. r.; *Merc.;* Nit. ac.; Stram.; Sul. See Dysphagia (Throat).

Sweating—Ant. t.; Chin. s.; *Hep.;* Mere. c.; *Merc. s.;* Nit. ac.; Op.; Phos. ac.; *Sep.;* Stram.; Ver. a.

Sweets—*Ant. c.; Arg. n.;* Ign.; *Lyc.;* Med.; Sang.; *Zinc. m.*

Talking—Ambra; Am. c.; Anac.; *Arg. m.;* Arum; Calc. c.; Can. s.; Chin. s.; *Cocc.;* Mag. m.; *Mang. ac.;* Nat. c.; *Nat. m.;* Phos. ac.; Rhus t.; *Selen.; Stann.;* Sul.; Verbasc.

Tea—*Abies n.; Cinch.;* Diosc.; Lob. infl.; Nux v.; Puls.; *Selen.;* Thuya.

Temperature, extremes of—Ant. c.; Ipec.; Lach.

Thinking of symptoms—Bar. c.; *Calc. p.;* Caust.; *Gels.; Helon.; Med.;* Nux v.; *Ox. ac.;* Oxytr.; Pip. m.; Sabad.; Staph.

Thunder storm, before, during—Agar.; Gels.; Med.; Meli.; *Nat. c.;* Petrol.; *Phos.;* Phyt.; Psor.; *Rhod.;* Sep.; Sil.

Tobacco chewing—*Ars.;* Ign.; Lyc.; Selen.; *Ver. a.*

Tobacco smoke—Acon.; Cic.; Cocc.; *Ign.;* Staph. See Smoking.

Touch—*Acon.;* Angust.; *Apis;* Arg. m.; *Arn.;* Asaf.; *Bell.;* Bor.; *Bry.;* Calc. c.; Camph.; Caps.; Carbo an.; *Cham.;* Cic.; *Cinch.;* Cocc.; *Colch.;* Col.; Commocl.; Cupr. ac.; *Cupr. m.;* Equis.; Euphorb. d.; Euphras.; Ferr. p.; Guaiac.; Helon.; *Hep.;* Hyos.; Ign.; *Kali c.; Lach.; Lil. t.;* Lob. infl.; Lyc.; Mag. p.; Mez.; Murex; *Nit. ac.; Nux v.;* Oleand.; *Ox. ac.;* Phos.; *Plumb. m.;* Puls.; *Ran. b.; Rhod.;* Rhus t.; Sab.; Sang.; Sep.; *Sil.; Spig.;* Staph.; *Strych.;* Sul.; *Tar. h.;* Tellur.; *Ther.;* Urt.; Zinc. m.

Touch of hat—Glon.

Traveling—Coca; Plat.

Twilight, to daylight—Aur.; *Merc.;* Phyt.; *Syph.*

Uncovering—Ars.; Bell.; Benz. ac.; Caps.; Dros.; Helleb.; *Hep.;* Kali bich.; *Mag. p.; Nux v.;* Rheum; *Rhus t.; Rumex; Samb.;* Sil.; Stront. c.

Vaccination, after—Sil.; Thuya.

Veal—Ipec.; *Kali n.*

Vital drains—Calc. c.; *Calc. p.;* Carbo v.; *Cinch.;* Con.; *Kali c.; Kali p.;* Nux v.; *Phos.; Phos. ac.;* Puls.; *Selen.;* Sep.; Staph.

Voice, using—Arg. m.; Arg. n.; Arum; Carbo v.; *Dros.;* Mang. ac.; Nux v.; *Phos.;* Selen.; *Stann.;* Wyeth.

Vomiting—Æth.; Ant. t.; *Ars.;* Cupr. m.; *Ipec.; Nux v.;* Puls.; Sil.

Waking—Ambra; Lach.; Nit. ac.; Nux v. See Sleep.

Warmth, heat—Acon.; Æth.; Agar.; Alum.; Ambra; Anac.; *Ant. c.;* Ant. t.; *Apis;* Arg. n.; Asaf.; Bell.; *Bry.;* Calc. c.; Camph.; *Cepa; Cham.;* Cinch.; Clem.; *Commocl.;* Conv.; *Dros.;* Euphras.; Ferr. m.; Fluor. ac.; Gels.; Glon.; *Graph.;* Guaiac.; Helianth.; Hyos.; Iberis; *Iod.;* Jugl. c.; Justicia; Kali iod.; *Kali m.;* Lach.; *Led.;* Lyc.; Med.; *Merc.; Nat. c.;* Nat. m.; Nit. ac.; Nux m.; Op.; *Puls.;* Sab.; *Sec.;* Stellar.; Sul. ac.; Sul.; Tab. See Weather, Hot.

Warmth of bed—Alum.; Apis; Bellis; Calc. c.; *Cham.;* Clem.; *Dros.; Led.;* Lyc.; Mag. c.; *Merc.;* Mez.; *Puls.;* Sab.; *Sec.; Sul.;* Thuya; Viscum.

Washing, water—*Am. c.; Ant. c.;* Ars. iod.; Bar. c.; Bell.; *Calc. c.;* Canth.;

Cham.; Clem.; *Crot. casc.;* Ferr. m.; Kreos.; Lil. t.; Mag. p.; *Merc.;* Mez.; *Nat. s.;* Nit. ac.; Rhus t.; Sep.; Sil.; Spig.; *Sul.;* Urt.

Water, drinks cold—Ant. c.; Apoc.; Arg. n.; *Ars.;* Calc. c.; *Canth.;* Clem.; Cocc.; *Crot. t.;* Cycl.; Dros.; Ferr. m.; Lob. infl.; Lyc.; Nux m.; *Rhus t.;* Sabad.; Spong.; Sul.

Water, drinks warm—Ambra; Bry.; *Lach.;* Phos.; *Puls.;* Sep.; Stann.

Water, seeing or hearing—Lyssin.

Water, working—*Calc. c.;* Mag. p.

Weather changes—*Am. c.;* Bry.; Calc. c.; Calc. fl.; *Calc. p.;* Chel.; Cinch.; *Dulc.;* Mang. ac.; Mag. c.; *Merc.;* Nat. c.; Nit. ac.; *Nux m.;* Phos.; *Psor.;* Ran. b.; *Rhod.;* Rhus t.; Ruta; Sticta; Stront. c.; Sul.; Tar h. See Dampness.

Weather changes, in spring—Ant. t.; Cepa; Gels.; Kali s.; Nat. s.

Weather, dry, cold—Agar.; Alum.; Apoc.; *Asar.;* *Aur.;* *Caust.;* Dulc.; Ipec.; *Kali c.;* Kreos.; Nit. sp. d.; *Nux v.;* Petrol.; Rhus t.; Viscum. See Air, Cold.

Weather, hot—*Acon.;* Æth.; Aloe; *Ant. c.;* *Bell.;* Bor.; *Bry.;* Croc.; Crot.; Crot. t.; *Gels.;* *Glon.;* Kali bich.; Lach.; *Nat. c.;* *Nat. m.;* Nit. ac.; Phos.; Picr. ac.; *Pod.;* Puls.; Sab.; Selen.; Syph. See Sun.

Weather, stormy—Nux m.; *Psor.;* Ran. b.; *Rhod.;* Rhus t.

Weather, windy, dry—*Acon.;* Arum; Cham.; Cupr. m.; *Hep.;* Lyc.; Mag. c.; *Nux v.;* Phos.; Puls.; *Rhod.*

Weather, windy, moist—Cepa; Dulc.; *Euphras.;* Ipec.; *Nux m.;* Rhod.

Weeping—Cham.; *Nat. m.;* Puls.; *Sep.;* Stann.

Wet application—*Am. c.;* *Ant. c.;* Calc. c.; *Clem.;* Crct.; *Merc.;* Rhus t.; *Sul.* See Washing.

Wet exposure—Am. c.; Ant. c.; Apis; Aran.; Ars.; *Calc. c.;* Caust.; Cepa; *Dulc.;* *Elaps;* Meli.; *Merc.;* Narcissus; Nat. s.; Nux m.; *Phyt.;* Picr. ac.; Ran. b.; Rhod.; *Rhus t.;* Ruta; Sep. See Dampness.

Wet feet—Calc. c.; Cepa; Puls.; *Rhus t.;* *Sil.*

Wine—*Alum.;* Ant. c.; Arn.; *Ars.;* Benz. ac.; *Carbo v.;* Con.; Fluor. ac.; Led.; Lyc.; *Nux v.;* Op.; Ran. b.; Selen.; Sil.; *Zinc. m.*

Yawning—Cina; *Ign.;* Kreos.; *Nux v.;* Rhus t.; *Sars.*

Yearly—Lach.; Rhus r.

AMELIORATIONS—Acids: Ptel.; Sang.

Air, cool, open—*Acon.;* *Æsc.;* Æth.; Aloe; *Alum.;* Ambra; Am. m.; *Amyl;* Ant. c.; Ant. t.; *Apis;* Arg. n.; Asaf.; Bar. c.; Bry.; Bufo; Cact.; Can. ind.; *Cepa; Cinch.;* Clem.; Coca; Commocl.; Conv.; Crat.; Croc.; Dig.; Diosc.; Dros.; Dulc.; Euonym.; Euphras.; Gels.; *Glon.;* Graph.; Iod.; *Kali iod.;* *Kali s.;* Lil. t.; *Lyc.;* *Mag. c.;* Mag. m.; Merc. i. r.; Mez.; Mosch.; Naja; *Nat. m.;* Nat. s.; Ol an.; Phos.; *Picr. ac.;* Plat.; *Puls.;* Radium; Rhus t.; *Sabad.;* Sab.; Sec.; *Sep.;* Stellar.; Strych. p.; Sul.; *Tab.;* *Tar. h.;* Vib. op. See Warmth (Aggravation).

Air, cool, must have windows open—*Amyl;* Arg. n.; Bapt.; Calc. c.; *Lach.;* Med.; *Puls.;* *Sul.* See Asthma (Respiratory System).

Air, warm—Aur. m.; Calc. c.; Caust.; Led.; Mag. c.; Merc.; Petrol.; Rhus t. See Warmth.

Bathing—Acon.; Apis; Ars.; *Asar.;* *Caust.;* Euphras.; *Puls.;* Spig.

Bathing, cold—Apis; Asar.; Bufo; Meph.; Nat. m.; Sep.

Bathing, vinegar—Vespa.

Bathing, warm—Ant. c.; Bufo; Radium; *Stront.;* Thea.

Bending, double—Aloe; Cinch.; *Col.; Mag. p.* See Pressure.

Bending, forward—Gels.; *Kali c.*

Boring into, nose, ears—Nat. c.; Spig.

Breakfast, after—Nat. s.; Staph. See Eating.

Carrying—Ant. t.; *Cham.*

Chewing—Bry.; Cupr. ac.

Coffee—Euphras.; Fluor. ac.

Cold—Bellis; Bor.; *Bry.;* Cepa; Fagop.; Iod.; *Led.;* Lyc.; Onosm.; Op. *Phos.; Sec.*

Cold applications, washing—Alum.; *Apis;* Arg. n.; Asar.; Bell.; Ferr. p.; Kali m.; Merc.; Phos.; *Puls.;* Sab. See Bathing.

Cold water—Agar. em.; Aloe; Ambra; *Bry.;* Camph.; Can. ind.; *Caust.;* Cupr. m.; Fagop.; *Led.; Phos.;* Picr. ac.; *Puls.;* Sep.

Colors, objects, bright—*Stram.;* Tar. h.

Combing hair—Formica.

Company—Æth.; *Bism.;* Kali c.; Lil. t.; Lyc.; *Stram.*

Consolation—Puls.

Conversation—Eup. perf.

Coughing—Apis; Stann. See Respiratory System.

Covering light—Sec.

Dark—Coca; Con.; *Euphras.;* Graph.; Phos.; *Sang.*

Day, during—Kali c.; Syph. See Aggravations.

Days, alternating—Alum.

Descending—Spong.

Discharges appearances of—*Lach.;* Mosch.; Stann.; *Zinc. m.*

Drawing limbs up—Sep.; Sul.; Thuya.

Drinks, cold—Ambra; *Cupr. m.*

Drinks, warm—Alum.; Ars.; Chel.; *Lyc.;* Nux v.; Sabad.; *Spong.* See Warm.

Eating—Acet. ac.; *Alum.;* Ambra; *Anac.;* Brom.; Cad. m.; Caps.; *Chel.;* Cim.; Cistus; Con.; Ferr. ac.; Ferr. m.; Graph.; *Hep.;* Homar.; *Ign.; Iod.; Kali p.;* Lach.; *Lith. c.; Nat. c.;* Nat. m.; Onosm.; *Petrol.;* Phos.; Pip. nig.; *Psor.;* Rhod.; Sep.; *Spong.;* Zinc. m.

Eructations—Ant. t.; *Arg. n.;* Bry.; *Carbo v.;* Diosc.; *Graph.;* Ign.; *Kali c.;* Lyc.; Mosch.; Nux v.; Ol. an.; Sang.

Evenings—Bor.; Lob. infl.; Niccol.; Nux v.; Stellar.

Excitement, pleasurable—Kali p.; Pall.

Exercise—Alumen; Brom.; Plumb. m.; *Rhus t.;* Sep. See Walking.

Expectoration—Ant. t.; Hep.; *Stann.;* Zinc. m. See Respiratory System.

Expulsion of flatus, per ano—Aloe; Arn.; Calc. p.; Corn. c.; Grat.; Hep.; Iris; Kali n.; Mez.

Fanned, being—*Arg. n.; Carbo v.;* Cinch.; Lach.; Med.

Fasting—Cham.; Con.; *Nat. m.*

Feet in ice water—*Led.;* Sec.

Food cold—Ambra; Bry.; Lyc.; Phos.; Sil.

Food warm—Kreos.; Lyc. See Aggravations.

Forenoon, in—Lil. t.

Head bent backward—Hyper.; Senega.

Head bent forward, while lying—Col.

Head, wrapped up warm—Hep.; Psor.; Rhod.; Sil.

Head elevated—Ars.; Gels.

Heat—*Ars.;* Caps.; Gymnocl.; Xerophyl. See Warmth.

Ice, holding in mouth—Coff.

Inland, mountains—Syph.

Inspiration—Colch.; Ign.; *Spig.* See Respiratory System.

Lemonade—Cycl.

Light—Stram.

Limb hanging down—Con.

Lying down—Acon.; Anhal.; Arn.; *Bell.;* Bellis; Brom.; *Bry.;* Calad.; Calc. c.; Coff.; *Colch.;* Equis.; Ferr. m.; *Mang. ac.; Nat. m.;* Nux v.; Onosm.; *Picr. ac.;* Pulex; *Puls.;* Radium; *Stann.;* Strych.; Symphor.

Lying, on back with shoulders raised—Acon.; Ars.

Lying, on left side—Ign.; Mur. ac.; Nat. m.; Stann. See Aggravations.

Lying, on painful side—Ambra; Am. c.; Arn.; Bor.; *Bry.;* Calc. c.; *Col.;* Cupr. ac.; Ptel.; *Puls.;* Sul. ac. See Pressure.

Lying, on right side—Ant. t.; Nat. m.; *Phos.;* Sul.; Tab. See Aggravations.

Lying, on right side, with head high—Ars.; Cact.; *Spig.;* Spong.

Lying, on stomach—*Acet. ac.;* Am. c.; Ant. t.; *Col.;* Med.; *Pod.; Tab.*

Lying, with head high—Petrol.; Puls.; Spig.

Lying, with head low—Arn.; Spong.

Magnetized—Phos.

Menses, between—Bell.; Bov.; Elaps; Ham.; Magnol.

Menses, during—Am. c.; Cycl.; *Lach.; Zinc. m.* See Female Sexual System.

Mental occupation—Ferr. m.; Kali br.; *Helon.;* Nat. c.

Midnight, after—Lyc. See Night.

Midnight, until noon—Puls.

Mind being diverted—Calc. p.; Helon.; Ox. ac.; Pip. menth.; Tar. h.

Mornings—Apis; Jugl. c.; Still.; Xerophyl.

Motion—Abrot.; Æsc.; *Alum.;* Arn.; Ars.; Asaf.; *Aur.;* Bell.; Bellis; Brom.; *Caps.;* Cinch.; Coca; Coccus; Commocl.; Con.; *Cycl.; Diosc.; Dulc.;* Euphorb.; *Ferr. m.;* Fluor. ac.; Gels.; *Helon.;* Homar.; Ign.; Indigo; Iris; Kali c.; Kali iod.; Kali p.; Kreos.; Lith. c.; Lith. lact.; Lob. infl.; Lyc.; *Mag. c.;* Mag. m.; Magnol.; Menyanth.; Nat. c.; Op.; Parth.; Pip. menth.; Plat.; *Puls.;* Pyr.; Radium; Rhod.; *Rhus t.;* Ruta; Sabad.; *Samb.; Sep.:* Stellar.; Sul.; Syph.; *Val.;* Ver. a.;; Xerophyl.; Zinc. m.

Motion, slow—Agar.; Ambra; Ferr. ac.; *Ferr. m.;* Plat.; Stann.; Zinc. m.

Mouth, covered—Rumex.

Music—Tar. h.

Night—Cupr. ac.

Oil applications—Euphorb. d.

Position, change of—Apis; Caust.; *Ign.;* Nat. s.; Phos. ac.; *Rhus t.;* Val.; Zinc. m.

Position, hands and feet—Eup. perf.

Position, semi-erect—Ant. t.; Apis; Bell. See Rest.

Pressure—*Arg. n.;* Asaf.; Bor.; *Bry.; Caps.;* Chel.; *Cinch.; Col.;* Con.; Cupr. ac.; *Diosc.;* Dros.; Euonym.; Formica; Guaiac.; *Ign.;* Indigo; *Lil. t.;* Mag. m.; *Mag. p.;* Menyanth.; Nat. c.; Nat. m.; Nat. s.; Nux v.; Picr. ac.; *Plumb. m.; Puls.;* Radium; *Sep.;* Sil.; *Stann.;* Ver. a.

Putting feet on chair—Con.

Rest—Æsc.; Ant. c.; Bell.; *Bry.;* Cadm. s.; Can. ind.; *Colch.;* Crat.; Gettysburg Water; Gymnocl.; Kali p.; Merc. c.; Merc. v.; *Nux v.;* Phyt.; Pulex; Scilla; Staph.; Strych. p.; Vib. op.

Riding in carriage—Nit. ac.

Rising—Ambra; Am. c.; *Ars.;* Calc. c.; Lith. c.; Parth.; Samb.; Sep.

Rocking—Cina; Kali c.

Room close, in—Euphorb. d. See Warmth.

Rubbing—Anac.; Calc. c.; *Canth.;* Carb. ac.; Diosc.; Formica; Indigo; *Mag. p.;* Nat. c.; Ol. an.; Phos.; Plumb. m.; *Pod.;* Rhus t.; Sec.; *Tar. h.*

Scratching—Asaf.; *Calc. c.;* Commocl.; Cycl.; *Jugl. c.;* Mur. ac.; Nat. c.; Phos.; Sul.

Sea, at—Brom.

Seashore, at—Med.

Shaving, after—Brom.

Sipping water—Kali n.

Sitting erect—Ant. t.; Apis; Bell.

Sitting up in bed—*Kali c.;* Samb.

Sleep—Calad.; Colch.; Merc.; Myg.; *Nux v.;* Phos.; *Sang.;* Sep.

Smoking—Aran.; Tar. c.

Standing erect—Ars.; Bell.; *Diosc.;* Kali p.

Stimulants—Gels.; Glon.

Stooping—Colch.

Storm, after—Rhod.

Stretching limbs—Amyl; Plumb. m.; Rhus t.; Sec.; Teucr.

Summer, during—Alum.; Aur. m.; Calc. p.; Ferr. m.; Sil. See Warmth.

Sweat—Acon.; Ars.; Calad.; *Cham.;* Cupr. m.; Franciscea; Rhus t.; *Ver. a.* See Fever.

Taking hold of anything—Anac.

Thinking of symptoms—*Camph.;* Helleb.

Touch—Asaf.; Calc. c.; Cycl.; Mur. ac.; Tarax.; Thuya.

Uncovering—Apis; Camph.; Lyc.; Onosm.; *Sec.; Tab.* See Aggravations.

Urination—*Gels.;* Ign.; *Phos. ac.;* Sil.

Vomiting—Helianth.

Warmth, heat—*Ars.;* Aur. m.; Bad.; Bell.; Bry.; Calc. fl.; Camph.; Caust.; Cim.; *Col.; Collins.;* Coff.; Coral.; Cupr. ac.; Cycl.; *Dulc.;* Formica; *Hep.;* Ign.; Kali bich.; Kali p.; Kreos.; Lach.; Lob. infl.; Lyc.; *Mag. p.;* Nux m.; *Nux v.;* Phos. ac.; Phyt.; Psor.; Rhod.; Rhus t.; *Rumex;* Sabad.; Sep.; Sil.; Solan. lyc.; Staph.; Stram.; Sul. ac.; Thea; Ver. a.

Warmth, heat of, applications—Ars.; Bry.; Calc. fl.; *Lach.; Mag. p ;* Nux m.; Radium; Rhus t.; Sep.

Warmth, of head—Bell.; Graph.; *Hep.; Psor.;* Sanic.; *Sil.*

Water, cold—Aloe; *Bry.;* Caust.; *Jatropha; Phos.;* Picr. ac.; Sep.

Water, hot—Spig.

Weather, damp, wet—Alum.; Asar.; *Caust.; Hep.;* Med.; Mur. ac.; Nux v.

Weather, damp, warm—Cham.; Kali c.; Sil.

Weather, dry—Am. c.; Calc. c.; Kali c.; Magnol.; Petrol.; Still. See Aggravations.

Weather, dry, warm—Alum.; *Calc. p.;* Nat. s.; Nux m.; Rhus t.; *Sul.* See Summer.

Wine—Coca.

Winter, during—Ilex.

INDEX TO REPERTORY
(Ninth Edition)

990   INDEX TO REPERTORY

THERAPEUTIC INDEX

THERAPEUTIC INDEX

Any attempt to select the proper homœopathic remedy for any case except by the study of the totality of symptoms must prove futile. In order to prescribe homœopathically, the essentials for so doing must be observed,—i. e., *to let the characteristic symptoms of the individual patient, largely independent of the pathological nature of the case, be paramount in selecting the remedy.*

Such characteristics are found especially—

(1) In the location or part affected;

(2) In the sensations;

(3) In the modalities.

The study of the repertory alone will give the indicated remedy. But throughout this work are found numerous suggestions for remedies based on clinical observations or deductions from partial provings, all of which may prove most valuable additions to our Materia Medica if further verified at the bedside. As many of them have no place as yet in our published repertories, I have thought it advisable to give them a place with others in this therapeutic index, in order to bring them to the attention and further study of the physician. At best, a clinical index is but suggestive.

Abortion, threatened.—Caulophyl; Viburnum.

Abscess.—Bellad.; Merc.; *Hepar;* Silica; Ananther.

Acidity.—Calc.; *Robin.;* Sulph. ac.; Nux.

Acne.—Kal. brom.; Cimicif.; *Berb. aquif.;* Led.; Hydrocot.; Antimon.; Kali brom.

——**Rosacea.**—Oophor.; Kreos.; Sulph.; Carb. an.; Radium.

Acromegaly.—Thyroid; Chrysarob.

Actinomycosis.—Nitr. ac.; Hippoz.; Hecla.

Addison's disease.—Adrenalin; Ars.; Phos.; Calc. ars.

Adenitis.—Bell.; Merc.; Cist.; Iod.

Adenoids.—Agraphis; Calc. jod.

Adiposity.—Phytolacca; Fucus.

Adynamia.—Phos. ac.; China.

After-pains.—Caulophyl; Magnes. phos.

Agalactia.—Lactuca; Agnus; Urtica.

Ague.—Nat. mur.; China; Cedron.

Albuminuria.—Ars.; Kalmia; Merc. cor.

Alcoholism.—Quercus; Avena; Capsic; Nux.

Alopecia.—Fluor. ac.; Pix. liq.

Amenorrhoea.—Puls.; Graph.; Nat. mur.

Anasarca.—Oxydend; Elater; Liatris.

Anaemia.—Fer. cit. Chin.; Nat. m.; Calc. phos.

——**Pernicious.**—Ars.; T. N. T.

Aneurism.—Baryt.; Lycop.

Angina pectoris.—Latrodect; Cactus; Glonoin.; Bryon; Hæm-
atox; Oxal. ac.; Spigel.

Angioma.—Abrotan.

Ankylostomiasis.—Carduus mar.

Anorexia.—*Nux; Hydrast.; China.*

Anthrax.—*Echinacea.*

Aortitis.—*Aurum ars.*

Antrum.—Hep.; Nit. ac.; K. bich.; Euphorb.; Amyg.

Aphasia.—Bothrops; Stram.; Kal. brom.

Aphonia.—Alumen; Arg. m.; Nit. ac.; Caust.; Oxal. ac.;
Spongia; Aurum.

Aphthæ.—Æthus.; *Borax; Merc.;* Nit. ac.; Kal. mur.; Hydr.
mur.

Apoplexy.—Op.; Phos.; Arnica; Bellad.

Appendicitis.—Echin.; Bellad.; Laches.; Iris tenax.

Arterial tension lowered.—Gels.

Arterial tension raised.—Verat. vir.; Viscum.

Arteriosclerosis.—Am. iod.; Plumb. iod.; Polyg. avic.; Baryta; Glonoin 2x; Aurum; Carduus; Sumbul.

Arthritis.—Arbut.; Sulph.; Bry.; Elater.

Ascarides.—Abrotan.; Sabad.; Cina; Spig.

Ascites.—Acet. ac.; Apocyn.; Helleb.; Apis; Ars.; *Dig.*

Asthenopia.—Nat. mur.; Ruta; Croc.; Senega.

Asthma.—Ipec.; Ars.; Eucalypt; *Adrenalin;* Nat. sulph.

——**Cardiac.**—Conval.; Iberis; Ars. jod.

Astigmatism (myopic).—Lilium.

Atrophy.—Ol. jecor.; Iod.; Ars.

Auricular Fibrillation.—Digital.; Quinidine.

Auto-intoxication.—Skatol; Indol.; Sulph.

Azoturia.—Caust.; Senna.

Backache.—Oxal. ac.; Æsc.; Rhus; Puls.; Kal. carb.; Cimicif.; Nux; Ant. tart.; Variol.

Balonitis.—Merc.

Barber's Itch.—Sulph. iod.; Thuja.

Bed-sores.—Fluor. ac.; Arn.; Sulph. ac.

Bell's Paralysis.—Am. phos.; *Causticum;* Zinc. pic.

Beri Beri.—Elater.; Rhus; Ars.

Bilharziasis.—Antimon. tart.

Biliousness.—Yucca; Euony.; Bry.; Pod.; Merc.; Sulph.; Nux; Nyctanthes; Chelidon.

Bladder (irritable).—*Eup. purp.;* Copaiv.; Ferr.; Nux; Apis; Sarsap.

——**Hæmorrhage.**—Amygd.; Hamam.; *Nit. ac.*

Blepharitis.—Puls.; Graph.; Merc.

Blepharospasm.—Agaric.; Physost.

Blood-pressure.—High—Baryta mur.; Glonoin.; Aurum; Viscum.

Boils.—Bellis; Calc. pic.; Ferr. iod.; Ol. myr.; *Bell.;* Sil.; *Hep.;* Ichthyol.

Bone Affections.—Aurum; Calc. phos.; Flour. ac.; Ruta; Mezer.; Silica; Symphyt.

Borborygmi.—Hæmatoxyl.

Bradycardia (slow pulse).—Abies nig.; *Digit.;* Kalm.; Apocn. can.

Brain, Softening.—Salamand; Phos.; Baryta.

Brain-fag.—Anhalon.; Zinc.; Phos.; Anacard.; Sil.

Bright's Disease.—Ars.; Phos. ac.; Apis; Merc. cor.; Tereb.; Kali cit.; Natrum mur.

Bromidrosis.—Silica; Calc.; Butyr. acid.

Bronchitis.—Acon.; *Bry.;* Phos.; Tart. e.; *Fer. phos.;* Sang.; Pilocarp.

——**(chronic)**—Ammoniac; Ars.; Seneg.; Sulph.; Antim. jod.

Broncho-pneumonia.—Kali bich.; Tart emet.; Tuberc.; Phos.; Squilla.

Bronchorrhœa.—Ammoniacum; Eucalyp.; *Bals. Peru;* Stan.; Bacillin.

Bulbar Paralysis.—Guaco; Plumb.; Botulin.

Bubo.—Merc.; Nit. ac.; Carb. an.; Phytol.

Burns—Cantharis; Urtica; Picric acid.

Bursæ.—Benz. ac.; Ruta; Sil.

Calculi (biliary).—China; Berberis; Chelidon.

——**(renal)**—Berberis; Pareira; Sarsap.

Cancer—(Bladder.)—Taraxac.

——**(Epithelial.)**—Acetic acid.

——**(Gastric.)**—Geranium.

——**(Rectal.)**—Ruta; Hydr.; Kal. cyan.

——**(Tongue.)**—Fuligo.

Cancer.—Semp. viv.; *Ars.;* Hyd.; Ant. chlor.; Galium.

——**Mammæ.**—Aster.; Con.; Plumb. iod.; Carcinosin.

——**Pains.**—Euphorb.

Cancrum Oris.—Secal.; Kreos.; Ars.; Baptis.

Capillary Stasis.—Capsic.; Echinac.

Carbuncles.—*Anthrac;* Ledum; Tar. cub.; *Ars.;* Lach.; Silic.

Cardiac Dropsy.—Adonis; Digit.

Cardiac Dyspnœa.—Acon. ferox.; Aspidos.

Cardialgia.—Fer. tart.

Cardio-vascular spasm.—Actæa spicata.

Caries.—Aur.; Asaf.; Sil.; Phos.

Car Sickness.—Coccul.

Caruncle, Urethral.—Thuja.

Catalepsy.—Curare; Hydroc. ac.; *Can. ind.*

Cataract.—Cineraria; *Phos.;* Platanus; Quass.; *Naphth.;* Calc. fluor.

Catarrh (chronic).—Anemopsis; Nat. sulph.; *Aur.; Eucaly.; Kal. bich.;* Puls.; Sang. nit.; Nat. carb.

Cellulitis.—Apis; Rhus; Vespa.

Cerebro-spinal Meningitis.—Cicut.; Zinc. cyan.; Cupr. acet.; Helleb.

Chancre.—Merc. bin iod.; Merc. prot.; Merc. sol.; Kali iod.

Checked Discharges.—Cupr.; Psorinum.

Cheyne-Stokes Respiration.—Grind.; Morphin.; Parthen.

Chicken-pox.—Tart. e.; Rhus; Kal. mur.

Chilblains.—Abrot.; *Agar.;* Tamus; Plantag.

Chloasma.—Sep.; Paull.

Chlorosis.—Ars.; Ferr.; Helon.; Cupr.; Puls.

Cholelithiasis.—Chionanth; Hydrast.

Cholera.—Camph.; *Verat.;* Ars.; Cupr.

Cholera Infantum.—Æthus.; Cuphea; Cal. phos.

Chordee.—Canth.; Salix; Yohimb.; Lupul.; Agave.

Chorea.—Absinth.; Agar.; Hippom.; Mygal.; Tanacet.; Tarant. hisp.; Ignat.; Zinc.; Cimicif.

Cicatrices.—Thiosin.; Graphites.

Ciliary Neuraglia.—Prunus; Spig.; Sapon.; Cinnab.

Cirrhosis of Liver.—Nasturt.; Nat. chlo.; *Merc.*

Climacteric Flushings.—Amyl nit.; *Lach.;* Sang.; Cimic.; Sep.

Coccygodynia.—Caust.; Silica.

Cold Sores.—Camphor; Dulcam.

Colic.—Cham.; Mag. phos.; Diosc.; Plumb.

Colic, Renal.—Eryng; Pareira.

Colitis.—Merc. dulc.; Aloes; Allium sat.

Collapse.—Camph.; Morph.; Verat.; Ars.

Color-blindness.—Benzin.; Carb. sulph.

Coma.—Opium; Pilocarp.; Bell.

Comedones.—Abrotan.; Æthiops.; Baryta.

Condylomata.—Cinnab.; Nat. sulph.; Nit. ac.; *Thuja.*

Conjunctivitis.—Acon.; Puls.; Euphr.; Guar.

Constipation.—Opium; *Hydr.;* Iris; Verat.; Mag. mur.; Nux; Paraf.; Lac defl.; Tan. ac.; Mag. phos.; Sulph.; Alumina; Veratrum.

——(**in children**)—Æsc.; Collins.; Bry.; Alumina; Paraf.; Psorin.

Convulsions.—Hydroc. ac.; Laburn.; *Cupr.;* Cicut.; *Bell.;* Œnanth.

Corns.—Ant. curd.; Graph.; Sil.

Coryza.—Cepa; Penthor.; *Nat. mur.; Quillaya; Gels.;* Euphras.; Acon.; Ars.; Kali hyd.

Cough (dry).—Alum.; Bell.; Hyos.; Lauro.; Con.; Mentha; Rumex; Spongia; Sticta.

——(**laryngeal**)—Nit. ac.; Brom.; Caps.; Caust.; Lach.

——(**hoarse**)—Bry.; Hep.; Phos.; Samb.; Spong.; Verbasc.

——(**loose**)—Kal. sulph.; Tart. e.; Ipec.; Merc.; Puls.; Squilla; Stannum; Coccus c.

——(**phthisical**)—All. sat.; Crotal.; Phelland.; Naja.

——(**nervous**)—Ambra; Ignat; Hyos.; Kali brom.

——(**spasmodic**)—Corall.; Dros ; Mephit.; Cupr.; Mag. phos.; *Bellad.;* Ipec.; Coccus c.

Cracked Lips.—*Condur.;* Graph.; Nat. mur.

1000

THERAPEUTIC INDEX

Croup.—*Acon.; Hep.;* Kaolin; *Spong.;* Brom.; Iod.; Kali bich.; Sang.

Cyanosis.—Tart. emet.; Carbo; Cuprum; Laches.; Laurocer.; Opium.

Cystitis.—Epigea; Saurur.; Popul.; *Canth.;* Chimaph.; Tereb.

Cysts.—Iod.; Apis.

Dandruff.—Kal. sulph.; Ars.; Lyc.; Badiaga.

Day-blindness.—Bothrops.

Deafness.—Calend.; Puls.; Hydr.; Graph.

Debility.—Chin.; Phos. ac.; Ars.; Curar; Kali phos.; Alfalfa.

——(after gout)—Cyprip.

Delirium.—Bell.; Hyos.; Agar.

Dentition.—Bell.; *Calc. phos.; Tereb.; Cham.*

——(drooling)—Trifolium; Mercur.

Diabetes.—Ars. brom.; Coca; Codein; Helleb.; Sizyg.; Phlorid.; Uran. nit.; Phosph.; Aur.

Diaphragmitis.—Cactus; Nux.

Diarrhœa.—Camph.; *Verat.; Ipec.; China;* Puls.; *Phos. ac.;* Merc.; Manzanita; Natrum sulph.; Sul.; Podophyl.

——(chronic)—Liatris; Chaparo; Coto; Natr. sulph.; Sulphur; Calcar.

——(teething)—Arundo; *Cham.;* Cal. phos.

Diphtheria.—Lach.; *Merc. cyan.;* Merc. bin iod.; Phyt.; Carb. ac.; Apis; Vinca; Nit. ac.; Echinacea.

——(nasal)—Am. caust.; *Kal. bich.*

Diplopia.—Bell.; Gels.; Oleand.; Hyos.

Dipsomania.—Capsicum.

Dissecting Wounds.—Crotal.; Ars.; Echinac.

Dropsy.—Apis; *Apocy. can.;* Cahinca; *Samb. can.;* Oxyd.; Helleb.; Dig.; Arsenic.

Dupuytren's Contraction.—Gels.; Thios.

Dysentery.—Asclep. t.; *Aloe;* Ipec.; *Merc. cor.;* Tromb.; Colocy.; Colchic.; Ars.; Canth.

Dysmenorrhœa.—Apiol.; Puls.; Caulop.; *Viburn.;* Mag. phos.; Aquilegia.

——(membranous)—Calc. ac.; Borax.

Dyspepsia.—*Nux;* Hyd.; Graph.; Petrol.; *Anacard.;* Puls.; Lycop.; Homar.; Carbo.

Dyspepsia—(Acid.)—Robinia.

——(Atonic)—Hydrastis.

——(Fermentative)—Salicyl. acid.

——(Nervous.)—Ignatia; Anacard.

Dysphagia.—Bell.; Lach.; Merc.; Cajap.; Curar.; Epilob.

Dyspnœa.—Apis; Ars.; Ipec.; Quebrach.; Spong.

Dysuria.—Tritic.; Fabian.; *Canth.;* Apis; Sarsap.; Camphor.; Bellad.

Ear-ache.—Bell.; Cham.; Mullein Oil.

Ear—(discharges).—Kal mur.

——(very offensive)—Elaps.

Ecchymosis.—Æthus.; *Arn.;* Rhus; Sulph. ac.

Eczema.—Arbut.; Clem.; Dulc.; *Rhus;* Sulph.; *Ars.;* Bovist.; Nat. ars.; *Anac.;* Oleand.; Petrol.; *Psorin.;* Alnus; Graphites.

Elephantiasis.—Elæis; Ars.; Hydrocot.; Lyc.

Emphysema.—Am. carb.; Ant. ars.; Lobel.

Empyemia.—Arnica.

Enteritis (acute).—Cinch.; Croton.; Podop.

——(chronic)—Ars.; Sulph.; Arg. nit.

Enuresis.—Benz. ac.; Caust.; Sulph.; Rhus ar.; Equiset.; Lupul.; Uran.; Physalis; Bellad.

Epididymitis.—Sabal; Puls.

Epilepsy.—Absinth.; Artem.; Sol. carol.; Fer. cyan.; Cupr.; Hyd. ac.; Sil.; Calc. ars.; *Œnanthe.*

Epistaxis.—Ambros.; Nat. nit.; *Arn.;* Ipec.; Bry.; Hamam.; Fer. phos.; *Nit. ac.;* Phosph.

Epithelioma.—Jequir.; Ars.; Thuj.; Chromic acid.

Erotomania.—Origan.; Phos.; Pic. ac.; Stram.; Plat.

Erysipelas.—Ananth.; Bell.; *Apis;* Canth.; Graph.; *Rhus;* Verat. vir.

Erythema.—Bell.; Mezer.; Antipyrin.

——nodosum—Apis; Rhus.

Eustachian Deafness.—Kal. sulph.; Rosa; Hydr.

Exophthalmic Goitre.—Lycopus; Pilocarp.

Exostosis.—Hekla; Calc. fluor.

Exudative Pleurisy.—Abrotan.

Eyes—(Inflamed).—Acon.; Euphras.; Ruta.

——(Detachment of retina)—Naphthalin.

Fever.—*Acon.;* Agrostis; Spiranthes; *Gels.;* Bapt.; Verat. vir.; Ferr. phos.

Fibroids.—Calc. iod.

Fibroma.—Trillium; Ergot; Lapis.

Fissures.—Ledum; Graph.; Petrol.

Fistula.—Fluor. ac.; Nit. ac.; Sil.

Flatulence.—Carb.; *Asaf.; Nux mos.;* Mosch.; Lycop.; China; Carbol. ac.; Cajup.; Argent. nit.

Framboesia.—Jatropha; Merc. nit.

Freckles.—Badiaga; Sepia.

Gallactorrhœa.—Salvia; Calc.

Gall-stones.—China; Calc.; Berber.; Chionanth.; Calculus 8-10x trit.

Ganglion.—Ruta; Benz. ac.

Gangrene.—Euphorb.; Lach.; *Secale;* Carbo.

Gastralgia.—Bism.; Carb.; Coccul.; Nux; Cup. ars.; Petrol.; Phosph.

——**(recurring)**—Graph.

Gastric Ulcer.—Geran.; Arg. nit.; Ars.; *Atrop.;* Kal. bich.; Uran. nitr.

Gastritis.—Ars.; Nux; Oxal. ac.; Phos.; Hydr.

Gastro-enteritis.—Arg. n.; Ars.

Glanders.—Hippoz.; Merc.

Glands, Swollen.—Bell.; Merc. jod.; Phytol.; Kali hyd.; Alnus.

Gleet.—Thuja; Sepia; Santal.; Pulsat.; Abies can.

Glossitis.—Laches.; Mur. ac.; Apis.

Globus hyst.—Ignat.; Asaf.

Gonorrhœa.—Cann. sat.; Gels.; Ol. Sant.; Tussilago; Petros.; Merc.

Gout.—Amm. benz.; Lycop.; Urtica; Formica; Colchic.; Ledum; Lithium; Fraxinus.

——**(Retrocedent)**—Cajuput.

Gravel.—Hydrang.; Solidago; Lycopod.; Berberis.

Growing Pains.—Phosph. ac.; Guaiacum; Calc. phos.

Gumboil.—Bell.; Merc.; Hecla; Phosph.

Hæmatemesis.—Ipec.; Ham.; Phos.; Millefol.

Hæmaturia.—Canth.; Ham.; Tereb.; Nit. ac.

Hæmoglobinuria.—*Pic. ac.; Phos.*

Hæmophilia.—Nat. sil.; Phos.

Hæmoptysis.—Acal.; Ferr. phos.; Ipec.; Millef.; **Ergot.**; Eriger.; Geran.; Hydr. mur.; Allium sat.

Hæmorrhages.—Adrenalin; Hydrasing; Ipec.; Chin.; Sabina; Hamam.; Millef.; Crotal.; Trill.

——**(chronic sequelæ)**—Stront.

Hæmorrhoids.—Negundo; Scrophul.; *Aloe; Mur. ac.; Hamam.;* Fluor. ac.; *Nux;* Æs.; Collins.

Hallucinations.—Antipyr.; Stram.; Bell.

Halophagia.—Nit. sp. d.; Ars.; Phos.

Hay-fever.—Ambros.; Aral.; Cup. acet.; Napth.; Arundo; Rosa; *Sabad.;* Linum; Phleum pretense.

Headaches.—(**anæmic)**—Chin.; Ferr. phos.

——**(bursting)**—*Usnea;* Glonoin.

——**(congestive)**—Acon.; Bell.; Glon.; Lach.; Melil.; Gels.

——**(nervous)**—Cimic.; Ign.; Coff.; Guar.; Cannab.; Zinc.; Niccol.

——**(sick)**—Iris; Sang.; Nux; Chionanth.

Heart Affections.—Acon.; *Cactus; Naja; Dig.; Cræt.;* Lycop.; Spig.; Spong.; Adon.; Conval.; Phaseol.

Heartburn.—Geran.; Carbo.

Heart Failure.—Strych. sulph., 1/60-1/30 gr.; Spartein Sulph., ¼ gr.; Agaricin, 1/10 gr.; hypodermically.

Hectic Fever.—Baptis.; Ars.; Chinin. ars.

Hemicrania.—Ol. an.; Onos.; Sep.; Stann.; **Coff.**

Hemiplegia.—Oleand.; Coccul.; Bothrops.

Hemopia (vertical).—Titan.

Hepatitis.—Bry.; Merc.; Lach.; Natr. sulph.

Herpes—(Circinatus).—Sep.; Tellur.

Herpes Labialis.—Caps.; Nat. mur.; Rhus.

——**(preputialis)**—Hep.; Nit. ac.

——**(pudendi)**—Calad.; Nat. mur.; Nit. ac.

——**Zoster.**—Carb. oxyg.; Mentha; Ran. bulb.; Rhus.

Hiccough.—Ginseng.; Ratanh.; Nux; Sulph. ac.

Hoarseness.—Acon.; Bry.; Dros.; Carb.; Phos.; Caust.

Hodgkin's Disease.—Ars. iod.; Phos.; Iod.

Homesickness.—Caps.; Ignatia.

Hookworm.—Chenopod.; **Thymol.**

Housemaid's Knee.—Sticta; Slag.

Hydrocephalus.—Helleb.; Iodof.; Zinc.

Hydrocyle.—Rhodod.; Graph.; Puls.

Hydrophobia.—Xanthium; Anagallis; Canth.

Hydrothorax.—Lactuca; Ran. bulb.; Kali carb.; Merc. sulph.; Fluor. ac.; *Adonis.*

Hyperchlorhydria.—Chin. ars.; Robin.; Orexine; Arg. nit.; *Atropin;* Anacard.; Iris.

Hysteria.—Aquileg.; Castor.; Mosch.; Pothos.; Plat.; Sumb.; Valer.; Ignat.; Asaf.

Hysterical Joint.—Cotyledon.

Ichthyosis.—Ars. iod.; Syphil.

Impetigo.—Ars.; Tart. e.; Mez.

Impotence.—Agnus; Calad.; Onos.; *Phos. ac.;* Con.; Lycop.; Selen.; *Yohimbin.*

Indurations.—Carb. an.; Plumb. iod.; Alumen.

Inflammations.—Acon.; Bell.; Ferr. phos.; Sulph.

Influenza.—Eryng.; Bap.; Eucalyp.; Lobel. cerul.; *Gels.; Rhus;* Eup. perf.; Bryonia; Arsenic.

Insomnia.—*Coff.;* Cyprip.; Daph. ind.; Ignat.; Passifl.; *Aquileg.*

——(delirium tremens)—Sumbul.

Intermittent Fever.—Helianth.; *Chin.; Ars.;* Ipec.; *Nat. mur.;* Caps.; Tela aranea.

Iritis.—Bell.; Merc.; Clemat.; Syph.; Dubois.; Sarcolact. ac.

Jaundice.—Chionanth.; Cholest.; Bry.; Chin.; Myric.; Podop.; Mercur.; Chelid.; Kali pic.; Nat. phos.

——(infantile)—Lupulus; Cham.

——(toxic)—Trotyl.

Keloid.—Fluor. ac.

Kidneys (congestive).—Bell.; Tereb.; Canth.

Lagophthalmus.—Physos.

Laryngitis (acute).—Acon.; Hep.; Spong.; Phos.; Caust.; Arum.

Lectophobia.—Cann. sat.

Leprosy.—Elæis; Hydrocot.; Crotalus; Pyrara.

Leucocythæmia.—Ars.; Pic. ac.; Thuj.

Leucoderma.—*Ars. sul. r.*
——(chronic)—Dros.; Selen.; Mang.; Argent.
Leucorrhœa.—Alum.; Calc.; Hyd.; Sulph.; Puls.; Kreos.;
 Sep.; Hydr.; Eucalyp.; Thuj.
——(in little girls)—Calc.; Cub.; Hyp.; Asperul.
Lithiasis.—Asparag.; Lycop.; Sep.
Liver (congestion).—Berb.; Bry.; Card.; Chel.; Lept.; *M*erc.;
 Mag. mur.; Pod.; Sulph.
Liver-spots.—Nat. hyposulph.
Locomotor Ataxia.—Zinc. phos.; Plumb.; Arg. nit.; Oxal. ac.;
 Chromium sulph.; *Aragallis.*
Lumbago.—Guaiac.; Hyos.; *Rhus;* Tart. em.; Macrot.; Phy-
 tol.; Kali oxal.
Lungs, Congestion.—Acon.; Verat. vir.; Fer. phos.
——Œdema.—Am. carb.; Tart. em.; Ars.
Lupus.—Am. ars.; Ars.; Hydrocot.; Thuja.
Lypothemia.—Ignatia; Nux mosch.

Malaria.—Alstonia; Am. pic.; Cornus.
Malnutrition.—Alfalfa; Calc. phos.
Mania.—Bell.; Hyos.; Stram.; Lach.
Marasmus.—Abrotan.; Iod.; Nat. mur.; Ars. iod.
Mastitis.—Bell.; Phytol.; Con.
Mastoid.—Caps.; Onos.; Hydr.
Measles.—Gels.; Puls.; Fer. phos.; Kal. mur.
Megrim.—Menisp.; Coff.; Sep.; Stan.
Meniere's Disease.—Carb. sulph.; Chenop.; Nat. sal.; Sal.
 ac.; Silica; Pilocarp. mur.
Meningitis (tubercular).—Bacil.; Cup. cyan.; Iodof.
Menorrhagia.—Chin.; Sabina; Croc.; Calc.; Plat.; Sedum;
 Tellur; Sanguisorba.
Menstruation.—(cessation)—Laches.; Puls.; Graph.; Sanguin.
——(delayed)—Puls.; Calc. phos.; Cauloph.; Nat. mur.
——(painful)—Bell.; Viburn. op.; Mag. phos.
——(profuse)—Cham.; Ipec.; Trill.; Bellad.; Sabina.
Metritis, Chronic.—Aur. mur. nat.; Mel. c. s.; Merc.
Milk-leg.—Bufo; Ars.; Puls.; Rhus; Hamam.
Miscarriage.—(repeated)—Syphilin.; Bacill.
——(threatened)—Sabina; Viburn. op.

Morning Sickness.—Amygdal.; Nux; Ipec.; Cucurb.; Coccul.; Apomorph.; Aletris.

Morphine Habit.—Avena.

Morvan's Disease.—Aur. mur.; Thuya.

Mountain Sickness.—Coca.

Mumps.—Bell.; Merc.; Pilocarp.; Rhus.

Muscæ Volitantes.—Caustic.; Cypriped.; China.

Mushroom Poisoning.—Absinth.

Myalgia.—Acon.; Bry.; Macrot.; Rhus.

Myelitis.—Ars.; Plumb.; Oxal. ac.; Secale; Dulc.

Myocardial Degeneration after Influenza.—Nux; Gels.

Myocarditis.—Dig.; Ars. iod.; Aur. mur.

Myositis.—Arn.; Mez.; Rhus.

Myxœdema.—Thyroid.

Nævus.—Fluor. ac.; Thuja.

Nephritis.—Meth. blue; Koch's lymph.; Berb.; Kali chlor.; Canth.; Merc. cor.; Phos.; Tereb.; Apis; Eucalyp.

Nephrolithiasis.—Pareira; Senecio aur.

Neuralgia.—Am. val.; *Acon.;* Bell.; *Spig.;* Kalm.; *Ars.;* Colocy.; Phos.; Zinc. val.

——**(lumbo-abdominal)**—Aran.

——**(periodic)**—Nic. sulph.; Ars.; Cedr.

——**(spermatic cord)**—Ol. an.; Oxal. ac.; Clemat.

Neurasthenia.—Anac.; *Zinc. pic.;* Stry. phos.; Physostig.

——**(gastric)**—Gentiana; Anacard.

Neuritis.—Stann.; Plumb.; Hyper.; Thallium; Ars.

Nictalopia.—Bell.; Helleb.

Night-sweats.—Acet. ac.; Nat. tell.; Popul.; Agaricus; Picrot.; Salvia; Pilocarp.

Nipples, Ulcerated.—Cast. eq.; Eup. ar.; Ratanh.

Nodosities of Joints.—Am. phos.

Nymphomania.—Robin.; Canth.; Hyos.; Phos.; Murex.

Obesity.—Am. brom.; Fucus; Calc.; Phyt.; Thyroid.

Oedema.—Apis; Ars.; Dig.

——**(of lungs)**—Tart. emet.

——**(pedum)**—Prunus.

Œsophagus.—Cajup.; Condur.; Bapt.

Onychia.—Silica; Psorin.

Orchitis.—Puls.; Bell.; Rhodod.; Spong.; Aur.

Osteitis.—Conchiolin.

Osteomalacia.—Phosph. ac.

Otitis Media (chronic).—Chenopod.; Cap.; Bell.; Merc.; Puls.; Calc.

Otorrhœa.—Kino; Merc.; *Calc.; Puls.;* Sulph.; Hydr.; Tellur.

Ovaralgia.—Zinc. val.; Apis; Lach.

Ovarian Cyst.—Oophor.; K. brom.; Apis.

Ovaritis.—Apis; Laches; Platina; Colocyn.; Sepia; Xanthox.

Oxaluria.—Senna; Nit. mur. ac.

Ozæna.—Alum.; Hippoz.; Aur.; Nit. ac.; Merc.; Hydr.; *Cadmium;* Sulph.

Panaritium.—Am. carb.; Fluor. ac.; Sil.

Pancreatic Troubles.—*Iris.*

Paralysis Agitans.—Aur. sul.; Hyos. hydrob.; Merc.

Paralysis.—(post-diphtheritic)—Gels.; Coccul.; Lach.; Aur. mur.; Arg. nit.

Paraplegia.—*Mang. ox.;* Kal. tart.; Lathyr.; Thall.; Hyper.; Anhalon.

Paresis.—Æsc. glab.; Badiag.

——(pneumo-gastric)—Grind.

——(respiratory)—Lobel. purp.

——(senile)—Aur. iod.; Phos.

——(spinal)—Irid.

——(typewriter's)—Stann.

Pellagra.—Bovista.

Pemphigus.—Caltha; Mancin.; Ran. scel.

Pericarditis.—Ant.; Ars.; Bry.; Colch.; Spig.; Dig.

Periostitis.—Asaf.; Aur.; K. bich.; Merc.; Phos.; Mez.; Sil.; Apis.

Peritonitis.—Apis; Bell.; Bry.; Colocy.; Merc. cor.; Sinapis; Sang. nit.; Wyeth.

Pharyngitis, follicular.—Æsc. hip.; Hydr.; Sang.; Wyethia.

——(sicca)—Dubois.

Phimosis.—Merc.; Guaiac.

Phlebitis.—Hamam.; Puls.

Phthisis.—Acalyph.; Gall. ac.; Nat. cacod.; Polyg. avic.; Silphium; Calc. ars.; Kreos.

——(laryngeal)—Dros.; Stan.; Selen.; Nat. selen.

Plague.—Ignatia; Operculina.

Pleurisy.—Acon.; *Bry.;* Squill.; Asclep.; Kal. c.

——(effusion stage)—Apis; *Canth.;* Ars.; Sulph.

Pleurodynia.—Bry.; Cimic.; Ran. bulb.

Plica Polonica.—Vinca; Lycop.

Pneumonia.—Bry.; Phos.; Sang.; Iod.; Chelid.; Lyc.; Pneu-mo-coccin.

Poison-oak.—Anac.; Xerophyl.; Grind.; Cyprip.; Rhus; Croton.; Graph.; Erecht.

Poliomyelitis.—Lathyrus; *Bungaris;* Kali phos.

Polychrome Spectra.—Anhalon.

Polypi.—Phos.; Calc.; Sang.; Thuj.

——(nasal)—Lemna; *Calc.; Teuc.*

Polyuria.—Arg.; *Phos. ac.;* Murex; Squill.; Uran.; Rhus aromat.

Porrigo capitis.—Calc. mur.

Portal congestion.—Æscul glabra.

Priapism.—Pic. ac.; Canth.

Proctitis.—Ant. crud.; Collins.; Aloe; Podop.

Prosopalgia.—Cactus; Verbas.; Kalmia; Puls.

Prostatic Hypertrophy.—Fer. pic.; Thuj.

Prostatitis.—Merc. dulc.; Sabal.; Pic. ac.; *Thuj.;* Tritic.; Staph.

Pruritus.—Antipyr.; Carbol. ac.; Dolich.; Fagop.; Sulph.; Rhus; Pulex.; Radium.

Psilosis.—Fragaria.

Psoriasis.—Kal. ars.; K. brom.; Thyroid.; *Ars.;* Graph.; *Borax;* Sulph.; Emetin ½ gr.

Pterygium.—Zinc.; Ratanh.; Sulph.

Ptomaine Poisoning.—Ars.; Kreos.; Pyrog.

Ptyalism.—Merc.; Iris; Iod.; Trifol.

Purpura.—Crotal.; Phosp.; Ars.; Hamam.; Naja.

Pyæmia.—Ars. jod.; Chinin.; Lach.; Pyrogen.

Pyelitis.—Merc. cor.; Hep.; Tereb.; Cup. ars.; Epigea; Juni-perus.

Pyorrhœa.—Emetin.; Staphis.; Plantago.

Pyrosis.—Gallic ac.; Bismuth.; Caps.

Rachitis.—Calc.; Iris; Phos.; Sil.

Ranula.—Thuja; Calc.; Fluor. ac.

Raynaud's Disease.—Ars.; Secale; Cactus tincture.

Rectal Pockets.—Polygon.

Respiration (Cheyne-Stokes).—Antipyr.

Rheumatism.—Colch.; Propyl.; Acon.; *Bry.;* Dulc.; Merc.; *Rhus;* Cimic.

——(chronic)—Stellar.; Ol. jecor.; *Sulph.;* Viscum.

——(gonorrhœal)—Irisin; Sarsap.; Thuja.

Rhinitis (atrophic).—Lemna.

Riggs' Disease.—Calc. renal.

Ringworm.—Sepia; Tellur.; Ars.; Bacillin.

Scarlatina.—Bell.; Rhus; Stram.

——(malignant)—Am. carb.; Mur. ac.; Lach.; Ailanth.; Crotal.; Baptis.; Nit. ac.

Sciatica.—Cotyled.; Viscum; *Colocy.;* Rhus; *Gnaph.*

Sclerosis, multiple.—Aur. mur.

Sclerotic Degeneration.—Baryt. m.; Plumb.; Aur. mur.

Scrofula.—Æthiops; Fer. iod.; Cistus; Merc.; Calc.; Sulph.; Therid.

Scurvy.—Acet. ac.; Agave; Phos.; Merc.

Seasickness.—Apomorph.; Petrol.; *Coccul.;* Nux; Tabac.

Seborrhœa.—Heracleum.; Ars.; Graph.; Vinca; Nat mur.

Senile Decay.—Oophor.; Baryta.

Sepsis.—Crotal.; Bapt.; Echin.; Ars.; Lach.

Sleeping Sickness.—Nux mosch.; Opium; Gelsem.; *Atoxyl.*

Sleeplessness.—Tela aran.; *Coff.;* Ign.; Cimicif.; Gels.; Opium (high); Daphne; Hyos. hydrob.

Snake-poison Antidotes.—Golond.; Cedr.; Gymne.; Sisyr.; Guaco; Salag.

Somnambulism.—Kali phos.; Kali brom.

Spermatorrhœa.—Salix; Chin.; Phos. ac.; Staphys.

Spleen Affections.—Ceanoth.; Quercus; Helianth.; Nat. m.; Polymnia.

Sterility.—Agnus; Nat. m.; Borax.

Stomach Dilatation.—Hydr. mur.

Stomatitis.—Borax; Arg. nit.; Kal. mur.; *Nit. ac.*

Subinvolution.—Fraxin.; Aur. mur. nat.; Epipheg.

Sycosis.—Asterias; Thuja; Natr. sulph.; Aur. mur.

Synovitis.—Apis; Bry.; Calc. fluor.

Syphilides.—Ars. s. fl.; K. hyd.; Nit. ac.

Syphilis.—Calotropis; Coryd.; Plat. mur.; Merc.; K. hyd.; Aurum.

——(latent)—Ars. met.; Syphil.

——(nodes)—Coryd.; Stilling.; K. hyd.

Tachycardia.—*Abies nig.;* Agnus.

Tape-worm.—Filix; Cina; Ioduretted Pot. iod.

Tetanus.—Strych.; Upas; Passif.; Physos.

Thrombosis.—Borthrops.; Lach.

Tinnitus.—Antipyr.; Cannab. ind.; Carb. sulph.; Sal. ac.

Tobacco-craving.—Daph. ind.

Tonsillitis.—Am. mur.; Guaiac.; Baryta. ac.; Bell.; Merc.; Phyt.

Toothache.—Plantago; Mag. carb.; Bell.; Chamom.

Torticollis.—Lachnant.

Traumatism.—Arnica; Bellis.

Trismus.—Linum.

Tuberculosis.—Ars. jod.; Phelland.; Tuberculin.; Calcar.

Tumors.—Calc. fluor.; Conium; Baryta mur.; Thuja; Merc. iod. rub.; Hydrast.; Phytol.; Plumb. jod.

Tympanitis.—Lycop.; Tereb.; Asaf.; Erigeron.

Typhoid.—Bapt.; Mur. ac.; Ars.; Phos. ac.; Bry.

——(diarrhœa)—Epilob.

Ulcers.—Nit. ac.; Sil.; Ars.; Comocl.; Kal. hyd.; Lach.; Pæon.; Calend.

Uræmia.—Am. carb.; Cup. ars.; *Morph.*

Urethral Caruncle.—Cann. sat.; *Eucalyp.*

Urethritis.—Acon.; Apis; *Canth.*

——(in children)—Doryph.

Uric Acid Diathesis.—Hedeom.; Ocim.

Urticaria.—Ant. c.; Antipyr.; Apis; Astac.; Bombyx; Copaiv.; Fragar.; Nat. mur.

Uterine Displacement.—Abies can.; Eupion; Heliot.; Sep.; Puls.; Fraxin.; Fer. iod.

——(induration)—Aur. mur.; Kalmia.

——(tumors)—*Aur. m. nat.*

Vaginismus.—Cactus; Plumb.; Bellad.
Varicose Veins.—Calc. fluor.; Hamam.; Puls.
Variola.—Ant. tart.; Saracen.
——(hæmorrhage)—Crotal.; Phos.; Ars.
Vascular Tension.—Acon.; Bell.; Ver. v.
——(with arterial lesion)—Adrenal.; Baryt. mur.; Tabac.; Plumbum.
——(rapid reducers)—Glon.; Amyl.; Nat. nit.; Trinitin.
Vertigo.—Gels.; *Granat.*; Phos.; Coccul.; Con.
Venous Stasis.—*Æsc. hip.*

Warts.—Ant. c.; Caust.; Nit. ac.; *Thuj.*; Salicy. acid.
Wens.—Thuja; Benz. acid.; Bacillin.
Whooping-cough.—Castan.; *Dros.*; Cupr.; Mag. ph.; Pertuss.
Worms.—Calc.; Cina; Santon.; Spigel.; Teuc.; Naphth.
Wrist Rheumatism.—Actea spic.; Viol. od.
Writers' Cramp.—Arg. m.; Sulph. ac.
Weil's Disease.—Chelid.; Phosph.

Yellow Fever.—Cadmium; Ars.; Crotal.

LIST OF REMEDIES
COMMON NAMES

LIST OF REMEDIES
COMMON NAMES

LIST OF REMEDIES
PHARMACEUTICAL
AND
LATIN NAMES

LIST OF REMEDIES

PHARMACEUTICAL AND LATIN NAMES

CPSIA information can be obtained
at www.ICGtesting.com
Printed in the USA
LVOW08s1244110617
537720LV00001B/71/P

9 780766 183889